Paediatric Library

Handbook

EIGHTH EDITION

Edited by

Kate Thomson, MBBS, FRACP
General Paediatrician
Department of Developmental Medicine
Emergency Department
Sunshine Hospital
Victoria, Australia

Dean Tey, MBBS
Allergy and Immunology Fellow
Royal Children's Hospital
Melbourne, Australia

Michael Marks, MBBS, MPH, MD, FRACP
Paediatrician
Department of General Medicine
Senior Lecturer
Department of Paediatrics
University of Melbourne
Victoria, Australia

ⓦWILEY-BLACKWELL

A John Wiley and Sons, Ltd., Publication

Library of Congress Cataloging-in-Publication Data

Paediatric handbook. – 8th ed. / [edited by] Kate Thomson, Dean Tey, Michael Marks.
    p. ; cm.
   Rev. ed. of: Paediatric handbook. 7th ed. / [by the staff of the Royal Children's Hospital, Melbourne, Australia];
editors, Georgia Paxton, Jane Munro; associate editor, Michael Marks.
   Includes bibliographical references and index.
   ISBN 978-1-4051-7400-8 (pbk.: alk. paper)
   1. Pediatrics–Handbooks, manuals, etc. 2. Children–Diseases–Handbooks, manuals, etc. I. Thomson, Kate, Dr.
II. Tey, Dean, Dr. III. Marks, Michael, Dr. IV. Royal Children's Hospital.
   [DNLM: 1. Pediatrics–Handbooks. WS 39 P1253 2008]
   RJ48.P277 2008
   618.92–dc22
                                                                                        2008022218

ISBN: 978-1-4051-7400-8

A catalogue record for this book is available from the British Library.

Set in 7.5 on 9.5 pt Frutiger Light by SNP Best-set Typesetter Ltd., Hong Kong
Printed & bound in Singapore by Utopia Press Pte Ltd

1 2009

Contents

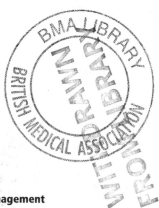

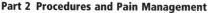

Contents

Appendices

Contributors

All authors are staff or associates of the Royal Children's Hospital (RCH) unless otherwise indicated.

George Alex, MBBS, FRACP, MMed, MRCP, PhD
Gastroenterologist
Department of Gastroenterology

Roger Allen, MBBS, FRACP
Paediatric Rheumatologist
Department of General Medicine

Peter Barnett, MBBS, FRACP, MSc, FACEM, MSpMed
Deputy Director
Emergency Department
Associate Clinical Professor
University of Melbourne
Victoria, Australia

Robert Berkowitz, MDBS, FRACS
Director
Department of Otolaryngology

Julie Bines, MBBS, FRACP, MD
Head of Clinical Nutrition
Murdoch Children's Research Institute
Victor Loti Smorgon Professor of
   Paediatrics
University of Melbourne
Victoria, Australia

Avihu Boneh, MD, PhD, FRACP
Head, Metabolic Service
Genetic Health Services
Victoria, Australia

Paul Brooks, MBBS (Hons)
Department of Cardiology

Jim Buttery, FRACP MSc
Infectious Diseases Physician
Department of General Medicine
NHMRC CCRE in Child and Adolescent
   Immunisation
Murdoch Children's Research Institute
Department of Paediatrics
University of Melbourne
Victoria, Australia

Fergus Cameron, B.Med.Sci, MBBS, DipRA-COG, FRACP, MD
Associate Professor
Deputy Director
Department of Endocrinology
   and Diabetes

George Chalkiadis, MBBS, DA(Lon), FANZCA, FFPMANZCCA
Staff Anaesthetist
Head, Children's Pain Management Service
Clinical Associate Professor
Department of Paediatrics
University of Melbourne
Murdoch Children's Research Institute
Parkville, Victoria
Australia

Tom Clarnette, MBBS, MD, FRACS
Consultant Paediatrician Surgeon

Noel Cranswick, MBBS, BMedSci, FRACP
Director, Clinical Pharmacology
Director, APPRU
Murdoch Children's Research Institute and
    the Royal Children's Hospital
Associate Professor
University of Melbourne
Victoria, Australia

Nigel Curtis, B.Arts, M.Arts, PhD Philosophy
MBBS, Dip Trop Med and Hygiene
Associate Professor
Head of Paediatric Infectious Diseases
    Unit
Department of General Medicine
Chair of Infectious Diseases
Department of Paediatrics
University of Melbourne
Victoria, Australia

Margot Davey, MBBS, FRACP
Director, Melbourne
Children's Sleep Unit
Monash Medical Centre
Clayton, Australia

Trevor Duke, MD, FRACP
Intensive Care Specialist
Associate Professor
Director, Centre for International

Child Health
Department of Paediatrics
University of Melbourne
Victoria, Australia

Daryl Efron, MBBS, FRACP, MD
Consultant Paediatrician
Department of General Medicine
Co-ordinator of Clinical Services
Centre for Community Child Health

James Elder, MBBS, FRANZCO, FRACS
Associate Professor
Director
Department of Ophthalmology

Susan Gibb, MBBS, FRACP
Paediatrician
Department of General Medicine

Kay Gibbons, BAppSc, FDAA
Manager, Nutrition Services
Murdoch Children's Research Institute
Melbourne, Victoria
Australia

H. Kerr Graham, MD, FRCS (ED), FRACS
Orthopaedic Surgeon
Professor, Department of Paediatrics
University of Melbourne and Murdoch
Children's Research Institute

Sonia Grover, MBBS, FRANZCOG, MD
Director, Department of Paediatric
    and Adolescent Gynaecology
Consultant Gynaecologist
Mercy Hospital for Women
    and Austin Health
Heidelberg, Victoria
Australia

Contributors

Michael Harari, MBBS, FRACP
Paediatrician
Department of General Medicine and
    Continence Clinic

Simon Harvey, MD, FRACP
Neurologist
Department of Neurology

John Heath, MBBS, BVSc (Hons), MD, PhD
Consultant Physician
Clinical Associate Professor
University of Melbourne
Victoria, Australia

Rod Hunt, FRACP, PhD, MMed, MRCP (UK),
BMBS
Consultant Neonatologist

John Hutson, MD, MB, DSc, FRACS, FAAP
Urology and General Surgery
    Departments
Chair of Paediatric Surgery
Department of Paediatrics
University of Melbourne
Victoria, Australia

Jenny Hynson, MBBS, FRACP
Consultant Paediatrician
Victorian Paediatric Palliative Care
    Program

Colin Jones, MBBS, FRACP, PhD
Associate Professor
Director, Department of Nephrology

Julian Kelly, MBBS, FRACP
Paediatrician
Department of General Medicine
Senior Lecturer
University of Melbourne
Victoria, Australia

Nicky Kilpatrick, BDS, PhD, FDS, RCPS,
FRACDS (Paed)
Associate Professor
Director, Department of Dentistry
Leader, Oral Health Research
    Unit
Murdoch Children's Research Institute
Parkville, Victoria
Australia

Andrew Kornberg, MBBS (Hons), FRACP
Director of Neurology

Lionel Lubitz, MBChB (UCT), DCH, MRCP,
FRACP
Consultant Paediatrician
Department of General Medicine

Mark Mackay, MBBS, FRACP
Paediatric Neurologist
Department of Neurology
Research Affiliate
Murdoch Children's Research Institute
Parkville, Victoria
Australia

Wirginia Maixner, MBBS, FRACS
Director
Department of Neurosurgery

Michael Marks, MBBS, MPH, MD, FRACP
Paediatrician
Department of General Medicine
Senior Lecturer
Department of Paediatrics
University of Melbourne
Victoria, Australia

Catherine Marraffa, MBBS, FRACP,
FRCPCH
Deputy Director
Developmental Medicine

John Massie, FRACP, PhD
Respiratory Physician
Clinical Associate Professor
University of Melbourne
Victoria, Australia

Zoë McCallum, MBBS, FRACP
Paediatrician
Department of General Medicine
Department of Clinical Nutrition
Senior Lecturer
Department of Paediatrics
University of Melbourne
Victoria, Australia

Maria McCarthy, B. Appl Sci. M. Appl. Sci.
Coordinator, Psycho-Oncology Program and
   Family Therapist
Children's Cancer Centre

Peter McDougall, MB, BS, FRACP, MBA
Chief of Medicine
Director of Neonatology

Michele Meehan, RN, RM.Dip.CHN. Dip.Hlth
Ed.
Clinical Nurse, Consultant
Maternal and Child Health

Paul Monagle, MBBS, MSc, MD, FRACP,
FRCPA, FCCP
Director, Department of Haematology
Department of Pathology
University of Melbourne
Victoria, Australia

Jane Munro, MBBS, FRACP, MPH
Paediatric Rheumatologist
Department of General Medicine

Mary O'Toole, BA, BSW, Grad Dip.
Creative Arts Therapy
Bereavement Services Coordinator

Ed Oakley, MBBS, FRACME
Staff Specialist
Department of Emergency Medicine

David Orchard, MBBS, FACD
Dermatologist
Department of Dermatology

Greta Palmer, MBBS, FANZCA, FFPMAVZCA
Clinical Associate Professor
Specialist Anaesthetist and Pain
   Management Consultant
Murdoch Children's Research Institute
University of Melbourne
Victoria, Australia

Georgia Paxton, MBBS, BMedSci, MPH,
FRACP
General Paediatrician
Department of General Medicine

Dan Penny, MD, PhD, FRACP
Professor
Director of Cardiology

Rod Phillips, MBBS, FRACP, PhD
Consultant in Paediatric Skin Disease
Department of General Medicine

Chidambaram Prakash, MBBS, DPM,
FRANZCP, Cert. Child Psychiatry (RANZCP)
Integrated Mental Health Program

Sarath Ranganathan, MBChB, MRCP,
FRCPCH, FRACP, PhD
Consultant Respiratory Physician

Andrew Rechtmann, MBBS
Clinical Pharmacology Fellow

Dinah Reddihough, MD, BSc, FRACP,
FAFRM
Director, Developmental Medicine

Contributors

Sheena Reilly, B.App.Sc., PhD, MRCSLT, MSpAA
Director, Department of Speech Pathology
Professor of Paediatric Speech Pathology
Department of Paediatrics
University of Melbourne
Director, Healthy Development Theme
Murdoch Children's Research Institute
Parkville, Victoria
Australia

Jenny Royle, MBBS, FRACP
Paediatrician
Immunisation Service
Department of General Medicine

Matthew Sabin, MRCPCH (UK), PhD
RCH Foundation Clinical Research Fellow

Chris Sanderson, BSc (Hons), MBBS, FRACP
Consultant Paediatrician
Visiting Medical Officer
Barwon Health
Geelong, Victoria
Australia

Susan Sawyer, MBBS, MD, FRACP
Director, Centre for Adolescent Health
Chair of Adolescent Health
Department of Paediatrics
University of Melbourne
Victoria, Australia

Joanne Smart, BSc, MBBS, PhD, FRACP
Clinical Immunologist/Allergist
Department of Allergy and Immunology

Anne Smith, MBBS, FRACP
Medical Director
Victorian Forensic Paediatric Medical
    Service

Mike Starr, MBBS FRACP
Paediatrician
Infectious Diseases Physician
Consultant in Emergency Medicine

Mimi Tang, MBBS, PhD, FRACP, FRCPA
Director, Allergy and Immunology
    Department
Group Leader – Allergy and Immune
    Disorders
MCRI, Associate Professor
Department of Paediatrics
University of Melbourne
Victoria, Australia

Russell G. Taylor, MBBS FRACS
Director of General Surgery

Dean Tey, MBBS
Allergy and Immunology Fellow
Department of Allergy and Immunology

Kate Thomson, MBBS, FRACP
General Paediatrician
Department of Developmental Medicine
Emergency Department
Sunshine Hospital
Victoria, Australia

James Tibballs, BMedSc(Hons), MB BS, MEd, MBA, MD, MHlth&MedLaw, GDipArts(Fr), FRANZCA, FJFICM, FACLM
Intensive Care Physician and Resuscitation
    Officer
Principal Fellow
Australian Venom Research Unit
Department of Pharmacology
University of Melbourne
Principal Fellow
Department of Paediatrics
University of Melbourne
Victoria, Australia

Garry Warne, MBBS, FRACP
Senior Endocrinologist
Director, RCH International
Professor, Department of Paediatrics
University of Melbourne
Victoria, Australia

George Werther, MD, FRACP, MSc (Oxon)
Director, Department of Endocrinology and
    Diabetes and Centre for Hormone
    Research

Murdoch Children's Research Institute
Professor, Department of Paediatrics
University of Melbourne
Victoria, Australia

Joshua Wolf, MBBS, BA
Advanced Trainee in Paediatric Infectious
    Diseases

Margaret Zacharin, MBBS, FRACP
Paediatric and Adult Endocrinologist

Editorial committee

Daryl Efron, MBBS, FRACP, MD
Consultant Paediatrician
Co-ordinator of Clinical Services Centre for
    Community Child Health

Michael Marks, MBBS, MPH, MD, FRACP
Paediatrician
Department of General Medicine
Senior Lecturer
Department of Paediatrics
University of Melbourne
Victoria, Australia

Jane Munro, MBBS, FRACP, MPH
Paediatric Rheumatologist
Department of General Medicine

Georgia Paxton, MBBS, BMedSci, MPH, FRACP
General Paediatrician
Department of General Paediatrics

Chris Sanderson, BSc (Hons), MBBS, FRACP
Consultant Paediatrician
Visiting Medical Officer
Barwon Health, Geelong
Victoria, Australia

Mike South, MBBS, DCH, MRCP (UK), FRACP,
FJFICM, MD
Director, Department of General
    Medicine
Paediatric Intensive Care Physician
Professor and Deputy Head of Paediatrics
University of Melbourne
Victoria, Australia

Dean Tey, MBBS
Allergy and Immunology Fellow
Department of Allergy & Immunology

Kate Thomson, MBBS, FRACP
General Paediatrician
Department of Developmental Medicine
Emergency Department
Sunshine Hospital
Victoria, Australia

Foreword

Over the past four decades the *Paediatric Handbook* has provided a valuable source of up-to-date, practical clinical information as a guide to clinicians who care for infants, children and adolescents. Produced by the staff of the Royal Children's Hospital, Melbourne, the handbook has become a highly respected source of advice developed from evidence-based practice as well as a wealth of clinical experience. The *Paediatric Handbook* reflects the Hospital's longstanding commitment to improving the health care of children, young people and their families through the provision of clinical services, research and the education and training of healthcare professionals.

In this eighth edition of the handbook, all chapters have undergone comprehensive revision with major updates in resuscitation, pain management, the management of stroke and immunisation reflecting recent advances in clinical practice. Emerging areas of child and adolescent clinical practice, including obesity, sleep disorders and continence problems, have become the focus of new chapters.

To enhance the accessibility of the handbook, the online supplement has been extensively revised with updates and links to key websites to facilitate pathways to further information. For the busy clinician, the electronic PDA version provided with the handbook will provide a terrific user-friendly companion to assist clinical decision-making.

The Royal Children's Hospital and its staff are justifiably proud of the eighth edition of the *Paediatric Handbook* and hope that their contribution may benefit the health of children and adolescents.

Julie Bines MBBS, MD, FRACP
Victor and Loti Smorgon Professor of Paediatrics,
University of Melbourne, Australia

Head of Clinical Nutrition, Department of Gastroenterology and Clinical
Nutrition, Royal Children's Hospital, Melbourne, Australia

Head, Intestinal Failure and Clinical Nutrition Group, Infection, Immunity
and Environment Theme, Murdoch Children's Research Institute,
Melbourne, Australia

Preface

The fascinating field of paediatrics and child health continue to move forwards rapidly. Clinical assessment and management of illnesses in children have benefited enormously from an ever-advancing body of evidence and research. With this in mind, we are proud to present the eighth edition of the *Paediatric Handbook*, which contains new and revised chapters and will be available in a PDA version. We aim to provide primary healthcare providers, junior hospital medical staff and medical students with concise, management-focused information regarding important paediatric conditions.

Some of the exciting new features of this eighth edition include:

- New chapters on sleep, continence, slow weight gain (failure to thrive) and obesity.
- Extensively revised chapters on renal conditions, pain management and immigrant health.
- New topics, including continuous subcutaneous insulin infusion (pumps), cystic fibrosis, stroke and management of illicit drug poisoning.
- Links to useful websites, indicated by a symbol in the text margins.
- A new handbook supplementary website at www.rchhandbook.org.

Putting this handbook together has been a monumental task for the staff of the Royal Children's Hospital. The handbook represents the invaluable cumulative experience of these clinicians, and we thank them for their dedication and contribution. Those named in the eighth edition have been actively involved for two years in this most recent incarnation; however, they had the good fortune to begin with chapters that have been built over time by successive generations of authors. To all these previous authors, we extend our heartfelt thanks.

We are grateful to Professor Frank Shann for allowing us to include large parts of his drug doses book. The PDA version of this reference will be available separately for purchase at www.drugdoses.net.

Thanks also to our artists: Bill Reid for many of the illustrations, and Nicholas Mansfield (aged 10 years, from Ascot Vale Primary School, Melbourne, Victoria) for his fantastic design which has been adapted for the cover of this new edition.

The editorial committee have debated long and hard over some major and some minor details. 'Best practice' is a moveable feast and it is sometimes challenging to reach a consensus (follow-up investigation for children with first presentation urinary tract infection is a good example). Hence, we encourage our readers to continually familiarise themselves with the most current published literature on each topic. In the case of medications, it is essential that drug dosage and product information is checked before administration.

Thank you for allowing us to share this handbook with you. We hope that you find it an invaluable tool in the delivery of high-quality, empathic health care for children and young people, wherever you are.

Best wishes

Kate Thomson
Dean Tey
Michael Marks
(*Editors*)

CHAPTER 1

Medical emergencies

James Tibballs
Ed Oakley

Cardiorespiratory arrest

Cardiorespiratory arrest may occur in a wide variety of conditions that cause hypoxaemia or hypotension, or both. Examples include trauma, drowning, septicaemia, sudden infant death syndrome, asthma and congenital anomalies of the heart and lung.

The initial cardiac rhythm discovered during early resuscitation is usually severe bradycardia or asystole. Although the spontaneous onset of ventricular fibrillation in children is approximately 10%, it may occur more frequently with congenital heart conditions or secondary to poisoning with cardioactive drugs. In hospital, respiratory arrest alone is more common than cardiorespiratory arrest.

Diagnosis and initial management

- Cardiorespiratory arrest may be suspected when the patient becomes unresponsive or unconscious, is not moving or breathing normally or appears pale or cyanosed. Call for help.
- Assess airway and respiration by observing movement of the chest, as well as listening and feeling for expired breath while positioning the head and neck to open and maintain an airway. Movement of the chest without expiration indicates a blocked airway.
- Assess circulation by palpation of the carotid, brachial or femoral pulse and by other signs of circulation (adequate breathing, movement, consciousness).
- Whenever possible, manage in a treatment room. Carry the patient there if necessary. If this is not possible, fetch the resuscitation trolley from a treatment room.
- Cardiopulmonary resuscitation (CPR) must commence with basic techniques and be continued using advanced techniques (Fig. 1.1).

Airway maintenance and ventilation

- If airway obstruction is present, quickly inspect the pharynx. Clear secretions or vomitus by brief suction using a Yankauer sucker.
- Maintain the airway with backward head tilt, chin lift or forward jaw thrust.
- If adequate spontaneous ventilation does not resume, ventilate the lungs mechanically with a self-inflating resuscitator (e.g. Laerdal, Ambu, Air-viva) with added oxygen 8–10 L/min. If ventilation cannot be achieved with the resuscitator, use a mouth-to-mask technique. Give two initial breaths.

Paediatric Handbook, 8th edition. By Kate Thomson, Dean Tey and Michael Marks. Published 2009 by Blackwell Publishing, ISBN: 978-1-4051-7400-8.

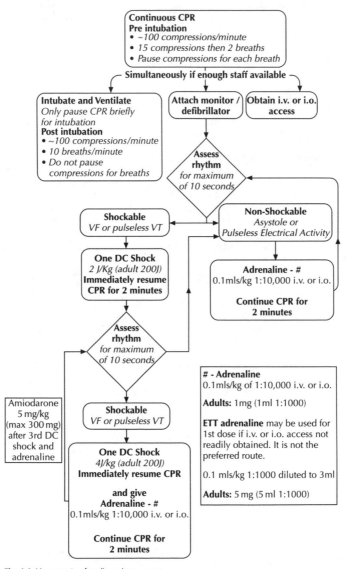

Continuous CPR
Pre intubation
- ~100 compressions/minute
- 15 compressions then 2 breaths
- Pause compressions for each breath

Simultaneously if enough staff available

Intubate and Ventilate
Only pause CPR briefly for intubation
Post intubation
- ~100 compressions/minute
- 10 breaths/minute
- Do not pause compressions for breaths

Attach monitor / defibrillator

Obtain i.v. or i.o. access

Assess rhythm
for maximum of 10 seconds

Shockable
VF or pulseless VT

Non-Shockable
Asystole or Pulseless Electrical Activity

One DC Shock
2 J/Kg (adult 200J)
Immediately resume CPR for 2 minutes

Adrenaline - #
0.1mls/kg 1:10,000 i.v. or i.o.
Continue CPR for 2 minutes

Assess rhythm
for maximum of 10 seconds

Amiodarone
5 mg/kg
(max 300 mg)
after 3rd DC
shock and
adrenaline

Shockable
VF or pulseless VT

One DC Shock
4J/kg (adult 200J)
Immediately resume CPR
and give
Adrenaline - #
0.1mls/kg 1:10,000 i.v. or i.o.
Continue CPR for 2 minutes

 # - Adrenaline
0.1mls/kg of 1:10,000 i.v. or i.o.

Adults: 1mg (1ml 1:1000)

ETT adrenaline may be used for 1st dose if i.v. or i.o. access not readily obtained. It is not the preferred route.

0.1 mls/kg 1:1000 diluted to 3ml

Adults: 5 mg (5 ml 1:1000)

Fig. 1.1 Management of cardiorespiratory arrest

Note: Self-inflating bags (e.g. Laerdal) have a one-way valve and will provide no gas flow to the patient unless they are compressed cyclically.

- **Whatever technique is used, ensure that ventilation expands the chest adequately.**
- Intubate the trachea via the mouth if possible, but do not cause hypoxaemia by prolonged unsuccessful attempts. Select the tube and insert it at a depth appropriate to the patient's age in years.

Endotracheal tube (ETT) size and position

- Tube size (internal diameter) = (age/4) + 4 mm (for patients over 1 year of age)
- Depth of insertion is approximately (age/2) + 12 cm from the lower lip

Neonates: see Table 32.1 p435

Secure the tube with cotton tape around the neck or affix it firmly to the face with adhesive tape to avoid endobronchial intubation or accidental extubation.

External cardiac compression

Start external cardiac compression (ECC) over the lower sternum if:

- A pulse is not palpable within 10 s.
- A pulse is less than:
  - 60 beats/min (for infants)
  - 40 beats/min (for older children).
- Other signs of circulation (adequate ventilation, movement, consciousness) are absent.

Place the patient on a firm surface and depress the lower sternum one third the depth of the chest:

- Newborn infant or an infant (<1 year) – two-thumb technique in which the hands encircle the chest.
- Small child (1–8 years) – the heel of one hand.
- Larger child (>8 years) and adult – the two-handed technique.
  Avoid pressure over the ribs and abdominal viscera.

Compression–ventilation rates and ratios

The rates and ratios recommended for healthcare rescuers by the Australian Resuscitation Council (*www.resus.org.au*) are shown in Table 1.1.

When using bag-to-mask ventilation or mouth-to-mask ventilation, the rescuer giving compressions should count aloud to allow the rescuer giving ventilation to deliver effective breaths during pauses between compressions with minimal interruption in compressions. Compression may be commenced at the end of inspiration.

The *rate* of compression is 100/min, that is one compression every 0.6 s, aiming to give approximately 80–100 actual compressions each minute.

If ventilation is given by bag and ETT, ECC may be continued during ventilation provided lung expansion can be achieved. In this circumstance, restrict the number of ventilations to about 10/min.

Management of cardiac dysrhythmias

Determine the cardiac rhythm with defibrillator paddles or pads or chest leads.

Table 1.1 Compression–ventilation ratios (from the Australian Resuscitation Council)

	Give 2 initial breaths, then	
	One rescuer (expired air resuscitation) Compression : breaths	**Two rescuers (bag–mask ventilation) Compression : breaths**
Newborn infants	3 : 1	3 : 1
Infants (<1 yo)	30 : 2	15 : 2
Small children (1–8 yo)	30 : 2	15 : 2
Larger children (>8 yo)	30 : 2	15 : 2
Adults	30 : 2	30 : 2

- Give DC shock if ventricular fibrillation or pulseless ventricular tachycardia is present. See Table 1.2 and Fig. 1.1 for energy doses in DC shock.
- Give adrenaline if any other pulseless rhythm is present (see Fig. 1.1). The dose is:
  - i.v. and intraosseous: 10 mcg/kg (0.01 mL of 1 : 1000 solution)
  - endotracheal tube (ETT): 100 mcg/kg (0.1 mL of 1 : 1000 solution)
- Insert an i.v. cannula. Although this is the preferred access to the circulation, do not waste time (>90 s) with repeated unsuccessful attempts, as access can be achieved with the alternative techniques of:
  - *Intraosseus administration* (see Procedures, chapter 3, p. 39): all i.v. drugs and resuscitation fluids can be given.
  - *ETT administration*: only adrenaline, atropine and lignocaine (lidocaine) can be given; this is the least effective method, with some evidence suggesting possible adverse effects on the circulation.
- A quick reference guide to drug doses and fluid volume is provided in Table 1.2 and Fig. 1.1.

Other drugs
Calcium
This is a useful inotropic and vasopressor agent but it has no place in the management of a dysrhythmia, unless it is caused by hypocalcaemia, hyperkalaemia or calcium channel blocker toxicity. It is not useful and probably harmful for asystole, ventricular fibrillation or electromechanical dissociation. The i.v. dose is 10% calcium chloride (0.2 mL/kg) or 10% calcium gluconate (0.7 mL/kg). Do not administer calcium via ETT and do not mix it with bicarbonate.

Adenosine
This is the preferred drug treatment (200 mcg/kg i.v.) for supraventricular tachycardia (SVT). See management of SVT in Cardiac conditions, chapter 21, p. 256.

Table 1.2 Table of drugs, fluid volume, endotracheal tubes and direct current shock for paediatric resuscitation

Age	0	2 months	5 months	1 year	2 years	3 years	4 years	5 years	6 years	7 years	8 years	9 years	10 years	11 years	12 years	13 years	14 years
Bodyweight (kg)*	3.5	5	7	10	12	14	16	18	20	22	25	28	32	36	40	46	50
Height (cm)*	50	58	65	75	85	94	102	109	115	121	127	132	138	144	151	157	162
Adrenaline 1:1000 (mL)																	
10 mcg/kg	0.035	0.05	0.07	0.10	0.12	0.14	0.16	0.18	0.2	0.22	0.25	0.28	0.32	0.36	0.4	0.46	0.5
100 mcg/kg	0.35	0.5	0.7	1	1.2	1.4	1.6	1.8	2	2.2	2.5	2.8	3.2	3.6	4	4.6	5
Adrenaline 1:10000 (mL)																	
10 mcg/kg	0.35	0.5	0.7	1	1.2	1.4	1.6	1.8	2	2.2	2.5	2.8	3.2	3.6	4	4.6	5
100 mcg/kg	3.5	5.0	7.0	10	12	14	16	18	20	22	25	28	32	36	40	46	50
Lignocaine (lidocaine) 1% (mL)																	
1 mg/kg	0.3	0.5	0.7	1.0	1.2	1.4	1.6	1.8	2.0	2.2	2.5	2.8	3.2	3.6	4.0	4.6	5.0
Sodium bicarb. 8.4% (mL)																	
1 mmol/kg	3.5	5	7	10	12	14	16	18	20	22	25	28	32	36	40	46	50
Fluid volume (mL)																	
20 mL/kg	70	100	140	200	240	280	320	360	400	440	500	560	640	720	800	920	1000
Endotracheal tube																	
Size (mm) Age/4 + 4	3	3.5	3.5	4	4.5	4.5	5	5	5.5	5.5	6	6	6.5	6.5	7	7	7.5
Oral length (cm) Age/2 + 12	9.5	11	11.5	12	13	13.5	14	14.5	15	15.5	16	16.5	17	17.5	18	18.5	19
Direct current shock (J) Unsynchronised																	
VF, VT 2 J/kg	7	10	20	20	20	30	30	30	50	50	50	50	70	70	70	100	100
VF, VT 4 J/kg	10	20	30	50	50	50	70	70	70	100	100	100	150	150	150	200	200
Direct current shock (J) Synchronised																	
SVT 1 J/kg	3	5	7	10	10	10	20	20	20	20	30	30	30	30	50	50	50

* 50th percentiles.

Source: Oakley, P., Phillips, B., Molyneaux, E. & Mackway–Jones, K. (1993) Updated standard reference chart. *BMJ* 1993; **306**, 1613.

Post-resuscitation care
- Ensure adequate ventilation and normocarbia.
- Maintain adequate blood pressure with infusion of fluids and inotropic support as needed.
- Do not actively rewarm and if unconsciousness remains after resuscitation, cool to 33–34 °C within 6 h for 2–3 days.

Anaphylaxis
See also Allergy and immunology, chapter 19.

The life-threatening clinical manifestations are:
- Hypotension due to vasodilatation and loss of plasma volume due to increased capillary permeability.
- Bronchospasm.
- Upper airways obstruction due to laryngeal or pharyngeal oedema.

Immediate treatment
- Vasopressor and bronchodilator therapy: give adrenaline 10 mcg/kg (0.01 mg/kg) at 0.01 mL/kg of 1 : 1000 solution by **intramuscular (i.m.)** injection or 0.01 mg/kg (i.e. 0.1 mL/kg of 1 : 10 000 solution) by slow i.v. injection (over 10 min). A continuous infusion (0.1–1.0 mcg/kg per min) may be required if manifestations are prolonged. **Note**: Do *not* use subcutaneous adrenaline, as absorption is less reliable.
- Oxygen by mask: mechanical ventilation may be required.
- I.v. volume expander: give 0.9% saline at 20 mL/kg. Give repeat boluses of 10–20 mL/kg until the blood pressure is restored.
- Bronchodilator therapy with salbutamol: continuous nebulised (0.5%) or i.v. 5 mcg/kg per min for 1 h, then 1 mcg/kg per min thereafter. Secondary therapy with a steroid, aminophylline and an antihistamine may be helpful for prolonged bronchospasm and capillary leak.
- Relief of upper airway obstruction: mild to moderate oedema may respond to inhalation of nebulised 1% adrenaline (1 mL per dose diluted to 4 mL) or 5 mL of nebulised 1 : 1000 solution, but intubation of the trachea may be required.
- Anaphylaxis can be biphasic and the patient may deteriorate again over the next few hours.
- All patients with anaphylaxis should be observed carefully for at least 12 h, followed up for allergen testing, provided with self-injectable adrenaline and a Medi-alert bracelet.

Allergic oedema causing acute larygeal obstruction
Treat with nebulised 1% adrenaline 1 mL per dose diluted to 4 mL, or 5 mL of 1 : 1000 solution. Refer to an intensive care specialist or anaesthetist for endotracheal intubation, or an ENT surgeon for tracheostomy.

Haemorrhagic shock
The normal circulating blood volume is 70–80 mL/kg. A child may lose a substantial volume of blood without developing hypotension. Cardiac output and blood pressure are preserved by tachycardia and vasoconstriction, so hypotension is a late sign of blood loss.

- Control external haemorrhage by direct wound pressure, arterial vessel pressure or a tourniquet and elevation of the injured area.
- Administer oxygen by mask.
- Insert a large-bore i.v. cannula, preferably in the upper limb. Two cannulae are usually required.
- Withdraw blood for group and cross-match.
- Infuse rapidly by pressure 20 mL/kg of 0.9% saline solution. This may also be administered rapidly by syringing with the aid of a three-way tap. Titrate additional volume to the heart rate, blood pressure and other indices of perfusion. Further boluses of 10–20 mL/kg 0.9% saline solution may be given.
- **If exsanguinating, transfuse urgently** with (in order of preference):
  - crossmatched blood, or
  - un-crossmatched blood of the same group as the patient, or
  - un-crossmatched O negative blood.
- Warm the blood.
- Monitor blood pressure, heart rate, oxygenation and urine output.
- Measure the central venous pressure, serum calcium, serum potassium, coagulation and acid–base status if a massive transfusion is required. Calcium (10% calcium chloride 0.2 mL/kg) and fresh frozen plasma are usually needed after 1–2 blood volumes have been transfused.
- Investigate and surgically explore internal haemorrhage if necessary.

Septicaemic shock

Hypotension is due to vasodilatation, (early) leakage of fluid from capillary beds and depression of myocardial contractility.

- Collect blood for culture, but do not delay administration of an **antibiotic** if a blood sample cannot be collected. If no information is available regarding the source of pathogen, give flucloxacillin 50 mg/kg (max 2 g) i.v. 4 hourly and cefotaxime 50 mg/kg (max 2 g) i.v. 6 hourly. For particular circumstances consult the Antimicrobial guidelines. For shock due to meningococcaemia, which is usually accompanied by a purpuric rash, give cefotaxime 50 mg/kg (max 2 g) i.v. 6 hourly. Give benzylpenicillin 60 mg/kg (max 3 g) i.v./i.m. 4 hourly if cefotaxime not available.
- Treat shock with **0.9% saline solution**, 20 mL/kg initially – further boluses of 10–20 mL/kg may be needed.
- Give **oxygen** and monitor blood gases. Mechanical ventilation may be required.
- Commence infusion of an **inotropic agent**. Dopamine (5–20 mcg/kg per min) is preferred. Administration via a central vein is preferred but it may be given via a peripheral vein as a dilute solution (e.g. 15 mg/kg in 500 mL at 10–40 mL/h = 5–20 mcg/kg per min). Dobutamine (5–20 mcg/kg per min) may be administered into a peripheral vein.
- Defer lumbar puncture, if indicated, until the child has been stabilised.

Near drowning

There is a global hypoxic–ischaemic injury often associated with lung damage from aspiration of water and gastric contents. The differences between freshwater and saltwater drowning are not usually clinically important.

- Adequate oxygenation and ventilation are of paramount importance. Mechanical ventilation is required for severe lung involvement, circulatory arrest or loss of consciousness. Lung hypoxic–ischaemic injury is compounded by pulmonary oedema or aspiration of water or gastric contents.
- Decompress the stomach, which is usually distended with air and water.
- Support the circulation with i.v. infusion of colloid (e.g. 4% albumin) or 0.9% saline solution and infusion of an inotropic agent (e.g. dopamine 5–20 mcg/kg per min into a central vein).
- If signs of cerebral oedema are present (i.e. a depressed conscious state) administer mannitol 0.25–0.5 g/kg i.v. once.
- Correct electrolyte disturbances; hypokalaemia is common.
- Administer benzylpenicillin 60 mg/kg (max 3 g) i.v. 6 hourly if ventilation is required (to prevent the complication of pneumococcal pneumonia).
- If CPR is required, prevent hyperthermia and induce controlled hypothermia (33–34 °C) for 72 h for cerebral protection.

Acute laryngeal obstruction

The most common cause is laryngotracheobronchitis (croup) and occasional causes are epiglottitis, an inhaled foreign body, allergic oedema and trauma. The hallmark of obstruction is stridor, which when accompanied by a barking cough suggests croup, or when accompanied by dysphagia/drooling suggests epiglottitis. Severe obstruction stimulates forceful diaphragmatic contraction that results in a retraction of the rib cage, tracheal tug and abdominal protrusion on inspiration. Cyanosis and irregular respiratory effort are terminal signs.

Epiglottitis

See also Respiratory conditions, chapter 36, p. 513.
- Complete obstruction may occur in just a few hours. In general, tracheal intubation under anaesthesia is required. Arrange promptly.
- Keep the child as calm as possible in a seated position and administer oxygen by mask.
- If complete obstruction is imminent, summon immediate help from an intensivist or anaesthetist. If inexperienced, do not attempt intubation unless the child becomes comatosed. Intubate orally initially with a relatively small endotracheal tube. It may be hard to see the larynx because of secretions in the pharynx and the swollen epiglottis. Be prepared to aspirate the pharynx with a Yankauer sucker. Cricoid pressure is very helpful to visualise the vocal cords.
- If intubation proves to be impossible, attempt to ventilate with bag–valve–mask; a good technique may achieve adequate oxygenation and ventilation. If ventilation is impossible, perform cricothyrotomy or tracheostomy (see below).
- Antibiotic therapy: Ceftriaxone 100 mg/kg (max 2 g) i.v. followed by 50 mg/kg (max 2 g) 24 h later.

Croup

See also Respiratory conditions, chapter 36, p. 515.

- Avoid any examination that may distress the child.
- In severe obstruction, give an inhalation of nebulised 1% adrenaline 1 mL per dose diluted to 4 mL, or 5 mL of 1:1000 solution to obtain temporary relief.
- Give corticosteroid i.m./i.v. (e.g. dexamethasone 0.6 mg/kg).
- Obtain intensive care or anaesthetic help with a view to endotracheal intubation. If this is not available, intubate when the child is going into respiratory failure. Use an introducing stylet in an endotracheal tube of size 0.5–1 mm smaller than usually calculated by age in years; i.e. (age/4 + 4 mm).
- Children admitted to a general paediatric ward should **not** be administered oxygen. Decreased saturations are a marker of obstruction requiring medical review and often further adrenaline. Giving oxygen masks this.

Aspirated foreign body
See also Respiratory conditions, chapter 36, p. 518.
- Give first aid (back slaps, chest thrusts) if obstruction occurs, otherwise allow the child to cough. Do not instrument the airways if the child is coping, but summon an anaesthetist and ENT surgeon. Give oxygen.
- If complete obstruction occurs, attempt removal of an impacted laryngeal foreign body with forceps – if this is unsuccessful, perform cricothyrotomy or tracheostomy (see below).
- If respiratory failure is due to a foreign body lodged in the lower trachea or bronchi, attempt ventilation via an endotracheal tube while organising endoscopic removal.

Emergency relief of a totally obstructed upper airway
- Adequate oxygenation (but not normal ventilation) can be obtained by inserting a 14-gauge i.v. cannula percutaneously into the trachea via the cricothyroid membrane (which lies between the thyroid and cricoid cartilage); the patient should be lying straight, with the cannula in the midline and angled towards the feet. Remove the needle of the i.v. cannula; connect the cannula to a resuscitator or a bagging circuit using a connector from a 3.0 mm endotracheal tube. Oxygenate with sustained 100% oxygen inspirations. Alternatively, connect the cannula to the compressed wall oxygen supply via a three-way i.v. tap (to allow expiration) and a length of plastic tubing. A length of plastic tubing that has a side hole cut may also be used to allow expiration. Aid intermittent expiration by lateral chest compression.
- Alternatively, perform cricothyrotomy. Identify and maintain stabilisation of the thyroid–cricoid region with one hand. Incise the skin over the cricothyroid membrane. Bluntly dissect into the trachea with forceps in the midline or incise vertically with scalpel. Insert a small tracheostomy or endotracheal tube.
- Alternatively, perform percutaneous mini-tracheostomy.

Status asthmaticus
See also Respiratory conditions, chapter 33.

Critical asthma

Children unresponsive to intermittent inhalation of salbutamol should receive:

- Continuous inhalation of undiluted 0.5% salbutamol solution nebulised with oxygen.
- Methylprednisolone 1 mg/kg i.v. (max 50 mg) 6 hourly.
- Nebulised ipratropium may be added as 250 mcg/dose diluted to 2–3 mL every 20 min × 3 and then 4–6 hourly (beware anticholinergic effects).
- I.v. salbutamol load 5 mcg/kg per min for 60 min followed by infusion 1–2 mcg/kg per min (beware hypokalaemia). Discuss with nearest paediatric ICU or retrieval service at this stage.
- Aminophylline (subject to prior theophylline use and serum level) 10 mg/kg (max. 500 mg) i.v. over 1 h. This can be followed by an infusion: 1.1 mg/kg per hour (age 1–9 years) or 0.7 mg/kg per hour (10 years to adult) or 6 hourly doses (each over an hour). Check level following loading dose.
- $MgSO_4$ 0.1 mmol/kg infused over 30 min.
- Refractory critical asthma – manage in ICU.

Status epilepticus

See also Neurologic conditions, chapter 33, p. 453.

A convulsion involving the respiratory musculature and upper airways that does not cease within a few minutes may cause hypoventilation with hypoxaemia and hypercarbia. Refer to Fig. 1.2 for proposed algorithm on acute seizure management.

- Administer oxygen.
- Be prepared to give mechanical ventilation, particularly if the child has meningitis.
- Check blood glucose, electrolytes, blood gas and septic screen.
- Some initial i.v. anticonvulsant choices include:
  - Diazepam: 0.2–0.4 mg/kg (max 10–20 mg) i.v. May be given per rectum if there is no i.v. access.
  - Midazolam: 0.1–0.15 mg/kg i.v. or 0.15–0.2 mg/kg (i.m.) effective i.m. within 5–10 min.
  - Clonazepam: 0.25 mg (<1 year); 0.5 mg (1–5 years); 1 mg (>5 years) i.v.
  - Phenobarbitone: 20–30 mg/kg over 30 min; repeat doses 10–15 mg/kg every 15–30 min up to 100 mg/kg in 24 h (beware of hypotension) if required (adults – max 600 mg/d).
  - Phenytoin: 15–20 mg/kg (max 1.5 g) i.v. over 1 h to avoid negative inotropic effect. Slow onset. Infuse under ECG monitoring.
  - Thiopentone: titrate dose slowly to effect (usually 2–5 mg/kg). Beware of hypotension and be ready to control the airway and breathing before administration. This is usually undertaken with ICU support.
- Consider i.v. ceftriaxone if meningitis suspected.

Prolonged convulsions may require large and repeated doses of anticonvulsant drugs or infusions and, consequently, mechanical ventilation. Repeated doses of a single anticonvulsant such as phenobarbitone (where the serum level correlates with the effects) are preferable

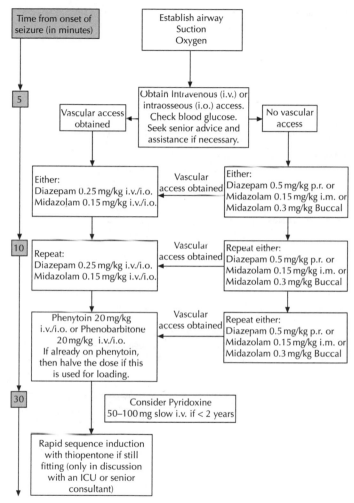

Fig. 1.2 Acute seizure management. (From NSW Heath Acute Paediatrics Clinical Practice Guidelines.) Reproduced with permission, NSW Department of Health from its publication *Acute management of seizures in children* (December 2004).

to using multiple anticonvulsants. Suspect hyponatraemia as the cause of convulsions in meningitis and severe gastroenteritis-related dehydration.

Raised intracranial pressure

Acute intracranial hypertension threatens the blood supply and may cause herniation of the brain. It is recognised (in approximate sequence) by:

- Headache, vomiting, papilloedema, deterioration in the conscious state with diminution of spontaneous limb movements.
- Ipsilateral pupillary dilatation and contralateral hemiparesis, limb hypertonicity and spasm if there is uncal herniation into tentorial hiatus with supratentorial lesion. These can be bilateral with an extensive lesion.
- Alteration in pattern of respiration (hyperventilation; irregular respiration), bradycardia and hypertension are near-terminal events due to medullary herniation into the foramen magnum.

Common causes

- Acute brain swelling due to cerebral oedema caused by trauma, infection, ischaemia or hypoxaemia.
- Space-occupying lesion, such as an intracerebral haemorrhage, tumour or abscess.
- Obstruction of cerebrospinal fluid circulation.

Management

- A neurosurgeon should be contacted immediately where indicated, e.g. in cases of trauma.
- If it is impossible to treat the cause immediately, reduce the intracranial blood volume by using mechanical hyperventilation to lower the P_{CO_2} and cause cerebral vasoconstriction. (*Note*: prolonged or excessive hyperventilation to P_{CO_2} of <25–35 mmHg may be harmful.)
- Mannitol may be used to reduce cerebral oedema (0.25–0.5 g/kg i.v.). Fluids should be restricted to avoid cerebral oedema, but not at the expense of causing hypotension. Blood pressure may be maintained with a vasopressor (e.g. dopamine up to 10 mcg/kg/min).
- Hypoxaemia and hypotension must be avoided.
- A lumbar puncture should **not** be done in the presence of intracranial hypertension because of risk of brain stem herniation (coning). A guide to the role of lumbar puncture and chemotherapeutic agents in the undiagnosed unconscious patient is given in Fig. 1.3.

USEFUL RESOURCES
- *www.resus.org.au* – Australian Resuscitation Council. Voluntary co-ordinating body which fosters uniformity in the practice of resuscitation.

Consider: post-ictal state, infection (meningitis, encephalitis), trauma (including non-accidental injury), poisoning (drugs, toxins), metabolic conditions, hydrocephalus, hypertension, hepatic or renal failure and Reye's syndrome

Look for: bruises, fundal haemorrhages, blood pressure, urinalysis and blood sugar (reagent strip)

Initial investigations may include: full blood examination, urea and electrolytes, glucose, liver function test, arterial blood gas, drug screen, urine antigens, culture of blood and urine, and ammonia

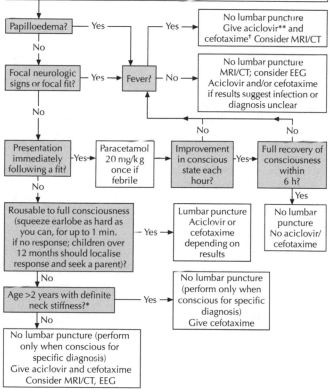

* Neck stiffness is not a reliable sign of meningism in children <2 years
** Aciclovir 10 mg/kg i.v. 8 hourly (age 2 weeks–2 years)
500 mg/m² i.v. 8 hourly (age 2–12 years)
† Cefotaxime 50 mg/kg (max 2 g) i.v. 6 hourly

Fig. 1.3 A guide to the role of lumbar puncture and use of chemotherapeutic agents in the child unconscious due to unknown cause

CHAPTER 2
Poisoning and envenomation

James Tibballs

Poisoning
Background

Poisoning during childhood occurs mainly among 1–3 year-olds and tends to follow the ingestion of one of a wide variety of agents improperly stored in the home. It should be considered in any child presenting with symptoms that cannot be explained, such as altered conscious state, tachy- or bradycardia and unusual behaviour.

Other circumstances of poisoning are iatrogenic (particularly in infants) and the deliberate self-administration of substances by older children for their recreational use or to manipulate their psychosocial environments. Increasingly, the intention is suicidal and this should be considered, even in young children. See also chapter 15, Adolescent health and chapter 16, Child psychiatry.

Although poisoning in childhood is frequently minor in severity and mortality is low, serious illness may be caused by prescription and over-the-counter drugs and non-pharmaceutical products, including complementary medications (see p. 546, chapter 39, Prescribing for children).

Prevention

- Action should be taken according to the circumstance of poisoning to prevent recurrence.
- Parents should be encouraged to store all medicines in childproof cabinets and toxic substances in places inaccessible to young children.
- Urgent psychosocial help should be organised for children who have poisoned themselves intentionally.
- Steps should be taken to ensure that iatrogenic poisoning is not repeated. Institutions should develop programmes to detect and prevent drug errors.

General management

See Fig. 2.1. The principles of management for all poisonings are:
- Resuscitate the patient and remove the poison if indicated.
- Administer an antidote if one exists (see Table 2.1).

In Australia, call Poisons Information on **13 11 26** – a 24-hour nationwide service.

Paediatric Handbook, 8th edition. By Kate Thomson, Dean Tey and Michael Marks. Published 2009 by Blackwell Publishing, ISBN: 978-1-4051-7400-8.

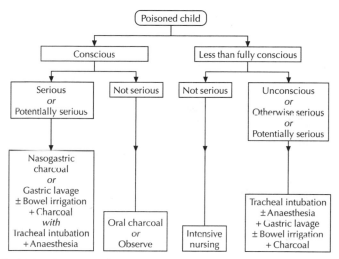

Fig. 2.1 General management of the poisoned child

Recovery is expected in the majority of cases if vital functions are preserved and the complications of poisoning and its management are avoided.

A decision to remove the poison from the body should be dependent on the severity of the poisoning and the likelihood of success in removing the poison without further endangering the patient. Most poisonings in childhood are minor and observation alone or non-invasive treatment is indicated.

The severity of poisoning may be assessed by the:
- Established and expected effects.
- Quantity of the poison(s).
- Preparation of the poison.
- Interval since exposure.

Removal from the body usually involves gastrointestinal decontamination but occasionally other methods, such as dialysis, exchange transfusion, charcoal haemoperfusion, plasmapheresis or haemofiltration are required.

Gastrointestinal decontamination

If the conscious state is depressed, all methods of gastrointestinal decontamination carry a substantial risk of aspiration pneumonitis, even if the patient is intubated. Hence, the most important factor determining the technique of decontamination is the conscious state. A guideline for the general management of poisoning using these techniques according to severity of poisoning is shown in Fig. 2.1. The most commonly used method is with activated

Table 2.1 Antidotes to poisons

Poison	Antidotes and doses	Comments
Amphetamines	Esmolol 0.5 mg/kg i.v. over 1 min, then 25–200 mcg/kg per min i.v. Labetalol 0.15–0.3 mg/kg i.v. or phentolamine 0.05–0.1 mg/kg i.v. every 10 min.	Treatment for tachyarrhythmia. Treatment for hypertension.
Benzodiazepines	Flumazenil 5 mcg/kg i.v. repeated at 1 min then 2–10 mcg/kg per h by i.v. infusion.	Specific antagonist at receptor. Titrate to effect. Caution: may precipitate convulsions or arrhythmia in multi-drug ingestion, especially with tricyclics.
Beta blocker	Glucagon 7 mcg/kg i.v. then 2–7 mcg/kg per min i.v. infusion. Isoprenaline 0.05–2 mcg/kg per min i.v. Beware b₁ hypotension. Noradrenaline 0.05–0.5 mcg/kg per min i.v.	Stimulates non-catecholamine cAMP production. Preferred antidote.
Calcium blocker	Calcium chloride 20 mg (0.2 mL of 10%)/kg i.v.	
Carbon monoxide	Oxygen 100%	Hyperbaric oxygen may be required.
Cyanide	Dicobalt edetate 7.5 mg/kg (max 300 mg i.v.) over 1 min, then repeat at 5 min if no effect. Sodium nitrite 3% i.v. (0.33 mL/kg over 4 min), *then* sodium thiosulphate 25% i.v. 1.65 mL/kg (max 50 mL) at 3–5 mL/min.	Chelates. Give 50 mL 50% glucose after each dose. Nitrites form methaemoglobin-cyanide complex (beware excess methaemoglobinaemia – restrict to <20%) Thiosulphate forms non-toxic thiocyanate from methaemoglobin-cyanide.
Digoxin	Digoxin Fab. Dose: acute ingestion 1 vial/2.5 tablet (0.25 mg); in steady state vials = serum digoxin (ng/mL) × BW (kg)/100.	

Ergotamine	Sodium nitroprusside infusion 0.5–5 mcg/kg per min. Heparin 100 units/kg i.v. then 10–30 units/kg i.v. per h according to clotting.	Treats vasoconstriction. Monitor BP continuously. Treatment of coagulopathy.
Lead	If symptomatic or blood lead >2.9 µmol/L dimercaprol (BAL) 75 mg/m² i.m. 4-hourly 6 doses then calcium disodium edetate (EDTA) 1500 mg/m² i.v. over 5 days. If asymptomatic and blood lead 2.18–2.9 µmol/L infuse calcium disodium edetate 1000 mg/m² per day for 5 days.	
Heparin	Protamine 1 mg/100 units heparin i.v.	Heparin half-life 1–2 h.
Iron	Desferrioxamine 15 mg/kg per h 12–24 h if serum iron >90 µmol/L or >63 µmol/L and symptomatic.	Beware anaphylaxis.
Methanol, ethyleneglycol, glycol ethers	Ethanol, infuse loading dose 10 mL/kg 10% diluted in glucose 5% i.v. and then 0.15 mL/kg per h to maintain blood level at 0.1% (100 mg/dL).	
Methaemoglobin e.g. 2° to drug treatment	Methylene blue 1–2 mg/kg i.v. over several min.	
Opiates	Naloxone 0.01–0.1 mg/kg i.v., then 0.01 mg/kg per h as needed.	
Organophosphates and carbamates	Atropine 20–50 mcg/kg i.v. every 15 min until secretions dry. Pralidoxime 25 mg/kg i.v. over 15–30 min, then 10–20 mg/kg per h for 18 h or more. Not for carbamates.	Restores cholinesterase.
Paracetamol	N-acetylcysteine. I.v.: 150 mg/kg over 60 min, then 10 mg/kg per h for 20–72 h. Oral: 140 mg/kg then 17 doses of 70 mg/kg 4 hourly (total 1330 mg/kg over 68 h).	Give for >72 h if still encephalopathic.
Tricyclic antidepressants	Sodium bicarbonate i.v. 1 mmol/kg to maintain blood pH >7.45.	

charcoal, with gastric lavage and whole-bowel irrigation having limited roles. There is no role for induced emesis in the hospital setting.

Activated charcoal

Activated charcoal is more efficacious than induced emesis or gastric lavage and is currently regarded as a 'universal antidote'. It adsorbs most poisons but not metals, corrosives or pesticides. Like other techniques, however, it is contraindicated in the less than fully conscious patient or if ileus is present. If aspirated, charcoal may cause fatal bronchiolitis obliterans. Constipation is relatively common. Addition of a laxative decreases transit time through the gut but does not improve efficacy in preventing drug absorption. It may also upset fluid and electrolyte balance. The initial dose is 1–2 g/kg. Repeated doses of activated charcoal enhance elimination of many drugs, particularly slow-release preparations. A suitable regimen is 0.25 g/kg per hour for 12–24 h.

Gastric lavage

Although gastric lavage appears to be a logical therapy for ingested poisons, it has a limited place in management. Problems include
• Poor efficacy in preventing absorption when done >60 min after ingestion.
• Risk of aspiration pneumonitis in the less than fully conscious patient and to a lesser extent in the conscious child.
• In the conscious young child, it is psychologically traumatic and difficult to do.

If it is undertaken, care should be taken to avoid water intoxication and intrabronchial instillation of lavage fluid.
• Gastric lavage is **contraindicated** after ingestion of corrosives, hydrocarbons or petrochemicals.
• Gastric lavage is **indicated** in serious poisoning when a child is already intubated for airway protection and ventilation. The child should be in the lateral position during lavage. If potentially serious effects are expected, gastric lavage should only be done after rapid sequence induction of anaesthesia and tracheal intubation.

Whole bowel irrigation

Whole bowel irrigation is done with a solution of polyethylene glycol (30 mL/kg per hour for 4–8 h) and electrolytes administered by nasogastric tube. It is useful in delayed presentations and for the management of poisoning by slow-release drug preparations, substances not adsorbed by activated charcoal (e.g. iron) or substances which are irretrievable by gastric lavage.

Induced vomiting

Syrup of ipecacuanha is no longer routinely recommended. Its usefulness in the hospital setting is extremely limited – perhaps only to a case of serious poisoning presenting very early after ingestion when no other effective treatment is possible. It was previously used as a first aid measure in the home, but it does not reliably empty the stomach and is contraindicated where conscious state is impaired (risk of aspiration pneumonitis) and when the ingested substance is corrosive, hydrocarbon or petrochemical.

Poisoning with unknown or multiple agents

- Suspect poisoning on presentation with convulsions, depression of the conscious state, hypoventilation, hypotension or an illness that is not otherwise readily explained. A urinary drug screen may be useful for diagnosis.
- Multiple poisons may have been ingested. Determine blood levels if there is any possibility of ingestion of paracetamol, iron, salicylate, theophylline, methanol, digoxin or lithium. Blood levels may influence clinical management.
- Contact the Poisons Information hotline for advice; see p. 14.

Individual poisons

Thousands of poisons exist. The most common serious poisons in young children presenting to the Royal Children's Hospital have been paracetamol, rodenticides, eucalyptus oil, benzodiazepines, tricyclic antidepressants and theophylline.

Only the most common serious poisonings, or poisonings peculiar to children are considered here briefly. Some have antidotes (see Table 2.1). **The general principles of management apply to all individual poisons** (see Fig. 2.1). Details of effects of specific poisons and suggested management should be obtained from a Poisons Information Centre and from appropriate, up-to-date references.

Consider the possibility of intentional drug ingestion. These children are often at 'high risk' for multiple psychological and social reasons. See also chapter 15, Adolescent health.

Paracetamol (acetaminophen)

Paracetamol is the most common pharmaceutical poisoning.

Effects

The liver metabolises it to a toxic product, N-acetyl-p-benzoquinoneimine, which causes hepatic necrosis unless neutralised by the hepatic antioxidant, glutathione. Multi-organ failure and death may occur after 3–4 days if the ingested quantity exceeds 150 mg/kg or with smaller amounts with prior hepatic dysfunction, alcohol or anticonvulsants. Early symptoms are anorexia, nausea and vomiting.

Specific management

N-acetylcysteine (NAC) is an effective antidote if given before hepatic necrosis occurs. Its use is associated with adverse reactions (e.g. rash, bronchospasm and hypotension) that occur more frequently when administered i.v. If reactions occur, cease NAC temporarily and give promethazine 0.2–0.5 mg/kg i.v. (max. 10–25 mg) and recommence the NAC infusion at a reduced rate.

Since the outcome is related to serum levels of paracetamol measured 4–20 h after ingestion, a decision to administer NAC after a single overdose may be made according to time-related plasma levels. Administer if the level exceeds 1000 μmol/L at 4 h, 500 at 8 h, 200 at 12 h, 80 at 16 h, or 40 at 20 h (μmol/L × 0.15 = μg/mL).

- I.v. NAC: 150 mg/kg in 5 mL/kg of glucose 5% over 60 min, then 10 mg/kg per hour for 20 h or longer if the child is encephalopathic, or presentation is 10–36 h after ingestion or
- Oral NAC: 140 mg/kg, then 17 doses of 70 mg/kg (4 hourly).

Note:
- Serum levels >18 h after a single ingestion are unreliable predictors of risk.
- These recommendations do not apply to multiple smaller ingestions (seek expert advice).
- Presentation <1 h after significant ingestion may be treated with gastric lavage (see p. 18).
- Monitor liver function tests and serum potassium.

Iron
Small quantities (<20 mg/kg) of elemental iron may be toxic. This is usually ingested as iron tablets/capsules, mixtures or multivitamin preparations.

Effects
- Immediate: Nausea, vomiting, abdominal pain and possible gastric erosion.
- At 6–24 h: Hypotension, hypovolaemia and metabolic acidosis.
- At 12–24 h: Multi-organ failure – gastrointestinal (ileus, gastric erosion), CNS, cardiovascular, hepatic and renal.
- At 4–6 weeks: Pyloric stenosis.

Specific management
- Serum iron level (mcg/dL × 0.1791 = μmol/L). Note: Absorption may be slow.
- Abdominal radiograph may reveal the quantity ingested.
- Whole bowel irrigation (not if ileus, obstruction or erosion are present). Activated charcoal is ineffective.
- Infusion of desferrioxamine no faster than 15 mg/kg per hour for 12–24 h is indicated if:
  - Patient is clinically hypotensive or has depressed consciousness.
  - >60 mg/kg elemental iron has been ingested.
  - Iron level is >90 μmol/L.
  - Iron level is >63 μmol/L and patient is symptomatic.

Tricyclic antidepressants
Sudden death may occur.

Effects
The life-threatening effects are:
- CNS depression: coma, convulsions.
- Non-cardiogenic pulmonary oedema.
- Cardiac depression: hypocontractility, hypotension and sudden dysrhythmias (conduction blocks and ventricular ectopy, including tachycardia/fibrillation).

Specific management
- ECG monitoring: assess heart rate, QRS duration and QT interval.
- Alkalisation of blood to pH 7.45–7.50 with sodium bicarbonate infusion or hyperventilation, or both.
- Anticonvulsant therapy with diazepam 0.1–0.4 mg/kg (max 10–20 mg).
- Antidysrhythmia therapy: give phenytoin slowly (over 30 min). Beware of hypotension.

- Treatment of hypotension with an alpha-agonist (noradrenaline 0.01–1 mcg/kg per min). Avoid beta-agonists and drugs with mixed alpha and beta actions.
- Treatment of ventricular tachycardia/fibrillation with DC shock, amiodarone (5 mg/kg i.v.) or lignocaine (lidocaine) (1 mg/kg, then 10–50 mcg/kg per min) and a beta-blocker.
- Treatment of *torsade de pointes* with DC shock, magnesium sulfate (0.1–0.2 mmol/kg i.v.) or lignocaine (lidocaine) as above.

Salicylates
Toxicity is expected if >150 mg/kg is ingested.

Effects
- Coma, hyperpyrexia and respiratory alkalosis followed by metabolic acidosis.
- Cardiac depression, pulmonary oedema and hypotension.
- Hepatic encephalopathy (Reye syndrome) with chronic use.

Specific management
- Serum salicylate level, blood glucose, serum potassium and blood pH.
- Correction of dehydration.
- Correction of acidosis and maintenance of urine pH >7.5 (with sodium bicarbonate) and correction of hypokalaemia.
- Haemodialysis/haemoperfusion if the serum level is >25 mmol/L (mcg/mL × 0.0724 = μmol/L).

Theophylline
Toxicity is related to serum levels and may be delayed with slow-release preparations.

Effects
- Gastrointestinal: nausea, protracted vomiting, abdominal pain.
- Metabolic:
  - Hypokalaemia due to migration into cells, diuresis and vomiting.
  - Metabolic acidosis.
  - Hyperglycaemia, hyperinsulinaemia and hypomagnesaemia.
- CNS: seizures, agitation, coma (uncommon).
- Cardiovascular: atrial and ventricular ectopy, hypotension.

Specific management
- Prolonged observation if a slow-release preparation is ingested.
- Serum level (anticipate seizures at approximately 300 μmol/L and the need for charcoal haemoperfusion or plasmapheresis at approximately 550 μmol/L, or less if there is protracted vomiting).
- Anti-emetic therapy with metoclopramide 0.15 mg/kg (max 10–15 mg) i.v. 6 hourly.
- ECG monitoring. Beware of early hypokalaemia and late hyperkalaemia when potassium re-enters the blood.

Eucalyptus and essential oils
Effects
- Initial coughing, choking.
- Rapid onset (30 min, occasionally delayed) CNS depression (convulsions and meiosis are rare).
- Vomiting and subsequent aspiration pneumonitis.

Specific management
- Exclude pneumonitis (perform chest radiograph and measure oxygenation).

Amphetamines
Effects
- Amphetamine and derivatives, e.g. methamphetamine ('ice') and 3,4-methylenedioxymethamphetamine (Ecstasy), are strong stimulants of the CNS, but may also induce convulsions, hyperthermia (with secondary coagulopathy and rhabdomyolysis), hypertension, cardiovascular collapse and adult respiratory distress syndrome.

Specific management
Treatment is largely supportive and may include sedatives (benzodiazepine), anticonvulsants, beta- and alpha-blockade, dantrolene, mechanical ventilation, inotropic and renal support.

Petroleum distillates
Inhaling the fumes of petrol, kerosene, lighter fluid, lamp oils, solvents and mineral spirits is often referred to as 'chroming' or 'sniffing.' There are significant social and cognitive effects of long-term abuse and these children are at high risk because of multiple psychosocial reasons. See also chapter 15, Adolescent health.

Effects
- CNS obtundation, convulsions, vomiting or hepatorenal toxicity.

Specific management
- Exclude pneumonitis (perform chest radiograph and measure oxygenation).

Button or disc batteries
- Ingestion may cause electrolysis, corrosion, the release of toxins or pressure effects.
- Impaction in the oesophagus is an emergency – it may cause perforation or an oesophagotracheal fistula and must be removed endoscopically as soon as possible. Surgical follow-up is essential.

Caustic substances
- Automatic machine dishwashing detergents, caustic soda, drain cleaners are strong alkalis and cause burns to the gastrointestinal tract when ingested.

- Significant oesophageal damage may occur in absence of proximal injury.
- Arrange surgical oesophagoscopy and follow-up.

Envenomation

The Australian Venom Research Unit (*www.avru.org*) provides a 24-hour advisory service on 1300 760 451.

Snake bite

This section applies to bites by Australian snakes of the family *Elapidae*. Snake bites by species in other countries cause different effects and are not outlined in this handbook. Refer to local publications.

Although not all snakes are venomous and envenomation does not always accompany a bite by a venomous snake, **every snake bite should be regarded as potentially lethal**. In young children a history of snake bite is often uncertain.

Of the many species of snakes in Australia, the principal dangerous species are from the genera of:

- Brown snakes
- Tiger snakes
- Taipans
- Death adders
- Black snakes
- Copperheads
- Several marine genera.

Venom from these species contain:

- **Neurotoxins** which cause neuromuscular paralysis and subsequent respiratory failure.
- **Procoagulants** that cause disseminated intravascular coagulation (DIC) via depletion of clotting factors, resulting in subsequent haemorrhage (death adders do not contain significant procoagulant).
- **Rhabdomyolysins** which cause delayed destruction of skeletal muscle (not present in brown snake or death adder venoms).

Other less important components are haemolysins and anticoagulants.

Symptoms and signs of envenomation

The bite site may be identifiable by fang or scratch marks surrounded by bruising or oedema. However, note that a bite site may be undetectable and occasionally unnoticed by a victim.

- Headache, nausea, vomiting and abdominal pain may occur within an hour of envenomation.
- Early neurotoxic signs include ptosis, diplopia, blurred vision, facial muscle weakness, dysphonia and dysphagia.

Emergencies

- Advanced neurotoxic signs include weakness of limb, trunk and respiratory muscles.
- Spontaneous haemorrhage may occur from mucous membranes, occasionally into solid organs and from needle puncture sites.
- Hypotension secondary to haemorrhage and respiratory failure.
- Renal failure may occur, secondary to hypotension, haemolysis and rhabdomyolysis, particularly if treatment with antivenom is delayed.

The syndrome culminates in respiratory and cardiovascular failure within several hours after envenomation, but may be accelerated in a small child or after multiple bites.

Suspected envenomation
If there is a suspicious history of snake bite but the patient is asymptomatic, the patient should be observed closely for approximately 12 h.
- Test blood coagulation, as it is both a sensitive and reliable indicator of envenomation by major species except death adders.
- Apply a pressure-immobilisation first-aid bandage (Fig. 2.2). It can be removed after ensuring that antivenom is available.
- Perform a venom-detection test (see below). A positive test of a swab from the bite site or of a biological sample (urine or blood) indicates which antivenom to administer, if clinically indicated.

Definite envenomation
A number of measures may be required, depending on the severity of envenomation (see Fig. 2.3):
- Resuscitation with mechanical ventilation, oxygen therapy and fluid volume restoration.
- Application of a pressure-immobilisation first-aid bandage (Fig. 2.2) if not already in place. Do not remove an existing first-aid bandage until antivenom has been administered. Cut a hole in the existing bandage to obtain a bite site swab if needed and then reinforce.
- Perform a venom test of urine (preferred), blood and/or bite site swab.
- Administer antivenom (i.v.).
- Administer coagulation factors (fresh frozen plasma) after antivenom. Occasionally blood transfusion is needed.

Antivenom therapy
Specific antivenoms are available against the brown snake, tiger snake, black snake, taipan, death adder and beaked sea snake. A polyvalent preparation contains all the above-named antivenoms except the beaked sea snake. All are given i.v.
- Antivenom is required for clinical envenomation or for significant asymptomatic coagulopathy that may result in serious (e.g. intracranial) haemorrhage. A mild coagulopathy may resolve but requires repeat testing.
- Monovalent preparations are preferred because of a lower incidence of adverse reaction compared with polyvalent antivenom.
- **Always premedicate the patient with adrenaline 0.005–0.01 mg/kg (i.e. 0.05–0.1 mL/kg of 1:10000 s.c. or 0.005–0.01 mL/kg of 1:1000 for larger patients).**

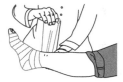

Apply a broad pressure bandage over the bite site as soon as possible. Do not remove clothing, as the movement in doing so will promote the entry of venom into the blood stream. Keep the bitten limb still.

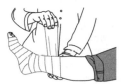

The bandage should be as tight as you would apply to a sprained ankle.

Note: Bandage upwards from the toes or fingers of the bitten limb to help immobilisation. Even though a little venom may be squeezed upwards, the bandage will be far more comfortable than if applied from above downwards; and may be left in place longer.

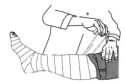

Extend the bandages as far up the limb as possible.

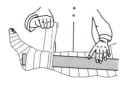

Apply a splint to the leg to immobilise joints on either side of the bite.

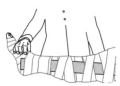

Bind it firmly to as much of the leg as possible. Bring transport to the patients.

Hospital Staff:
Please note that first aid measures are usually removed soon after the patient is seen in hospital. Do not leave on for hours.

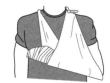

Bites on the hand or forearm
1. Bind to elbow with bandages.
2. Use splint to elbow.
3. Use sling.

Fig. 2.2 Pressure-immobilisation first-aid bandage

- This is required only for the first dose of antivenom to prevent or decrease the severity of anaphylaxis.
- A course of prednisolone 1 mg/kg orally, daily for 2–5 days may prevent serum sickness, which may occur after polyvalent antivenom or after multiple doses of monovalent antivenom.
- Selection of antivenom should be based on the result of a venom-detection test or on reliable identification of the snake, as there is little cross-reactivity between antivenoms. Do not rely upon the victim's or witness's identification unless they are an expert.
- If antivenom therapy is required urgently before species identification, administer antivenom according to location. In Victoria give both brown and tiger snake antivenom, in Tasmania give tiger snake antivenom, and elsewhere give polyvalent antivenom. All bites by marine species can be treated with beaked sea snake or tiger snake antivenom.
- Brown snake, taipan, death adder and black snake antivenoms are only effective against those species, whereas tiger snake antivenom is effective against tiger snakes, copperheads, red-bellied black snake and many minor species.
- Dilute with crystalloid and infuse i.v. over 30 min (faster in life-threatening envenomation).
- The dose of antivenom cannot be predetermined because the amount of venom injected and the patient's susceptibility to it are unknown. In moderate envenomation, initially administer at least 4 ampoules of brown snake antivenom or 1 ampoule of other types and titrate additional doses against the clinical and coagulation status. Larger number of ampoules may be required in moderate and severe envenomation.
- Administer antivenom before giving blood or coagulation factors to forestall further DIC.

Venom detection kit

The venom detection kit (VDK) is a bedside or laboratory three-step enzyme immunoassay, able to detect venom in urine, blood or from a swab of the bite site in very low concentration. It takes about 25 min to perform. If positive, it indicates which antivenom to administer (if clinically indicated), but not necessarily the species of snake.

Spider bite
Red-back spider

The venom of this spider contains a neurotoxin that causes release of neurotransmitters. Although potentially lethal, the syndrome of envenomation (latrodectism) develops slowly over many hours, and no deaths have been recorded since an antivenom has been available. A similar syndrome is caused by many species of the genus *Latrodectus* worldwide (Australia, *L. hasselti*; New Zealand, *L. katipo*, *L. hasselti*).

Symptoms and signs

- Severe persistent local pain, often worsened with movement and referred elsewhere.
- Local erythema, oedema, pruritus, sweating and regional lymphadenopathy.
- Systemic effects may include distal limb and abdominal pain, hypertension, sweating, vomiting, fever and headache.
- Myalgia, muscle spasms, arthralgia, paraesthesia and weakness may last many weeks.

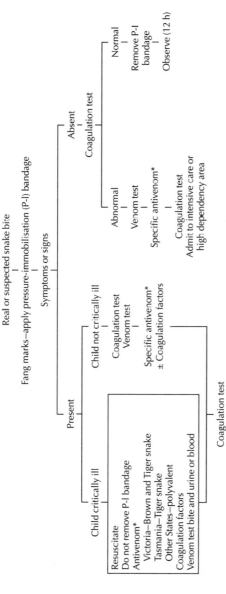

Fig. 2.3 Management of snake bite

Management
- Do **not** use a pressure-immobilisation bandage. The symptom onset is slow and immobilisation may exacerbate pain.
- If the effects remain mild and localised up to 24 h after a bite, treatment may be symptomatic but pain should be treated with antivenom.
- Severe local and systemic effects or prolonged mild effects warrant administration of antivenom i.m. (occasionally i.v.). Sometimes several ampoules are needed. Antivenom has been effective even when administered months after envenomation.
- Although the rate of adverse reactions is low (<0.5%), premedication with promethazine may be used. In all cases, adrenaline should be at hand to treat anaphylaxis (see chapter 1, Medical emergencies).

White-tailed spider
Contrary to popular belief, bites by this spider are rarely troublesome, but severe local inflammatory reaction or skin necrosis may occasionally occur.

Funnel-web spiders
Several large aggressive species can threaten life with a venom that releases neurotransmitters and catecholamines. Several dangerous species exist in NSW and Queensland. In some other states (including Victoria) funnel-web species exist but are not known to be dangerous. Envenomation does not always accompany a bite.

Symptoms and signs
Envenomation is indicated by (in approximate sequence):
- Local muscle fasciculation, piloerection, vomiting, abdominal pain, profuse sweating, salivation and lacrimation.
- Hypertension, tachyarrhythmias and vasoconstriction develop.
- The syndrome culminates in coma, respiratory failure and terminal hypotension.

Management
- Apply a pressure-immobilisation bandage.
- Administer funnel-web spider antivenom i.v.
- Provide mechanical ventilation, airway protection, atropine and cardiovascular therapy as required.

Jellyfish stings
Chironex box jellyfish
This is the world's most venomous animal. It has a cuboid body, approximately 30 cm in diameter, numerous trailing tentacles and inhabits shallow northern Australian coastal waters. Stings are most common from October to May, but have been recorded throughout the year. Contact with the tentacles leads to the discharge of millions of nematocysts that fire barbs through the epidermis and blood vessels, releasing venom that contain myotoxins, haemolysins, dermatonecrotic toxins and possibly a neurotoxin. Severity of envenomation is related to the length of tentacles contacting the skin.

Symptoms and signs
Severe pain and possible cardiorespiratory arrest due to direct cardiotoxicity and possible neurological effects causing apnoea.

Management
- Rescue the victim from water to prevent drowning.
- Cardiopulmonary resuscitation may be required on the beach.
- Dowsing of adherent tentacles with vinegar/acetic acid to inactivate undischarged nematocysts (supplies of vinegar are stocked at popular beaches).
- Analgesia: parenteral for extensive stings, cold packs for minor stings.
- Antivenom i.v. (3 ampoules for life-threatening signs, 1–2 ampoules for analgesia or to prevent skin scarring).

Prevention is most important. Envenomation is prevented by light clothing. Unguarded waters must not be entered when jellyfish are inshore. Beach warning signs should not be ignored.

Irukandji jellyfish
This small tropical jellyfish has a bell measuring 2 × 2.5 cm and four tentacles – one from each corner, a few trailing up to 75 cm. It is almost transparent and difficult to see.

Symptoms and signs
Although the sting is only moderately painful, it is followed by a variable period of:
- Nausea, vomiting, profuse sweating, agitation and muscle cramps.
- Vasoconstriction and severe systemic and pulmonary hypertension (due to release of catecholamines). This may cause acute heart failure.

Management
- Mechanical ventilation and vasodilators may be required.

USEFUL RESOURCES
- *www.avru.org* – Australian Venom Research Unit. World-renowned Melbourne University unit.
- *www.toxnet.nlm.nih.gov* – Toxicology Data Network. American database containing useful information on toxicology, hazardous chemicals, environmental health, and toxic releases.
- *www.toxinology.com* – Excellent clinical toxinology resource from the Women's & Children's Hospital, Adelaide, Australia.
- *www.museumvictoria.com.au/bioinformatics/snake* – Images and ecological data on Victorian Snakes.

CHAPTER 3

Procedures

Georgia Paxton
Peter Barnett

Procedures can be pain- and anxiety-free with good planning and procedural pain management. It is easier to perform any procedure with a calm child and family. Ideally, procedures should be carried out in a designated procedure room, with equipment ready before the child enters the room. Procedural pain management includes both non-pharmacological techniques such as distraction, presence of a parent, and pharmacological techniques with analgesia and sedation as required. Sedation itself does not provide pain relief. Suggested analgesia is included for procedures in this chapter, further details are included in Pain management, chapter 4, p. 61. Universal precautions should be taken during any procedure. Gloves and protective eyewear should be worn and a hard plastic container should be within easy reach for the disposal of sharps. Procedures should be documented in the medical record.

Venepuncture
Sites
- Cubital fossa.
- Dorsum of the hand.
- Others, as dictated by availability or necessity.

Suggested analgesia
- Topical local anaesthetic, e.g. amethocaine or EMLA (lignocaine [lidocaine], prilocaine), can be used for any age except preterm neonates.
- Sucrose in infants <3/12 (max 2 mL, 0.5 mL in infants <1500 g).
- Consider nitrous oxide in children >4 years.
- Consider sedation, e.g. midazolam oral 0.5 mg/kg (max 15 mg) intranasal/buccal 0.3 mg/kg (max 10 mg).

Refer to chapter 4, Pain management.

Equipment
Needle (straight or butterfly), syringe, alcohol wipe, tourniquet, cotton ball, band-aid/tape, blood collection tubes.

Paediatric Handbook, 8th edition. By Kate Thomson, Dean Tey and Michael Marks. Published 2009 by Blackwell Publishing, ISBN: 978-1-4051-7400-8.

Technique

- In adolescents and older children, blood can be collected with a needle and syringe, as in adults. In infants and small children, a 23-gauge butterfly needle offers more stability.
- Wash the site with an alcohol preparation and allow to dry. Using a tourniquet around the limb, insert the needle into a vein and aspirate gently; once enough blood is collected, release tourniquet and apply local pressure with a cotton ball on the puncture site.
- Some visible veins are too small to be used to take blood. A palpable vein is more likely to be successful than a visible but non-palpable vein.
- With small children, an assistant can hold the limb still and provide a tourniquet at the same time.
- An alternative technique is to insert a 21- or 23-gauge needle into a vein and allow the blood to drip out directly into collection tubes. Several millilitres can be collected this way.

Blood culture collection

- Strict asepsis is required.
- Use alcoholic chlorhexidine or 70% alcohol-based preparations for skin preparation and wait at least 1 min before taking blood. Do not touch the venepuncture site after skin preparation.
- Most paediatric blood culture bottles require 1–4 mL of blood; take as close to 4 mL as possible for optimal sensitivity.
- Consider anaerobic blood cultures (as well as aerobic) in neonates where there has been prolonged rupture of membranes or maternal chorioamnionitis, poor dentition, severe mucositis, sinusitis, abdominal sepsis, perianal infections, bite wounds or in immunosuppressed patients.
- In patients with central venous access devices take paired peripheral and central line cultures.
- There is no need to change needles between venepuncture and injecting the blood culture bottles. Inject blood culture bottles first (before dividing blood into other specimen tubes).

Intravenous cannula insertion

Sites

- Dorsum of the non-dominant hand is preferred.
- Alternative sites include the anatomical snuffbox, volar aspect of the forearm, dorsum of the foot, great saphenous vein or cubital fossa.
- The site usually requires splinting and this should be taken into consideration (e.g. foot in a mobile child is less desirable).
- Scalp veins should only be used when there are no other possibilities.

Suggested analgesia

- As for venepuncture above.
- Consider injectable local anaesthetic in older children, e.g. lignocaine (lidocaine) 1%, 1–2 mL.

Equipment
Dressing pack, antiseptic solution, i.v. cannula, blood collection tubes and syringe if needed, 0.9% saline flush, three-way tap/connection tubing (primed with 0.9% saline), tourniquet, splint, tapes, bandage.

Technique
- Be patient and look carefully for the best option. Ensure the child is warm and there is adequate light.
- If using the back of the hand in infants, grasp the wrist between the index and middle fingers with the thumb over the patient's fingers, flexing the wrist. This achieves both immobilisation and tourniquet (see Fig. 3.1).
- Insert the cannula just distal to and along the line of the vein at an angle of 10–15°. When a large vein is entered, a 'flash' of blood will enter the hub of the needle.
- Advance the cannula a further 1–2 mm along the line of the vein, then remove the needle while advancing the cannula along the vein. If the cannula is in the vein, blood will flow back out along the cannula.
- Safety i.v. cannulae have a clip or mechanism which covers the needle tip when the needle is retracted fully from the cannula. It may be necessary to insert the cannula (with needle *in situ*) slightly further into the vein initially, as the safety mechanism often produces a backward movement as it retracts and may dislodge the cannula.
  - When trying to cannulate a small vein, there may not be a flashback of blood. Insert the cannula and when it is likely to be in the vein, partially remove the needle and watch for blood moving slowly back along the cannula. Advance the cannula along the vein gently. With safety cannulae it is not possible to remove the needle and reinsert.
- Take required blood samples at this stage. In neonates and young infants, blood can be collected by allowing it to drip directly into collection tubes (without a syringe).
- Connect a primed three-way tap/connector and tape the cannula. Place tape over the cannula, then a clear plastic dressing and further tape over the top.

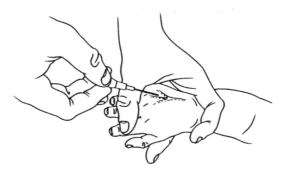

Fig. 3.1 Intravenous cannula insertion

- Flush the cannula with saline to confirm i.v. placement. Connect the i.v. tubing and splint the arm to an appropriately-sized board. Wrap the entire distal extremity in a bandage.

Long line insertion
Indications
- Prolonged venous access.
- Central venous placement for parenteral nutrition.

Sites
- Basilic and cephalic veins in older children.
- Basilic, cephalic and saphenous veins in neonates and infants.

Suggested analgesia
- See i.v. cannula insertion.

Equipment
Sterile drapes and gloves, dressing pack, antiseptic solution, silastic long line kit, i.v. cannula or butterfly needle, syringe with 0.9% saline flush, three-way tap/connection tubing, tourniquet, steristrips, clear adhesive dressing, bandage.

Technique
- Strict asepsis is required.
- Measure the distance from the site of insertion to the desired location of the catheter tip (e.g. axilla).
- Prime silastic line and three-way tap with sterile saline. Insert the introducer needle or i.v. cannula into the vein until free-flowing blood return is obtained. Release the tourniquet. If using an i.v. cannula, remove the needle leaving the cannula *in situ*.
- Using smooth forceps, grasp the catheter very close to the tip and feed the catheter through the introducer needle/cannula to the desired length (see Fig. 3.2a).
- Place a finger over the vein proximally and slowly withdraw the needle/cannula keeping it parallel to the skin, leaving the silastic line in position. When the needle clears the skin, secure the catheter by trapping it with a gloved finger at the skin exit site (see Fig. 3.2b). Attach the catheter to the appropriate i.v. line connections and flush the catheter.
- Secure silastic line in place with steristrips, followed by a sterile transparent dressing.
- If the line is used for central access, confirm catheter tip placement radiologically. This may be aided by the injection of 0.3 mL of a contrast agent.

Accessing central venous catheters
Types
- Catheter devices, e.g. Hickman or Broviac catheters, are central venous access devices that are tunnelled subcutaneously before they enter a central vein. They may be either single or double lumen. The external part of the line has a clamp and a connector which is accessed.

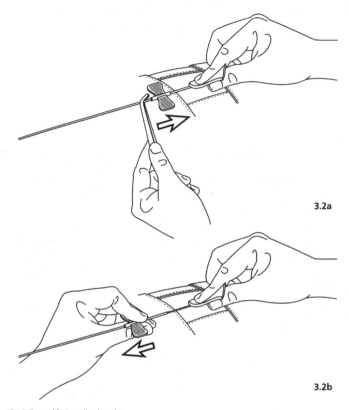

3.2a

3.2b

Fig. 3.2a and b Long line insertion

- Infusaports are placed completely under the skin so no part is exposed. They consist of a small chamber placed subcutaneously on the chest wall attached to a catheter that is placed in a central vein. The chamber can be accessed through the skin.

Suggested analgesia
- Topical local anaesthetic, e.g. amethocaine or EMLA (lignocaine [lidocaine], prilocaine), for Infusaport access.
- Consider sedation and nitrous oxide in children >4 years.
- A procedural pain management plan should be developed for all children requiring a central access device.

Equipment

Sterile gloves, dressing pack, alcohol-based chlorhexidine, Huber point needle (90° bend) for Infusaport, short three-way tap or minimum volume extension tubing, giving set, sterile adhesive strips, syringe with sterile 0.9% saline flush, additional syringes/blood collection tubes, gauze, occlusive clear plastic dressing × 2.

Technique
Generic (Hickman, Broviac, Infusaport)

- Strict asepsis is required.
- Central venous access devices are flushed with heparin-containing solutions when not in use.
- For short-term disconnection use 50 units heparin/5 mL 0.9% saline.
- For long-term disconnection (e.g. on discharge) use 1000 units heparin/1 mL 0.9% saline ×1 mL diluted to 10 mL with 0.9% saline (i.e. 100 units heparin/1 mL final concentration).
- For both types of flush use 4–5 mL volume. Stop backflow immediately by clamping catheter devices and in Infusaports by turning tap to off (short term flush) or removing needle (long-term flush).
- Catheter devices require weekly flushing; Infusaports require monthly flushing.
- Catheter devices require dressing changes weekly. The exit site is washed with antiseptic solution (applied radially from centre outwards) and the tubing is also washed. The solution is allowed to dry, then two clear adhesive dressings are used to 'sandwich' the tubing. The distal tubing is then taped to the child's chest wall and the remainder safety-pinned to clothing to avoid pulling on the line. In younger children tape the clamp and tap to avoid little fingers exploring.

Infusaport specific

- Wash the site with antiseptic preparation and allow it to dry.
- Attach Huber point needle to minimum volume extension tubing connected to a three-way tap and prime the line with 0.9% saline.
- Insert Huber point needle into the centre of the port chamber. Aspirate 5 mL of blood back through three-way tap (may be used for blood cultures), then take other bloods using a second syringe as required. Ensure tap is turned to 45° to avoid backflow when connecting/disconnecting syringes. Flush line with 5 mL 0.9% saline.
- Make a pillow of gauze under the Huber point needle and secure with sterile adhesive strips then apply airtight adhesive clear plastic dressing.

Umbilical vein catheterisation
Indications

Used in neonates up to 7–10 days of age for:
- Emergency vascular access for resuscitation.
- I.v. access for exchange transfusion.
- Venous access in low-birthweight infants (preferred initial access in infants <800 g).

Equipment

- Sterile drapes, gown, mask and gloves, sterile instrument pack (gauze, forceps, needle holder, scalpel holder), umbilical tape (or rolled gauze), scalpel blade, antiseptic solution, umbilical catheter (baby <1000 g 3.5 FG, >1000 g 5.0 FG), syringe with 0.9% saline flush, three-way tap/connection tubing, suture.
- If no umbilical catheter is available, a sterile 5 FG feeding tube can be used for umbilical vein access in an emergency.

Site

- Measure the distance of a line drawn from the tip of the shoulder to the level of the umbilicus.
- Using Fig. 3.3 determine the catheter length needed to place **the tip between the diaphragm and the right atrium in the inferior vena cava (IVC)**. Add the height of the umbilical stump to obtain the total length.
- In an emergency, short-term access can be obtained with the UVC tip inserted 3–5 cm past the mucocutaneous junction (will not be in portal circulation)

Technique

- Strict asepsis is required.
- Attach a three-way tap to the catheter and flush with sterile saline then close the three-way tap. Throughout insertion the catheter and connection must be kept filled with fluid to prevent air embolism.
- Drape and prepare the skin. Loosely tie a sterile umbilical tape or rolled gauze around base of the cord. Cut through the cord with a scalpel horizontally 1.5–2 cm from the skin; tighten the tape/gauze to prevent bleeding if necessary.
- Stabilize the cord with artery forceps. Identify the single large thin-walled vein and two smaller thick-walled arteries. Clear any thrombi with forceps, gently dilate the vein with curved iris forceps and insert the catheter.
- Gently advance the catheter to the pre-measured distance. Do not force. Aspirate to check position (blood should fill the cannula easily).
- Secure the catheter with both a purse string suture around the cord and a tape bridge. Radiologically confirm that the catheter tip lies above the diaphragm in the IVC; it is not acceptable within the liver.

Umbilical artery catheterisation

Indications

Used in low-birthweight neonates for:
- Monitoring blood pressure and arterial blood gases.
- Access and infusion site.

Equipment

As for umbilical vein access. In addition, blood pressure transducer and heparin solution.

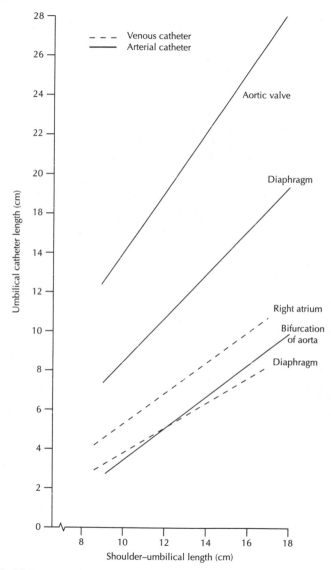

Fig. 3.3 Determining umbilical vein and artery catheter length

Site
- Measure the distance of a line drawn from the tip of the shoulder to the level of the umbilicus. Use Fig. 3.3 to determine the catheter length needed:
  - High line position: between T6–T9; tip above the diaphragm (proximal to the origin of renal and mesenteric arteries).
- The catheter length may also be calculated by formula: (weight (kg) × 3) + 9 cm.

Technique
- Strict asepsis is required.
- Flush the catheter and three-way tap, prepare skin and cord and cut cord as above.
- Identify the arteries, clear any thrombi and dilate the artery with curved iris forceps. Initially one tip of the forceps is inserted, then both, with the tips allowed to spring gently open.
- Insert catheter and advance gently. Aim tip towards the feet. Avoid excessive pressure or repeat probing. Aspirate to check position (blood should fill the cannula easily and pulsations will be seen) then flush line. Arterial lines are heparinised (see Pharmacopoeia).
- Secure the catheter as above and confirm tip position radiologically.
- Check for any complications caused by catheter placement, especially blanching or cyanosis of lower extremities. Nurse infant supine for 24 h after the procedure.

Arterial puncture
Indications
Suspected hypoxaemia, hypercapnia or severe acidosis with poor peripheral perfusion.
   Note: Acid–base status can also be assessed by capillary or venous collection.

Sites
Radial artery.
   Note: The femoral artery is used only in emergencies when no other arteries are palpable.
Never use the ulnar artery.

Suggested analgesia
- Sucrose in infants <3/12.
- Topical local anaesthetic or injectable local anaesthetic, e.g. lignocaine (lidocaine) 1%, can be used, but does not prevent pain caused by puncturing the artery.

Equipment
Alcohol wipe, 23 or 25 FG needle (straight or butterfly), syringe (2 mL pre-heparinised syringe for blood gas), cotton ball, band-aid/tape, blood collection tubes.

Technique
- Clean the skin with an alcohol wipe.
- Pierce the skin at a 15–30° angle directly over the artery. On entering the artery, blood will fill the hub; however, gentle aspiration is usually required to fill the syringe.
- If there is no flashback at full depth or when the bone is contacted, withdraw the needle very slowly while aspirating. Blood will often be obtained at this point if the artery has been transfixed. If no blood is aspirated check position of pulse and repeat.

- Only 0.5 mL of blood is required for arterial blood gas, sodium, potassium and haemoglobin measurements.
- After obtaining a specimen, remove the needle quickly and apply firm pressure to the puncture site for 3–5 min.

Intra-arterial cannula insertion
Indications
Invasive blood pressure monitoring and frequent blood sampling in the intensive care setting.

Sites
Radial, posterior tibial and dorsalis pedis arteries.

Suggested analgesia
- Sucrose in infants <3/12.
- Topical local anaesthetic or injectable local anaesthetic, e.g. lignocaine (lidocaine) 1%, can be used, but does not prevent pain caused by puncturing the artery.

Equipment
Dressing pack, antiseptic solution, i.v. cannula, blood collection tubes and syringe if needed, 0.9% saline flush, three-way tap/connection tubing (primed with 0.9% saline), pressure transducer, heparin solution, splint, tapes, bandage.

Technique
- Do not use a tourniquet. Feel for the pulse of the artery to be cannulated and insert the cannula at an angle of 15–30° to the skin. Once a flashback of blood is obtained reduce the angle (to 10–15°) and advance the cannula gently with the needle *in situ* so it is clearly within the artery before the needle is removed.
- Place a finger proximally over the pulse when withdrawing the needle and attach (primed) connector tubing and transducer quickly.
- Take bloods if required, flush slowly and watch for blanching around the site and distally.
- Arterial lines require continuous heparin infusion.

Intraosseous cannula insertion
Indications
For emergency vascular access when efforts to cannulate a vein are unsuccessful.

Sites
Preferred sites of insertion are:
- Proximal tibia (depending on size, 1–3 cm inferomedial to tibial tuberosity).
- Distal femur (approximately 3 cm above the condyles on anterolateral surface) (see Fig. 3.4).
- Avoid fractured bones and limbs with proximal fractures.

Suggested analgesia
Performed in emergency situations. Injectable local anaesthetic (lignocaine [lidocaine] 1%) if patient is conscious.

Equipment
Intraosseus needle (if not available a short large-bore lumbar puncture needle or bone marrow aspiration needle are alternatives), syringe with 0.9% saline flush, three-way tap/connection tubing (primed with 0.9% saline), alcohol wipe, syringe, blood collection tubes.

Technique
- Prepare the insertion site.
- Insert the needle at 90° to the skin (see Fig. 3.4). Apply downward pressure with a rotary motion to advance the needle. When the needle passes through the bony cortex into the marrow cavity, resistance suddenly decreases. The needle should stand without support (except in a very young infant).
- Remove the stylet and attach a syringe; aspirate to confirm that the needle is in the bone marrow (this is not always possible). Flush the needle with saline to confirm correct placement and connect i.v. tubing. Often fluids will not flow by gravity into the marrow – a three-way tap and syringe or pressure infusion may be needed.
- Watch the infusion site for fluid extravasation, or the calf becoming tense. A pair of artery forceps clamped around the base then taped along the limb (with appropriate padding underneath) can provide stability. The needle should be removed once i.v. access has been obtained.
- Any fluid or drug that can be given i.v. can be administered through the intraosseous route.

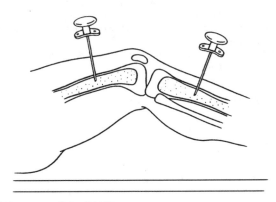

Fig. 3.4 Intraosseous needle insertion sites

Suprapubic aspiration (SPA)
Indications
Sterile urine collection for suspected urinary tract infection (UTI) as part of septic workup.

Note: Not recommended in age >12 months (unless the bladder is palpable or percussible).

Site
• Midline in the skin crease above the symphysis pubis.

Suggested analgesia
Topical local anaesthetic.

Equipment
• Alcohol wipe, 23-gauge needle and 2 or 5 mL syringe, cotton ball, adhesive tape, sterile urine collection pot.
• Bladder ultrasound if available

Technique
• If multiple procedures are planned, aim to **perform the SPA first** as the child may void whilst having a venepuncture or lumbar puncture.
• Wait at least 30 min after the last void.
• Use a bladder ultrasound if possible; attempt SPA only if >20 mL urine present.
• Position the patient with legs either straight or bent in the frog-leg position. Have a sterile bottle handy for a midstream clean catch in case the child voids.
• Prepare the skin with an alcohol wipe. Insert a 23-gauge needle attached to a 2 or 5 mL syringe perpendicular to the abdominal wall (see Fig. 3.5). Pass almost to the depth of the needle and then aspirate while withdrawing. If urine is not obtained, do not remove the needle completely. Change the angle of the needle and insert it again, first angling superiorly and then inferiorly.

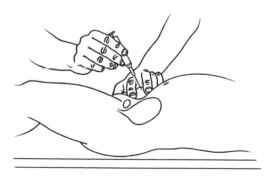

Fig. 3.5 Suprapubic aspiration

- In the event of obtaining no urine, either: (1) perform urethral catheterisation; or (2) wait 30 min, giving the child a drink during this time. Repeat the SPA. It is a good idea to put a urine bag on to determine if the child has voided before proceeding with a further SPA.

Urethral catheterisation
Indications
- Suspected UTI where midstream specimen is not possible.
- Acute urinary retention.

Suggested analgesia
- Local anaesthetic topical gel (e.g. lignocaine [lidocaine] 2% gel) – takes 10 min for full effect.
- Consider nitrous oxide.

Equipment
- Sterile drapes and gloves, water-based antiseptic solution, catheter, catheter bag and syringe with 0.9% saline (if indwelling catheter), sterile urine collection pot, and bowl/kidney dish (to hold urine).
- For diagnostic catheterisation, use a 5 FG feeding tube (depending on age). For indwelling catheters, use a silastic catheter with an inflatable balloon. Appropriate sizes are: 0–6 months 6 FG, 2 years 8 FG, 5 years 10 FG, 6–12 years 12 FG; this may vary with the size of the patient. Lubricants will aid insertion.

Technique
- The child lies with legs apart in the frog-leg position. Prepare and drape the area, apply local anaesthetic gel and wait.
- Using a sterile technique, locate the urethral orifice (in girls: see Fig. 3.6). In boys the foreskin need not be retracted for successful catheterisation. Gently advance the catheter posteriorly until urine is obtained.
- For indwelling catheters: inflate balloon **only** when urine has been obtained, attach catheter to collection device and tape catheter securely to leg.

Lumbar puncture
Indications
- A febrile, sick infant or child with no focus of infection.
- Fever with meningism.
- Prolonged seizure with fever.
See also Fig. 1.3, p. 13.

Contraindications
- Coma.
- Focal neurological signs.

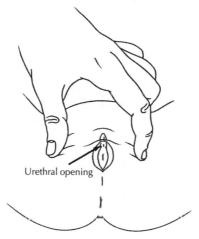

Fig. 3.6 Urethral orifice in girls

- Focal seizures, recent seizures (within 30 min) or prolonged seizures (>30 min).
- Signs of raised intracranial pressure (ICP): altered pupil responses, decerebrate or decorticate posturing, papilloedema (unreliable and late sign in meningitis).
- Cardiovascular compromise/shock.
- Respiratory compromise.
- Thrombocytopenia/coagulopathy.
- Local superficial infection.
- Strong suspicion of meningococcal infection (typical purpuric rash in ill child).

Note: Coma – reduced conscious state and absent or non-purposeful responses to painful stimuli. Elicit by squeezing the earlobe hard for up to 1 min. Children should localise response and seek a parent. If in doubt, do not proceed with lumbar puncture.

Note: Drowsiness, irritability, vomiting and isolated tonic–clonic, myoclonic, absence or atonic seizures are not in themselves contraindications. A bulging fontanelle in the absence of other signs of raised ICP is not a contraindication.

Suggested analgesia
Topical local anaesthetic plus:
- Sucrose in infants <3/12.
- Injectable local anaesthetic (lignocaine [lidocaine] 1%).
- Consider nitrous oxide.

- Consider sedatives (e.g. midazolam), although this may complicate assessment of conscious state.

Equipment

- Sterile drapes, gown, mask and gloves, antiseptic solution, sterile dressing pack, specimen collection tubes, cotton ball, band-aid/adhesive dressing.
- A lumbar puncture needle with introducing stylet should be used. A 22 or 25 FG needle is usually appropriate. The correct needle length is:
  - 20 mm for preterm infants
  - 30 mm for <2 years old.
  - 40 mm for 2–5 year olds.
  - 50 mm for 5–12 year olds.
  - 60 mm for older children.
- Longer needles may be required in large adolescents.

Insertion site

- The iliac crests are at the level of L3–4. Use this space or the space below (see Fig. 3.7).
- At birth the conus medullaris finishes near L3, but in adults it finishes at L1–2.

Technique

- Using a strict aseptic technique, cleanse the skin and drape the patient.
- Positioning of the patient is crucial and an assistant is needed. Restrain the patient in the lateral position on the edge of a flat surface. A line drawn between the iliac crests should be perpendicular to the table surface. Maximally flex the spine without compromising the airway. In small babies flex from the shoulders only; neck flexion can cause airway obstruction.
- Anaesthetise the area until the proximity of the dura (i.e. about 2/3 the length of the appropriate lumbar puncture needle).
- Grasp the spinal needle with the bevel facing upwards. With the needle perpendicular to the back, insert it through the skin between the spinous processes slowly, aiming towards the umbilicus (i.e. slightly cephalad). Continue advancing the needle until there is decreased resistance (having traversed ligamentum flavum), or the needle has been inserted half its length. Remove the stylet and advance the needle about 1 mm.
- Wait at least 30 s for CSF to appear in the hub. Rotation of the needle 90–180° may allow CSF to flow. Advance 1 mm at a time if no CSF has appeared. If no CSF is obtained when bone is contacted or the needle is fully inserted, withdraw the needle very slowly until CSF flows, or the needle is almost removed. Reinsert the stylet, recheck the patient's position and needle orientation, and repeat the procedure.
- Collect 0.5–1 mL of CSF in each of two tubes, for microbiological and biochemical analysis. Remove the lumbar puncture needle swiftly. Press on the puncture site with a cotton ball for about 30 s. Cover with a light dressing.

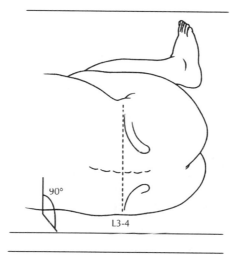

Fig. 3.7 Position for lumbar puncture

Nasogastric tube insertion
Indications
- Oral rehydration.
- Administration of medication (e.g. charcoal, bowel washout solutions).
- Decompression of stomach (e.g. bowel obstruction, abdominal trauma).

Suggested analgesia
Topical anaesthetic spray (e.g. cophenylcaine) and lubrication with lignocaine (lidocaine)-containing lubricant.

Equipment
- Nasogastric tube, tape or adhesive dressing, litmus paper.
- Select the correct tube size (size may vary depending on the use of the nasogastric):
  8 FG for newborns
  10–12 FG for 1–2 year olds
  14–16 FG for adolescents.

Technique
- Measure the correct length of insertion by placing the distal end of the tube at the nostril and running it to the ear and to the xiphisternum. Add a few centimetres. Mark the tube with permanent marker at this point so the position can be checked.

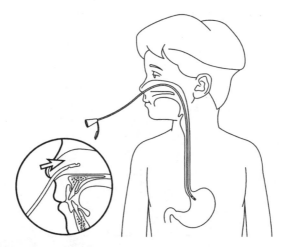

Fig. 3.8 Nasogastric tube insertion

- If the tube is too pliable, stiffen it by immersing in cold water or freezing briefly.
- Grasp the tube 5–6 cm from the distal end and insert it posteriorly. Advance it slowly along the floor of the nasal passage (see Fig. 3.8). Firm pressure is needed to pass the posterior nasal opening.
- If the child is cooperative, once the tube is in the naso/oropharynx, ask the child to flex their neck and swallow.
- If the child coughs and gags, their voice becomes hoarse or the tube emerges from the mouth, pull the tube back into the nasopharynx and start again.
- Once the tube has been passed to the measured length, check position by aspirating fluid and testing for an acid pH. Confirm position with radiograph if necessary.
- Secure the tube to the side of the face using adhesive tape.

Gastrostomy tube replacement
Indications
- Burst balloon/malfunctioning parts.
- Displacement/extrusion of tube.

Suggested analgesia
Nitrous oxide or sedation (e.g. midazolam).

Equipment

Gastrostomy tube, syringe and sterile water, lubricant. When a replacement gastrostomy tube is not available, a sterile indwelling urinary catheter can be used as a temporary measure to keep the stoma patent.

Technique

- Check the balloon of the new tube by injecting 3–5 mL of air into the side port. Deflate the balloon fully.
- Slide the skin flange on the new tube to the 8–10 cm mark. Close off the feeding ports and apply a small amount of lubricant to the tube.
- If the old tube is still *in situ*, attach an empty syringe to the side port and deflate the balloon by removing the water. *Note:* There is usually less than the expected 4 or 15 mL of water left in the balloon.
- Gently pull on the tube and rotate it slowly until it is removed.
- Place the tip of the new tube at the opening of the stoma. Hold the distal end of the tube and slowly put pressure on the tube to push it into the hole.
- The new tube should insert easily. Insert it to 6–8 cm.
- Inflate the new tube to either 4 or 15 mL (i.e. not to full capacity) with water. Slowly pull back on the tube until resistance is felt.
- Slide the skin flange down until there is a snug fit, but not too tight. This is usually at the 2–4 cm mark.
- In the case of a MIC key, the correct tube for that patient should be inserted to its full depth before inflating the balloon.
- Gastrostomy buttons or Malecot catheters need introducers and should only be replaced by experienced staff.

Note: If there is any difficulty inserting the tube, a radiographic study (i.e. contrast through the tube) should be performed to check correct positioning.

Tuberculin skin test (intradermal injection)
Indications

Tuberculosis (TB) screening in children.

Sites

By convention: volar surface of left forearm at junction of upper and middle thirds.

Equipment

- Alcohol wipe, short (10mm) 26-gauge beveled needle, 1 mL syringe, cotton ball, tape.
- Protective eyewear is essential.
- Dose of 5 TU = 0.1 mL purified protein derivative (PPD).

Contraindications

- Past history active TB or history large reaction.
- Within 3 months of another tuberculin skin test (TST).

- Within 4 weeks of MMR or varicella vaccine (can result in false negatives).
Note: Not reliable in children aged <6/12.

Technique

- TST can only be given by accredited providers. Contact the relevant TB screening programme.
- Stretch the skin between a finger and thumb and insert the bevel (facing upwards) 2 mm into the dermis. It will be visible through the epidermis. Inject slowly; there will be considerable resistance. The injection will raise a blanched bleb of about 7 mm with the appearance of peau d'orange. Cover with adhesive dressing/cotton ball and tape and advise not to scratch.
- The test should be read at 48–72 h (up to 5 days). Measure induration (not erythema) in the transverse axis of the forearm. It is helpful to use a pen to draw towards the induration at the same level on either side – it will stop at the edge of the induration and the distance between the points can be measured.
- A large reaction may take days–weeks to disappear.
- For interpretation, see chapter 10, Immigrant child health.

Immunisation

See chapter 9, Immunisation.

BCG vaccination is given by intradermal injection (technique as above); by convention it is given in the left upper arm, in the skin over the site of insertion of deltoid into the humerus.

Wound management

Assessment

Lacerations are common in childhood. Most are superficial and tend to occur on the face, scalp and extremities. When assessing a wound consider:

- Is the wound contaminated or could it contain a foreign body (e.g. glass)?
- Are there likely to be other associated injuries?
- Is there injury to deeper structures?
- Is blood supply impaired or is this an area of end-arteriolar supply? Do **not** use local anaesthetic with adrenaline on such wounds.

Cleaning wounds

- Superficial wounds can be cleansed with normal saline or aqueous chlorhexidine.
- Adequate analgesia is required for complete examination, cleaning and repair of all but the most superficial wounds.
- Radiograph if there is a possibility of a foreign body (particularly glass).

Suggested analgesia

Topical local anaesthetic
- LAT (lignocaine [lidocaine] 4%, adrenaline 1 : 2000 and tetracaine 2%) or ALA (adrenaline/lignocaine [lidocaine]/amethocaine). Dose = 0.1 mL/kg bodyweight.

- Apply on a piece of gauze or cotton wool placed **inside** the wound and held in place with an adhesive clear plastic dressing.
- Leave for 20–30 min. An area of blanching (~1 cm wide) will appear around the wound. Anaesthesia lasts about 1 h.
- Test the adequacy of anaesthesia by washing and squeezing the wound: if pain free, suturing will usually be painless.
- The sensations of pulling and light touch are preserved. This should be explained to the child and parent.

Injectable local anaesthetic (lignocaine [lidocaine] 1%)

Injectable lignocaine [lidocaine] 1% (max 0.4 mL/kg (4 mg/kg)) can be used:

- Where LAT/ALA are contraindicated (e.g. areas of end-arteriolar supply).
- In adolescents.
- To supplement topical local anaesthetic if adequate anaesthesia has not been achieved.

There are several ways to decrease the pain from injecting local anaesthetic:

- Use topical anaesthesia first.
- Use 27 FG needles.
- Inject slowly.
- Place the needle into the wound through the lacerated surface, not through intact skin.
- Pass the needle through an anaesthetised area into an unanaesthetised area.
- Use 1% lignocaine (lidocaine) rather than 2%.
- Buffer lignocaine (lidocaine) with sodium bicarbonate (10:1 dilution).

Sedation/other

- Nitrous oxide or sedation (e.g. midazolam).
- Ketamine may be used in children >12 months by staff experienced in its use.

Regional blocks

- Regional blocks provide excellent analgesia. See p. 51.

Wound closure
Tissue adhesive glues

- Tissue glue (e.g. Dermabond) is an alternative to suturing in wounds that are small (<3 cm), straight, easily approximated and under no tension. It must not be used on mucosal surfaces.
- Topical anaesthesia will reduce bleeding from the wound and the discomfort of gluing.
- Clean the wound with normal saline or aqueous chlorhexidine and let dry. Hold the edges firmly together and apply a small amount of glue (~0.05 mL) to the line of the laceration. Do not allow glue to enter the wound itself.
- Hold the wound edges together for 30 s. Steristrips should be applied (using tincture of benzoin) to prevent the child picking the glue off.
- The wound should be kept dry for 3–4 days. It then can be washed. The scab will come off in 1–2 weeks.

Suturing
- Rapidly absorbable sutures (e.g. fast catgut, Vicryl rapid) are appropriate for use on areas where the cosmetic advantages of non-absorbable sutures are not required (e.g. scalp and hand). Using absorbable sutures avoids the stress and potential pain of suture removal.
- Non-absorbable sutures (e.g. nylon and polypropylene) are used in areas where cosmetic appearance is important.
- Deep sutures (absorbable) should be used to close deep tissues; this reduces cavitation and dead space, which increase the risk of infection.
- The size of suture and timing of suture removal depends on the area affected:
  - Scalp: 4/0–5/0, 5–7 days.
  - Face: 5/0–6/0, 5–7 days.
  - Arm/hand: 4/0–5/0, 7–10 days.
  - Trunk/legs: 4/0–5/0, 10–14 days.
Note: Areas of stress (e.g. over joints) need longer.
- Splint any sutured wound that is under tension (e.g. across joints or on the hand), for at least 1 week. This decreases pain and promotes healing.

Special circumstances
Lips
- Accurate approximation of vermilion border and skin is essential.
- May need general anaesthesia and plastic surgical repair in small or uncooperative children.
- Sutures: mucosa/muscle 4/0 gut, skin 6/0 nylon.
- Lacerations of the inner lip rarely need intervention, but degloving to the gum margin requires specialist referral (see chapter 22, Dental conditions).

Palate
- Rarely requires suturing unless laceration is wide, extends through posterior free margin or is actively bleeding.
- Beware retropharyngeal injury (needs specialist opinion: see chapter 24, Ear, nose and throat conditions).

Tongue
- Small lacerations do not require suturing.
- Plastic surgical opinion is required if the laceration is large, bleeding actively, extends through the free edge or is full thickness.

Finger tips
- Areas of skin loss up to 1 cm^2 are treated with dressings and heal with good return of sensation. Greater areas require specialist referral.
- Involvement of the nail bed requires plastic surgical consultation.

Scalp
For small lacerations suitable for tissue adhesive glue; use hair from each side of the laceration to approximate the wound: twist hair together, pull across the wound and glue over the hair.

Other
Lacerations involving cartilage (e.g. nose, ear) require specialist opinion.

Tetanus prophylaxis
See *The Australian Immunisation Handbook*, 9th edition.
- For clean minor wounds, if the patient has had a:
  - Tetanus course (≥3 doses), last dose within the past 10 years: no requirement.
  - Tetanus course (≥3 doses), last dose >10 years ago: give tetanus toxoid.
  - Unimmunised/incomplete/unknown treatment: give tetanus toxoid.
- For tetanus-prone wounds, if the patient has had a:
  - Tetanus course (≥3 doses), last dose within the past 5 years: no requirement.
  - Tetanus course (≥3 doses), last dose >5 years ago: give tetanus toxoid.
  - Unimmunised/incomplete/unknown treatment: full three-dose course and tetanus immunoglobulin.

Note: Tetanus toxoid: give DTPa/DT/Td/dTpa as appropriate.
- Dose of tetanus immunoglobulin is 250 IU <24 h, 500 IU >24 h intramuscular injection (21 FG needle).

Antibiotics
- Antibiotics are not indicated for simple lacerations. They are usually given for bites and wounds with extensive tissue damage, but are of secondary importance to the initial decontamination of the wound.
- Recommended antibiotics are amoxicillin clavulanate (400/57 mg per 5 mL), 12.5–22.5 mg/kg/dose, 12 hourly for 5 days.

Femoral nerve block
Indication
- Pain relief for femoral fractures (in addition to other techniques including splinting the fractured leg).
- It may be appropriate to use nitrous oxide or sedation when giving a femoral nerve block.

Equipment
Dressing pack, antiseptic solution, 23-gauge needle and syringe × 2, local anaesthetic solution, adhesive tape.

Technique
- After skin preparation, palpate the femoral artery below the inguinal ligament. Raise a wheal just lateral to the artery with local anaesthetic, e.g. lignocaine (lidocaine) 1%.

- Introduce a short bevelled needle (such as a lumbar puncture needle or a 23-gauge needle) through this wheal and advance downwards perpendicular to the skin. A characteristic 'pop' or loss of resistance is felt as the needle goes through the fascia lata and again as it penetrates the fascia iliaca (if using a lumbar puncture needle).
- Aspirate to ensure that the needle is not in a blood vessel. Inject local anaesthetic solution (usually bupivacaine 0.5% 2 mg/kg). The anaesthetic should inject smoothly without sub-cutaneous swelling. Paraesthesia need not be elicited.

Bier's block
Indication
Children over 5 years with forearm fractures requiring manipulation. Consider also intranasal fentanyl (1.5 mcg/kg, half in each nostril) for long bone fractures (see chapter 4, Pain Management, p. 63).

Equipment
Dressing pack, antiseptic solution, i.v. cannula × 2 (and associated equipment), lignocaine (lidocaine) 1%, monitored tourniquet system, equipment for plaster application.

Technique
- Keep child nil orally and give adequate pain relief.
- Two trained staff must be present and full resuscitation equipment available. Radiology should be notified.
- Insert an i.v. cannula into a distal vein on each hand.
- Elevate the affected arm above the level of the heart while compressing the brachial artery for 1 min.
- Inflate the tourniquet cuff to 200 mmHg. This reading should be maintained throughout the procedure.
- Infuse lignocaine (lidocaine) 0.5% 3 mg/kg (0.6 mL/kg, max 40 mL). Full anaesthesia takes 5–10 min.
- Release tourniquet cuff **at least** 20 min after lignocaine (lidocaine) infusion, after procedure is complete and position confirmed radiologically.

Digital/proximal nerve block
Indication
Anaesthesia of finger for minor surgical procedures (e.g. suturing, drainage of paronychia).

Equipment
Dressing pack, antiseptic solution, 25-gauge needle and syringe, local anaesthetic.
Note: Use local anaesthetic, e.g. lignocaine (lidocaine) 1%. Do **not** use adrenaline.

Technique
Digital nerve block
- With the palm facing up, insert a 25-gauge needle at the base of the finger on either medial/lateral side at a 45° angle to the vertical (see Fig. 3.9).
- Inject when needle hits periosteum.

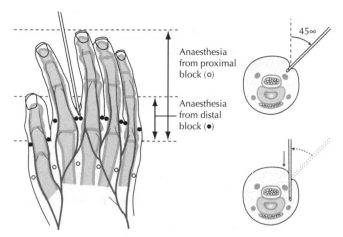

Fig. 3.9 Digital nerve block

- Rotate needle to vertical and inject along the side of the finger to at least 3/4 of the depth of the finger.
- Remove needle and repeat on the other side.

Proximal nerve block
- Insert a 25-gauge needle between the fingers at the interdigital fold in line with the web space (see Fig. 3.9).
- Insert until needle tip is level with the head of the metacarpal bone.
- Inject 1–2 mL at this level.
- Repeat on the other side, or for index/fifth finger; inject half ring wheal around the outer side of the finger.

USEFUL RESOURCES
- *www.rch.org.au/clinicalguide* [Suprapubic Aspirate Guideline] – Includes video of procedure and flowchart of using a bladder ultrasound.
- *www.rch.org.au/clinicalguide* [Lumbar Puncture Guideline] – Includes video of procedure, interpretation of CSF and patient information handouts.
- *www.rch.org.au/clinicalguide* [Intraosseous Access]
- *www.netsvic.org.au/nets/handbook* [Umbilical Artery/Vein Catheterisation] – Excellent website from the Newborn Emergency Transport Service (NETS) of Victoria.

CHAPTER 4

Pain management

George Chalkiadis
Greta Palmer
Jane Munro

Numerous misconceptions contribute to under-treatment of paediatric pain, including:
- Neonates and children do not experience pain or remember painful events.
- Children tolerate pain better than adults as their nervous systems are immature.
- All children are 'sensitive' to analgesics.
- Opioids are addictive or too dangerous to use in children.

These myths lead to poor pain prevention and management in neonates, children and adolescents. If unrelieved or inadequately treated, pain has negative physiological, psychological and emotional consequences.

Assessment of acute pain
Pain scores are important! They are the fifth vital sign on patients' observation charts. Pain assessment includes a combination of the following:

History
- Including site, onset, duration, quality, radiation, triggers and relievers, impact on functioning (including sleep disturbance and other activities), treatments tried and their effectiveness.
- In developmentally normal children, ask the child directly about their pain using appropriate tools.
- In neonates, pre-verbal children and cognitively impaired children, parents and regular caregivers are often best equipped to interpret the child's pain reliably.

Examination
- Behavioural observation (e.g. vocalisation, facial grimacing, posturing, movement).
- Physiological parameters (e.g. heart rate, respiratory rate, blood pressure) and physical signs (e.g. muscle spasm).
- Functional effects: for example, the ability to move (e.g. sitting up after laparotomy) and the tolerance of touch of the painful area usually signify adequate analgesia, whereas a child lying still and withdrawn may be in severe pain.

Paediatric Handbook, 8th edition. By Kate Thomson, Dean Tey and Michael Marks. Published 2009 by Blackwell Publishing, ISBN: 978-1-4051-7400-8.

Use of pain-rating scales

Observe trends of change in an individual's pain score or function (e.g. ability to turn in bed comfortably, ability to walk to the toilet) rather than the 'raw' pain score.

- Verbal children:
  - FACES scales for children >4 years, e.g. Wong–Baker FACES Pain Rating Scale (Fig. 4.1) or Bieri revised.
  - Visual analogue scale (e.g. 100 mm ruler).
  - Verbal numerical rating scale (e.g. 'out of 10 . . .').
- Non-verbal children including neonates and cognitively impaired are particularly vulnerable (see Pain in children and adolescents with disabilities, p. 70).
  - FLACC: Face, Legs, Activity, Cry and Consolability.
  - PATS (for neonates): Pain Assessment Tool Score.

Analgesics for acute pain

Multimodal analgesia (MMA) involves the use of more than one drug and/or method of controlling pain to obtain additive beneficial effects, reduce side effects, or both.

MMA use is ideal for acute pain management including pain due to surgery, trauma or cancer, as it allows analgesia to be optimised and directed according to the multiple sources of pain (somatic, visceral and/or neuropathic).

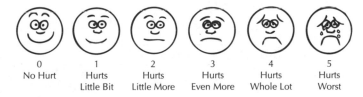

| 0 | 1 | 2 | 3 | 4 | 5 |
| No Hurt | Hurts Little Bit | Hurts Little More | Hurts Even More | Hurts Whole Lot | Hurts Worst |

Instructions

Explain to the child that each face is for a person who feels happy because they have no pain (hurt) or sad because they have some pain or a lot of pain.

Face 0 is very happy because it doesn't hurt at all.

Face 1 hurts just a little bit.

Face 2 hurts a little more.

Face 3 hurts even more.

Face 4 hurts a whole lot more.

Face 5 hurts as much as you can imagine, although you don't have to be crying to feel this bad.

Ask the child to choose the face that best describes how they are feeling.

Fig. 4.1 Wong–Baker FACES Pain Rating Scale. (Reproduced with permission from Hockenberry MJ, Wilson D, Winkelstein ML: Wong's Essentials of Pediatric Nursing, ed. 7, St. Louis, 2005, p. 1259. © Mosby.)

Procedures and Pain Management

Drug options include paracetamol, NSAIDs, COX-2 inhibitors, muscle relaxants (e.g. buscopan for smooth and diazepam for skeletal muscle spasm), tramadol and neuropathic analgesics (such as gabapentin, amitriptyline, clonidine and ketamine).

Drugs can be administered by various routes. Specialised infusions (e.g. local anaesthetics, ketamine and opioids) can be via bolus and/or continuous infusion.

Use an analgesic ladder approach to manage acute pain (see Table 4.1). The progress up or down the steps varies according to:

- the intensity of pain experienced
- its anticipated duration
- the expected recovery period.

Each step up employs all the analgesics listed in the steps below. Once pain is controlled, wean back to the previous step. This varies with the speed of resolution of the painful condition and the number of breakthrough or rescue agents that are required in the higher category. If pain is poorly responsive to these measures, get consultant assistance.

See Table 4.2 for dosing.

Examples of patients with severe pain and suggested management
Femoral fracture
- Single shot local anaesthetic femoral nerve block.
- Diazepam.
- Place in back slab or traction.
- Give other agents according to need.

Table 4.1 Analgesic ladder approach

Degree of pain and setting	Analgesic 'steps'
Severe pain inpatient	Add specialised infusion, e.g. ketamine, epidural local anaesthetic
	Add parenteral opioid by infusion (nurse or patient controlled)
outpatient or emergency presentation	Add parenteral opioid by bolus or regular oral opioid (consider controlled release when long duration)
	Consider parenteral tramadol, NSAID, paracetamol
	Address sleep impairment and anxiety if present

Moderate pain	Add one (or combination) of:
	    strong opioid e.g. oral morphine, oxycodone
	    'non-opioid': tramadol
	    mild opioid: codeine
	Address environmental/psychosocial contributors

Mild pain	Begin with paracetamol and/or NSAIDs

Table 4.2 Analgesic medication

Drug	Dose	Route(s)	Indications	Side effects	Special notes/Contraindications
Paracetamol	**Short-term oral total daily maximum:** 90 mg/kg per day for 48 h **Chronic or unsupervised community setting oral dosing:** limit to 60 mg/kg per day *Oral,rectal:* 15 mg/kg per dose 4 hourly prn or 30 mg/kg per dose nocte as stat dose *Rectal:* 20–40 mg/kg as a one-off dose, rounded to appropriate suppository strength *I.v.:* 15 mg/kg 6 hourly	Oral: syrup or tablets Oral is preferred to rectal administration as absorption is more reliable and has an earlier peak concentration (oral 30–60 min vs rectal 2–3 h) I.v. (onset 15 min)	Effective for mild to moderate pain Also has antipyretic effects **but** physical measures are better	Hepatotoxicity Otherwise well tolerated	Hepatotoxicity has been reported in children. Use with caution in patients with severe liver disease, jaundice, malnutrition, glutathione depletion, dehydration and long-term ingestion Significant opioid sparing effects

(Continued)

Table 4.2 *Continued*

Drug	Dose	Route(s)	Indications	Side effects	Special notes/Contraindications
Opioid					
Codeine	0.5–1 mg/kg 4 hourly	Oral (onset 40–60 min) Combination preparations include codeine with ibuprofen or paracetamol ± antihistamine	Effective for moderate pain in combination with paracetamol and/or NSAIDs Weak opioid	Same as for morphine: itch, nausea, vomiting, dizziness, constipation, sedation, respiratory depression	Some patients are unable to convert codeine (via CYP2D6) to its active metabolite, morphine Non-converters still experience side effects Increased dose results in increasing opioid side effects, with ceiling analgesic effect
Oxycodone	0.1–0.2 mg/kg 4 hourly	Oral tablet (onset 30–60 min) Also available in SR form	Stronger opioid	As above Less itch than morphine or codeine	Cost is only slightly greater than codeine and no metabolism issues Avoids morphine stigma
Morphine	0.25–0.5 mg/kg 4 hourly	Oral (onset 40–60 min) Also available in CR form	Stronger opioid	As above	Stigma
Tramadol	1–2 mg/kg 6 hourly	Oral; 50 mg capsules, IR (onset ~30–60 min) Also available in: SR tablet I.v. form (onset same as i.v. morphine)	For moderate to severe pain	Nausea and vomiting, dizziness, sedation Not constipating and less itch and respiratory depression than opioids	Off-licence use in <12 y requires anaesthetist-only prescription or Drug Usage Committee approval at RCH Use with caution if active seizures Mechanism of action via serotonin, noradrenaline reuptake and opioid receptors Opioid effect by metabolite M1 (requires CYP2D6 for conversion)

(Continued)

Table 4.2 _Continued_

Drug	Dose	Route(s)	Indications	Side effects	Special notes/contraindications
Fentanyl	1.5 mcg/kg (half into each nostril)	Intranasal (initial studies have used a specially designed atomiser)	Short-term analgesia		Initial emergency department studies have used 300 mcg/mL concentration. Studies validating the use of 100 mcg/2mL are pending
NSAIDS					
Ibuprofen	5–10 mg/kg tds–qid	Oral: Syrup 100 mg/5 mL 200 mg tablets (large)	For mild to moderate pain Particularly for muscular, bony or visceral pain	Gastrointestinal Renal Platelet inhibition (bleeding)	Caution in low volume status, poor urine output, bleeding and asthma Avoid in severe asthma with nasal disease (because of NSAID/aspirin-ERD) Can be used in mild asthma Generally NSAIDs are avoided in infants <6 months in Australia and <12 months in USA
Diclofenac	1 mg/kg bd–tds	Oral and rectal 25 and 50 mg tablet Rectal suppositories available at RCH			
Piroxicam	0.2–0.4 mg/kg (adult 10–20 mg) daily	Oral tablet			

Table 4.2 *Continued*

Drug	Dose	Route(s)	Indications	Side effects	Special notes/Contraindications
Indomethacin	0.5–1.0 mg/kg per dose (adult 25–50 mg) 8 hourly (max. 6 hourly)	Oral tablet			
Ketorolac	0.2 mg/kg i.v. (**not** i.m.)	I.v. available for anaesthetists to use at RCH			Off-licence use <16 years
COX-2 inhibitor					
Celecoxib	1.5–3 mg/kg bd	Oral capsule		No platelet inhibition	COX-2s are OK in NSAID-ERD Off-licence use <18 years
Local anaesthetics					
Lignocaine (lidocaine) 1–2% (1 mL of 1% = 10 mg)	Maximum doses: Lignocaine (lidocaine) with adrenaline: 7 mg/kg Without adrenaline: 3 mg/kg	Injectable	Wound infiltration Nerve blocks/infusion	Neurological Cardiac	**Do not** inject adrenaline into 'end organs' such as fingers, toes, penis, nose or ears due to the risk of ischaemia
Bupivacaine 0.25–0.5%	Maximum dose 2–2.5 mg/kg e.g. <0.5 mL/kg of 0.5%				
Levobupivacaine 0.25–0.5%					

COX, cyclooxygenase; CR, controlled release; ERD, exacerbated respiratory disease; IR, immediate release; NSAIDs, non-steroidal anti-inflammatory drugs; SR, slow release.

Bowel obstruction requiring large laparotomy

The patient will be nil orally and will universally require parenteral analgesia for severe pain. The following are suggested options. It is important that analgesia be commenced even if the child is to be transferred to a larger centre.

- Regular parenteral NSAID and paracetamol **and**
- Postoperative epidural local anaesthetic infusion; **or**
- Opioid via patient-controlled analgesia (PCA) and ketamine infusion.

Metastatic cancer with bony metastases and large intraabdominal mass

- Will benefit from regular dosing with a long acting opioid such as MSContin or fentanyl patch (applied every 3 days).
- Manage breakthrough pain with immediate release morphine, fentanyl lozenges, sufentanil nasal/buccal spray or ketamine lozenges.
- See also Haematology and Oncology, chapter 29, p. 377.

Procedural pain management

See Procedures, chapter 3.

Everyday events such as blood collection, cannula insertion, port cannulation, lumbar puncture and suturing are often a source of fear and anxiety for children. The aims of treating procedure-related pain are to prevent or minimize pain and distress.

Children with illnesses that require multiple painful procedures should be treated with care and sensitivity from the outset to avoid unnecessary psychological trauma. Anticipation by staff and preparation of patients and their parents are of key importance. Consider:

- The patient: age, previous experiences, emotional and physical condition of the child.
- The procedure: is it needed and how urgently, the level of expected pain and duration.
- The proceduralist: availability of appropriately skilled staff.

Always combine pharmacological and non-pharmacological techniques.

- Behavioural strategies (e.g. calico dolls, play therapy) can be used before all painful procedures.
- Analgesic and sedative drugs are added when required.
- Remember that sedatives alone are not analgesics.
- It is difficult to assess pain and the effects of analgesia and sedation in neonates and children with cognitive impairments.

Before the procedure

General principles – preparation is the key

- Prepare yourself and the other staff involved.
- Ensure parents and the child understand what the procedure involves. Ideally, prepare the child <6 years immediately before the procedure and >6 years 1 week before.
- Avoid medical jargon; explain what is going to happen and in what order.
- Obtain consent from the parents (verbal or written as required).

Procedures and Pain Management

- Set up your equipment before the child enters the procedure room.
- Encourage the parents to play an active role during the procedure by involving them in distraction techniques and comfort strategies. Avoid asking them to restrain their child.
- Children may be assisted to develop their own personal procedure routine, comfort or distraction strategies, e.g. counting backwards from 100.
- An explanatory video may be helpful in preparing the child and their parent for the procedure.
- If considering sedation, ensure adequate staffing and resources are available.

Pharmacological
- Topical anaesthetics (e.g. AnGel, EMLA for intact skin; Laceraine for wounds).
- Oral paracetamol, and/or NSAIDs and/or opioids e.g. oxycodone.

During the procedure
General principles
- Give the child some feeling of control (choice of hand for i.v., sitting up or lying down).
- Prompt the child to use the previously planned coping methods.
- Monitor the pain and effectiveness of pain management techniques during a procedure.
- If the child is not coping well, consider changing pain control measures or aborting the procedure.
- Consider sedation, depending on the procedure involved and the child's previous experience.

Comfort techniques
- Position for comfort (i.e. infants on parents' lap with physical/eye contact with parent).
- Have parents comfort child with gentle massage/touch or holding hands.
- Calm breathing.
- Swaddling for infants (<6 months).

Distraction techniques
- Choosing and playing a music CD or watching a favourite DVD.
- Playing with developmentally appropriate toys.
- Counting objects in the room or looking at posters on the wall or ceiling.
- Reading interactive storybooks.
- Visual imagery (e.g. ask the child to imagine a place where they would like to be and to tell you about it).

Pharmacological techniques
- *Sucrose:* for infants (2 mL of 33% sucrose). Give 0.25 mL 2 min before the start of a procedure onto the infant's tongue. Offer a dummy if it is part of the infant's care. Give the remainder of the sucrose slowly during the procedure.
- *Topical local anaesthetic* (e.g. EMLA or AnGel).

- i.v. cannulation, lumbar punctures and blood sampling are all potentially distressing for children.
- Apply local anaesthetic cream 60–90 min before soft tissue needling procedures (this ensures skin analgesia a few millimetres deep).
- Creams remain effective for up to 4 h after application.
- EMLA is a mixture of prilocaine 2.5% and lignocaine (lidocaine) 2.5%, and often vasoconstricts the area under application (onset 60–90 min).
- AnGel (amethocaine 1%) has a faster onset than EMLA (60 min). If amethocaine is left on for >1 h, erythema and itch can occur.
- *Peripheral nerve block.*
- *I.v. regional anaesthesia* (e.g. Bier's block).
- *Local anaesthetic infiltration* (lignocaine [lidocaine], ropivacaine, bupivacaine or levobupivacaine).
  - The skin and subcutaneous tissues can be effectively infiltrated with local anaesthetic solutions.
  - Lignocaine (lidocaine) stings as it is injected. Stinging may be reduced by adding 1 mL 8.4% sodium bicarbonate to 9 mL of lignocaine (lidocaine) solution.
  - The addition of adrenaline 1:200000 or 1:400000 (or 5–10 mcg/mL) may increase the duration of action, slows systemic absorption by up to 50% and reduces bleeding, **but adrenaline should not be used in 'end organs' such as fingers, toes, penis, nose or ears because of the risk of ischaemia.**
- *Nitrous oxide.*
  - Useful inhalational analgesic agent which provides potent short-term analgesia for painful procedures such as wound dressings and the removal of catheters.
  - Rapid onset and offset.
  - Side effects may include sedation, nausea and vomiting. Bone marrow depression can occur with prolonged exposure (>12 h) – consider in the child requiring daily repeat procedures.
  - Do not use in patients with head injuries, pneumothorax, cardiac disease and those who are obtunded.
  - The person administering nitrous oxide should have adequate airway management skills.
  - Fast patient before administration (2 h for solids and liquids, or longer as clinically appropriate for more complex patients).
  - Methods of delivery include:
    Entonox (a mixture of 50% nitrous oxide and 50% oxygen).
    Quantiflex (variable demand delivery system of nitrous oxide and oxygen).
- *Intranasal fentanyl*
- Has been used in Australian emergency departments in the initial pain management of long-bone fractures.
- A more concentrated solution of 300 mcg/mL was initially used, administered via an atomiser at a dose of 1.5 mcg/kg, given into one nostril only (where the child is >50 kg or if the less concentrated solution is used, give half the dose into each nostril).
- This has been administered prior to cannulation for subsequent opioid analgesia to be given intravenously.

- *Note*: the role of this agent via this route as the neat standardly available solution (100 mcg/2 mL) in procedural sedation requires further delineation.

Anxiolytics and sedatives

Procedural sedation should only be undertaken by accredited staff members, with appropriate monitoring and equipment and line-of-sight nursing until return to baseline sedation score. Midazolam oral 0.5 mg/kg (usual max. 15 mg) 20–30 min before treatment. Intranasal delivery stings and is now avoided at RCH.

- Sedation is not analgesia!
- Sedation alone is useful for non-painful procedures, e.g. diagnostic ultrasound.
- For painful procedures, analgesia is also necessary.
- **Cautions:**
  - Observe the child in department or ward (line-of-sight nursing) until return to baseline sedation score.
  - Usually recovery occurs by 60 min after oral/intranasal administration and 30 min after i.v. administration.
  - Midazolam potentiates the sedative effects of other drugs, e.g. opioids.
  - Be prepared for a paradoxical reaction (agitation secondary to benzodiazepines).
  - Midazolam should not be given to children with pre-existing respiratory insufficiency or neuromuscular disease (such as muscular dystrophy).

After the procedure

- Encourage the parent to remain with their child.
- Provide ongoing analgesia as needed.
- Document pain management techniques used and perceived success in minimising pain.
- Depending on the procedure, the child may need the opportunity to debrief. For example, staff and parents should focus on the helpful things the child did during the procedure. Staff may also like to suggest alternative techniques for any further procedures that may be planned.

Chronic or persistent pain management

Acute and chronic pain are distinct entities that require vastly different diagnostic and management skills; see Table 4.3.

Assessment
General principles

- Integrated multidisciplinary assessment and management is vital.
- Assess the physical and psychosocial causes for the child's presentation.
- The factors maintaining persistent pain will determine specific treatment.
- An integrated approach with good communication between the involved healthcare providers is ideal.

Table 4.3 Comparison of the qualities and clinical course of acute versus chronic or persistent pain

Acute pain	Chronic or persistent pain
• Tangible and understandable by the patient, family, friends and the treating doctor • Usually brief, evoked by a recognised noxious stimulus and associated with an adaptive biological significance (e.g. protection of injured part to encourage healing) • Usually improves rapidly and is associated with functional improvement and pain score reduction on a daily basis • Usually related to the nature and extent of tissue damage • Responds to pharmacological intervention	• Often nothing to see and minimal evidence of tissue damage • Often presents for prolonged duration • May be evoked by minor trauma • Improves slowly over time with an undulating course • Improvement and deterioration may be linked to life stresses • Not necessarily related directly to the nature and extent of tissue damage • Does not always respond to pharmacological intervention • Often associated with secondary gains (e.g. school, sport or chore avoidance)

History

- Is the pain:
  - Nociceptive (arising from peripheral or visceral nociceptors)?
  - Neurogenic (arising at any point from the primary afferent neurone to higher centres in the brain)?
  - Psychogenic (occurs in the absence of any identifiable noxious stimulus or injurious process)?
- Fixed factors (age, cognitive level, previous pain experience, witnessed examples of how other family members react to pain).
- Situational factors (social and academic functioning at schools, learned pain triggers, independent pain-reducing strategies).
- Suffering (fear, anxiety, anger, frustration, depression).
- Pain behaviour (overt distress, secondary gain, consultation with multiple health professionals factors, moaning, splinting, complaining of pain). Pain behaviour is exacerbated where the following factors are present:
  - Pain is central to communication (e.g. to receive a diagnosis or treatment).
  - Similarly, there is an absence of reinforcement for non-pain communication.
  - The child is fearful of increased pain (e.g. with movement).
  - The meaning of pain is fear-inducing.
  - The child and their parents may hold unhelpful beliefs and inadvertently maintain suffering, disability and dependency. The parents or child may obtain significant secondary gain from the child's maintained pain.

- Assess for:
  - Unhelpful belief systems of child and/or family (e.g. if pain were cured the other problems would not exist).
  - Unrealistic expectations (e.g. it is others' responsibility to fix the problem).
  - Functional disability (e.g. inability to play sport, socialise with peers, attend school).

Examine the painful site:
- What is causing the pain?
- Are there signs of complex regional pain syndrome? (see p. 69).
- Is there secondary deconditioning (e.g. muscle wasting, joint stiffening, tendon shortening)?
  - These can occur rapidly, especially when fear of touch or movement exists.

Treatment

The goals are to eliminate pain, restore function and reduce pain behaviour. It is desirable to identify the cause of pain, treat and eliminate it; however, this is not always possible. Therefore management aims to achieve a more active and fulfilling lifestyle, less constrained by pain.

Coordinate outpatient appointments to facilitate achieving these goals and minimising school absenteeism, time off work for parents and discouraging adoption of the sick role.

When to refer to a multidisciplinary pain clinic

A multidisciplinary team should ideally include a pain medicine specialist, physiotherapist, clinical psychologist, occupational therapist and child psychiatrist. The team should have access to an orthopaedic surgeon, neurosurgeon, paediatrician, paediatric rheumatologist and a rehabilitation specialist.

Refer when:
- Pain is more intense or persists longer than anticipated (e.g. after an injury).
- Character of pain is different to that expected.
- Pain responds poorly to medication.
- Loss of function results in secondary deconditioning (e.g. muscle wasting).
- Pain interferes with sleep, socialising with peers, school attendance and leisure activities.
- Pain behaviour manifests.
- Complex regional pain syndrome (CRPS) is present.
- Pain is neuropathic.

Non-pharmacological techniques in chronic pain management

- Pain education:
  - Help the patient understand that stress, anxiety and anger may contribute to pain. Identifying these stressors (often school or family) and managing these feelings more effectively may reduce or eliminate pain.

- Help the patient understand that pain does not always mean damage, and that pain is not a hindrance to return to function.
- Provide illness information (if one has been identified) outlining implications for the future. This can minimise anxiety.
- Cognitive behavioural techniques address the (often unhelpful) thoughts that maintain pain and disability.
  - Thought stopping or challenging techniques.
  - Behaviour modification techniques: based on modifying the consequences of the child's pain experience and pain behaviour by rewarding positive behaviour.
- Pain coping strategies include
  - Relaxation techniques: muscle relaxation via body awareness techniques, meditation, self-hypnosis or biofeedback.
  - Distraction techniques: art, play or music therapy.
- Physiotherapy reconditioning programmes:
  - Involve gradual return to function.
  - Utilise: muscle stretches, postural exercises, reconditioning programmes and stress loading (e.g. 'scrub and carry' techniques for the upper limbs, weightbearing for lower limbs).
  - Ultrasound treatment.
  - Heat/cold treatment.
  - Transcutaneous electrical nerve stimulation (TENS): activates large, myelinated primary afferent fibres (A fibres) that act through inhibitory circuits within the dorsal horn to reduce nociceptive transmission through small unmyelinated fibres (C fibres). TENS is more likely to be effective if pain responds to heat or cold.
- Pacing activity with reasonable goals.
- Management of setbacks.
- Sleep management.
- Family therapy:
  - Addresses how family dynamics may maintain pain.
  - Addresses how pain affects the rest of the family (e.g. lack of attention for well siblings).
- Parental counselling:
  - Parents may inadvertently support illness and ignore non-pain activities.
  - Addresses parental feelings of helplessness and loss of control.
  - Equips parents with strategies to manage pain behaviour.
- Assertiveness training.
- School liaison:
  - Address bullying.
  - Modifications to allow return to school despite disability.
  - Equip teachers with strategies to deal with pain behaviour.
  - Graded return-to-school programmes with involvement and education of teachers.
- Vocational counselling.
- Hydrotherapy.
- Acupuncture.

Pharmacological techniques in chronic pain management
Paracetamol
Limit the dose for long-term administration to 60 mg/kg per day.

Steroids
- Triamcinolone used for joint injections, trigger point injections, tendon sheaths and neuralgias.
- Dexamethasone administered by iontophoresis for soft tissue injuries.
- Epidural steroid administration for localised nerve root irritation due to disc herniation without motor weakness.

NSAIDs
- Topical gels (diclofenac, piroxicam, ibuprofen).
- Oral and rectal preparations (described in Table 4.2).

Anti-neuropathic medications
Tricyclic antidepressants (TCADs)/newer noradrenergic and serotonergic reuptake inhibitors
Improve pain even if depression is not present by suppressing pathological neural discharges. Provides more effective analgesia, usually within days, once appropriate dose reached.

Indications:
- Severe unremitting pain, especially if neuropathic.
- Complex regional pain syndrome (CRPS).
- Associated depression.
- Poor sleep.

Amitriptyline is the most commonly used TCAD, starting at 0.2 mg/kg per day increasing over 2 weeks to 2 mg/kg per day. Administer as a single dose before bed to take advantage of sedative properties. Increase dosage until the desired treatment goal is achieved or side effects become unacceptable, e.g. dry mouth, morning somnolence.

Anticonvulsants (e.g. gabapentin or carbamazepine)
Indicated for neuropathic pain and CRPS.

Dosage should be in the therapeutic anticonvulsant range, although there is no evidence of any relationship between analgesic effect and the plasma level. Some recommend increasing the dosage to the point of side effects or analgesia. Gabapentin is not licensed for use in pain and incurs an out-of-pocket cost.

Opioids
- Only partially modulate central sensitisation.
- Usually ineffective in controlling neuropathic pain or pain secondary to CRPS.
- Indicated in cancer pain and nociceptive pain.
- Tramadol may be useful.

Other techniques can include ketamine, baclofen, clonidine, sympathetic and peripheral nerve blocks. Surgical techniques are rarely used in paediatrics.

Complex regional pain syndrome (CRPS), types I and II

This condition is of unknown aetiology and is more common in paediatrics than is generally realised. The diagnosis is clinical and treatment is easier when the condition is recognised early.

- **Type I** was formerly known as reflex sympathetic dystrophy (RSD). It often occurs after a noxious stimulus to the affected limb (e.g. minor trauma or surgery). Symptoms are disproportionate to the inciting event.
- **Type II** was formerly referred to as causalgia. It differs from type I because it occurs after peripheral nerve injury.

Clinical manifestations

The affected area, usually a limb, manifests autonomic, sensory and motor symptoms consisting of:

- Pain:
  - Regional non-dermatomal distribution.
  - Hyperaesthesia (diffuse pain exacerbated by touch).
  - Allodynia (pain elicited by a stimulus that is not usually painful).
- Temperature change (affected limb often colder).
- Changes in skin blood flow – often red/purple colour change.
- Abnormal sweating.
- Oedema.
- Loss of function/reduced range of motion
- Motor dysfunction – weakness, tremor, dystonia.
- Abnormal hair growth, skin and/or nail atrophy.

Investigations

- Acute phase markers – normal.
- Bone scan often abnormal – increased or decreased uptake.
- Plain radiograph – osteopenia in prolonged cases.
- MRI – diffuse marrow infiltration is sometimes present.

Management

- Management requires early identification, skilful physical therapy, avoidance of immobilisation and multidisciplinary pain team input.
- Consider psychiatric assessment, pharmacological and interventional techniques.

Neuropathic pain

- Typified by continuous burning with an intermittent electric shock, stabbing or shooting-type discomfort.

- May be paroxysmal or spontaneous.
- Pain in an area of sensory loss.
- Pain in the absence of ongoing tissue damage.
- Associated with dysaesthesia (unpleasant, abnormal sensation, e.g. ants crawling on skin), allodynia and hyperalgesia (increased pain in response to noxious stimuli).
- Increased sympathetic activity may be present.
- Causes include CRPS type II, tumour, spinal cord injury, nerve damage (e.g. neuropraxia or avulsion, neuroma).
- Usually poor response to opioid medication.
- Consider the use of anti-neuropathic medications and early referral to a pain specialist and/or multidisciplinary pain management team if prolonged or refractory.

Pain in children and adolescents with disabilities

See also chapter 14, Developmental delay and disability, p. 170.

Pain assessment in individuals with cerebral palsy, cognitive impairment and/or communication difficulties can prove challenging.

- No simple pain assessment tool exists.
- Caregivers are best placed to distinguish pain from 'normal' behaviour in the individual.
- Pain may manifest as crying, screaming, frequent waking, grimacing, arching, muscle spasm or self-injurious behaviour, but some individuals with cerebral palsy or intellectual disability may exhibit these behaviours without experiencing pain.
- Differential diagnosis includes seizures, muscle spasm, anxiety, depression and anger.
- A thorough search for the cause of pain will guide treatment options.

Night waking

- Occurs frequently and has implications for the functioning of the whole family.
- Most settle with re-positioning.
- Tricyclic antidepressants, via their analgesic and sedative effects, may be useful in reducing the frequency of waking.

USEFUL RESOURCES
- *www.rch.org.au/anaes/pain* – RCH Acute Pain Management Service Clinical Practice Guidelines. Links to many topics including: morphine by intermittent bolus guideline; opioid by infusion and patient controlled analgesia (PCA) .
- *www.rch.org.au/rchcpg* [Procedural Pain Management] – RCH guidelines for procedural pain management.
- *www.rch.org.au/clinicalguide* [Analgesia & Sedation] – RCH Clinical Practice Guidelines including links to Nitrous Oxide and Ketamine Guidelines.
- *www.pediatric-pain.ca* – Pediatric Pain Research Lab. Site created by a Canadian research group, devoted to the topic. Contains useful downloadable pamphlets and protocols.

CHAPTER 5

Fluid and electrolyte therapy

Julian Kelly
Trevor Duke

Sick children should be given enteral feeds where possible, as this provides nutrition. If oral fluids are not tolerated, consider feeds via a nasogastric (NG) or nasojejunal (NJ) tube. Clear i.v. fluids provide no nutrition.

There are marked differences between children and adults in fluid and electrolyte composition (Table 5.1), as well as maintenance fluid requirements (Table 5.2). Maintenance fluid requirements are the daily water needs in a disease-free state. This is high (per kg of body-weight) in infancy and gradually decreases throughout childhood.

Hypovolaemic shock

Dehydration without shock can generally be managed with oral rehydration fluid and solids. Children with shock (hypotension and acidosis) caused by hypovolaemia should be given parenteral fluid immediately: **administer 20 mL/kg repeatedly until plasma volume is restored** (20–100 mL/kg may be required). Fluid can be given i.v. or into the bone marrow (see p. 39); NG or intraperitoneal fluid is not effective in shock.

Use 0.9% saline to restore intravascular volume in hypovolaemic shock. Do not use albumin or Haemaccel (polygeline). Dextrose solutions may cause hyperglycaemia if infused rapidly and hyponatraemia if they contain <0.9% saline.

In states of hyponatraemia or hypernatraemia, the correction of serum sodium should not occur at a rate >0.5 mmol/L per hour.

Replacement and maintenance therapy

Four basic aspects are considered:
- Existing deficit.
- Losses during therapy.
- Maintenance requirements.
- Principles of safe fluid management.

Existing deficit
Fluid deficit
The fluid deficit is most reliably estimated from the loss of body weight if a recent pre-illness weight is available. Otherwise the degree of dehydration can be estimated by the following:

Paediatric Handbook, 8th edition. By Kate Thomson, Dean Tey and Michael Marks. Published 2009 by Blackwell Publishing, ISBN: 978-1-4051-7400-8.

Table 5.1 Fluid distribution

	Total body water (mL/kg)	Intracellular fluid (mL/kg)	Extracellular fluid (mL/kg)	Blood volume (mL/kg)
Neonate	750	350	400	85
Infant	700	400	300	80
Child	650	400	250	70
Adult	600	400	200	60

- Decreased perfusion (pallor or reduced central capillary return; hypotension is a late sign).
- Deep (acidotic) breathing – not useful in diabetic ketoacidosis.
- Decreased skin turgor.
- Increased thirst.

Weak markers of mild–moderate dehydration include a history of oliguria, restlessness, lethargy, sunken eyes, dry mouth, sunken fontanelle and the absence of tears.

Hence, if the bodyweight loss is

- <3–4%: no clinical signs
- 4–6%: clinical signs are present and the number and severity is a guide to the degree of dehydration
- ≥7%: hypotension and acidosis may be present.

In general, fluids to replace the existing deficit are given over the first 24 h. But, for hypernatraemic or hyponatraemic dehydration, they should be given over at least 48–72 h.

Electrolyte deficit

The type and degree of electrolyte deficit depends on the diagnosis. For example, in gastroenteritis, the loss of base leads to acidosis; in pyloric stenosis, the loss of acid and chloride leads to hypochloraemic alkalosis.

The rate of infusion of potassium should rarely be >0.2 mmol/kg per hour (and never >0.4 mmol/kg per hour). Concentrations of potassium >40 mmol/L should be used with extreme caution, generally only through a central line. Infusions of potassium at concentrations of ≥60 mmol/L should only be given in the intensive care unit. ECG monitoring should be considered in massive potassium replacement and infusions of concentrated solutions should be controlled with the use of a pump.

Continuing losses

Fluid balance charts should accurately record volumes of vomitus, gastric aspirates, drainage from fistulae, diarrhoea, urine output and other fluid losses. These parameters will determine both the volume and type of fluid and electrolyte replacement (see Table 5.5). Weights should be measured at least daily, as they are an important marker of ongoing losses.

Maintenance requirements

Maintenance fluid requirement is the daily water requirement for well children to excrete an iso-osmotic urine. The volumes required to achieve this in disease states are different from those in well children. See Tables 5.2 and 5.3.

Many acutely ill children have high levels of antidiuretic hormones (ADH), resulting in reduced free water excretion. This is termed Syndrome of 'Inappropriate' ADH secretion (SIADH), occurring particularly in postoperative children and those with brain or lung disease (meningitis, encephalitis, bronchiolitis, pneumonia). Hence, the total fluid required to maintain normal intravascular volume in these children is reduced (note that the aim is **not** to 'dry out' the patient). If these children are given standard maintenance fluid i.v., tissue oedema and hyponatraemia may occur. Hence, in these children give a total fluid intake (TFI) of about 60% of the usual maintenance volumes in Tables 5.2 and 5.3.

In contrast, some sick children will have increased fluid requirements (e.g. those with high fever, ongoing vomiting and diarrhoea, capillary leak or third-spacing of fluid into the abdomen). These children may need more than the standard maintenance fluid to maintain normal intravascular volume. Prescribing fluid volumes can be complex; some ill children have clinical features that imply a need for increased *and* decreased fluids. These children need regular assessments to ensure adequate hydration is achieved.

Principles of safe fluid management
Calculate the total fluid intake

At least once a day the TFI in mL/h and in mL/kg per day should be calculated. The prescribed TFI should include all fluid intake the child receives: i.v. deficit replacement + maintenance + estimation of continuing losses.

As the total fluid volume **must not** be exceeded, remember to factor in the following:
- i.v. fluid for drug lines
- blood products
- enteral feeds
- other.

Table 5.2 Daily maintenance intravenous fluid requirements

Bodyweight	Requirements
3–10 kg	100 mL/kg per day
10–20 kg	1000 mL + (50 mL/kg per day for each kg over 10 kg)
20 kg and over	1500 mL + (20 mL/kg per day for each kg over 20 kg)

Table 5.3 Hourly maintenance intravenous fluid requirements

Weight (kg)	4	6	8	10	12	14	16	20	30	40	50	60	70
mL/h	16	24	32	40	45	50	55	65	70	80	90	95	100

Fluids and Nutrition

Table 5.4 Adjustments to maintenance intravenous fluid requirements

Condition	Adjustment to fluid intake
Renal failure	×0.2 + urine output
Basal state	×0.7
High ADH (e.g. brain injury, meningitis)	×0.7
Breathing humidified gas	×0.75

Table 5.5 Composition of some body fluids in children

Fluid	Na^+ mmol/L	K^+ mmol/L	Cl^- mmol/L	HCO_3^- mmol/L	Other
Gastric fluid	20–80	10–20	100–150	0	H^+ 30–120
Ileal fluid	50–150	3–15	20–120	30–50	
Diarrhoeal fluid	10–90	10–80	10–110	20–70	
Sweat Normal Cystic fibrosis	 10–30 50–130	 3–10 5–25	 10–35 50–110	 0 0	
Burn exudate	140	5	110	20	Protein 30–50 g/L

Hospitalised children on i.v. fluids often receive more than intended because other fluids (as listed above) have not been included in the calculation. The balance of enteral and parenteral fluid should be adjusted around this prescribed TFI. See Tables 5.2–5.5.

Regular monitoring

The key to good fluid management is regular clinical monitoring. Signs of dehydration should be corrected, but signs of overhydration, such as rapid weight gain and eyelid oedema, avoided.

- **Children receiving i.v. fluids must be weighed every day.** An increase in weight of 5% or more over 24 h indicates fluid overload. Manage by stopping i.v. fluids, measure serum sodium and consult senior medical staff. A decrease in weight of 5% or more indicates dehydration. Children receiving deficit replacement fluid should be weighed every 6 h.
- **Assess for oedema every day.** Check for eyelid and lower limb swelling. If either is present, stop i.v. fluids and consult senior medical staff.

- **Children receiving i.v. fluids should have serum electrolytes checked at least daily.** Senior medical staff should be consulted if:
  - serum sodium is ≤130 mmmol/L or has fallen by >5 mmol/L
  - serum sodium is ≥150 mmol/L or has risen by >5 mmol/L.
- For infants receiving i.v. fluids, consider measuring blood glucose every 6 h. If BSL is <3 mmol/L, increase glucose concentration of i.v. fluid from 5% to 10%.

Acid–base problems

The maintenance of pH within narrow limits is a result of two mechanisms:

- Buffer systems: the bicarbonate system is quantitatively the most important in plasma (70% of total).
- Excretory mechanisms: via the kidneys and lungs.

Acidosis (low pH) and alkalosis (high pH) may be respiratory or metabolic in origin. Respiratory disorders result from changes in the excretion of volatile carbon dioxide and, consequently, in the levels of carbonic acid. Metabolic disorders occur with changes in concentrations of non-volatile acids and, consequently, in the concentration of buffer base – mainly bicarbonate.

The four primary disorders are:

- **Metabolic acidosis.** This arises from increased production of non-volatile acid (e.g. ketoacids and lactic acid), failure of the kidney to excrete non-volatile acid or conserve base, or excess loss of buffer base (e.g. gastroenteritis or intestinal fistula).
- **Metabolic alkalosis.** This arises from excess loss of non-volatile acid (e.g. pyloric stenosis), excess intake of buffer (e.g. bicarbonate infusion), or potassium depletion where an extracellular alkalosis occurs as hydrogen ions are lost in the urine (e.g. renal tubular syndromes, pyloric stenosis or diuretic therapy).
- **Respiratory acidosis.** Hypercapnia is the result of alveolar hypoventilation from any cause (e.g. central, neuromuscular or pulmonary).
- **Respiratory alkalosis.** This is caused by hyperventilation.

Indicators of acid–base status

pH

This reflects the actual hydrogen ion concentration and alters in response to both respiratory and metabolic changes.

P_{CO_2} (partial pressure of carbon dioxide)

In arterial and capillary blood samples, this represents the P_{CO_2} in blood leaving the lungs. Alterations reflect disturbance in the respiratory component of the acid–base state. Changes may also reflect respiratory compensation for primary metabolic acidosis or alkalosis.

Base excess

This is an estimate of the change in total buffer base that would be present if the P_{CO_2} was normal (40 mmHg). Change in the base excess reflects disturbance in the metabolic component of the acid–base status (not respiratory). In metabolic alkalosis the total buffer base is increased, and thus the base excess is positive. Other calculated measures of the metabolic component are the standard bicarbonate and the total buffer base.

Actual bicarbonate

This is the plasma concentration of bicarbonate; it is influenced by both metabolic and respiratory components.

In practice, isolated metabolic and respiratory disorders are uncommon. Most disorders have a metabolic and a respiratory component. Usually one is the primary disorder and the other occurs secondarily and tends to correct the change in pH. However, sometimes primary metabolic and respiratory disturbances occur together; e.g. in respiratory distress syndrome, acidosis is contributed by both hypoxia leading to lactic acid accumulation and subsequent metabolic acidosis, whilst carbon dioxide retention results in respiratory acidosis (see Tables 5.6 and 5.7).

The interpretation of changes in base excess and P_{CO_2} as primary or secondary changes must be made clinically.

Correction of metabolic acidosis

Metabolic acidosis often resolves rapidly once the cause has been corrected and administration of bicarbonate is usually not required. Consider giving bicarbonate if there is marked metabolic acidosis (large base deficit, normal P_{CO_2}) with a pH of <7.10. Give bicarbonate for metabolic acidosis with a pH <7.15 caused by bicarbonate loss, which is characterised by a normal anion gap of <12 mmol/L (anion gap = Na − bicarbonate − Cl).

- The amount of bicarbonate required is guided by:
  - mmol of HCO_3 required = base deficit (mmol/L) × weight (kg) × 0.3
- It is usual to give only **half** the amount of bicarbonate suggested by this formula, then repeat the blood gas measurement before giving more.
- The factor (weight × 0.3) represents the volume of extracellular fluid through which the base deficit (negative base excess) is distributed.

Table 5.6 Changes in arterial capillary blood (before compensation)

	pH (mmol/L)	P_{CO_2} (mmHg)	Base excess (mmol/L)	Actual bicarbonate (mmol/L)
Normal reference range	7.36–7.44	36–44	−5 to +3	18–25
Metabolic acidosis	Decrease	Normal	Decrease	Decrease
Metabolic alkalosis	Increase	Normal	Increase	Increase
Respiratory acidosis	Decrease	Increase	Normal	Increase
Respiratory alkalosis	Increase	Decrease	Normal	Decrease

Table 5.7 Change in indicators of acid–base status seen in combined disorders

	pH (mmol/L)	P_{CO_2} (mmHg)	Base excess (mmol/L)	Actual bicarbonate (mmol/L)
Normal reference range	7.36–7.44	36–44	−5 to +3	18–25
Primary metabolic acidosis + compensatory respiratory alkalosis (e.g. gastroenteritis, diabetic ketosis)	Decrease or normal	Decrease	Decrease	Decrease
Primary metabolic alkalosis + compensatory respiratory acidosis (e.g. pyloric stenosis)	Increase or normal	Increase	Increase	Increase
Combined primary respiratory and metabolic acidosis (e.g. respiratory distress syndrome)	Decrease	Increase	Decrease	Normal

- In babies <5 kg, the factor is weight × 0.5 because of the greater percentage of extra-cellular fluid.

The rate of administration of bicarbonate will be determined by the cause of the metabolic acidosis and the clinical state of the patient; e.g. in cardiac arrest infuse bicarbonate rapidly; if acidosis has been present for >6 h, the correction should usually be undertaken over at least 6 h (and mild to moderate acidosis will resolve with rehydration alone). Rapid correction of metabolic acidosis will cause a fall in extracellular potassium.

The principles of correction of metabolic alkalosis are discussed in the following section on pyloric stenosis.

Management of some special conditions
Pyloric stenosis
All infants with pyloric stenosis should have their acid–base and electrolytes measured. Persistent vomiting results in predominantly hydrogen and chloride loss, with consequent hypochloraemic alkalosis. Losses of potassium in vomitus and urine can lead to significant hypokalaemia. In severe hypokalaemia, potassium is conserved in the kidneys preferentially to hydrogen ions, leading to paradoxical aciduria.

The duration and severity of vomiting will, to a large extent, determine the degree of fluid and electrolyte imbalance.

Assessment
All patients require biochemical assessment, but not all require i.v. therapy preoperatively. Any child who is clinically dehydrated or has significant biochemical derangement requires i.v. fluids.

I.v. therapy

- In severe dehydration (≥7%), commence with 0.9% saline until adequate circulation has been established and continue with 0.45% saline and 5% dextrose (see Table 5.11).
- In moderate dehydration (4–6%), commence with 0.45% saline and 5% dextrose (see Table 5.11).
- In mild dehydration, await electrolyte results before commencing therapy.
- Adequate potassium and chloride replacement is necessary to correct the acid–base abnormality. As soon as urine flow is established, potassium chloride is given up to a maximum of 0.4 mmol/kg per hour. Usually 20–40 mmol/L is adequate.

Acute oliguria and anuria

Severe oliguria is a urine output of <0.5 mL/kg per hour.

Initial management

Three clinical situations occur:

- Sudden and complete anuria should arouse suspicion of urinary obstruction. Ensure the catheter is correctly placed and not blocked.
- Renal hypoperfusion causing oliguria should be suspected in the presence of clinical dehydration or septicaemia leading to hypotension; the urinary sodium is usually <20 mmol/L. Blood volume expansion is necessary.
- Renal tissue injury (e.g. acute poststreptococcal glomerulonephritis or secondary to hypoperfusion or nephrotoxin). Urinary sodium is usually >40 mmol/L. Give i.v. frusemide (1–2 mg/kg) and, if there is no response, institute treatment for continuing anuria.

Continuing anuria

Fluid intake is restricted to the previous 24 h urine output and any abnormal losses; approximately 20% of normal maintenance requirements must also be given to replace insensible water loss.

At least 20% of full energy requirements is given as carbohydrate to spare tissue protein from catabolism for energy, which accentuates the rise in blood urea. I.v. 10–20% glucose, oral Caloreen or Polyjoule are suitable.

Peritoneal dialysis or haemofiltration will be required for hyperkalaemia, severe uraemia (blood urea ≥50 mmol/L), acidosis, or water overload leading to hyponatraemia, oedema or hypertension. It should also be considered if anuria persists for >24 h.

Hyperkalaemia

The management of hyperkalaemia depends on the underlying cause. Serum potassium is increased by acidosis and reduced by alkalosis. In acute oliguric renal failure, if urine is not formed after i.v. frusemide (see above), the presence of hyperkalaemia (≥7.0 mmol/L) is an indication for dialysis. High values (up to 7.0 mmol/L) not requiring treatment may be found in the neonatal period. Obtain an urgent 12-lead ECG – peak T waves suggest that treatment is needed, especially if the QRS complex is widened.

If cardiac arrhythmias are present, rapid but temporary benefit may be achieved by giving (while arranging dialysis):

- I.v. sodium bicarbonate 2 mmol/kg.
- Short-acting (regular) insulin 0.1 unit/kg given with 2 mL/kg of i.v. 50% dextrose.
- I.v. calcium gluconate 10% 0.5 mL/kg, given slowly.
- Rectal or NG sodium polystyrene sulfonate (Resonium) 1 g/kg.

Hypokalaemia

Metabolic alkalosis may cause hypokalaemia, but this resolves if alkalosis is treated. Severe hypokalaemia causes long QT interval, often with prominent U waves. Management is usually sufficient with supplementation of oral potassium or by adding it to i.v. maintenance fluid. Potassium should rarely be given faster than 0.2 mmol/kg per hour and never faster than 0.4 mmol/kg per hour even in ICU. Concentrated potassium infusions can cause chemical burns if extravasation occurs, hence the need for reliable central line access.

Hypernatraemia

If the patient is 'shocked', provide volume resuscitation with 0.9% saline as required in 20 mL/kg boluses. The aim is to lower the serum [Na^+] slowly at a rate of no faster than 12 mmol/L in 24 h (0.5 mmol/L per hour). **If sodium is corrected too rapidly in hypernatremia, cerebral oedema, seizures and permanent brain injury may occur.** Monitor and manage for concurrent hyperglycaemia and hypocalcaemia.

Moderate hypernatraemic dehydration, [Na^+] 150–169 mmol/L

After initial resuscitation, replace the deficit plus maintenance **over 48 h**.

- Use nasogastric oral rehydration solution (Gastrolyte), but remember that Gastrolyte has a sodium concentration of 60 mmol/L.
- If needing i.v. rehydration use **0.45% NaCl + 5% dextrose or 0.9% NaCl + 5% dextrose**. Add maintenance KCl once urine output established.

Daily volume (mL) = Daily maintenance fluids (mL) + remaining fluid deficit (mL)/2
Rate (mL/h) = Daily volume (mL)/24(h)

- Check urea, electrolytes and glucose 1 hourly – if serum sodium is falling faster than 1 mmol/h, slow down rate of infusion by 20%. Recheck the serum sodium in 1 h.
- If after 6 h of rehydration therapy the sodium is decreasing at a steady rate then check the U&Es and glucose 4 hourly.
- If there are persistent neurological signs, consider cerebral imaging.

Severe hypernatraemic dehydration, [Na^+] > 169

- Consider admission to intensive care.
- After initial resuscitation, replace deficit and maintenance with **0.9% NaCl + 5% dextrose over 72–96 h**.

> Daily volume (mL) = Daily maintenance fluids (mL) + remaining fluid deficit (mL)/3
> Rate (mL/h) = Daily volume (mL)/24(h)

Hyponatraemia

A low serum sodium should be corrected slowly, especially if the abnormality is long-standing. It should never be increased faster than 0.5 mmol/L per hour and usually at 0.25 mmol/L per hour or less. To increase the sodium by 0.25 mmol/L per hour, infuse saline at a rate of (mL/h) = Wt (kg)/(% saline infused).

If sodium is corrected too rapidly in hyponatremia, cerebral (especially pontine) demyelination and permanent brain injury may occur.

Other conditions

See acute infectious diarrhoea (p. 401), haemorrhagic shock (p. 6), burns (p. 247), diabetes mellitus (p. 298) and meningococcal septicaemia (pp. 7 and 388).

The newborn

This section should be read in conjunction with chapter 32, Neonatal conditions, p. 431 and the section relating to newborns in chapter 6, Nutrition, p. 85.

Babies are different from older children because they have:

- Proportionately more body water in all compartments (see Table 5.8).
- Greater insensible water losses.
- Reduced renal capacity to compensate for abnormalities.
- Less integrated and responsive endocrine controls.

These differences are of practical importance only in sick babies, i.e. those requiring inpatient care in level 2 or level 3 nurseries.

This section highlights major practical differences between the sick newborn and older age groups. However, any baby needing i.v. therapy should be in a level 2 or level 3 nursery.

Insensible water losses can vary from around 20–30 mL/kg per day at term to >60–80 mL/kg per day at <27 weeks' gestation.

The newborn kidney is less efficient at concentrating and diluting urine, as well as retaining and excreting Na^+, K^+ and H^+ loads.

Table 5.8 Neonatal body water distribution

	<28 weeks	Term
Total body water	85% (of bodyweight)	75%
Extracellular water	55%	45%
Circulating blood volume	90–100 mL/kg	85 mL/kg

Intermediate gestations lie between these figures.

Water requirements

Babies' water and milk requirements are different. For normal nutrition, babies need 150–200 mL/kg per day of milk. This is substantially more than their water requirements (see Table 5.9). This difference is of greatest importance in babies suffering illnesses that are made worse by excess water administration, e.g. acute and chronic lung disease, heart failure or renal impairment. Newborns who are fasted should not be given the volumes required for milk nutrition as i.v. fluid, as this invariably leads to water overload.

Water requirements depend on:

- *Gestational age*: the earlier the gestation, the greater the skin losses and the poorer the renal concentration.
- *Postnatal age*: skin losses decrease and renal function improves steadily from day 1.
- *Nursing condition*: dressed babies lose least; naked babies under radiant heaters lose most. Humidified respiratory circuits (e.g. ventilators) reduce respiratory losses.

Before 27 weeks' gestation, requirements are too variable to tabulate: start at 60 mL/kg and modify 6–12 hourly according to clinical status, serum Na^+ and urine osmolality.

Sodium

Babies are less able to conserve sodium and excrete excess loads. Usual daily requirements are 2–4 mmol/kg; the earlier the gestation, the higher the need (e.g. up to 8 mmol/kg per day if <1000 g).

Hyponatraemia (serum Na^+ <132 mmol/L)

This may be due to excess water administration, inadequate sodium administration, excess sodium loss or high ADH secretion. It is important to assess and treat the underlying cause.

It is easy to overload sick babies with water in the first days after birth. This is a common cause of hyponatraemia. In general, i.v. rates >60 mL/kg per day in sick mature babies will provide excessive water in the first 48 h.

When the cause is water overload, serum Na^+ correction by water restriction alone is often effective in the newborn. The serum sodium should be rechecked in 4–6 h. As serum Na^+ ≤125 mmol/L can result in seizures and injury to the CNS, it should be treated with Na^+ administration if water restriction is not successful, even when the primary cause is water overload. The dose required can be calculated as follows:

Table 5.9 Water requirements in well newborn babies

	Water requirement (mL/kg per day)		
	Days 0–1	Days 2–3	Days 4–7+
Mature 35 weeks	60 mL/kg per day	80–100	100–120
Immature 27 weeks	80–100	100–140	100–120

* NB: in sick and/or ventilated term babies fluid requirements are usually 20 ml/kg per day less. In very preterm babies fluid requirements may be 20–40 mL/kg per day higher.

dose of Na^+ (mmol) = bodyweight $\times$ 0.8 $\times$ (140 − current serum Na^+)

Once serum Na^+ is ≥125 mmol, further correction should continue slowly over 36 h. Serum Na^+ should be checked every 4–6 h: if correction is occurring rapidly, Na^+ administration can be ceased once the serum levels are safe.

Hypernatraemia (serum Na^+ >154 mmol/L)
This may be due to excess Na^+ administration, inadequate water administration or disproportionate loss of water in relation to sodium.

It is easy to overload sick babies with sodium-containing i.v. fluids. For example, 1 mL/h of normal saline = 4 mmol Na^+/24 h; this is the entire Na^+ requirement of a 1000 g baby and more than half the daily requirements of a 2000 g baby. The use of sodium bicarbonate for correction of acidosis also often leads to sodium overload.

Na^+ should be added to i.v. maintenance fluids from the beginning of day 2, taking into account separate sodium administration as sodium bicarbonate or heparinised saline.

Potassium
- Potassium requirement is 2–4 mmol/kg per day. Serum K^+ does not reflect body K^+. With high or low levels the cause should be defined.
- Except with anuria, K^+ should be added to maintenance i.v. fluids from day 2.
- With diuretic therapy, Na^+ and K^+ losses are much greater in babies than in older age groups.

Glucose
Both hypoglycaemia and hyperglycaemia are associated with adverse outcomes. Glucose requirement for neonates is around 6–8 mg/kg per minute. 10% dextrose solutions at 2 mL/kg per hour provide only 3.3 mg/kg per minute, so on the first or second day of life, a higher concentration glucose solution may be required to maintain the blood glucose above 2.2 mmol/L. Blood glucose should be measured at admission for all sick neonates and then every 4–24 h depending on severity of illness, risk factors for hypoglycaemia, clinical signs of hypoglycaemia and changes made to glucose infusions.

Infants at high risk of hypoglycaemia include infants born to diabetic mothers (hyperinsulinaemia) and those with intrauterine growth restriction (low glycogen stores). Infants of diabetic mothers who are feeding well by 12 h of age with no hypoglycaemia are unlikely to

Table 5.10 Glucose delivery on infusions of different concentrations and rates

I.v. fluid infusion rate (mL/kg/hour)	Daily fluid volume given (mL/kg/day)	Amount of glucose received (mg/kg/min)		
		10% dextrose	15% dextrose	20% dextrose
2	48	3.3	5	6.7
3	72	5	7.5	10
4	96	6.7	10	13.3

develop hypoglycaemia; blood glucose should then only be checked if symptoms occur. In some babies with hyperinsulinaemia, glucose infusions of 10–15 mg/kg per minute may be required. Concentrations >5% should be given through central venous access.

Table 5.10 outlines the amount of glucose a baby receives on infusions of different concentrations and rates.

Acid–base problems

Metabolic acidosis is the most common acid–base disturbance in sick babies. Management should be tailored to the underlying cause, including consideration of a fluid bolus. Correction with sodium bicarbonate is controversial: it may be reasonable to correct a pH <7.10 over 30–60 min or pH 7.10–7.20 over 2–4 h, after discussion with senior medical staff.

mmol of HCO_3 required = base deficit (mmol/L) × weight (kg) × 0.5

The acid–base status is usually assessed after half of this correction is given, before administration of further bicarbonate. 8.4% sodium bicarbonate needs to be diluted to 4.2% (with sterile water or saline) before administration if being given via a peripheral vein. Remember to also check the serum Na^+. Other measures to control acidosis (e.g. volume expansion) should be instituted at the same time.

Commonly used intravenous solutions

There are many types of i.v. fluids. In general it is better to use isotonic solutions (i.e. fluids that contain sodium concentrations similar to that of serum) along with avoidance of over-hydration with i.v. fluids. This reduces the risk of iatrogenic hyponatraemia. Never use 5% dextrose in water or 0.18% NaCl as routine maintenance or resuscitation fluid as there is a high risk of hyponatraemia. See Table 5.11 for commonly used i.v. fluids.

Table 5.11 Commonly used intravenous solutions

	Na^+ (mmol/L)	Cl^- (mmol/L)	K^+ (mmol/L)	Lactate (mmol/L)	Ca^{2+} (mmol/L)	Glucose (g/L)
0.9% NaCl (Isotonic or normal saline)	150	150	–	–	–	–
0.45% NaCl with 5% glucose	75	75	–	–	–	50
0.18% NaCl with 4% glucose	30	30	–	–	–	40
0.18% NaCl with 4% glucose and KCl 20 mmol/L	30	30	20	–	–	40
Hartmann's solution	130	110	5	30	2	–
Hartmann's solution with 5% glucose	130	110	5	30	2	50

4% Normal serum albumin (NSA)

This solution contains human albumin 40 g/L, sodium 140 mmol/L, chloride 128 mmol/L and octanoate 6.4 mmol/L. It has an osmolality of 260 mOsm/kg and a pH of 6.7–7.3. It should **not** be used for rapid correction of hypovolaemia (use 0.9% saline).

Albumin (20%)

This solution contains albumin 200 g/L, sodium 46–58 mmol/L and octanoate 32 mmol/L. It has an osmolality of 80 mmol/kg and a pH of 7.0. Dose (mL/kg) = 0.25 × (increase in serum albumin in g/L).

> It is important to explain to parents that NSA and albumin are blood products and risks of transfusions are associated with their use.

Additives

- Molar potassium chloride (0.75 g in 10 mL) = 1 mmol/mL of K^+ and Cl^-.
- 20% sodium chloride = 3.4 mmol/mL of Na^+ and Cl^-.
- Molar sodium bicarbonate (8.4%) = 1 mmol/mL of Na^+ and HCO_3^-.
- Calcium gluconate 10% = 0.22 mmol/mL of Ca^{2+}, which is 8.9 mg/mL of Ca^{2+}.
- Magnesium chloride for injection (0.48 g anhydrous in 5 mL) = 1 mmol/mL of Mg^{2+}.

Formulae and definitions

Conversion factors

- Sodium chloride 1 g contains 17 mmol Na^+ and 17 mmol Cl^-.
- Potassium chloride 1 g contains 13 mmol K^+ and 13 mmol Cl^-.
- Sodium bicarbonate 1 g contains 12 mmol Na^+ and 12 mmol HCO_3^-.

Molarity

Osmolality is the number of osmotically active molecules in a solution per kg of solute (usually mmol/kg of water). Osmolarity is the number of osmotically active molecules in a solution per litre of solute (usually mmol/L of water).

Useful formulae

- Anion gap = $Na^+ - (HCO_3^- + Cl^-)$; normal <12.
- Number mmol = mEq/valence = mass (mg)/mol. wt.
- Sodium deficit: mL 20% NaCl = wt × 0.2 × (140 − serum Na^+).
- Water deficit (mL) = 600 × wt (kg) × [1 − (140/Na^+)] (if body Na^+ normal).
- Non-catabolic anuria: urea rises 3–5 mmol/L per day.
- Bicarbonate dose (mmol) = base excess × wt × 0.3 (give 1/2 this).
- Osmolality serum = 2Na^+ glucose + urea (normal 270–295 mmol/L).

USEFUL RESOURCES
- *www.rch.org.au/clinical guide* [Intravenous Fluids] – Includes useful links to fluid calculator, neonatal fluid requirements, hyponatremia and hypernatremia guidelines.

CHAPTER 6
Nutrition

Julie Bines
Kay Gibbons
Michele Meehan

Breast-feeding

Breast-feeding is the best means of feeding babies, and all efforts should be made to promote, encourage and maintain it. Exclusive breast-feeding is recommended for the first 6 months of life. Breast-feeding can be continued for as long as mother and baby prefer (see Table 6.1).

Normal variations of breast-feeding
Frequency of feeds

Breast-fed infants usually feed every 2–5 h from both breasts each feed. Young babies feed frequently but demand feeding (i.e. feeding when hungry) will usually have the baby settle into a fairly predictable pattern of feeds. The frequency of feeds is determined by the baby's appetite and gastric capacity, as well as the amount of mother's milk available.

Length of feeds

The duration of the feed is determined by the rate of transfer of milk from the breast to the baby, which, in turn, depends on the baby's suck and the mother's 'let down'. This may vary from 5 to 30 min. Young infants tend to feed for longer. It is the cessation of strong drawing sucks and the appearance of shorter-duration bursts of sucking that indicate the 'end' of the feed – not the time.

If the mother feels the baby is on the breast 'all the time', rather than focusing on the sucking alone, it is more important to look for longer duration of pauses between bursts of sucking. At this point, either take the baby off the breast or swap to the other side.

Appetite spurts

Babies seem to experience appetite spurts at 2 weeks, 6 weeks and 3 months. It is crucial that parents are aware of this or the baby's natural increase in feed frequency may be mistaken for diminution of milk supply. This is especially true at 6 weeks when breasts are no longer carrying extra fluid and the supply is settling to the demands of the baby. Unfortunately, many women wean at this time through poor advice. Let the baby feed on demand, even 2 hourly, and this should settle in 48 h.

Paediatric Handbook, 8th edition. By Kate Thomson, Dean Tey and Michael Marks. Published 2009 by Blackwell Publishing, ISBN: 978-1-4051-7400-8.

Fluids and Nutrition

Table 6.1 How to assess good breast-feeding

	Good	Problem
Baby's body position	On side – chest to chest	On back – angled away from mother
Mouth	Open wide	Lips close together
Chin	Touching or pressing into the breast	Space between chin and breast
Lips	Flanged out	Tucked in, inverted
Cheeks	Well rounded	Dimpled or sucked in
Nose	Free of or just touching the breast	Buried in breast, baby pulls back
Breast in mouth	Good mouthful, more of bottom part of breast in mouth	Central, little breast tissue in mouth or only nipple in mouth
Jaw movement	Rhythmic deep jaw movement	Jerky or irregular shallow movement
Sounds	Muffled sound of swallowing milk	No swallowing, clicking sounds
Body language of the baby	Peaceful, concentrated	Restless, anxious
Body language of the mother	Comfortable, relaxed	Tense, hunched, awkward
Awareness of feelings during feed	Pain free, may feel a drawing feeling deep in breast or 'let down'	Nipple or breast pain
Nipple, post-feed	Nipple elongated, well shaped	Not elongated, compressed 'stripe' or blanched

Source: Murray S., *Breast Feeding Information and Guidelines for Paediatric Units*, Royal Children's Hospital, Melbourne, Australia 1992.

Qualities of breast milk

Breast milk is naturally thinner in consistency than an artificial formula and may have a bluish tinge – this is normal, healthy and nutritious. The composition of breast milk varies during the feed. The fat content of milk varies diurnally: it is lowest at about 6 am and gradually increases to its peak at about 2 pm. At any one feed, the highest concentration of fat is at the end of the feed in the 'hind milk'. The change in concentration is a gradual merging over the feed and is part of the feeding process. Hind milk is not 'better' than the early 'fore milk'; fore milk is higher in water and lactose and provides liquid to quench the baby's thirst and a quick surge of energy.

The presence of blood in the milk may cause a red or pinkish-brown discoloration. If this is present when the mother first starts expressing colostrum it may be due to duct hyperplasia. This gradually disappears and is of no significance. The most common cause of blood-stained milk (usually first noticed when the baby possets) is trauma to the nipple.

Bowel actions

The motions of breast-fed infants are normally bright yellow and soft to loose. The baby may have a bowel action with every feed (strong gastrocolic reflex) or once every 5–8 days.

Mastitis is a common reason for early weaning. Any reports of pain by the mother should be actively addressed (see chapter 32, Neonatal conditions, p. 450).

Temporary cessation of breast-feeding

If the feeding pattern is interrupted because of illness, a planned fast for a procedure or the mother's absence, the mother will need to express to maintain milk supply.

- Milk can be expressed by hand or by pump.
- Express as often as the baby would normally feed (i.e. 6–8 times a day). Several volumes of expressed milk can be added to the same bottle or storage bag (available from commercial pharmacies), but a new container should be used every 24 h.
- Milk may be kept in the freezer section of the refrigerator for 2 weeks or in the deep freeze for 3 months.
- To thaw frozen milk, place a bag/bottle in a container of cool water and run in hot water until the bag/bottle is standing in hot water. When the milk is thawed, it will be cold; continue to heat in hot water or place in the fridge until required for a feed.
- Thawed milk should be used within 24 h.

How much milk to express?

If the mother wants to express to give a feed by bottle or to substitute a feed as she is weaning, how much will the baby need?

Daily requirements of milk are:
- From 0–6 months: 150 mL/kg.
- >6 months: 120 mL/kg.

Divide this amount by the usual number of feeds to calculate the amount required per feed.

Growth in breast-fed infants

Growth patterns differ between breast-fed and artificially fed infants. Average weights of breast-fed babies are similar to or higher than formula-fed babies until 4–6 months, after which breast-fed babies slow significantly in their weight gain. Length and head circumference remain similar.

Growth charts are now available for fully breast-fed infants, although these are not in standard use. The naturally slower weight gain of breast-fed infants should not be taken in isolation as abnormal.

Maternal illness

When the mother is unwell, breast-feeding should continue. In the case of maternal infection, antibodies will pass through the breast milk to protect the baby.

Maternal drugs

If the mother has to take medication, the risk–benefit ratio should be weighed carefully by the prescriber. The mother should continue to breast-feed unless use of the drug is absolutely contraindicated during lactation and there is no safe alternative. There are very few such drugs and almost all have a safe alternative. If the mother is concerned about continuing breast-feeding, even if the drug is safe, suggest taking the drug after a feed to minimise the concentration or dividing the dose if possible.

Vitamin D

Vitamin D deficiency is increasingly recognised in Australia. Women who wear coverings (hejab), are dark-skinned or have limited sunlight exposure are at highest risk. They should be prescribed oral supplementation with vitamin D at 1000 IU/day during pregnancy. Their infants are at risk of vitamin D deficiency due to low hepatic stores and the paucity of vitamin D in breast milk. Exclusively breast-fed infants of vitamin D-deficient mothers should be screened or treated empirically e.g. with Penta-Vite 0.45 mL/day.

Formula feeding

If breast milk is not available, either from the breast or as expressed milk, a commercially prepared formula should be chosen. These are based on cow's milk, modified to lower the protein, calcium and electrolytes to levels better suited to the human infant and contain added amino acids, vitamins and trace minerals. See tables of formula composition at *www.rchhandbook.org*, Nutrition, chapter 6. A 'from-birth' formula should be selected for infants from birth to 6 months. For infants >6 months, follow-on formulas may be used. They have a higher protein and renal solute load and are not suitable for infants <6 months of age.

The introduction of some formula (e.g. when returning to work, low milk supply) need not mean the end of breast-feeding. A combination of breast and formula may be quite suitable for the infant.

Cow's milk-based formulas

- The range of formula options has increased in recent years, with options now including specifically modified proteins, long-chain polyunsaturated fatty acids (LCPUFA) and probiotics. All formulas meet the Australian Food Standards code and are suitable, although some are more expensive.

- Changes between types of formula are made for a variety of reasons, including irritability, poor sleep and possetting. In the normal thriving infant there is little indication to change the type of formula.
- Care should be taken when changing between formulas to use the correct scoop and dilution (as these vary between brands). A history for a formula-fed infant with possible feeding problems should include a review of formula preparation.

Soy formulas
If a soy-based feed is required, an infant formula should be chosen. These are nutritionally adequate for infants, but are suggested for specific indications (such as lactose intolerance) rather than as a regular feed option. Follow-on soy formulas are available.

Antiregurgitation formulas
Thickened formulas are aimed at reducing regurgitation. Their use should be limited to the stepwise treatment of gastro-oesophageal reflux (see chapter 27, Gastrointestinal conditions page 345). They are not recommended in healthy infants without regurgitation.

Low-lactose formulas
Infant formulas with low-lactose content are recommended only in cases of proven lactose intolerance (see chapter 27, Gastrointestinal conditions page 340).

Hypoallergenic formulas
Based on partially hydrolysed protein in place of whole cow's milk protein, this formula group is intended as part of a preventive programme for infants who are not being breast-fed and are at high risk of developing allergy. Breast-feeding continues to be the feed of choice in infants at high risk of developing allergy. Hypoallergenic formula is **not** to be used as a treatment formula for an infant with diagnosed cow's milk allergy.

Number of feeds
Babies <6 weeks of age usually feed every 3 h; however, they may take more each time and feed 4 hourly. Babies rarely sleep through the night before 6–8 weeks. When they miss a night feed (usually sleeping 5–6 h straight) they will have five feeds and consequently take more milk at each feed. Babies who sleep longer in the day (e.g. 5 h between feeds) often need to feed overnight to maintain adequate intake. Parents may need to wake the baby after 4 h in the daytime. There is no need to wake a baby overnight if intake and weight gain are adequate.

Introduction of whole cow's milk
The introduction of cow's milk products as part of an expanding diet is appropriate, but the main milk intake should be breast milk or formula until 12 months of age because of the

risk of iron deficiency. Small amounts can be used on cereal, in custard and yoghurt from about 7–8 months.

Full-cream dairy products should be used for children up to 2 years; reduced-fat milk can be used from 2 years. Skim milk (essentially no fat) should not be used for children under 5 years.

Introduction of solids

Breast milk (or formula) will meet all nutrient needs until infants are 6 months old. This also corresponds to the age when most infants develop head control and oropharyngeal function sufficient to allow introduction of solids. From around 6 months solids can be introduced, to increase the intake of nutrients, such as iron, and as part of the educational process of learning to eat.

Solids can be iron-fortified baby cereal, smooth vegetables or fruits, followed by meat and chicken. Foods should be introduced one at a time to allow observation of tolerance. Texture should be increased so that by about 8–9 months the infant is managing lumps and varying textures, and is starting to manage finger foods.

By about 12 months, most family foods can be offered. Increasing intake of solids should result in a reduction of milk intake to about 600 mL/day by 12 months. Higher intake of cow's milk limits the intake of other foods and is associated with iron deficiency.

Iron deficiency and associated anaemia is the most common nutrient deficiency in children in Australia. It is associated with the early introduction of cow's milk, high intake of cow's milk in the second year and low intake of iron-rich foods, such as meat and pulses.

Weaning

There is no set rule for weaning time. Solids should be introduced at around 6 months and cup-drinking of breast milk, formula or water should start by 7–9 months. There is no need for the baby to be weaned to a bottle – if they are old enough they can go straight to a cup. Most babies can manage adequate fluid from a cup by 12–15 months.

Sudden cessation of breast-feeding leaves the mother at risk of developing mastitis. Ideally, weaning is achieved by reducing the feeds by one a week. Start by offering a drink in a cup or bottle instead of a breast-feed at midday, and gradually increase these other drinks. Many mothers retain the early morning feed or the last feed at night for longer.

Persistent difficulty in weaning usually requires someone to support the mother, giving the baby a feed and allowing the baby some time away from the mother to help with mutual separation. Both need to be ready to let go. Specialist lactation advice may be needed.

Toddlers who will not eat

An assessment of the toddler who refuses food includes the following steps:
- Plotting weight and height to assure the parents of the child's normal growth.
- Using the growth chart to demonstrate that the growth rate normally slows in the second year.

- Linking this to a lessened need for food and subsequent drop in appetite.
- Emphasising developmental progress.

Advise parents that:
- A healthy child will eat when hungry – *quit the fight!*
- Avoid arguments over food. Remember: 'It's the mother's job to offer food, it's the child's job to eat it!'
- Showing independence is an important part of toddler development – choosing and refusing food is an expression of independence.
- Serve small portions – lower expectations.
- Include limited healthy options and allow the child to choose among the options.
- Include some healthy food choices that they like. Offering cereal at lunch is okay! A lack of variety is not a major worry at this age.
- Avoid filling up on milk and juice – large volumes of milk (>600 mL a day) can make the child feel full. Juice is not necessary in the child's diet.
- Give the child time to enjoy the meal without comment. Remove the food after 30 min or if they dawdle or lose interest.
- Learning to eat is fun. Switch to finger food if they refuse to be fed.
- Do not use food as a punishment or reward. It only increases its potential power.

Daily food needs of preschoolers

The following is a guide to the quantities suitable for 2–5 year olds. Many parents are surprised at how little children of this age need. However, because total needs are small there is relatively little place for high-fat, high-sugar extras such as savoury snack foods and soft drinks.
- **Milk group:** 2 servings
  - 1 serving = 250 mL of milk, 200 g of yoghurt or 35 g of cheese.
  - Full-cream products are recommended up to 2 years; from 2 years reduced fat products can be included.
- **Bread and cereal group:** 4–5 servings
  - 1 serving = 1 slice of bread, 1/2 cup of pasta or 2 cereal wheat biscuits.
- **Vegetable and fruit group:** 4 or more servings
  - 1 serving = 1 piece of fruit or 2 tablespoons of vegetables – focus on variety of different vegetables and fruits rather than quantity.
- **Meat or protein group:** 2 servings
  - 1 serving = 30 g of lean meat, fish or chicken, 1/2 cup of beans or 1 egg.

Feeding the sick infant and child
Nutritional assessment

A thorough nutritional assessment should be undertaken taking into account:
- Medical history:
  - Type and duration of illness.

- Degree of metabolic stress.
- Treatment (medications or surgery, or both).
- Dietary assessment:
  - 24 h dietary recall.
  - 3 day food record.
- Physical examination:
  - General assessment: wasting, oedema, lethargy and muscular strength.
  - Specific micronutrient deficiencies: pallor, bruising, skin, hair, neurological and ophthalmological complications.
  - Anthropometry – weight, length, head circumference – serial measurements plotted. Correct for age for preterm infants.
  - Growth velocity.
  - Skinfold thickness, mid-arm circumference.
- Fluid requirements:
  - Take into account i.v. and enteral fluids.
  - Any restrictions as per medical team.
- Laboratory data:
  - Assessment of GI absorptive status – stool microscopy, pH and reducing sugars.
  - Protein status: albumin, total protein, pre-albumin, urea, 24 h urinary nitrogen.
  - Fluid, electrolyte and acid–base status: serum electrolytes and acid–base, urinalysis.
  - Iron status: serum ferritin and full blood examination.
  - Mineral status: calcium, magnesium, phosphorus, alkaline phosphatase, bone age and bone density.
  - Vitamin status: vitamins A, C, B_{12}, D, E/lipid ratio, folate and INR.
  - Trace elements: zinc, selenium, copper, chromium and manganese.
  - Lipid status: serum cholesterol, HDL cholesterol and triglycerides.
  - Glucose tolerance: serum glucose, HbA1c.

Establishing a nutrition treatment plan
Calculating nutritional requirements
Energy

Estimated energy requirements for the sick infant or child can be calculated by using either:
- The requirements of a normal well child of the same sex and age, or
- An estimate of basal requirements with additional stress and activity factors.

Less common, but the most accurate method to calculate energy requirements in very sick infants and children, is via measurement of energy expenditure using indirect calorimetry.

Energy requirements can be expressed as kilocalories (kcal) or as kilojoules. The conversion equation is: $kJ = kcal \times 4.2$.

Recommended energy and protein requirements for healthy infants and children are based on nutrient reference values (NRVs) for use in Australia and New Zealand. A full statement of the NRVs can be found at *www.nhmrc.gov.au/publications/subjects/nutrition.htm*

Energy requirements are increased in the following conditions:
- Very low birthweight (VLBW) infants.
- Chronic lung disease.
- Cardiac defects.
- Cystic fibrosis.
- Diseases causing malabsorption i.e. liver, SBS, allergic enteropathy.
- Burns.
- Tumours.

Energy requirements are decreased in:
- Critically ill patients who are ventilated.

Protein
Increased protein intake is recommended in:
- Protein-losing states i.e. enteropathy and nephrotic syndrome.
- Chronic malnutrition.
- Burns.
- Renal dialysis.
- HIV.
- Haemofiltration (~2 g/kg per day).

Reduced protein intake is recommended in:
- Hepatic encephalopathy (0.3 g/kg per day).
- Severe renal dysfunction (not dialysed).

Fat
- Concentrated source of energy and essential for transport of fat-soluble vitamins and hormones.
- Deficiency can occur rapidly in neonates and is evidenced by reduced growth rate, poor hair growth, thrombocytopenia, susceptibility to infection and poor wound healing.

Micronutrients
Special consideration is needed when estimating the micronutrient requirements of sick children (see Table 6.2).

Feeds for infants
See Table 6.3.
- Breast milk, including expressed breast milk (EBM).
- Infant formulas, including 'low birthweight' formulas.
- Specialised feeds for specific disease states, e.g. inborn errors of metabolism, renal, complex malabsorption and liver conditions.

Breast milk
Breast-milk feeding should be the primary aim for very sick babies. When babies are too ill or too premature to suckle at the breast, most mothers can establish lactation by expression. EBM can be fed via a tube until the baby is well enough to be placed on the breast. In this

Table 6.2 Diseases that increase micronutrient requirements

Disease	Increased requirement
Burns	Vitamins C, B complex, folate, zinc
HIV/AIDS	Zinc, selenium, iron
Renal failure: dialysis	Vitamins C, B complex, folate (reduce or omit copper, chromium, molybdenum)
Haemofiltration	Vitamins C, B complex, trace elements
Protein–energy malnutrition	Zinc, selenium, iron
Refeeding syndrome	Phosphate, magnesium, potassium
Short bowel syndrome, chronic malabsorption states	Vitamins A, B_{12}, D, E, K, folate, zinc, magnesium, selenium
Liver disease	Vitamins A, B_{12}, D, E, K, zinc, iron (reduce or omit manganese, copper)
High fistula output, chronic diarrhoea	Zinc, magnesium, selenium, folate, B complex, B_{12}
Pancreatic insufficiency	Vitamins A, D, E, K
Inflammatory bowel disease	Folate, B_{12}, zinc, iron

way breast-milk feeding can be achieved in extremely premature babies and those with major malformations, birth defects and other serious illnesses. The only situations in which breast-milk feeding is not possible are:

- When an informed mother chooses not to express.
- Specific inborn errors of metabolism, which require exclusion formulas.
- Some complex malabsorption syndromes.

Breast-milk fortifiers

Breast-milk fortifiers are available to add to EBM to increase its content of protein, energy and other nutrients. The addition of fortifier should be delayed until feeds are fully established (i.e. 150–200 mL/kg), unless babies have a condition requiring fluid restriction, e.g. congestive cardiac failure or chronic lung disease.

Babies who may benefit from fortifiers are those with increased nutritional requirements (e.g. VLBW babies) and those requiring fluid restriction (as listed above).

In addition, VLBW babies may require folate, iron, sodium and vitamins C, D and E. Iron should not be started until 12 weeks of age. VLBW babies who receive multiple blood transfusions may not need supplemental iron.

Infant formulas

When breast milk is not available an infant formula is required. Low birthweight (LBW) formulas are designed for very premature (<32 weeks) babies. In general, these contain more energy, protein, calcium, phosphorus, trace elements and certain vitamins than standard formula. They include LCPUFA as part of their fat content, based on evidence that this improves the developmental outcomes in premature infants. Generally LBW formulas are used until a weight of 2.5 kg is achieved. Babies are then fed with a standard infant formula which can be fortified if necessary.

Fortification of standard infant formulas

Standard formulas provide approximately 280 kJ/100 mL (20 kcal/30 mL) and 1.5 g protein/100 mL. Fortification should only be implemented under the supervision of a paediatrician or dietician.

- To increase energy to 350 kJ/100 mL (25 kcal/30 mL):
  - Use *additional* formula powder, i.e. for formulas where the standard dilution is 1 scoop/30 mL of water, use 1 scoop/25 mL of water, or for formulas where the standard dilution is 1 scoop/60 mL of water use 1 scoop/50 mL of water.
  - This will also increase protein and other nutrient intakes.
  - Care should be taken in infants with renal or liver impairment.
- To increase energy to 420 kJ/100 mL (30 kcal/30 mL):
  - Use additional formula powder as above with the addition of either glucose polymer or fat emulsion.
  - Concentrate the formula further with additional powder (e.g. 1 scoop/30 mL to 1 scoop/20 mL). This provides an improved energy/protein ratio and additional nutrients which can be beneficial in fluid restricted infants and those with high catch up growth requirements. Use of this formula needs to be monitored carefully due to its higher renal solute load (RSL) and osmolality.

Specialised feeds can also be fortified in similar ways to the above.
- **Infants and young children who develop an intercurrent gastroenteritis must have all fortification ceased until vomiting and diarrhoea resolve, to avoid the potential complication of hypernatraemic dehydration.**
- VLBW babies require 180–200 mL/kg per day of EBM or standard formula, or 150–180 mL/kg per day of fortified EBM or LBW formula, starting at 20–30 mL/kg per day at birth and increasing by 30 mL/kg per day as tolerated. Regimes should be modified according to condition and stability in VLBW infants. Initial feed frequency should be 1–2 hourly. Hourly feeds may be necessary in babies <1000 g.
- Orogastric tubes should be used in babies <1250 g, as nasogastric tubes cause significant airways obstruction. Continuous intragastric infusion of feed rather than intermittent boluses may help if reflux, gastric distension or apnoea is persistent.
- Term infants require 150 mL/kg per day. This is usually reached over 5–7 days, starting at 30–40 mL/kg per day and increasing by 30 mL/kg per day as tolerated. Feed frequency should be 3–4 hourly, although with reflux or abdominal distension, smaller volume and more frequent feeds may help.

Table 6.3 Appropriate feeds for infants

Normal gut function	EBM ± breast milk fortifier/formula **or** Standard infant formula or follow-on formula ± fortification	
Impaired gut function	Choice of formula dependent on type and degree of impairment	
	Lactose-free infant formula, e.g. Delact, S26 Lactose Free	For use after gastroenteritis when lactase is temporarily reduced
	Hydrolysed infant formula, e.g. Peptijunior, Alfaré	Suitable for cow's milk allergy, malabsorption, liver disease, CF
	Elemental infant formula, e.g. Neocate, Elecare	Suitable for multiple food allergy and malabsorption

Table 6.4 Oral or enteral feeds for children 1–6 years (8–20 kg)

Normal gut function	Concentrated infant formula
	Standard paediatric formulas, e.g.
	Nutrini, Pediasure, Resource for Kids (added fibre also available)
	    4.2 kJ/mL (1 kcal/mL)
	Nutrini Energy, Pediasure Plus (added fibre also available)
	    6.3 kJ/mL (1.5 kcal/mL)

Impaired gut function	Lactose-free formula, e.g Digestelact Concentrated hydrolysed infant formula Hydrolysed formula, e.g. MCT Peptide 1+, Vital HN Elemental formula, e.g. Neocate Advance, Elecare, Paediatric Vivonex

Feeds for children

Young children often maintain oral intake when they are ill. In some cases additional energy needs to be added to oral feeds to maintain nutritional status.

These include:

- Energy supplements, e.g. glucose polymers or fat emulsions added to normal foods and fluids to increase energy intake
- Complete supplements, e.g. Pediasure, Fortisip or Sustagen drinks, which can be used in addition to usual foods to increase energy, protein and nutrient intake.

Enteral feeding

Enteral nutrition is the provision of nutrients to the alimentary tract through a feeding tube. It can be used to provide the total nutritional needs of a patient (either short or long term), or to provide additional nutrients when voluntary oral intake is inadequate. See nutritional support algorithm, fig. 6.1.

Enteral feeding has certain advantages over parenteral nutrition:

- Less risk of infection.
- Less risk of metabolic abnormalities.
- Nutrients provided to the alimentary tract enhance intestinal growth and function.
- Inexpensive.

Administration

The most commonly used route is nasogastric, its main benefit being ease of insertion. When long-term feeding is required, a gastrostomy tube may be indicated. It is generally placed endoscopically rather than surgically.

When gastric motility is poor or when gastric residues are persistently high, a nasojejunal tube may be of benefit.

Feeding method

When choosing a method consider the feeding route, the expected length of time the feed will be required and the type of feeding regime to be used (see Table 6.6). The introduction of hyperosmolar feeds should be gradual.

Selection of feed

A full nutritional assessment (current nutritional status, current intake, requirements and the consideration of medical condition/fluid restrictions) should be carried out by a paediatric dietician to establish which feed will be optimal. See Tables 6.4 and 6.5 for appropriate feeds to use with different age groups.

It is **inappropriate** to administer puréed foods down feeding tubes as the amount of fluid required to achieve a suitable consistency dilutes the energy and nutrient content, while increasing the risk of microbial contamination and tube blockage.

Monitoring enteral nutrition

When monitoring patients on enteral feeds, mechanical, metabolic, gastrointestinal, nutritional and growth parameters must be assessed routinely. In the early stages of feeding, the patient's tolerance of the feeding regimen is critical to the success of feeding.

Once the feeding plan has been fully implemented, regular assessment of the patient's nutrient requirements is needed to ensure that nutritional support has been adequately maintained and to indicate when enteral feeding can be possibly ceased.

From enteral to oral feeding

Once the patient is able and willing to eat by mouth, enteral feeds can be reduced in proportion to the amount consumed orally. Transition from continuous feeds to overnight

Table 6.5 Oral or enteral feeds for children 6 years+ (>20 kg)

Normal gut function	Standard paediatric formula (as above) Standard adult formula, e.g.: Osmolite, Nutrison Standard, Ensure, Jevity, Resource (added fibre available) 4.2 kJ/mL (1 kcal/mL) Ensure Plus, Nutrison Energy, Resource Plus, Fortisip (added fibre available) 6.3 kJ/mL (1.5 kcal/mL) Novosource 2.0, TwoCal HN 8.4 kJ/mL (2 kcal/mL)
Impaired gut function	Hydrolysed formula, e.g. MCT Pepdite 1+, Vital Elemental formula, e.g. Elemental 028, Paediatric Vivonex, Vivonex TEN

Table 6.6 Types of enteral feeding regimens

	Advantages	Disadvantages
Bolus feedings	Most closely mimics physiological feeding Increases patient mobility Little equipment is needed Volume given can be precisely measured	Can be time-consuming for caregiver May decrease voluntary oral intake
Gravity drip	Little equipment needed Feeding most likely to be tolerated	Rate of delivery cannot be closely monitored
Pump-assisted continuous	Feeding can be delivered while patient sleeps Larger volumes can be tolerated than if given by bolus method	Requires feeding pump

feeds may help establish oral intake while ensuring the patient is not nutritionally compromised.

Home enteral feeding

The decision to provide home enteral feeding should take into consideration the patient's medical needs and the practical, social and psychological factors that influence the family's ability to cope with a home feeding programme.

Children on home enteral feeding, especially those who have minimal or no voluntary oral intake, require close monitoring of their growth and need their feeding regimens altered appropriately.

Common problems

- **Gastrointestinal disturbance.** This is the most common problem (diarrhoea, cramping, nausea and vomiting). It can be minimised by correct formula selection and review of medications. High gastric residues should be treated by reducing the rate of feeds given, feeding smaller volumes, continuously reassessing the concentration of feed and assessing GI function. Directing feed into the jejunum alleviates the problems caused by slow gastric emptying.
- **Food aversion.** Young children who have been fed enterally during infancy or for long periods of time may miss important developmental steps in self-feeding. Non-nutritive sucking and mouth contact or taking small amounts of appropriate food/fluid orally will help establish or maintain eating and feeding skills. A speech pathologist may be of assistance.
- **Malnutrition** is associated with major changes in electrolyte balance. Enteral feeding should be initiated with caution in patients with significant and long-standing undernutrition. Serum phosphate, potassium, magnesium and glucose levels should be assessed regularly (see Refeeding syndrome, p. 99).

Parenteral nutrition

General indications for parenteral nutrition:
- Recent weight loss of >10% of usual body weight and a non-functional GI tract.
- No oral intake for >3–5 days in a patient with suboptimal nutritional status and a non-functional GI tract.
- Anticipated need for parenteral nutrition for a minimum of 3–5 days.

Medical/surgical conditions that may require parenteral nutrition
- Patients unable to tolerate enteral feeding because of GI dysfunction; i.e. postoperative neonates, extensive short-bowel syndrome or severe malabsorption.
- Patients with increased metabolic requirements that may not be adequately treated with enteral therapy; i.e. severe burns, cystic fibrosis or renal failure.

 For ordering and monitoring parenteral nutrition, refer to *www.rchhandbook.org*, Nutrition, chapter 6.

Refeeding syndrome

After a period of prolonged starvation, aggressive nutritional therapy may precipitate a cascade of potentially fatal metabolic complications. These include:
- Hypokalaemia.
- Hypophosphataemia.
- Hypomagnesaemia.
- Glucose intolerance.
- Cardiac failure.
- Seizures.
- Myocardial infarction/arrhythmias.

At particular risk are patients with:
- Anorexia nervosa.
- Classical marasmus.
- Kwashiorkor.
- No nutrition for 7–10 days in adolescents (much less in infants and children) with significant metabolic stress.
- Acute weight loss of ≥10–20% of usual body weight and possibly metabolic stress, or >20% of usual body weight.
- Morbid obesity with massive weight loss (i.e. postoperative).

Management
- Identify risk and chronicity.
- Identify and treat metabolic stress if present (e.g. infection).
- Establish baseline status: weight, height/length, head circumference, fluid status, electrolytes, urea, creatinine, calcium, phosphate and magnesium, prior to commencing nutritional rehabilitation.

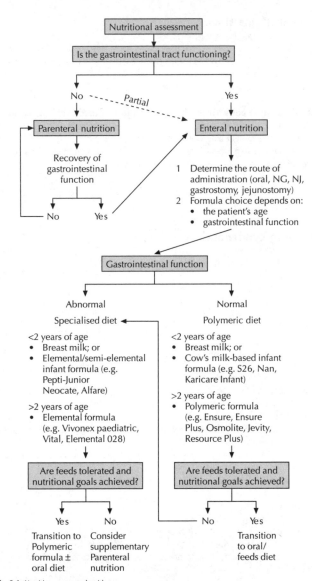

Fig 6.1 Nutrition support algorithm

- Establish modest nutritional goals initially (e.g. basal requirements until stability is assured), then aim to provide for catch-up growth. During the first week of nutritional therapy, weight gain may not be seen or, if present, may reflect fluid gain rather than muscle or fat gain.
- Monitor closely over the first week until a nutritional plan is established with: pulse rate, fluid balance, weight, caloric intake, glucose, electrolytes, urea, creatinine, phosphate and magnesium. Bloods are required daily for the first 3 days.
- Administer vitamin and mineral supplements.

USEFUL RESOURCES

- *www.breastfeedingbasics.org* – Breastfeeding Basics. Academic, web-based short course on breast-feeding fundamentals. Aimed at the medical practitioner, with useful revision of anatomy and physiology and a number of case studies.
- *www.lalecheleague.org* – LaLeche League. International breast-feeding advocacy/support group. Excellent FAQs for breast-feeding mothers.
- *www.raisingchildren.net.au* – Raising children network. Commonwealth government parenting site – contains comprehensive information.
- *www.goforyourlife.vic.gov.au* – Victorian government information on nutrition and physical activity.
- *www.rch.org.au/nutrition* – RCH Nutrition Department. Resources section contains useful fact sheets and links.

CHAPTER 7
Slow weight gain

Michael Harari

Slow weight gain (SWG; also known as failure to thrive) is arbitrarily defined as being <3rd percentile for weight or dropping ≥2 percentile tracks. It implies failure to gain weight, with height and head circumference being initially well preserved. Short stature is discussed in chapter 25, Endocrine conditions. Most cases do not have an organic cause. Clues to the cause usually lie in history and examination of the child, along with assessment of growth patterns of other family members. Investigations should be limited and focused.

Is this weight *normal* or is it *slow weight gain*?

Growth charts identify children who are lean. However, crossing percentiles or being in the lower echelons of the percentile chart does not necessarily mean the child has a problem. The charts may not distinguish between those who are sick/undernourished (i.e. true SWG) and those who are lean simply because they are meant to be (i.e. normal).

Birthweight percentile does not predict future weight and perfectly healthy children may cross percentile lines. In the first year of life, deceleration of growth may be normal, until infants equilibrate to their 'true' growth channels. Later in childhood, some children will be in the lower percentile for weight because of genetic or constitutional factors. These children are lean because they are meant to be. They will appear healthy, with good muscle bulk, adequate subcutaneous fat, normal activity and development.

Children who are lean because they are undernourished are usually apathetic and withdrawn with poor muscle bulk. Reference to the family's growth parameters may be helpful. Further evidence of adequate growth can be sought in anthropometric measurements such as skinfold thickness.

Categories of slow weight gain

- Poor caloric intake – nutritional, chronic illness.
- Increased caloric losses – vomiting, malabsorption.
- Poor utilisation.
- Increased metabolic requirements.

Paediatric Handbook, 8th edition. By Kate Thomson, Dean Tey and Michael Marks. Published 2009 by Blackwell Publishing, ISBN: 978-1-4051-7400-8.

Causes

Non-organic slow weight gain

This accounts for >50% of SWG in Australia.

- Inadequate food intake – careful dietary history.
- Psychosocial factors in parent or child – includes maternal depression, deprivation and neglect of the child.
- Rumination.

Organic slow weight gain

This may also have a non-organic component.

- Poor intake: numerous causes.
- Renal disease: UTI, renal tubular acidosis, chronic renal insufficiency.
- Cardiorespiratory: chronic upper airway obstruction, congenital heart disease, cardiomyopathy, bronchopulmonary dysplasia, cystic fibrosis (CF).
- Gastrointestinal: cleft lip and palate, Pierre Robin syndrome, gastro-oesophageal reflux, pyloric stenosis, coeliac disease, pancreatic insufficiency (CF, Shwachman syndrome), inflammatory bowel disease (IBD), Hirschsprung disease.
- Endocrine: hyper- and hypothyroidism, adrenal insufficiency, diabetes insipidus.
- CNS: congenital and acquired CNS or muscle disease may cause inadequate feeding.
- Tumours: including diencephalic syndrome.
- Chronic infection: immune deficiency, tuberculosis.
- Genetic, chromosomal or intrauterine causes: intrauterine growth retardation, trisomy syndromes.
- Metabolic: galactosaemia, phenylketonuria, acrodermatitis enteropathica, amino and organic acidopathies, hypercalcaemia.

History

History should focus on intake and losses. Also consider familial patterns of weight gain and growth, psychological and developmental assessment.

- Intake: what is consumed, how it is made up, when were solids commenced.
- Output: amount and colour of vomit, stool frequency and consistency.
- Birth: weight, gestation, complications.
- Past history: chronic illness, recurrent infections.
- Family history: possible maternal depression, growth pattern of other family members, illnesses and consanguinity.

Examination

Examination should focus on growth parameters and nutritional status (see chapter 6, Nutrition). Happy, outgoing children with good muscle bulk in thighs and buttocks are unlikely to have significant undernutrition. Look for signs of macro/micronutrient deficiency and evidence of system-based disease.

Investigations

Avoid random tests. The history and examination should guide the direction and tempo of investigation. If the cause of SWG is not readily apparent after history, examination and limited investigations (e.g. FBE, urine M/C/S), further investigations and management should be in consultation with a specialist.

Second line investigations might include liver function, renal function, thyroid stimulating hormone, inflammatory markers, faecal microscopy, screening for coeliac disease, rickets, occult infection, immune dysfunction and a sweat test.

Management

The underlying cause will determine the treatment. Admit to hospital for:

- Severe undernutrition.
- Failed outpatient management.
- Child abuse or neglect.
- Extreme parental anxiety or depression that requires time to allow a constructive patient–doctor relationship to develop.

Admission may facilitate further assessment of feeding technique, the parent–child interaction and allow the involvement of a multidisciplinary team.

CHAPTER 8

Obesity

Kay Gibbons
Zoë McCallum
Matthew Sabin

Obesity is increasingly prevalent among Australian children – up to 25% are now either overweight or obese. Over the last three decades the prevalence of overweight and obesity have doubled and trebled, respectively.

Childhood obesity is associated with important short- and medium-term complications, in addition to leading to adult obesity with an increased long-term risk of mortality and morbidity, independent of adult weight.

Complications of obesity

- **Psychosocial:** Body dissatisfaction, depression, bullying/teasing, school avoidance and low self-esteem.
- **Cardiovascular:** Dyslipidaemia and hypertension, metabolic syndrome.
- **Endocrine:** Glucose intolerance, insulin resistance, type 2 diabetes, accelerated linear growth and bone age, earlier onset of puberty, polycystic ovary syndrome and menstrual abnormalities.
- **Orthopaedic:** Blount's disease and slipped capital femoral epiphysis.
- **Renal:** Obesity-related glomerulopathy.
- **Respiratory:** Obstructive sleep apnoea ± possible links to asthma.
- **Gastrointestinal:** Non-alcoholic fatty liver disease (NAFLD).
- **Dermatological:** Intertrigo, furunculosis and acanthosis nigricans (marker of insulin resistance).
- **Neurological:** Idiopathic intracranial hypertension.

Aetiology

Many factors contribute to the development and maintenance of childhood obesity, although parental obesity appears to be one of the strongest risk factors for persistence of obesity in children. This underpins the need for family-based change if successful weight management is to be achieved in the child.

Obesity occurs because energy intake exceeds energy requirement. Our understanding of factors that influence this energy balance equation is incomplete, but important considerations include:

Paediatric Handbook, 8th edition. By Kate Thomson, Dean Tey and Michael Marks. Published 2009 by Blackwell Publishing, ISBN: 978-1-4051-7400-8.

- **Lifestyle factors** include increased sedentary activities such as watching television and computer gaming, less time partaking in physical activities and increased access to energy-dense foods (such as those containing high levels of sugar and/or fat).
- **Genetic factors** (susceptibility genes) may contribute to the development of obesity, although given that the gene pool changes slowly, lifestyle changes are more likely to be responsible for the recent increases in obesity prevalence. Single-gene disorders (e.g. leptin deficiency) are extremely rare.

Children with exogenous (non-medical) obesity are usually of normal intellect and either of normal or tall stature.

- **Hormonal and metabolic factors:** Endocrine causes are rare and are usually associated with growth failure (see chapter 25, Endocrine conditions page 319).
- **Syndromal causes** are often recognised by the presence of a significant developmental/intellectual disability and less frequently by dysmorphic features. Clues to syndromal or endocrine causes of obesity include
  - Height <50th centile (or less than genetic potential)
  - Dysmorphic features
  - Developmental/intellectual disabilities
  - Hypogonadism.

Assessment
Definition
A simple, clinically useful definition that reflects excess body fat is the body mass index (BMI). However, it does not reflect body composition and thus very well-muscled individuals may have a high BMI. This is usually clinically apparent.

$$\text{BMI (kg/m}^2) = \text{weight (kg)/height}^2 \text{ (m}^2)$$

In children, BMI changes with normal growth; an initial rise in BMI over the first year is followed by a nadir before gradually increasing to normal adult levels (see growth charts, Appendix 1). The initial rise after the nadir is termed the **adiposity rebound** and usually occurs around the age of 6 years. The timing of the adiposity rebound may be important for later risk of obesity.

Plot BMI on a BMI centile chart, now included in standard growth charts:
- **Overweight** is defined as a BMI between 85th and 95th centile for age and sex.
- **Obesity** is defined as a BMI >95th centile for age and sex.

Once obesity is diagnosed, the aim is to identify:
- Contributing factors for that individual
- Any underlying medical causes
- Individuals at high risk of associated disease
- Complications and co-morbidities.

History

A detailed personal, family, developmental and past (including perinatal) history, comple-mented by a thorough dietary history, activity history and a detailed physical examination, is sufficient in most cases.

Clues in a standard history may suggest an underlying cause for the obesity such as poor postnatal feeding and hypotonicity during infancy (Prader–Willi syndrome) and medications (e.g. long-term steroid use).

Explore risk factors suspicious of associated co-morbidities, document family history of obesity, heart disease, diabetes, hypertension, dyslipidaemia and other complications of obesity. Ethnicity is also important as children from certain ethnic backgrounds (e.g. Australian indigenous peoples, Pacific islanders, Asians and Indians) have a higher tendency for weight gain and display greater levels of co-morbidity for a given level of obesity.

An age-appropriate developmental approach is required. Parents can be the exclusive agents of change for preschool children, whereas adolescents should be offered the chance to be seen separately from their parents. It is important to address body image and ensure the young person has realistic, appropriate healthy weight goals.

Examination

- Plot height, weight and BMI on percentile charts.
- Document pubertal and developmental status.
- Assess the body build, posture and distribution of adiposity.
- Measure the waist circumference (at midpoint between lowest ribs and iliac crests – be sure to include any apron of abdominal fat).
- Measure the blood pressure with an appropriate-sized cuff.
- Look for acanthosis nigricans (velvet pigmentation on the neck and/or axilla).
- Look for clues to a syndromal/endocrine cause:
  - Height <50th centile (or less than genetic potential)
  - Dysmorphic features
  - Cushingoid features (including abdominal striae)
  - Developmental/intellectual disability
  - Hypogonadism.

Investigations

- For aetiology.
- For underlying cause, if clinically indicated (see chapter 25, Endocrine conditions).
- For complications:
  - Hyperlipidaemia – full lipid profile
  - Type 2 diabetes – formal oral glucose tolerance testing is preferred although fasting glucose and insulin provide useful information if this cannot be performed.
  - Hepatic steatosis – liver function tests ± liver ultrasound scan.

Screening for complications should be considered in children where obesity is resistant to lifestyle change and where there are risk factors for these conditions. These include a positive family history of type 2 diabetes and particular ethnic groups. Puberty is associated with a significant reduction in insulin sensitivity in normal individuals and investigation for type 2 diabetes is therefore further warranted in these children.

Other investigations, such as sleep studies in those with significant obstructive sleep apnoea, should be performed as clinically indicated.

General approach

The goal is to diminish morbidity and mortality risk, rather than to achieve an ideal body weight. Emphasis should be on improved fitness, health and social functioning rather than an aesthetic ideal. The primary objective is usually to maintain weight over time so that with normal longitudinal growth, the weight falls back into the healthy weight range. The exception to this is children and adolescents with severe obesity where a degree of actual weight loss may be required.

Successful maintenance of a healthy weight is best achieved through long-term family-based interventions that include a component of behavioural change. The aim is a shift in the child's energy balance. Ideally, the following should be provided by a multidisciplinary team.

- Provision of professional input which is:
  - Encouraging, empowering and understanding.
  - Non-judgemental and avoids use of pejorative language: consider not using the word 'obese', but rather 'above the child's healthiest weight'.
- Education of families about:
  - Medical complications of obesity – current and future health risks.
  - The concept of energy balance.
  - Healthy eating and interpreting food labels (see below).
  - Appropriate physical activities (see below).
- When approaching the family:
  - Identify the family's readiness to change – this will guide whether the goal of the consultation is just to raise awareness or actually explore behaviour change.
  - Explore ways to involve all family members and caregivers.
- Aim for permanent lifestyle changes, as opposed to short-term diets or exercise programmes that are aimed at rapid weight loss:
  - Severely energy-restricted diets are contra-indicated in the majority of obese children/adolescents.
  - Self-monitoring of diet and physical activities help maintain these changes.

Specific approaches
Physical activity

Any increase in activity is an improvement!
- Aim for 'lifestyle' exercise: using the stairs, walking to school, walking the dog.
- Involve the whole family (everyone can benefit, regardless of weight status).

- Use after-school time to get outdoors and be active.
- Decrease screen-based activities (TV, computer, electronic games).
- Have bikes, helmets and balls ready to go, right beside the door.

Nutrition

Not forgetting drinks!

- Water is the best drink for kids: cut out cordial, soft drink, fruit juice.
- Better to eat fruit rather than drink fruit juice.
- Low-fat (2% fat) milk (<500 mL/day) is preferred for children >2 years of age.
- Importance of breakfast, regular meals and healthy snacks.
- Basic food label reading and awareness of the 'traps' e.g. 'no fat' might mean large amounts of sugar and therefore the same number of kilojoules.
- Serving sizes – does the 5 year old get served as much as mum or dad? (see chapter 6, Nutrition, p. 91).
- Planning ahead, avoiding regular take-away meals.

Referral to a specialist

This may be indicated when there is:

- Suspicion of a pathological cause.
- Presence of complications.
- Lack of progress in weight maintenance.
- Severe and progressive, or early-onset, obesity.
- Parental or patient request.

Some specific medical therapies are now beginning to be assessed for their use in obese children:

- **Metformin** may be useful in reducing obesity-associated insulin resistance.
- Studies assessing **orlistat** and **sibutramine** in adolescent populations are under way and they may be used more in this population in the future, particularly in those with severe or resistant obesity. They should only be prescribed from specialist centres and must be used in conjunction with an ongoing lifestyle-modification intervention.
- **Gastric banding** is also being trialled in adolescents and this may become a useful tool in the future to aid weight loss in severely obese adolescents or those with major obesity-related co-morbidities.

USEFUL RESOURCES
- *www.iaso.org* – International Association for the Study of Obesity. Useful general information.

CHAPTER 9

Immunisation

Jenny Royle
Jim Buttery

Immunisation is one of the most cost-effective public health measures available. Modern vaccines are safe and effective. They prevent clinical manifestations of disease or substantially reduce severity. In Australia, vaccinations are not compulsory; they are recommended, with incentives including childcare payments and linkage of school entry to reporting of vaccination status. As a disease becomes less common through a successful immunisation programme, the occurrence and perception of side effects assume greater relative importance. Healthcare providers may need to explain the risks of the diseases themselves and inform parents clearly that disease complications far outweigh the potential vaccine side effects. With explanation, the vast majority of parents feel comfortable about immunising their children.

Health professionals have a responsibility to know the immunisation status of patients in their care and to offer due or overdue vaccinations. Use every healthcare visit as an opportunity.

> The Australian Childhood Immunisation Register (ACIR) can be used to check vaccination status for children up to 7 years of age (1800 653 809).

 For each dose of scheduled vaccine administered, notify ACIR and update the parent-held Child Health Record. The Australian Commonwealth Government website (*www.immunise. health.gov.au*) has extensive information including the online ACIR, *The Australian Immunisation Handbook* (9th edition, downloadable), the Australian Immunisation Schedule and parent fact sheets.

Vaccination technique

- It is important to minimise anxiety, distress and pain associated with injected immunisations.
- Use age-appropriate pain-reduction techniques; refer to chapter 4, Pain, p. 61. These might include:
  - Distraction techniques: passive (watching a toy) or active (blowing bubbles).
  - Rewards (stickers or new book).
  - A variety of pharmacological agents have been shown to attenuate immunisation pain (oral sucrose in infants, topical anaesthetic agents, etc.).

Paediatric Handbook, 8th edition. By Kate Thomson, Dean Tey and Michael Marks. Published 2009 by Blackwell Publishing, ISBN: 978-1-4051-7400-8.

- Use a new syringe and needle for each injection.
- Use a 23-gauge needle, 25 mm in length. Smaller gauge needles (25-gauge) may be used for the 2 month injections for premature babies; for subcutaneous injections into the upper arm; or for intradermal (e.g. BCG) vaccinations.
- All intramuscular vaccines should be injected deep into a muscle. Insert needle at an angle of 70–90° into the anterolateral thigh and pointing towards the knee (<12 months of age) or into the deltoid pointing towards the shoulder (≥12 months of age).
- Multiple vaccines: two injectable vaccines can be given into the same limb, separated by >25 mm.
- Ensure safe and efficient vaccination:
  - **Cold chain:** Never use a vaccine if there is any doubt about its safe cold chain storage. Vaccines should be kept in a refrigerator reserved for vaccine/medicine storage at 2–8°C and never frozen.
  - **Prevent immunisation errors:** Always maintain a high standard of systematic checking to reduce the chance of errors.
  - **Post-vaccine observation:** Recipients of any vaccine should remain in the vicinity of medical care for approximately 15 min. Although anaphylaxis is very rare, it can occur with any vaccine. I.m. adrenaline must be available and given urgently in this situation; refer to chapter 1, Medical emergencies, p. 6.

Common misconceptions for missing vaccinations

Children may be under-immunised for their age when health professionals miss opportunities to vaccinate, when parents forget/miss appointments or when parents actively oppose vaccination. Only 1–2% of parents refuse vaccination for their children because they oppose vaccination. Some common misconceptions about vaccination include:

- Natural infection is the best way to achieve immunity.
- Vaccination weakens the immune system.
- 'Homeopathic immunisation' is safer and more effective.

It is essential to address parents' concerns, to emphasise the well-established risks associated with not vaccinating their child and to provide reassurance about vaccine safety. The back cover of *The Australian Immunisation Handbook* has an invaluable table for immunisation providers and parents comparing the effects of vaccines and diseases. This table compares the range and rate of disease effects, and the range and rate of vaccine side effects. This table also appears on the back of the parent-checklist sheet that is given to each family when their child is having a vaccine.

Contraindications to vaccination: true and false

See Tables 9.1 and 9.2.

Table 9.1 False contraindications to vaccination

Usually, children **should** still be vaccinated, even if they:
- Have a cold, or low-grade fever (<38.5°C).
- Have a family history of any reactions following vaccination.
- Have a family history of convulsions.
- Have a history of pertussis-like illness, measles, rubella or mumps infection.
- Are premature (vaccination should not be postponed).
- Have a stable neurological condition such as cerebral palsy or Down syndrome.
- Have been in contact with an infectious disease.
- Have asthma, eczema, or hay fever.
- Are on antibiotics.
- Are on locally acting (inhaled or low-dose topical) steroids.
- Have a pregnant mother.
- Are being breast-fed.
- Have had recent or imminent surgery.
- Are of low weight but otherwise healthy.

(Adapted from *The Australian Immunisation Handbook*, 9th edition).

Table 9.2 Contraindications to vaccination

All vaccines	Acute febrile illness (if fever >38.5°C, postpone vaccination) Previous anaphylaxis contraindicates further dosage of the same vaccine
DTPa	Encephalopathy within 7 days of previous DTP vaccination*
Live vaccines (e.g. MMR, varicella)	Usually contraindicated in immunosuppressed children, e.g. chemotherapy or high-dose corticosteroids (2 mg/kg per day for >1 week). MMR and varicella vaccines should be deferred if <3 months after injection of a blood product (immunogenic response may be diminished) MMR and varicella should be given on the same day or separated by 1 month (this does not apply to any killed vaccines)
Other vaccines	Severe adverse reactions (extremely rare)

* defined as severe acute neurological illness with prolonged seizures and/or unconsciousness and/or focal signs not due to another identified cause.

Table 9.3 Current vaccines, their abbreviations and available forms with trade names

Disease	Vaccine	Available products
Hepatitis B	hepB	Engerix-B, H-B VaxII
Diphtheria, tetanus, pertussis, hepatitis B, *Haemophilus influenzae* type B, polio	DTPa-hepB-Hib-IPV	Infanrix-hexa
Diphtheria, tetanus, pertussis, polio	DTPa-IPV dTpa-IPV	Infanrix-IPV Boostrix-IPV
Diphtheria, tetanus, pertussis	dTpa	Boostrix, Adacel
Diphtheria, tetanus	dT	ADT Vaccine
Haemophilus influenzae type B	Hib (PRP-OMP) Hib (PRP-T)	Pedvax HIB Hiberix
Haemophilus influenzae type B, hepatitis B	Hib (PRP-OMP)-hepB	Comvax
Poliomyelitis	IPV	IPOL
Measles, mumps, rubella	MMR	MMR II, Priorix
Measles, mumps, rubella, varicella	MMR, VZV	ProQuad, Priorix-Tetra
Varicella	VZV	Varilrix, Varivax
Influenza	Influenza vaccine	Vaxigrip, Fluvax, Fluad, Fluarix, Fluvirin, Influvac
Pneumococcal disease	23-valent pneumococcal polysaccharide vaccine (23vPPV) 7-valent pneumococcal conjugate vaccine (7vPCV)	Pneumovax 23 Prevenar
Meningococcal C disease	Meningococcal C conjugate vaccine (MCCV)	Meningitec, Neis-Vac, Menjugate
Meningococcal disease A, C, W, Y	Meningococcal vaccine polysaccharide	Mencevax, Menomune

Table 9.3   *Continued*

Disease	Vaccine	Available products
Human papillomavirus	HPV 4-valent vaccine HPV bivalent vaccine	Gardasil Cervarix
Rotavirus	Rotavirus vaccine	Rotarix, RotaTeq

The Australian standard vaccination schedule 2008

Table 9.3 indicates current vaccines, their abbreviations and available forms with trade names. The NHMRC recommends an antigen-based vaccination schedule. Although vaccine antigens to be given are the same throughout Australia, the schedule differs slightly in different states of Australia as states purchase different combination vaccines. The Australian schedule, at March 2008, is shown in Table 9.4. Schedules applicable to other states are available in *The Australian Immunisation Handbook*, 9th edition.

- Premature infants born <32 weeks and infants born <2000 g require an additional HepB vaccine at 12 months.
- Premature infants born <28 weeks, infants born >28 weeks with chronic long disease and children with specific underlying medical conditions (see Pneumococcal vaccines, p. 116) require a fourth conjugate pneumococcal vaccine at 12 months and 23-valent polysaccharide pneumococcal vaccine at 4 years.
- Varicella vaccine is funded for infants aged 18 months. It can be given at 12 months of age on the same day as MMR vaccine or 4 weeks later.
- Catch-up varicella vaccine is given to students in Year 7 who have not had chickenpox or varicella vaccine.
- Adolescents aged 11–15 years who have not previously had hepatitis B vaccine are given 2 doses 4–6 months apart (using adult formulation).
- Influenza vaccine can be given to any infant ≥6 months. Children in certain risk groups are highly recommended annual influenza vaccine. Children <9 years require two doses in the first year they receive the vaccine. Doses vary according to age: 6 months–3 years = 0.25 mL, ≥3 years = 0.5 mL.
- One brand of oral rotavirus vaccine (RotaTeq) has a third dose given at 6 months.

Catch-up doses

When infants and children have missed scheduled vaccine doses, a 'catch-up' schedule should be recommended. Never miss an opportunity to provide overdue immunisations or at least institute a written catch-up plan. Sometimes the catch-up schedule is relatively simple to devise, e.g. the 2, 4 and 6 month vaccines can be given 1 month apart, hence a late 2 month vaccine given at 3 months can be followed by the routine 4 month vaccines just 1 month later at 4 months. Catch-up schedules for newly arrived immigrants can be complex; see chapter 10, p. 127 and the RCH website. Comprehensive catch-up doses according to the overdue vaccine are clearly covered in *The Australian Immunisation Handbook*, 9th edition.

Table 9.4 Australian Immunisation Schedule (from 1 March 2008)

Birth	hepB				
2 months	DTPa-hepB-IPV-Hib	Rotavirus[a]	7vPneumococcal		
4 months	DTPa-hepB-IPV-Hib	Rotavirus	7vPneumococcal		
6 months	DTPa-hepB-IPV-Hib	Rotavirus (RotaTeq only)	7vPneumococcal		[b]
12 months	Hib			MMR	MenC[c]
18 months				Varicella[d]	
4 years	DTPa-IPV			MMR[e]	
School Year 7	(HepB[f])	HPV[g] 3 doses		(Varicella[h])	
School Year 10	dTpa				

[a] RotaTeq, 2 mL at 2, 4 and 6 months of age. Rotarix, 1 mL at 2 and 4 months only. Minimum interval between doses is 4 weeks. Oral rotavirus vaccine is not recommended beyond the following age limits owing to limited safety data at older ages: RotaTeq 1st dose by 12 weeks of age and 3rd dose by 32 weeks of age, Rotarix 1st dose by 14 weeks of age and 2nd dose by 32 weeks of age.

[b] Influenza vaccine can be given to infants ≥6 months. Children in certain risk groups are highly recommended annual influenza vaccine. Children <9 years require two doses in the first year they receive the vaccine spaced ≥4 weeks apart. Doses vary according to age: 6 months–3 years 0.25 mL, >3 years 0.5 mL.

[c] Meningococcal C conjugate vaccine can be given <1 year but is not funded (2–6 months 3 doses; 6–12 months 2 doses).

[d] Varicella vaccine is funded for infants aged 18 months. It can be given at 12 months of age on the same day as MMR vaccine or 4 weeks later.

[e] MMR vaccine second dose can be given at 18 months.

[f] Catch-up hepatitis B vaccine is given to adolescents aged 11–15 years who have not had hepatitis B vaccine. Two doses 4–6 months apart (using adult formulation).

[g] Catch-up HPV vaccine is funded for girls aged 12–26 years until mid-2009. The funding will then be ongoing for girls in Year 7. Three doses spaced 0, 2 and 6 months.

[h] Catch-up varicella vaccine is given to students in Year 7 who have not had chickenpox or varicella vaccine.

The RCH immunisation service

Healthcare providers often encounter problems as the immunisation schedule changes regularly, catch-up doses can be difficult to work out and families sometimes have complex questions. The RCH Immunisation Service assists doctors, immunisation providers and parents through its telephone service (03 9345 6599) and weekly outpatient clinics for discussion of individual cases. There is a drop-in centre at the hospital to assist in provision of opportunistic immunisations for inpatients and outpatients.

Vaccines in the Australian schedule – further information
DTPa-IPV vaccine
Completing the first three doses on time
There is almost no clinical protection against pertussis following the first DTPa-IPV dose at 2 months. This fully killed combination vaccine is highly effective once the three-dose primary course is completed. If there has been a delay in the first DTPa dose, the second dose can be given 1 month after the first dose.

Targeting adolescents and adults to protect young children: pertussis booster vaccine
Although the pertussis vaccine is highly effective, it does not provide lifelong immunity against disease. Adults can contract pertussis 5–10 years after their most recent pertussis vaccine and spread it to infants, causing serious illness. Target immunisation of adults is important as they have been shown to be the major source of the disease in the community. Booster pertussis vaccine, dTpa (Adacel, Boostrix), is registered in Australia for use in adults and children >8 years old. This vaccine is given to all adolescents as part of the routine immunisation programme. It is highly recommended for healthcare workers working with young infants who are not old enough to have completed their three-dose infant vaccine schedule. The vaccine should be considered for parents, close contacts and childcare workers who are in contact with infants <6 months of age. Further data is needed to determine whether repeat boosters may be required in adults to maintain adequate immunity.

Hepatitis B vaccine
Neonatal and infant schedule
The first dose should be given within 7 days of birth. Infants born to mothers who are positive for hepatitis B surface antigen should receive passive protection with 100 IU hepatitis B immunoglobulin (0.5 mL) preferably within 12 h of birth. Their active hepatitis B vaccination should be commenced at the same time. This is not a live vaccine.

Three further doses of hepatitis B vaccine are required for all infants in the first year.

Preterm infants
Preterm babies do not mount as strong an antibody response to hepatitis B-containing vaccines as term babies. Consequently, as well as being immunised at 0, 2, 4 and 6 months of age, infants born at <32 weeks gestation or <2000 g should have:
- anti-HBs titre measured at 7 months of age and a booster given at 12 months of age if it is <10 mIU/mL, **or**
- a booster given at 12 months of age without measuring the antibody titre.

Adolescent schedule
See Table 9.5.

Pneumococcal vaccines
Background
Streptococcus pneumoniae is an important cause of infections in children, particularly those <2 years of age. Infections include meningitis, septicaemia, pneumonia and otitis media.

Table 9.5 Adolescent immunisation schedule for HepB vaccine

	Children and young adults (<20 yo)	Adolescents (11–15 yo)	Adults (>20 yo)
Vaccine strength	Paediatric	Adult	Adult
2nd dose (months after 1st dose)	1 month	4–6 months	1 month
3rd dose (months after 2nd dose)	2–5 months	No third dose required	2–5 months

Note: A two-dose adolescent schedule is used at 11–15 years. In Victoria, these are given as part of the school-based programme which is expected to continue until the neonatal schedule has vaccinated all children up to 13 years.

A 7-valent killed conjugate pneumococcal vaccine (7vPCV) was licensed for use in Australia in December 2000. This vaccine is almost 100% effective against invasive pneumococcal disease caused by the seven vaccine serotypes (responsible for approximately 60–80% of cases in Australia). The vaccine is also safe and effective over the age of 2 years, though the risk of invasive pneumococcal disease declines in this age group.

Schedule

Conjugate pneumococcal vaccine is given routinely at 2, 4 and 6 months of age. A booster (fourth dose) is not currently considered necessary for all infants in the second year of life and research is currently assessing this in more detail.

Children in certain risk groups are given an additional fourth dose of 7vPCV at 1 year of age. These children have underlying medical conditions predisposing them to invasive pneumococcal disease. A full list of the children who are given additional doses of pneumococcal vaccine is available in *The Australian Immunisation Handbook*, 9th edition. It includes those with: chronic lung disease, trisomy 21, insulin-dependent diabetes, nephrotic syndrome, impaired immunity and premature infants born before 28 weeks gestation. These children are also given a 23-valent polysaccharide pneumococcal vaccine at 4–5 years of age.

Aboriginal and Torres Strait Islander children in Northern Territory and Central Australia are given 7vPCV at 1 year and a booster of the 23-valent-polysaccharide pneumococcal vaccine (23vPPV) between 18 and 24 months. The recommendations for indigenous children living in other areas of Australia vary; refer to *The Australian Immunisation Handbook*, 9th edition, for details.

Meningococcal vaccines
Background

There are at least 13 meningococcal serogroups. Groups B and C are the most common in Australia. A vaccine against serogroup B is not yet available apart from a strain-specific vaccine designed for the local New Zealand strain.

Conjugate C vaccine

There are three brands of protein-conjugated group C meningococcal vaccine in Australia. Each brand is safe and effective at preventing group C meningococcal disease at all ages, including young infants. The killed conjugate vaccine provides long-term immunity. Ongoing research will provide information on whether a booster dose is needed later in life.

Who should be vaccinated?

A single MenC vaccine is given to all 1 year olds. Meningococcal C disease is particularly rare under the age of 1 year. Families can choose to purchase the vaccine for infants from 6 weeks of age. Infant doses at 2 and 4 months or 2, 4 and 6 months still require the booster dose at 1 year of age to provide lasting immunity equivalent to infants vaccinated at 1 year of age.

Catch-up

Catch-up vaccine is available for children born after 1 January 2002. Catch-up vaccine for other ages should be discussed with a doctor. Newly arrived refugees are given catch-up meningococcal C vaccine. See chapter 10 for further details on this group of patients.

Meningococcal polysaccharide vaccine

A short-acting polysaccharide meningococcal vaccine, which is particularly useful for travel, has been available for many years. This offers protection for up to 3–5 years against serogroups A, C, Y and W135. This unconjugated vaccine is ineffective in infants <2 years, except for serogroup A. It is used in patients with poor immunity against polysaccharide antigens (e.g. asplenia) and as a travel vaccine.

MMR vaccine
Two doses

Two doses of live-attenuated MMR vaccine are given to improve seroconversion and long-term protection. Until mid-2008 the two doses were given at 12 months and 4 years. The second dose will soon be changed on the schedule from 4 years to 18 months. When MMR-V (MMR and varicella vaccine) is more readily available it is anticipated this vaccine will be incorporated into the schedule at 1 year and 18 months of age.

Egg allergy

The MMR vaccine is safe for children with egg allergy, even in those with past anaphylaxis, as the vaccine is produced in chicken fibroblast cell cultures, not eggs. There is no evidence to suggest that children with egg allergy have an increased risk of anaphylaxis following MMR vaccine compared to the general community rate of 1/250 000.

Does MMR vaccine cause inflammatory bowel disease or autistic spectrum disorder?

There is no link between MMR vaccination and inflammatory bowel disease or autistic spectrum disorder. Families with further concerns about this topic should discuss them with a specialist.

Co-administration with other vaccines

The MMR vaccine can be given on the same day as the varicella vaccine, at a separate site. If MMR is not given on the same day as the varicella vaccine, they should be spaced at least 4 weeks apart.

Post-exposure prophylaxis

The MMR vaccine can be administered to susceptible contacts >9 months of age within 72 h of exposure to measles as post-exposure prophylaxis, **or** immunoglobulin given within 7 days of contact. Immunoglobulin can also be used for subjects with contraindications to MMR such as immunosuppression.

Previous proven measles, mumps or rubella

Children require protection from all components of MMR. Monovalent measles vaccine is not available in Australia. As vaccination of children who have been previously infected with any of the three components of this vaccine is not dangerous, MMR should be given to all children.

Varicella vaccine
Background

Chickenpox disease used to be considered a childhood rite of passage. A few children die each year in Australia from chickenpox. The most common complication is secondary bacterial infection of varicella skin lesions, but more severe sequelae include pneumonitis and encephalitis.

One or two doses for infants

Varicella vaccine is a live attenuated vaccine, highly effective against severe varicella disease. When a single dose is used the chance of mild breakthrough cases is about 7% in the next 10 years. The USA introduced a two-dose schedule in 2006 to reduce the rate of breakthrough varicella from 7% to 2%. Australia is considering the same.

Who should be given varicella vaccine?

- According to the 2008 schedule a single varicella vaccine at 18 months of age is recommended for all immunocompetent children who do not have a definite history of varicella. Families can purchase this dose earlier (e.g. at 1 year).
- Varicella vaccine should be spaced at least 4 weeks apart from the MMR if it is not given on the same day.
- It is highly recommended for non-immune healthcare workers and family members who are in contact with immunosuppressed subjects.
- Individuals ≥14 years of age without a definite history of chickenpox and those with serologically proven non-immunity are recommended two doses, at least 4 weeks apart.
- Healthcare workers with a negative or uncertain history of varicella should be serotested and vaccinated if negative. Serotesting after vaccination is not necessary.
- Non-immune women immediately postpartum or women planning a pregnancy should be given two doses of varicella vaccine ≥4 weeks apart and should not become pregnant for 1 month after a varicella vaccine dose.

Note: Approximately 40% of adults who do not think they have had chickenpox are found to be immune on serology and do not need vaccination. However, there is no known harm giving the vaccine to immune subjects.

Catch-up doses
Unimmunised children aged 1–13 years without a definite history of chickenpox can be given the vaccine without serological testing. Catch-up varicella vaccine is provided in Victoria as a school-based programme in Year 7.

Varicella vaccine rash
Rash and/or fever can occur in 2–5% of vaccinees during a period of 5 days–3 weeks after the vaccine. This can occur over the injection site or be generalised and the appearance is either maculopapular or vesicular. Although rare, varicella vaccine virus can be spread from vesicular rash lesions. If vaccinees develop a rash they should avoid contact with immuno-compromised persons for the duration of the rash. If a healthcare worker develops a vesicular rash following the vaccine, they should be reassigned to duties that do not require patient contact or placed on sick leave for the duration of the rash (not for 4–6 weeks as the product information states). The duration of the rash is likely to be <1 week. Florid vesicular rash after the vaccine is highly suspicious of wild-type varicella.

Post-exposure prophylaxis
Varicella vaccine is effective in preventing varicella in those already exposed if used within 3–5 days, with earlier administration preferable. It is not 100% effective but, as with pre-exposure vaccination, if breakthrough varicella occurs it is usually milder.

Oral rotavirus vaccine
Background
Rotavirus is the leading cause of severe childhood gastroenteritis in children <5 years. There are at least four main serotypes. Infection with any two of the natural strains provides broad protection to most children. There are two oral live attenuated vaccines licensed: Rotarix (two doses) and RotaTeq (three doses).

At what age should oral rotavirus vaccine be given?
The oral rotavirus vaccine should be given at the same time as the routine 2- and 4-month immunisations. If the three-dose vaccine (RotaTeq) is used, the third dose should be given with the 6-month immunisations. A previous rotavirus vaccine was temporally associated with intussusception, especially in infants who were over 3 months at the time of the first dose. The two new vaccines have demonstrated safety in trials, but can only be recommended for use in children within the specified age ranges that were used in their trials. For RotaTeq, recommended ages are first dose by 12 weeks and third dose by 32 weeks. For Rotarix, first dose is recommended by 14 weeks and second dose by 24 weeks. The vaccine is not licensed or funded for use beyond these age limits and hence infants late for the routine immunisation doses may miss out on a rotavirus vaccine dose. Knowledge of this should encourage parents and immunisation providers to have the 2-, 4- and 6-month immunisations on time. Families of infants >14 weeks requesting a first dose need to understand the current lack of safety data of this vaccine beyond the recommended ages.

Who can't have oral rotavirus vaccine?

There are some groups of infants for whom this live attenuated vaccine is **contraindicated**:
- Infants with significant immunosuppression, e.g.
  - Infants with severe combined immunodeficiency (SCID)
  - Infants on ≥ 2 mg/kg per day of prednisolone.
- Infants who have had surgery following necrotising enterocolitis may also be excluded from receiving oral rotavirus vaccine. Recommendations on these patients will need to be assessed on an individual basis.

The following group of patients **can** have the oral rotavirus vaccine:
- Infants with a minor degree of immunosuppression (e.g. low-dose steroids).
- Premature infants.
- Inpatients.

Human papillomavirus (HPV) vaccine
Background

HPV is responsible for most cervical carcinoma in females, as well as anogenital warts in both sexes. There are multiple strains. The high-risk types 16 and 18 are responsible for approximately 70% of cervical carcinoma. The low-risk types 6 and 11 are responsible for 90% of genital warts. Two killed vaccines are licensed in Australia, derived from inactive virus-like particles. Gardasil contains types 6, 11, 16, and 18, and Cervarix contains types 16 and 18.

Who should be vaccinated?

In Australia HPV vaccine is recommended and funded for all females between the ages of 12 and 26 years. HPV vaccine is registered for boys between the ages of 9 to 15 years but is not yet funded. Results of further research on the use of HPV vaccine in boys should be available soon. The HPV vaccination is most effective when it is given before exposure to HPV. Even if young people have already begun to have sexual contact, the HPV vaccine will provide excellent protection against whichever of the four vaccine types each person has not been infected with. The three doses are usually given within a 6-month period: second dose 1–2 months after the first dose, third dose 4–6 months after the first dose.

Influenza vaccine
Who should have annual influenza vaccine?

It is recommended that children with medical conditions that predispose them to an increased risk of influenza-related complications have annual influenza vaccine. This includes children with chronic illnesses requiring regular medical follow-up, but also specifically those with chronic suppurative lung disease, congenital cardiac disease and those receiving immunosuppressive therapy. Actually, the group of children who could benefit from protection against influenza disease is much broader and these recommendations are discussed in *The Australian Immunisation Handbook*, 9th edition. Healthcare workers and family members of those at increased risk of severe influenza disease are highly recommended to be vaccinated to reduce risk of transmission to at-risk individuals.

Vaccine dose varies according to age

Children >9 years and adults are given a single annual dose. Children <9 years are given 2 doses, ≥1 month apart, in the first year they receive the vaccine. Subsequent single annual doses are then given. The dose depends on age and was altered in 2007:

- 6 months–3 years: 0.25 mL
- >3 years: 0.5 mL.

Other influenza vaccine facts

The current influenza vaccines are grown in the allantoic cavity of embryonated eggs. When influenza vaccine is indicated in a child who has egg allergy, vaccination should only be considered following assessment by a paediatric immunologist.

Influenza vaccine is a killed vaccine and can be administered concurrently with any of the scheduled childhood vaccinations. Influenza vaccination is carried out during a season where it is common to have regular intercurrent illness. Symptoms post vaccine may be due to the killed vaccine dose or may be due to a coincidental intercurrent illness. The current injected influenza vaccines do not contain live virus and cannot cause influenza disease.

Adverse events associated with vaccinations

The vast majority of adverse events experienced after the scheduled vaccinations are minor (e.g. fever, local redness, swelling or tenderness) and do not contra-indicate further doses of the vaccine. Parents who have questions regarding potential adverse events should discuss these with their vaccine provider.

All vaccines are medications and all medications have side effects, just like aspirin and paracetamol. For each individual vaccine there are a known list of fairly common relatively minor symptoms and an important small list of significant major side effects. It is helpful for families to understand the risks and benefits of immunisations to feel comfortable and confident with their decision to vaccinate their young child. A summary of potential vaccine side effects compared with the effects of diseases is tabled on the back cover of *The Australian Immunisation Handbook*, 9th edition. There are parent information sheets at the RCH immunisation website on each scheduled vaccine that clearly discuss vaccine side effects.

SAEFVIC: Surveillance of Adverse Events Following Vaccinations in the Community

When symptoms occur in the hours or days after a vaccination, they may be directly due to the vaccine or totally unrelated and coincidental in nature. Adverse events following immunisations should never be dismissed and often require individual assessment to provide accurate advice for the family about the actual adverse event and about options for further doses of the same vaccine. Maintaining confidence in immunisations following an adverse event is very important. Notifying significant or unexpected adverse events is also very important to assist with safety monitoring of vaccines used in Australia.

SAEFVIC was established in 2007 to assist immunisation providers and families with advice when vaccine adverse events occur. This surveillance service provides telephone advice, out-patient clinic appointments and immunisation under supervision following certain adverse events. The unit records Victorian data on immunisation adverse events and reports to the national Adverse Drug Reactions Advisory Committee (ADRAC). SAEFVIC is located within RCH, The Murdoch Children's Research Institute and is funded by DHS.

SAEFVIC

Notifications of vaccine adverse events can be made to SAEFVIC by phone (1300 882 924), fax (03 9345 4163) or by email (saefvic@mcri.edu.au).

Immunisation guidelines for special groups
Immunosuppressed or immunodeficient children

Live vaccines (e.g. varicella vaccine, MMR, BCG, oral rotavirus vaccine) should not, as a general principle, be given to immunosuppressed individuals. The MMR vaccine can be given to some children with HIV; the safety of this should be assessed in each individual.

Children who have recently received high dose oral steroid therapy (prednisolone 2 mg/kg per day for >1 week, or 1 mg/kg per day for >1 month) should delay live vaccine administration until at least 3 months after therapy has stopped. The use of inhaled steroids is not a contraindication to vaccination with either live or inactivated vaccines.

Children who have recently received immunoglobulin products subsequently have reduced effectiveness of live vaccines. Varicella vaccine should be delayed for 3 months in children who have received zoster immunoglobulin and children who received i.v. immunoglobulin (IVIG) are recommended a 9-month delay in both MMR and varicella vaccines to avoid reduced effectiveness of the vaccine.

Children who have received bone marrow transplants may require booster doses or complete revaccination, depending on their serological and clinical status. Children who receive cancer chemotherapy require booster doses 6 months after completion of therapy.

Inactivated vaccines (such as pertussis), modified toxins (such as diphtheria and tetanus vaccines) and subunit vaccines (such as Hib and hepatitis B vaccines) can be safely given to children receiving immunosuppressive therapy, but may be less effective.

Influenza vaccine is an important safe vaccine for children with immunosuppression, even though it may not work optimally because of the reduced immune function. For further details of immunisation in immunosuppressed children refer to *The Australian Immunisation Handbook*, 9th edition.

Functional or anatomical asplenia

All splenectomised individuals should receive pneumococcal and meningococcal vaccinations in addition to the vaccinations of the standard schedule, as well as annual influenza vaccine. In cases of elective splenectomy, the vaccinations should ideally be given at least 2 weeks before the operation. A detailed immunisation protocol for children with asplenia is available from the RCH immunisation service website.

Household contacts of children with immune deficiency
Siblings and close contacts of immunosuppressed children should be given MMR, varicella and influenza vaccines. Immunisation will ensure that they have less chance of infecting their immunosuppressed siblings.

Premature infants
Preterm babies should be immunised with the recommended schedule according to their actual (not corrected) age, provided they are well and that there are no other contra-indications. Some preterm babies do not respond as well to the pneumococcal and hepatitis B vaccines and may require an extra dose of each at 1 year (see Table 9.6). For details see *The Australian Immunisation Handbook*, 9th edition.

Vaccination of newly arrived immigrants to Australia

See chapter 10, Immigrant child health, and the RCH Immigrant Health Resources (*www. rch.org.au/immigranthealth/resources.cfm?doc_id=10813*).

Table 9.6 Extra vaccines required for premature infants on the Australian schedule

Gestation	At 1 year	At 4 years
<28 weeks	7v conjugate pneumococcal HepB	23v polysaccharide pneumococcal
28–32 weeks	HepB	

USEFUL RESOURCES
- *www.rch.org.au/genmed/clinical.cfm* – RCH immunisation resources.
- *www.ncirs.usyd.edu.au* – National Centre for Immunisation Research and Surveillance of Vaccine Preventable Diseases website includes fact sheets related to specific vaccines, vaccine-preventable diseases and vaccine safety.
- *www.immunise.health.gov.au* – Immunise Australia Program website where *The Australian Immunisation Handbook* (9th edition, 2008) is downloadable. Also contains useful fact sheets and links to State and Territory Health Department websites.

CHAPTER 10

Immigrant child health

Georgia Paxton
Jim Buttery

Australia accepted 14 000 humanitarian entrants in the year 2005–06. Approximately 1/3 of them arrived as refugees under the United Nations High Commission for Refugees (UNHCR) resettlement programme and 2/3 under the Special Humanitarian Programme where they were sponsored by someone (typically a family member) living in Australia. One-third of the humanitarian entrants are aged <15 years. The current intake is predominantly from African countries of origin, notably Sudan. The demographic changes yearly. Families are often large and there may be many children in a family group.

People of a refugee background:
- Are usually resourceful and resilient.
- Will have experienced conflict and transitions with migration and resettlement.
- Will have experienced disruption to schooling, community and routines.
- May have experienced prolonged periods of dislocation with uncertainty about the future.
- May be separated from immediate family members.
- May have witnessed or experienced physical or sexual violence, including torture and severe human rights violations.
- May have been exposed to life-threatening situations or seen family members killed.
- May have spent long periods in refugee camps.
- Usually come from countries where health facilities and programmes are minimal or have been disrupted
- May not have had access to health care overseas
- Are more likely to have been exposed to communicable and vaccine-preventable diseases.
- Are at increased risk for mental health problems.
- Have higher rates of dental disease.
- May be less familiar with preventive health care.
- May be worried about or feel threatened by medical consultations.

Pre-departure screening
Pre-departure screening and treatment is limited for children and early adolescents. It varies with refugee camp, port of departure and services available. It includes:
- Medical assessment and height and weight.
- Rapid diagnostic test (RDT) for malaria (varies with country of origin).

Paediatric Handbook, 8th edition. By Kate Thomson, Dean Tey and Michael Marks. Published 2009 by Blackwell Publishing, ISBN: 978-1-4051-7400-8.

- A full ward test of urine in those aged ≥5 years.
- A chest radiograph (CXR) in those aged ≥11 years, or younger if clinical features suggest tuberculosis (TB) or if there is a history of contact with TB. A diagnosis of active TB delays issue of a visa until reassessment after treatment.
- HIV screening in those aged ≥15 years, younger if there is a history of blood transfusion or other clinical indication.
- A single dose of albendazole (varies with country of origin).
- Unaccompanied refugee minors are also screened for hepatitis B.

In some states of Australia (including Victoria) there are no routine post-arrival health checks. Access to health services is variable. People arriving as refugees have greater settlement support than those arriving under the Special Humanitarian Programme, where the onus is on the sponsor to facilitate access to health care. Healthcare visits need to be handled sensitively, and an interpreter will be needed with a majority of families. It is never appropriate to use a family member as an interpreter. Establishing trust is essential. Recently arrived communities may be small, and even an 'independent' interpreter may be known to the family.

Health issues

Children and adolescents of a refugee background have typical paediatric health problems and also have health issues specific to their background. Common paediatric issues such as iron-deficiency anaemia or constipation may have a more complicated aetiology in refugee children. Assessment of newly arrived children and adolescents focuses on:

- Parental (or self-identified) concerns.
- Excluding acute illness.
- Immunisation status and catch-up.
- TB screening.
- Symptoms of parasite infection and malaria.
- Nutritional status and growth (including iron deficiency, vitamin D and bone health, vitamin A deficiency).
- Dental issues.
- Concerns about development, vision and hearing.
- Mental health issues.
- Previous severe/chronic childhood illness or physical trauma.
- Issues arising from resettlement in Australia.

Children and adolescents need a thorough physical examination. Particular features to note include growth parameters, anaemia, rickets, dental assessment, ENT disease, presence of a BCG scar (proximal forearm, deltoid, other, either side), respiratory examination, lymphadenopathy, hepatosplenomegaly and skin (scars, infections). There may be particular cultural practices such as absent/cut uvula. Some children have scarification and there may be a history of female circumcision (female genital mutilation, FGM).

Suggested initial screening investigations

Screening (e.g. neonatal screening, visual and hearing assessment) may have been limited or non-existent in the country of origin, and prior access to health care, dental care and education varies widely. It is important to explain the concepts of health assessment, screening and disease prevention; families need to understand the implications of health screening and give informed consent. This means explaining all tests, the conditions being tested for, the meaning of a positive test and the next step in management. Individual counselling and an explanation of the bounds of confidentiality will be required in adolescents.

The following list includes suggested first line investigations; additional investigations may be needed depending on the clinical scenario.
- Full blood examination and film.
- Ferritin.
- Vitamin D (calcium, phosphate, ALP, PTH and UEC if clinical rickets).
- Vitamin A.
- Malaria screen (RDT and thick/thin film).
- Hepatitis B screen (surface antigen and surface antibody).
- Schistosoma serology.
- Strongyloides serology.
- Faecal specimen (ideally fixed) for ova, cysts and parasites (OCP).
- Mantoux test.
- Sexually transmitted infection screen (see chapter 15, Adolescent health), depending on age and history. Establishing the need and informed consent demands sensitive, confidential discussions with the young person.

Recently arrived children who are febrile and unwell require further testing for malaria and other investigations. Consult an infectious diseases specialist.

The prevalence of HIV (and hepatitis C) in recently arrived children of a refugee background is currently very low (<1%). There is likely to be limited benefit and considerable extra costs in terms of counselling and stress if this is included in the initial screen. Children will need screening for syphilis or HIV if their parents are known to be positive, and some groups may need additional screening investigations depending on prevalence data from their country of origin.

Immunisation

Vaccine-preventable diseases are endemic and/or epidemic in countries of origin of refugee families. Immunisation records are not a pre-departure requirement and most refugees do not have them. If present, written records are considered reliable evidence of vaccination status. Specific information on catch-up vaccination information is on pp. 45–46 of *The Australian Immunisation Handbook*, 9th edition and a summary can be found in chapter 9, Immunisation.
- People of a refugee background should be vaccinated so they are up to date according to the Australian Immunisation Schedule.
- Catch-up vaccination is required unless written documentation of immunisation is provided. See *www.rch.org.au/immigranthealth/resources.cfm* [Immigrant health clinic guidelines > Immunisation catch-up schedule].

- Check for a BCG scar.
- Vaccination information for children aged ≤7 years should be entered into the Australian Childhood Immunisation Registry (ACIR) and can be cross-checked.
- Provide a written record and a clear plan for ongoing immunisations.
- Translated health information sheets are available at *www.health.vic.gov.au/immunisation/language*.

Nutritional issues

Nutritional issues are common; fussy eating and concerns about weight gain (too little or too much) may be a family priority. These are common paediatric concerns and are not specific to refugee families. Specific issues include vitamin D deficiency, vitamin A deficiency, iron deficiency and anaemia.

Monitor growth parameters and clarify the correct birth date/age first. Linear growth is similar in children aged <5 years worldwide. Growth must be considered in the context of parental height and pubertal status; children may have different growth parameters from their Australian-born peers and still have normal growth.

An early severe/prolonged nutritional insult or chronic disease during infancy will affect long-term growth and may affect final height ('stunting'). This history is usually easily elicited. In children/adolescents with poor growth also consider gastrointestinal and other infections (including TB), vitamin D deficiency, rickets and thyroid dysfunction. Once an initial screen has been completed and treatment initiated as necessary, a period of monitoring growth is often appropriate.

Fussy eating is often due to high caloric intake in the form of drinks/juices at the expense of solids/mealtimes; a good dietary history will elicit this. Consider organic disease early in children of a refugee background, including gastrointestinal infection (*Giardia*, other parasites, *Helicobacter pylori*) and other infections. The principles of healthy eating are universal and should be discussed with families (refer to chapter 6, Nutrition). Breast-feeding should be promoted. Encourage regular meat intake and limit milk intake after 12 months of age (to 600 mL/day) but ensure adequate calcium intake.

Anaemia

Anaemia is usually multifactorial in the paediatric refugee population. Contributors include malaria infection, iron deficiency and parasite infection/infestation. Iron deficiency is usually nutritional but there may be a component of gastrointestinal loss. Other causes of anaemia to consider include haemaglobinopathies (more common in African and Asian populations) and lead toxicity (reported in paediatric refugees). See Anaemia, p. 360 in chapter 29, Haematologic conditions and oncology.

Vitamin D

See also Hypocalcaemia, Endocrine conditions, chapter 25, p. 322.

Vitamin D is essential for normal bone growth and mineralisation, dental health, the immune response and other aspects of health. 'Vitamin D' refers to both D_3 (cholecalciferol, produced in the skin) and D_2 (ergocalciferol, the form in food).

1 mcg of vitamin D = 40 IU.

Most vitamin D is made in the skin from the action of sunlight. In people with dark coloured skin more sunlight is required to make adequate vitamin D. The amount of sunlight required in children is unclear. Vitamin D is not naturally available in any great quantity in diet. Risk factors for low vitamin D include

- Dark skin colour.
- Covering clothing.
- Duration of time since migration.
- Time spent indoors.
- Breast-fed infants of vitamin D-deficient mothers.
  Low vitamin D may cause:
- **Rickets**: Deformity in growing bones due to failure of mineralisation of osteoid (children/adolescents only, with peaks of incidence in infancy and at puberty).
- **Other osseus effects:** Delayed fontanelle closure, bossing, delayed dentition, enamel hypoplasia, myopathy and hypocalcaemia.
- **Non osseous effects:** Developmental delay, hypocalcaemic tetany and seizures.
- **Osteomalacia**: Accumulation of unmineralised osteoid at sites of bone remodelling (both adults and children).

The normal level for vitamin D is 50–160 nmol/L.
- Deficiency = levels < 25 nmol/L.
- Insufficiency = levels 25–50 nmol/L.
- Biochemical rickets is defined as a raised alkaline phosphatase (ALP) ± raised parathyroid hormone (PTH).
- Typically, low vitamin D is associated with high ALP, low Ca, secondary hyperparathyroidism and low phosphate – but this may vary.
- 60–90% of the recently arrived African population living in temperate areas will have low vitamin D. Ask about:
  - Low-grade bony and muscular pain and fatigue with exercise.
  - Dairy intake and symptoms of low calcium (muscle cramps).
- Children aged <6 months with low vitamin D may present with hypocalcaemic seizures or stridor.
- Look for features of rickets (bossing, swelling of wrists and ankles, bony deformity, expansion of ribs at costochondral junction).

Note: Deformity reflects the age/growth of the child when the onset of low vitamin D occurred; it can be in any direction.

Screening

- In children with risk factors: check vitamin D levels, calcium, phosphate and ALP; if the initial vitamin D level is normal, repeat at the end of the first winter in Australia.
- In children with clinical rickets: in addition check PTH and renal function, consider wrist radiograph.
- In children with low dietary calcium intake (even without bony deformity), or if vitamin D level <25 nmol/L: check PTH.

- Repeat levels 3 months after treatment if clinical rickets or levels in the deficient range (<25 nmol/L) initially.
- Levels at the start and end of winter can help guide dose frequency.
- Clinical photography can be useful to monitor bony deformity.
- There is limited value in repeating a wrist radiograph within 12 months.

Management

- Severe symptomatic hypocalcaemia with rickets (including tetany, stridor, seizures) requires hospital admission for vitamin D and i.v. calcium infusion. Do **not** give vitamin D in an outpatient setting to this group.
- RCH uses cholecalciferol (D$_3$) 100 000 IU/mL in olive oil. Treat low vitamin D with 150 000 IU oral (75 000 IU oral in age <12 months) then dosing 3–12 monthly depending on clinical situation.
- Ensure adequate dietary calcium intake continues after vitamin D is given. Calcium supplements may be needed in patients with low dairy intake and should be given in patients with hypocalcaemia.
- There is very limited longitudinal data; treatment is likely to be needed lifelong while in Australia, particularly at lower latitudes. Encourage parents (especially mothers) of vitamin D-deficient children to be tested and treated.

Note: Large doses of vitamin D are not given to pregnant women due to the risk of hypercalcaemia in the developing fetus; these women will be treated with 1000 IU daily instead.

- Although it is worthwhile recommending time outside, this may not ensure adequate levels in temperate climates.
- Although some low-fat milk is fortified with vitamin D (e.g. Physical, 50 IU/250 mL), this is not recommended if <2 years or if there are concerns regarding nutritional status. Normal milk intake should be limited to 500 mL/day in children >12 months.
- Promote breast-feeding and recommend Penta-Vite 0.45 mL containing 400 IU vitamin D/dose oral daily until 12 months of age for all breast-fed infants of mothers at risk of low vitamin D.
- Parents with low vitamin D will also need treatment.

Vitamin A

Vitamin A is required for vision, immune function, growth and maintenance of epithelial cells. Infants accumulate stores in the third trimester of pregnancy and rely on breast milk for supply. Vitamin A is contained in yellow/orange fruits and vegetables as well as butter/eggs/cheese/liver. WHO recommends vitamin A supplementation in infants, children and postpartum women. High-dose vitamin A is not recommended in pregnant women. Vitamin A deficiency is not uncommon in recently arrived children and should be treated.

---

1 unit vitamin A = 0.3 mcg retinal.

Management
- Promote breast-feeding.
- Promote foods containing vitamin A in the diet.
- Screen vitamin A in recently arrived children/adolescents.
  - Levels 0.3–0.7 µmol/L (or low for age):
    - <6 months: 50 000 IU single dose
    - 6–12 months: 100 000 IU single dose
    - >12 months: 200 000 IU single dose
  - Levels <0.35 µmol/L or eye signs:
    - treatment dose for age as above with repeat dose on the next day
    - then repeat at 2–4 weeks and follow-up levels.

Available high-dose formulations of vitamin A are gelatin capsules containing an oil-based solution that is well absorbed following oral administration, typically containing 50 000 IU. The contents can be aspirated using a needle and syringe for administration to younger children.

Risk factors for vitamin A deficiency should resolve with good health care and access to fresh food in Australia.

Tuberculosis

There are differences in the presentation, screening and diagnosis of TB in children and adolescents compared to adults.

Definitions
- **TB infection:** *Mycoplasma tuberculosis* has been transmitted.
- **Latent TB infection (LTBI):** presence of infection without evidence of disease. Diagnosed by excluding active disease.
- **TB disease:** Infection causing pathology. Can be pulmonary, non-pulmonary (e.g. abdominal) or disseminated.
  - Can occur at time of initial infection (primary disease)
  - After a period of latency (reactivation).

Screening and management
Ask about BCG status, past history, contact history (including family history), pre-departure screening, health undertakings (in the family) and symptoms – cough, fevers, night sweats, poor growth, nodal disease and bony pain. Often a contact history will emerge after initial screening results; it is often wise to repeat the entire history.
- The Mantoux test (tuberculin skin test, TST) is the appropriate first line screen.
  - It is not reliable in children aged <6 months.
  - It may be negative in active disease.
  - It is not reliable within 4 weeks after measles infection or MMR vaccination (suppressed response).

- Interpretation of the Mantoux test is complicated and depends on age, BCG status, timing and other risk factors. See the RCH immigrant health guidelines (*www.rch.org. au/immigranthealth*).

Latent TB infection
The lifetime risk of TB disease in children with LTBI is in the order of 5–15%.
- The risk of progression from infection to TB disease is highest in young children, particularly in the first years post migration.
- Adolescents also have a relatively increased lifelong risk of reactivation disease.
- In children/adolescents with LTBI the risk of reactivation can be reduced with 6 months of isoniazid (INH) therapy, which is well tolerated in this age group. There is an increased risk of hepatic dysfunction from INH in adults.
- Malnourished children treated with INH should also receive pyridoxine.

TB disease
- Children with TB disease are rarely infectious because of their pattern of disease (lack of cavitating lesions, low bacterial load) and lack of tussive force.
- Primary disease is the more common form in children; reactivation disease is the more common form in adolescents and adults.
- Children with TB disease are more likely to be asymptomatic.
- Pulmonary disease is the most common form of TB. However, compared to adults, children are more likely to have non-pulmonary TB and disseminated disease.
- Children with suspected TB infection require specialist management.
- Children with TB disease should be tested for HIV after informed consent (2/3 of new TB cases in sub-Saharan Africa are co-infected with HIV).

Hepatitis B
See Infectious diseases, chapter 30, p. 405.

Hepatitis B infection is endemic in Africa and south Asia. Hepatitis B vaccination is part of the routine schedule in Australia and many countries of origin including Sudan and Egypt (but not Kenya or Somalia). Hepatitis B vaccination of non-immune children and adolescents is a priority. Chronic infection results in chronic hepatitis, and cirrhosis occurs in up to 1/3 of affected individuals, who have an increased risk of hepatocellular carcinoma. Chronic infection is most likely to occur after exposure in early life.

Screening
- Screen for HBsAg (infection) and HBsAb (immunity – due either to past infection or immunisation).
- HBsAb >10 IU/L indicates adequate immunity.
- Children who are HBsAg positive need further tests (LFTs, HBcAb, HBeAg, HBeAb) and a screen for hepatitis A and C (immunise against hepatitis A if needed).
- STI screening may be needed depending on age and history.

Further management of children with chronic hepatitis B infection
- All acute cases with clinical illness need immediate discussion with gastroenterology.
- Explanation/education/counselling:
  - Advice about blood spills and infection risk – suggest gloves to clean blood spills and disinfection with diluted (1:10) household bleach.
  - Advice to notify their treating doctors when starting medications.
  - Advice about avoiding excess alcohol consumption.
- Screen and vaccinate household against hepatitis B.
- Commence hepatotoxic drugs cautiously – particularly anti-TB therapy.
- Hepatitis B is a notifiable disease.
- Other management depends on serology, LFTs and clinical status. The primary goal of therapeutic management in the individual is to eliminate or suppress hepatitis B.

Intestinal parasites
- Children are at increased risk for faecal/oral and horizontal transmission.
- Symptoms may be non-specific:
  - Ask about abdominal pain (which may be anywhere), constipation, diarrhoea, bloody diarrhoea and growth.
  - Ask about bladder symptoms and haematuria (seen in *Schistosoma haematobium* infection).
  - Macroscopically visible worms are likely to be tapeworms or ascarids.
- Parasite infections may last for years and have sequelae for nutrition, growth and function.
- *Strongyloides* infection should be regarded as persisting lifelong if not treated. Patients with untreated *Strongyloides* infections can develop hyperinfection syndrome if given immunosuppressant therapy, including short-course steroids. Hyperinfection syndrome has a high mortality, even with treatment.

Management
- Screening should be part of the initial assessment.
- In general treatment is usually short course (often single dose) and well tolerated.
- The following require treatment, and specialist advice may be helpful:
  - *Ascaris lumbricoides.*
  - *Giardia intestinalis (lamblia).*
  - *Ancylostoma duodenale* or *Necator americanus* (hookworms).
  - *Strongyloides stercoralis.*
  - *Schistosoma* spp.
  - *Taenia solium* or *T. saginata* (tapeworms).
  - *Trichuris trichuria* (whipworm).
  - *Rodentolepis nana* (dwarf tapeworm).

Human immunodeficiency virus (HIV)

See Infectious diseases, chapter 30, p. 417.

- Many children come from regions with high prevalence of HIV infection (e.g. sub-Saharan Africa, south-east Asia).
- Consider testing:
  - Children with symptoms of possible HIV infection (e.g. failure to thrive, chronic respiratory infections, persistent thrush, generalised lymphadenopathy).
  - Where parents are known or suspected to be HIV positive, regardless of pre-departure screening results.
  - Children with TB disease.
- Pre-test counselling for HIV is legally compulsory.

Dental disease

Assessment of dental health is particularly important in refugee patients, as the patient may have had limited access to dental care services and/or poor diet, or may have sustained injuries. A dental review should be recommended for all recent immigrants.

Development and mental health considerations

Development may be affected by any combination of biological, environmental, social and emotional factors. Considerations in children and adolescents of a refugee background include.

- **Biological:** Malnutrition, chronic disease, hearing impairment, visual impairment, family history, prematurity.
- **Environmental:** Living conditions, access to schooling, access to food, exposure to communicable diseases, language transitions.
- **Social:** Parenting roles, family disruption, changing roles and responsibilities.
- **Emotional:** Stress, trauma experiences, displacement, uncertainty around future, mental health issues.

Responses to trauma include depression, anxiety, post-traumatic stress, low self-esteem and guilt. These may manifest in a variety of ways including behavioural problems, problems with sleeping and eating, poor school performance, difficulty making friends and psychosomatic symptoms. Consider mental health in the broad family context, parents with mental health issues themselves will have reduced coping and parenting skills.

A thorough history and examination will establish risk factors and contributors. In reality, developmental and mental health surveillance will usually occur after the initial assessment. If developmental or learning concerns are elicited, organise vision and hearing assessment, screen for thyroid dysfunction and treat iron deficiency early. Consider mental health issues as a contributing factor or co morbidity.

Health screening is only one part of promoting health and well-being in new immigrants to Australia. Facilitating resettlement in terms of learning English, educational placement and gaining employment are also priorities and will promote physical and psychological health in families. Parents are likely to have their own health needs and will also warrant appropriate health assessment.

USEFUL RESOURCES
- *www.foundationhouse.org.au* – Victorian foundation for survivors of torture.
- *www.health.vic.gov.au/immunisation/language* – Translated health information sheets.
- *www.rch.org.au/immigranthealth* – RCH immigrant health clinic website.
- *www.refugeehealth.org.au* – NSW refugee health service.
- *www.mhcs.health nsw.gov.au* – NSW Multicultural Health Communication Service. Contains an excellent resources section with multilingual support.

CHAPTER 11

Common behavioural and developmental problems

Daryl Efron
Sheena Reilly

Concerns regarding children's behaviour are common and need to be assessed within a developmental framework. Many presentations are in fact normal behaviour (e.g. toddler tantrums), but parents need empathic support and practical management advice.

Child behaviour is the result of interaction between innate biological or temperamental characteristics and environmental influences including parenting style, socioeconomic status and available resources, nutrition, ethnic and cultural factors, and educational setting.

Developmental status must always be evaluated in a child who presents with behaviour disturbance. Developmental delays or disabilities may present in this way. Physical causes for behaviour disturbance must be excluded (e.g. iron deficiency causing irritability, nocturnal seizures causing sleep disturbance). Behaviour modification strategies must be pitched at a developmentally appropriate level.

Infant distress ('colic')

A common research definition of colic is crying for >3 h per day, for ≥3 days per week for >3 weeks. However, parental tolerance of infant crying varies and it is more useful clinically to define the problem in terms of the parents' concerns.

The typical clinical scenario is an extended period of distressed behaviour. The infant cries vigorously and the parents may interpret this as pain. There are usually repeated bouts with sudden onset. The legs are often drawn up and the face red. The worst period is typically in the late afternoon and early evening, but some infants seem to be irritable at any time of day.

It occurs equally in both sexes and in both breast-fed and formula-fed infants. It begins in the early weeks of life and abates by 3 months of age in 60% and by 4 months in >90% of infants.

The parents of infants who cry excessively are often exhausted and worried. Depression is common in mothers of irritable infants.

Paediatric Handbook, 8th edition. By Kate Thomson, Dean Tey and Michael Marks. Published 2009 by Blackwell Publishing, ISBN: 978-1-4051-7400-8.

Assessment

A detailed history should be taken, noting:

- Temporal associations with feeds.
- Variation with contextual or environmental factors.
- Parental response (both affective and practical).
- Supports for the parents.

A detailed physical examination is important; particularly to reassure the parents that identifiable organic causes have been excluded. Physical causes are rare if the infant is thriving and developing normally.

History and examination should rule out conditions such as otitis media, reflux oesophagitis (rare in the absence of vomiting) and raised intracranial pressure. Allergy to cow's milk protein usually has associated features including vomiting, diarrhoea (sometimes with blood and/or mucus), failure to thrive or eczema. However, it can occasionally present with distressed behaviour alone. Lactose intolerance causes frothy stools with perianal excoriation and abdominal distension. Stool analysis is confirmatory with a low pH and presence of reducing substances.

 Inquire about the mother's supports, and evaluate for depressive symptoms. The 10-item Edinburgh Postnatal Depression Scale (*www.dbpeds.org/handouts)* is a simple and well-validated screening instrument.

Management

- Reassurance that the infant is healthy is important and often extremely helpful.
- Explain that some infants appear excessively sensitive to both internal (e.g. overtiredness, hunger) and environmental stimuli in the early months of life, but that it will settle with maturation.
- Minimise environmental stimulation – low-level background noise, soft lighting and comfortable ambient temperature.
- Maintain predictable routines.
- Carrying the infant in a sling (snugly) is often helpful and allows the parents to free their hands. Patting, rocking, movement (e.g. swing, walking in pram), massage, warm baths, and a dummy may also be helpful.
- In persistent or severe cases a trial of cow's milk protein elimination may be indicated. Mothers of breast-fed infants must carefully exclude all cow's milk products from their diets and take calcium supplements. Formula fed infants can be given a 2–4 week trial of an extensively hydrolysed formula. Symptoms persist in a minority of highly allergic infants, in which case an elemental (amino acid based) formula can be tried. Refer also to chapter 19, Allergy and immunology, p. 231.
- A lactose-free formula can be tried in those infants with symptoms suggestive of lactose intolerance. Lactase tablets can be used for breast-fed infants, or expressed breast milk can be pre-treated with lactase drops.
- Medications such as antispasmodics and sedatives should not be used, and over-the-counter anti-colic preparations are rarely helpful. Antacids or ranitidine may be tried if the history suggests gastro-oesophageal reflux (see chapter 27, Gastrointestinal conditions, p. 345).

- Encourage contact and support from extended family, friends, maternal and child health nurse, etc.

Breath-holding spells

These are extremely frightening for parents, particularly initially. The peak incidence is at 1–3 years of age, although they generally begin in infancy and sometimes in the newborn period.

The most common type of breath-holding spell is a cyanotic spell. In response to relatively minor frustration or a painful stimulus (e.g. a knock to the head), the child cries briefly before involuntarily holding the breath in expiration and becoming rapidly cyanosed. In some cases, loss of consciousness or even a brief hypoxic seizure results.

Pallid breath-holding spells are less common. The precipitating event is similarly minor and the child holds the breath and becomes markedly pale and limp. This is due to an excessive vagal response resulting in bradycardia or transient asystole.

Management

- Breath-holding spells need to be distinguished from seizures and this is usually possible on history. In breath-holding spells, cyanosis occurs **before** loss of consciousness whereas in seizures cyanosis occurs **after** loss of consciousness and onset of seizure activity.
- Place the child on its side until spontaneous recovery, which is usually rapid.
- Do not provide the child with excessive attention, which may promote secondary gain.
- Minimise unnecessary struggles with firm consistent behaviour management.
- Ensure the child is not iron deficient (dietary history ± laboratory testing) as this is associated with breath-holding spells.

Temper tantrums

It is developmentally normal for toddlers to express frustration as they strive for autonomy and some control over their world. From the second year of life most children will have temper tantrums, often persisting through to the preschool years. These tend to be more prominent in children with delayed speech development and associated frustration.

Management

- Assess contextual factors, e.g. avoid overstimulation or excessive fatigue.
- Assess the parents' response.
- Behaviour modification techniques are most likely to be successful if applied consistently. This involves the same consequence being applied each time a particular behaviour occurs, across different environmental settings and caregivers.
- Consequences should be determined (with agreement of all caregivers) and explained to the child in advance. They should be applied immediately when the behaviour occurs, instituted as calmly as possible without discussion, negotiation or bargaining.
- Toddlers and preschool aged children generally respond to Pavlovian-style conditioning, i.e. positive reinforcement of socially acceptable behaviour and negative reinforcement of undesirable or unacceptable behaviour.
- Ignoring is effective for tantrums and other behaviours that don't harm others. It involves the parents withdrawing any feedback that may be a positive reinforcer of the tantrum

behaviour. The parent needs to stand some distance from the child, withdraw eye contact and not speak to the child at all. The parent should continue with what they were doing, or may need to walk away. Following the tantrum, acceptable behaviour should be praised. Some children may need reassurance after a period of prolonged or severe loss of control.When an ignoring programme is started the behaviour may escalate initially. However, if the parents can persist through this period, the frequency of tantrums will decrease.

Aggression/oppositional-defiant behaviour

Most children will exhibit some defiant and non-compliant behaviours as they negotiate progressive developmental stages. Parents may seek help when relationships within the family are strained or the child's behaviour is extreme, antisocial, or impairs learning and social development.

Symptoms vary with age and sex. Young children particularly display verbal and physical aggression when unhappy or frustrated. Underlying contributing factors such as developmental and learning disabilities, family and parenting problems and the influence of violent electronic media need to be considered in a biopsychosocial model.

Management
Positively reinforce acceptable behaviour

Parents should be encouraged to 'catch the child being good', noticing and rewarding acceptable behaviour. Encourage abundant use of praise.

Structured reward systems are often extremely helpful for children from about 2.5 to 5 years of age. An example of this is for the child to make a colourful 'Big Boy' or 'Good Boy' chart. The child is rewarded with stickers (0–2/day) and once they accumulate five stickers they earn a special surprise in the form of a lucky dip selected from a box. Do not use food or sweets as rewards. Healthy competition can be set up with the model sibling, to increase motivation. Stickers should not be removed from the chart as punishment (rewards and punishments should be separate).

Ignore minor irritating behaviours

In many families a great deal of energy is spent arguing about relatively inconsequential behaviours such as whingeing, nagging or not tidying up. This is not sustainable, as the parents usually become exhausted. It is preferable to save energy for serious indiscretions.

Serious oppositional behaviours

Serious behaviours, including hitting or kicking somebody or damaging property, must be managed with consistent consequences.

Toddlers and preschool age children generally respond very well to time out when used consistently. This involves calmly and immediately placing the child in a chair or in their room for a timed period of 1 min per year of age, for certain predetermined, defined behaviours. If they are calm at the end of the time they can come out, otherwise the clock starts again.

Most children learn to abide by time-out rules if used consistently, as they recognise they need containment.

For school-age children withdrawal of privileges (e.g. TV, video games) is generally the best strategy. Again this should be introduced immediately after the behaviour occurs and applied for a brief period only (e.g. 1–2 days).

Smacking should be discouraged as it models violence and is usually not effective. Serious antisocial or delinquent behaviours such as frequent high-level violence, cruelty to animals, arson or repeated stealing are indicators of a significant conduct disorder and warrant referral to a child and adolescent mental health service. It is important, however, to recognise that isolated incidents are common and not necessarily indicative of severe psychopathology.

Attention deficit hyperactivity disorder

Attention deficit hyperactivity disorder (ADHD) is the term currently applied to a range of childhood behaviours sharing the core features of poor impulse control and limited sustained attention to tasks, often with motor hyperactivity. Common associated features include oppositional defiant behaviour, anxiety, learning difficulties and tics.

The DSM-IV diagnostic criteria for ADHD are provided in Table 11.1. Most children with ADHD have the combined type. The predominantly inattentive subgroup often present later with academic difficulties, as they do not generally display disruptive behaviour.

Assessment

- **History:** A detailed history is critical, focusing on attachment, early development, social skills and academic progress. The timing and nature of initial concerns along with secondary effects such as depression, low self-esteem and social ostracism should be noted. It is important to identify the child's strengths as well as their weaknesses. Standardised behaviour rating scales, completed by parents and teachers (e.g. Connors, Achenbach), are helpful.
- **Physical examination:** Should focus on neurodevelopment assessment including fine and gross motor coordination, visual-motor integration, auditory and visual sequencing, etc.
- **School reports.**
- **Psychoeducational assessment:** Children with significant learning difficulties should be referred to an educational psychologist for a formal assessment to identify their learning strengths and weaknesses. This can be arranged through the education department (via the school) or privately.
- **Audiology** including auditory processing assessment is often helpful. Other investigations are not usually required.

Management

Children with ADHD have multiple special needs and difficulties and the priorities often change over time. The child, family and school need sustained and skilled support over many years. This requires the doctor to work in collaboration with other health, educational and community professionals. A multimodal strategy is required.

Table 11.1 DSM-IV diagnostic criteria for ADHD

A *Either 1 or 2*

   1. Inattention At least six of the following nine symptoms have persisted for at least 6 months to a degree that is maladaptive and inconsistent with developmental level:

- Often fails to give close attention to details or makes careless mistakes in school work, work or other activities
- Often has difficulty sustaining attention in tasks or play activities
- Often does not seem to listen when spoken to directly
- Often does not follow through on instructions and fails to finish schoolwork chores or duties in the workplace (not due to oppositional behaviour or failure to understand instructions)
- Often avoids or dislikes tasks (such as schoolwork or homework) that require sustained mental effort
- Often has difficulty organising tasks or activities
- Often loses things necessary for tasks or activities (e.g. school assignments, pencils, books, tools or toys)
- Often easily distracted by extraneous stimuli
- Often forgetful in daily activities

   2. Hyperactivity/Impulsivity At least six of the following nine symptoms of hyperactivity/impulsivity have persisted for at least 6 months to a degree that is maladaptive and inconsistent with developmental level:

Hyperactivity

- Often fidgets with hands or feet and squirms in seat
- Often leaves seat in classroom or in other situations in which remaining seated is expected
- Often runs about or climbs excessively in situations where it is inappropriate (in adolescents or adults may be limited to feelings of restlessness)
- Often has difficulty playing or engaging in leisure activities quietly
- Is often on the go and acts as if driven by a motor
- Often talks excessively

Impulsivity

- Often blurts out answers to questions before the questions have been completed
- Often has difficulty awaiting turn
- Often interrupts or intrudes on others (e.g. butts into conversation or games)

B Onset no later than 7 years of age

C Symptoms must be present in two or more situations (e.g. at school, at home and/or at work)

D The disturbance causes clinically significant distress or impairment in social, academic, or occupational functioning

E Does not occur exclusively during the course of a pervasive developmental disorder, schizophrenia, or other psychotic disorder, and is not better accounted for by a mood disorder, anxiety disorder, or dissociative disorder, or a personality disorder

Behaviour modification
- The methods described previously under aggression/oppositional-defiant behaviour (p. 139) are generally helpful.
- Parents and teachers need to apply structured behavioural modification strategies as consistently as possible. Predictable routines are required both at home and at school.

Educational strategies
- An individualised plan should be developed to optimise learning and promote appropriate behaviour.
- Classroom adaptations include seating the child at the front of the classroom near a good role model and using written lists and other visual prompts. Some children need individualised instructions and encouragement to complete tasks, with increased adult one-to-one supervision such as a teacher's aide. Frequent breaks with the opportunity to move around the classroom help the child remain on task. Tasks such as collecting lunch orders similarly break up the work and are also good for self-esteem.
- Clear rules and predictable routines are important. Positive reinforcement should be provided for acceptable behaviour.

Medication
Stimulants
Psychostimulant medication is the single most effective intervention for children with ADHD (see Table 11.2). It is effective in about 75% of cases, helping children to control antisocial verbal and physical impulses and sustain attention to tasks to enable work completion and academic success nearer their potential. Secondary benefits, including improved peer status, family functioning and self-esteem, accrue over time. Extended release stimulant preparations are now available, avoiding the need for a dosing at school (Table 11.2).

The main side effect of stimulants is appetite suppression. Weight, height and blood pressure need to be monitored regularly.

In most states of Australia the prescribing of stimulants is restricted to paediatricians, neurologists and child psychiatrists.

Other medications
A number of other medications are useful in some children with ADHD. These include:
- *Atomoxetine*, a selective noradrenaline reuptake inhibitor, which is given once daily.
- *Clonidine*, which can help smooth out explosive behaviour and assist with sleep onset. If clonidine is used in combination with a stimulant, twice-daily dosing is preferable and the total daily dose should not exceed 200 mcg.
- *Antidepressants (tricyclics, SSRI, SNRI)* are particularly beneficial if there is associated anxiety.

Other strategies
The parents of children with ADHD commonly try a range of unproven complementary therapies, including behavioural optometry, cerebellar training exercises, chiropractic, etc. There is

Table 11.2 Medications for ADHD

Trade name	Generic name	Formulation	Duration of action	Usual dosing times
Dexamphetamine	Dexamphetamine	5 mg tab	4–5 h	Morning and lunchtime
Ritalin 10	Methylphenidate	10 mg tab	2.5–4 h	Morning, lunchtime ± after school
Ritalin LA	Methylphenidate biphasic release	20, 30, 40 mg caps	6–8 h	Morning
Concerta	Methylphenidate extended release	18, 27, 36, 54 mg tabs	10–12 h	Morning
Strattera	Atomoxetine	10, 18, 25, 40, 60 mg caps	Steady state	Morning (occasionally given in evening)

Note: All items are available on the PBS via an authority prescription. If the main impairing symptom is inattention then medication may be needed only for school +/– activities outside of school with high concentration demands. Drug holidays (planned treatment interruption over school holidays) are not necessary for most children; consider if suboptimal linear growth.

no evidence that these interventions are helpful and some are expensive and/or potentially harmful. Anecdotally, elimination of synthetic food colourings and preservatives is beneficial in a small number of children.

Prognosis
Most children with ADHD will continue to have some difficulties through adolescence and into adulthood, although many develop good compensating strategies and function very well. A significant minority suffer long-term complications including academic underachievement, school drop-out, delinquency, vocational disadvantage and relationship difficulties. Children with ADHD treated with stimulant medication appear to be less likely to develop substance abuse in adolescence and adult life than those left untreated.

Learning difficulties
There are many reasons why a child may experience learning difficulties, and often multiple factors are involved. These include specific learning disabilities (commonly language–literacy based), intellectual disabilities, attentional deficits, sensory impairments (hearing, auditory processing, vision), emotional disturbance, chronic illness, family and social difficulties, and suboptimal teaching or educational environments. A specific learning disability is defined as a discrepancy between a child's intellectual ability and their academic achievement. See also chapter 14, Developmental delay and disability.

Assessment

- Obtain information from both parents and teachers.
- Obtain previous school reports.
- Formal educational psychology assessment.
- Neurodevelopmental assessment undertaken by a developmental paediatrician is important in identifying areas of difficulty such as visuomotor integration, short-term auditory memory, motor planning and coordination, and fine motor skills.

Management

- The doctor has an important role in excluding treatable contributing medical factors (e.g. sleep deprivation, iron deficiency, ADHD, depression, epilepsy), as well as advocating for the child.
- Liaise closely with the school to ensure appropriate assessments are undertaken and that an individualised educational plan is devised and reviewed periodically, taking into account the child's special needs.
- In severe cases an application for disability programme funded assistance should be made via the school to the education department.
- Some children benefit from remedial tuition either within or outside school hours. It is important for parents not to overburden children, who also need normal recreational time.
- Parents need support in understanding their child's potential and ways in which they can help optimise their child's learning. Identifying and enhancing the child's strengths is important in maintaining self-esteem.

Speech and language delay

Language delay/impairment can involve receptive skills (ability to understand spoken language), expressive skills (language production) or both (Table 11.3). Articulation/phonological problems may also occur, resulting in reduced speech intelligibility.

Background

- Approximately 20% of 2 year olds are considered late talkers, i.e. children with smaller than expected expressive vocabularies (<50 words and few or no word combinations).
- Children with language delay at 1 and 2 years are at risk of later language impairment, but only 5–8% of 4–5 year olds have language impairment.
- Although some children spontaneously recover or 'grow out' of their early delay, it is not possible to predict with any certainty which children will have persistent speech and language problems.
- Delay in speech development may be specific, or may coexist with more general language problems. Speech and language delays may also be isolated, or may reflect a delay in the child's cognitive development.
- Children with autism may present with concerns regarding speech and language development. These children have distinct early communicative, social and behavioural difficulties that differ from children with primary language impairment (see chapter 14, Developmental delay and disability, p. 172).

Prognosis

Preschool children with persistent speech and language impairment tend to have:

- Learning and social difficulties when starting formal schooling.
- Increased risk for later literacy problems.
- Increased rate of emotional and behavioural disorders.

These problems may persist into adolescence and adulthood and affect employment opportunities.

Factors raising concern about speech and language

- Parental report of concern regarding speech and language development.
- History of hearing loss.
- Family history of speech and language difficulties.
- Receptive and expressive language skills both delayed.
- Concern about other aspects of development and lack of developmental progress (Table 11.3).
- Autistic features, for example, poor social interactions, limited use of gesture/facial expressions, stereotypic and repetitive behaviours, 'in their own world'.

Table 11.3 Speech and language milestones: indicators of concern

Age (years)	Reason for concern
6 months	No response to sound, not cooing, laughing or vocalising
12 months	Not localising to sound or vocalising. No babbling or babbling contains a low proportion of consonant vowel babble (e.g. baba). Doesn't understand simple words (e.g. 'no' and 'bye'), recognise names of common objects or responds to simple requests (e.g. 'clap hands') with an action
18 months	No meaningful words except 'mum/dad'. Doesn't understand and hand over objects on request
2 years	Expressive vocabulary <50 words and no word combinations. Cannot find 2–3 objects on request
3 years	Speech is not understood within the family. Not using simple grammatical structures (e.g. tense markers). Doesn't understand concepts such as colour and size
4 years	Speech is not understood outside the family. Not using complex sentences (4–6 words). Not able to construct simple stories
5 years	Speech is not completely intelligible. Does not understand abstract words and ideas. Cannot reconstruct a story from a book

- Concern regarding general stimulation received.
- Parental report of regression in babbling or language.

Management

- Assess other areas of the child's development, if uncertain or concerned refer to a specialist. Formal cognitive assessment may be needed.
- Exclude hearing loss as a contributing factor by referral to an audiologist.
- Referral to a speech pathologist is recommended as early as possible. Don't delay! Speech pathologists may decide to 'watch and wait' but only after they have considered factors such as the child's speech and language profile, environmental factors, family history, developmental history and progress to date.
- In cases where regression in language is suspected, refer promptly to a paediatrician. In a child <2 years, a sign of regression may be losing a number of words that had been previously well-established, used spontaneously and frequently for at least 4 weeks.

Stuttering

Stuttering is a disorder that affects the fluency of speech production. It has a strong genetic link, with 50–75% of people who stutter having at least one relative who also stutters. Stuttering is now considered to be a developmental anomaly rather than a psychological disorder.

About 5% of children start to stutter, usually during the third and fourth year. Stuttering may occasionally appear for the first time in school aged children and even more rarely in adulthood. Stuttering in children is more amenable to treatment than stuttering in adults. The period of time that has lapsed since the onset of stuttering is a strong predictor, with little chance of natural recovery in children >9 years old. More girls recover naturally than boys. Family history of recovery may increase the child's chance of recovering naturally.

Speech is disrupted by abnormal repeated movements of the speech mechanism, such as '*I w-w-w-w-w-was saying . . .*', and fixed postures of the speech mechanism during which speech stops.

Many features of stuttering are superfluous behaviours, such as body tics and abnormal patterns of speech respiration.

Management

- Do not ignore the stutter.
- If stuttering persists for ≥6 months, refer to a speech pathologist. Treatment of preschool stuttering should be undertaken by speech pathologists trained in the Lidcombe programme, which has been shown to be efficacious in this age group.

USEFUL RESOURCES
- *www.dbpeds.org* – Developmental and Behavioral Paediatrics Online. Fantastic website linked with the American Academy of Paediatrics, with abundant helpful, practical information for doctors and families.

CHAPTER 12

Sleep problems

Margot Davey

Sleep physiology

Sleep is a major challenge to the respiratory system, because it causes changes in respiratory mechanics and control of breathing leading to:

- Decreased ventilation.
- Decreased functional respiratory capacity (loss of intercostal muscle tone).
- Increased upper airways resistance (hypotonia of dilating muscles of upper airway).
- Depression of respiratory drive (REM > NREM > awake).
- Decreased response to hypoxia and hypercarbia.

Sleep stages and architecture

- Rapid eye movements (REM) and non rapid eye movement (NREM) sleep. NREM sleep is further divided into four stages – NREM1 (light sleep) through to NREM4 (deep sleep).
- REM/NREM cycles occur at intervals of 60 min in the infant and lengthen to 90 min in the preschooler.
- Newborn infants sleep around 16 h/day, reducing to 14.5 h by 6 months and to 13.5 h by 12 months.
- Around 3 months of age the infant's circadian rhythm is emerging, with sleeping patterns becoming more predictable and most sleep occurring at night.
- By 6 months of age most full-term healthy infants have the capacity to go through the night without a feed.
- Towards the end of the first year of life, the child's sleep architecture becomes similar to that of an adult, with most of the deep sleep (NREM3/4) occurring in the first third of the night and REM sleep concentrated in the second half of the night.
- Infants who develop the ability to transition from sleep cycle to sleep cycle without parental assistance appear to sleep through the night.

Assessment

One-third of families will complain of difficulties with their child's sleeping patterns. Assessment should include:

- Detailed sleep history over 24 h, looking at how and where the child goes to sleep, frequency and character of wakings, snoring and daytime functioning.
- Sleep patterns during weekends/holidays and with different caregivers.
- A sleep diary may help clarify the situation (see Fig. 12.1).

Paediatric Handbook, 8th edition. By Kate Thomson, Dean Tey and Michael Marks. Published 2009 by Blackwell Publishing, ISBN: 978-1-4051-7400-8.

SLEEP DIARY

Name:______________________

Draw ↓ when your child is placed in the bed or cot
Draw ↑ when your child gets out of the bed or cot

Shade ■ when your child is asleep

Shade □ when your child is awake

Day	Date	Events Medications	MN	1 am	2 am	3 am	4 am	5 am	6 am	7 am	8 am	9 am	10 am	11 am	MD	1 pm	2 pm	3 pm	4 pm	5 pm	6 pm	7 pm	8 pm	9 pm	10 pm	11 pm	MN
Mon	19/5										↑					↓		↑						↓			
Tues	20/5											↑											↓				

Fig. 12.1 Sleep diary

- Family and social history to examine the presence of contributing problems, such as maternal depression, marital problems and drug or alcohol abuse.
- Exclude medical conditions contributing to disrupted sleep patterns such as obstructive sleep apnoea, asthma, eczema, nocturnal seizures, gastro-oesophageal reflux, otitis media with effusion, and nasal obstruction.

Bedtime struggles and night-time waking

For infants <6 months of age no interventions other than schedule manipulation (making sure the infant is not overtired and that adequate spacing between sleep times is provided) and anticipatory guidance are used. If parents want their infant to learn to settle by itself then they can try to leave the infant settled in its cot but leave before it is asleep. In the first 3 months of life some infants sleep better swaddled.

For older children, treatment plans must be individualised and adapted for each family.

Aetiology

- Sleep associations occur when a child learns to fall asleep in a particular way, so that every time the child has a normal arousal they wake up fully and are unable to put themselves back to sleep unless those particular conditions are set up again. Examples include rocking, feeding or falling asleep in the pram or car.
- Frequent feeding can cause wakings both by sleep associations and by the child developing a 'learned hunger' response. Some children can develop patterns that lead to consumption of large quantities of milk which affects not only their sleep patterns but eating during the day. Most healthy full-term babies can go without a night-time feed by 6 months.
- Erratic routine can contribute by inappropriate timing of naps and lack of a regular bedtime routine.
- Inconsistent limit setting in toddlers and preschoolers can exacerbate bedtime struggles and night-time wakings.

Management

- Detailed explanation about normal sleep and sleep cycles in a non-critical manner.
- Strategies to deal with inappropriate sleep associations all aim to provide the child with the opportunity to learn to fall asleep without parental assistance. Interventions range from extinction (letting the child cry it out), graduated extinction or controlled crying (checking the child at increasing periods of time until they fall asleep by themselves) to a more gradual approach whereby gradually all 'props' are removed.
- If frequent feeding is a problem discuss reducing the amount of fluid over 7–10 days and allowing the child to develop other ways to settle to sleep. Increasing the interval between breast-feeds, decreasing the amount of fluid in bottles or substituting water for milk/cordial/juices are all useful strategies that parents can adopt.
- A regular day–night routine need to be established. An age-appropriate enjoyable bedtime routine should be introduced to help the child learn to anticipate going to bed. Sometimes a gate is useful when the child has graduated to a bed and the newfound freedom creates bedtime struggles.

- Sedative medication is not recommended for children <2 years. Promethazine or trimeprazine as single night-time dose – each 0.5 mg/kg (max 10 mg) – may be used in conjunction with behavioural techniques over a short time period or for parental respite.

Night-time fears and anxiety
Aetiology
Night-time fears may present in the preschool and school-age child with bedtime struggles and refusal to sleep by themselves. There may be a precipitant (frightening movie, bullying at school) or it may be a manifestation of an anxiety disorder.

Management
- Address separation issues for the child, which may include the introduction of a transitional object.
- Camper bed technique: a camper bed and a parent are moved into the child's room. The parent spends the entire night in the child's bedroom for 2 weeks helping them overcome their fears and gaining confidence in their own bed and room. This is often used in conjunction with a reward/sticker chart. The parent then gradually moves out of the child's bedroom, once the child is sleeping through the night.
- Self-control techniques including relaxation, guided imagery and positive self-statements may also be used, again often in conjunction with reward/sticker chart.
- Make sure that the child is not in bed too early, allowing them the opportunity to further fuss and worry, which will interfere with sleep onset.

Night-time arousal phenomena and differentials
Aetiology
Sleepwalking and night terrors are disorders of arousal. They usually occur in the first third of the night during transition from NREM3/4 (deep sleep) to another sleep stage. They share common characteristics of the child being confused and unresponsive to the environment, retrograde amnesia, and varying degrees of autonomic activation (dilated pupils, sweating, tachycardia). See Table 12.1.
- **Sleepwalking** occurs at least once in 15–30% healthy children and is most common between 8 and 12 years. It can range from quiet walking, performance of simple tasks such as rearranging furniture or setting tables, to more frenetic and agitated behaviour.
- **Night terrors** are most common between 4–8 years and have a prevalence of 3–5%. They usually begin with a terrified scream and the child may either thrash around in bed or get up and run around the house. Efforts to calm the child often make the episode worse.

Differentials
- **Nightmares** generally occur during REM sleep and are thus more common in the second half of the night. They are vivid dreams accompanied by feelings of fear which wake the child up from sleep. They are most common in 3–6 year olds.

Table 12.1 Characteristics of night terrors, seizures and nightmares

Characteristic	Night terrors	Nightmares	Epilepsy
Sleep stage	NREM 3/4	REM	NREM2 but can occur all stages
Time of night	First 1/3	Last 1/2	Any time
Wakefulness	Unrousable	Easily aroused	Usually unrousable
Amnesia	Yes	No	Yes, or may have some recall
Return to sleep	Easy	Difficult	Easy
Family history	Yes	No	Possibly

- **Nocturnal frontal lobe epilepsy (NFLE).** This can present with brief repetitive stereo-typical movements ± vocalizations throughout the night which can be associated with awareness by the patient. Alternatively NFLE can present with bizarre complex stereotypic dystonic movements which typically last <2 min.

Management
- Obtain detailed history including the timing and duration of events, and the exact nature of movements (rhythmic or stereotypical) and behaviours.
- Completion of a sleep diary.
- A home video may be useful to aid diagnosis.
- All but NFLE are generally self-limiting. Explain, reassure and discuss safety issues.
- Avoid sleep deprivation as this can precipitate events. Ensure regular bedtime routines and sleep patterns.
- If events occur at a consistent time then scheduled awakening (waking the child 30 min before an event) may be useful.
- Sleep study may be required if events are very frequent, violent, atypical, or to assess contributing factors such as obstructive sleep apnoea.
- Medication is rarely needed. In situations where no aetiology has been found and there are very frequent and disruptive events, then low-dose clonazepam before bedtime may be useful for 4–6 weeks.

Snoring and sleep disordered breathing
- Sleep provides a physiological stress to breathing which can unmask respiratory difficulties that may not be apparent during wakefulness.
- Snoring is the most common symptom of sleep-disordered breathing in children and can be associated with primary snoring (PS) through to obstructive sleep apnoea (OSA).
- PS refers to snoring not associated with sleep or ventilatory disturbances; incidence up to 22% of children.

OSA

- OSA is defined as repeated episodes of partial or complete upper airway obstruction that disrupt normal ventilation and sleep.
- Incidence is 3% of children with peak incidence at 2–6 years due to adenotonsillar hypertrophy.
- Complications of severe OSA include growth failure and cor pulmonale, with milder OSA associated with impairment of behaviour and neurocognitive functioning.
- Symptoms include snoring, difficult or laboured breathing, apnoeas, mouth breathing, excessive sweating and restless or disturbed sleep. Children less commonly present with tiredness and lethargy.
- Increased risk of OSA is associated with:
  - Adenotonsillar hypertrophy
  - Obesity
  - Syndromes (e.g. Down syndrome, Prader–Willi)
  - Craniofacial abnormalities (e.g. Pierre–Robin, Apert)
  - Mucopolysaccharidoses
  - Achondroplasia and skeletal abnormalities
  - Neuromuscular weakness (e.g. Duchenne)
  - Hypotonia, hypertonia (e.g. cerebral palsy)
  - Prematurity
  - Previous palatal surgery (repaired cleft palate).
- Examination involves assessment of predisposing conditions and complications of OSA:
  - Growth: either failure to thrive or obesity
  - Craniofacial structure (retro/micrognathia, midface hypoplasia)
  - Mouth breathing
  - Nasal patency, septum, turbinates
  - Tongue, pharynx, palate, uvula, tonsils
  - Pectus excavatum
  - Right ventricular hypertrophy, pulmonary hypertension.
- Investigation by nasal endoscopy or lateral neck radiograph may have a place in assessing adenoidal size.

Management
- Although a decision regarding adenotonsillectomy is often made on history and examination, further investigations may be necessary and dependent on availability of local resources.
- Overnight oximetry is the most useful screening tool with the highest specificity. If there are repeated oxygen desaturations then a diagnosis of OSA can be made.
- Oximetry is limited in that it does not provide any information on the type of events associated with oxygen desaturations, CO_2 retention or sleep disruption.
- Negative oximetry does not exclude OSA, but may provide reassurance that the child is unlikely to have severe OSA while awaiting further assessment.
- Overnight polysomnography (sleep study) continues to be the gold standard for diagnosis of OSA and should be performed if uncertainty persists, in high-risk children and children <2 years of age.

- Adenotonsillectomy is the first line treatment, being curative in majority of children. The role of adenoidectomy alone is unclear.
- Adenotonsillectomy is associated with a 2 week recovery period and there is a 2–3% risk of secondary haemorrhage especially 5–10 days postoperatively.
- Non-invasive ventilation (nasal CPAP) may be used for residual OSA, if there is a delay in surgery, or if surgery is contraindicated.
- Medical treatments of mild OSA include treatment of allergic rhinitis (intranasal steroids) and management of obesity.

Polysomnography (sleep study)

Polysomnography involves the continuous and simultaneous recording of multiple physiological parameters related to sleep and breathing. Sleep studies are indicated for:

- Obstructive sleep apnoea; primary snoring vs sleep-disordered breathing.
- Monitoring non-invasive ventilation requirements.
- Excessive daytime sleepiness (include multiple sleep latency testing if narcolepsy suspected).
- Atypical night-time disruptions including very frequent or violent wakings.
- A full EEG montage is required if seizures are suspected.
- Periodic limb movement disorder.

USEFUL RESOURCES
- *www.rch.org.au/ccch/profdev.cfm* – [Professional development materials > Practice Resources Online] – RCH Community Child Health Centre. Evidence-based settling and sleep problems practice resource.
- *www.sleephomepages.org* – Extensive information and resource available to both clinicians and families.
- *www.kidshealth.org/parent/growth* – US online resource for parents with doctor-approved information about children.

CHAPTER 13
Constipation and continence

Susie Gibb
Michael Harari

Chronic constipation
Definition
At least two of the following problems within the previous 8 weeks:
- <3 bowel motions/week.
- >1 episode of faecal incontinence per week.
- Large stools in the rectum or palpable on abdominal examination.
- Passing of stools so large that they obstruct the toilet.
- Retentive posturing and withholding behaviour.
- Painful defecation.

Aetiology
In most children, chronic constipation (CC) is due to functional faecal retention (withholding of stool). Painful or fear of painful defecation are the most common triggers, leading to apprehension about defecation and a cycle of withholding and passage of hard retained stool.

Organic causes of CC are rare. They include:
- Cow's milk protein intolerance, which may manifest as constipation in the first 3 years of life.
- Hirschsprung's disease usually causes failure to pass meconium in the first 48 h of life, and virtually never causes faecal soiling.
- Slow colonic transit and motility (including neuronal intestinal dyplasia).
- Coeliac disease.
- Hypothyroidism.
- Hypercalcemia.
- Drugs (codeine, antacids).
- Spinal cord lesions.
- Anorectal malformations.

Lack of dietary fibre and poor fluid intake rarely contribute to childhood CC. Inappropriate emphasis on diet and fluid serve to lay blame on the child or parents, while deflecting attention from treatments that do work.

Paediatric Handbook, 8th edition. By Kate Thomson, Dean Tey and Michael Marks. Published 2009 by Blackwell Publishing, ISBN: 978-1-4051-7400-8.

Infants

Constipation of early infancy is not well understood. Dyschezia (a healthy infant, straining and crying before passing soft stool) is normal but can be mistaken for constipation. Common organic causes include anal fissures, weaning, and cow's milk protein intolerance. Treatment with laxatives and stool softeners should be undertaken with great caution.

Faecal incontinence

Defined as the passage of stool in an inappropriate place. The term faecal incontinence (FI) supersedes the terms encopresis and faecal soiling.

Aetiology

Most FI is functional and is associated with constipation (see above). Other causes include functional non-retentive FI (i.e not constipated), and organic causes from neurological damage or anal sphincter anomalies.

Associations with faecal incontinence

- Nocturnal enuresis and daytime detrusor overactivity. When all three occur together it is known as 'dysfunctional elimination syndrome' – perhaps linked through pelvic floor dysfunction. About 30% of children with FI also have nocturnal enuresis. Many have a family history of nocturnal enuresis.
- Behavioural problems are common but most are secondary to FI rather than the cause.
- Genetics: a family history of FI is common.

Pathophysiology

The majority of children with FI have significant faecal retention causing in turn, chronic rectal dilatation, hyposensitivity to stretching of the rectal ampulla, loss of the normal urge to pass stool and further retention. When the external anal sphincter relaxes, the stool accumulated in the rectal ampulla leaks. Unaware of the full rectum, the child may only sense the passage of stool by its contact with external skin, initiating an urgent rush to the toilet and a false impression that the child has 'waited until the last minute' – leading to inappropriate blaming.

Assessment of chronic constipation and faecal incontinence

History

- Timing of passing meconium stool (most <48 h).
- New onset of symptoms in child with previously normal bowel habit.
- Regression of motor skills.
- Painful or frightening precipitating events.
- Apprehensive behaviour such as toilet refusal, hiding while defecating.
- Faecal or urinary incontinence, day or night.
- Social/psychological impact of the problem.

Physical examination

- Abdominal examination for faecal loading.
- Growth – slow weight gain.
- Lower back, neurological assessment of lower limbs.
- Inspection of the anus and perianal skin for painful conditions (if it can be performed without adding to the child's apprehension).

Investigation
- Abdominal radiograph and rectal examination most often do not change management, and are rarely required.
- Abnormal neurological findings are rare but must be investigated urgently.

Management
- Empty the bowel, keep it empty and provide soft lubricated stools.
- This needs to be maintained for a long period in order for the child to overcome the apprehension about defecation.

Disimpaction (for severe symptoms or to kick-start long-term management)
Rectally instilled medication (suppositories or enemas) may add to the child's fearfulness. If using medications per rectum, consider sedation with nitrous oxide or midazolam (see Pain Management, chapter 4, p. 63).

Suggested medications (singly or in combination) include:
- *Stool softener*: paraffin oil (see notes below) 20–40 mL daily PO.
- *Osmotic laxative*: Macrogol 3350 (Movicol) sachets. One BD on day 1. Two BD day 2, three BD day 3, etc., increasing until desired result is achieved.
- *Microlax enema* 5 mL
- *Gut stimulant*, e.g. Senokot granules ½–1 teaspoon/day.
- For children refusing oral medication: *sodium sulfate (Colonlytely)* 1–3 L/day, via nasogastric tube.

Follow-on treatment
A long-term approach is needed, often spanning months to years. The physician, child and family need to work together and design an individualised treatment plan.

Behaviour modification is the mainstay of treatment. This involves regular sitting on the toilet and pushing, three times a day for 3–5 min. Use of a timer can be helpful to avoid arguments. Attention to the sitting position: feet supported, hips flexed and encourage 'bulging' of the abdomen. Reinforce desired behaviour with stickers on an age-appropriate chart. Reward achievable goals such as good compliance with sitting programme rather than clean pants.

Medications are an adjunct to a toileting regimen. Paediatricians usually start with a single agent, most commonly paraffin oil or movicol.
- Stool lubricants/softeners:
  - *Paraffin oil* 15–25 mL/d (see below).
- *Osmotic laxatives:*
  - Movicol 1 sachet/day.
  - Lactulose: <12 months, 5 mL/day; 1–5 years, 10 mL/day; >5–years, 15 mL/day.
- *Stimulants:*
  - Senokot: 2–6 years, ¼–½ tsp/day; >6 years, 1 tab/d (7.5 mg).
  - Bisacodyl: >4y – 1 tab/d (5 mg).

Paediatric follow-up is advisable. Consider referral to a sub-specialist continence clinic if combined faecal/urinary incontinence, suspected organic cause, complex or difficult cases.

Long-term use of most of these medications is safe and does not render the bowel 'lazy' or make the child 'dependent.' Only when defecation has been effortless for many months and toileting behaviour is consistent should one try to gradually withdraw adjunct medications.

Medication notes

- *Paraffin oil* is a stool lubricant that is colourless, odourless and almost tasteless. It is easily camouflaged in many foods. In liquids it will float and disperse into droplets without changing the taste of the liquid.
- *Parachoc* is paraffin oil with soluble fibre, flavour and sweeteners which children often find too sweet. *Agarol* is similar, but with flavourings that some will prefer. Parachoc carries a warning about risks of aspiration and lipoid pneumonia. Although this complication is not seen in practice it seems reasonable to avoid using Parachoc in children <6 months, and those with swallowing difficulty (lactulose may be a helpful alternative).

Nocturnal enuresis

Nocturnal enuresis (NE) is (arbitrarily) defined as bedwetting in a child ≥5 years of age. It affects 20% of 5 year olds, 5% of 10 year olds and up to 1% of adults. Bedwetting in the absence of daytime urinary symptoms is called 'monosymptomatic' nocturnal enuresis (MNE) whereas if day symptoms occur it is 'polysymptomatic' nocturnal enuresis (PNE). Primary NE refers to a child who has never been dry for at least 6 months. Secondary NE refers to children who have become wet after a period of at least 6 months of dryness. Although secondary NE may suggest an organic or psychological cause, in practice most secondary NE is simply NE that never fully resolved.

Aetiology and pathophysiology

NE is usually inherited as an autosomal dominant trait with variable penetrance. The pathophysiology involves a combination of:

- Poor arousal to stimulus of full bladder.
- Nocturnal polyuria – relative deficiency of vasopressin at night.
- Overactive bladder with reduced nocturnal functional bladder capacity.

Other factors may be involved in a way as yet unexplained. NE is more common in children with developmental delay, clumsiness, short stature or low birthweight. Most psychological problems in children with NE are likely to be the result of the wetting rather than the cause, and resolve with resolution of the wetting.

Children with PNE have daytime symptoms such as wetting, jiggling, urgency, frequent passage of small volumes of urine. Parents of such children often mistakenly think their child is lazy, preoccupied with other pursuits or simply habitually 'waits until the last minute'. In fact they have an overactive detrusor muscle (irritable bladder) resulting in a small functional bladder capacity and small urgently voided volumes. The jiggling represents tightening of pelvic floor muscles in an attempt to defend against the forceful bladder contraction, so that wetting may be prevented or minimised. These children often have NE that is refractory to alarms and desmopressin, and persists beyond 10 years of age. Some also develop faecal incontinence (see p. 155).

Rare physical causes include UTI, diabetes mellitus/insipidus, epilepsy, ectopic ureter, obstructive sleep hypoventilation, neurogenic bladder. Sexual abuse will occasionally first present as NE.

Management

The spontaneous remission rate is only 15% per year. Those least likely to resolve spontaneously are those with PNE. Treatment should be offered to children ≥6 years for whom wetting has become a problem. See Fig. 13.1 for management algorithm.

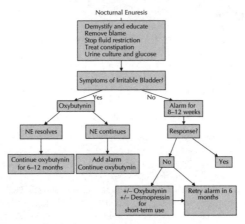

Fig. 13.1 Management algorithm for nocturnal enuresis

Monosymptomatic NE

Alarms

First line treatment is with a pad and bell alarm or personal (body-worn) alarm, used nightly for 8–12 weeks. Relapses may be minimised by 'overlearning' – using a fluid load before bed for the last 1–2 weeks of treatment. A wetting diary may help in motivation and monitoring. When symptoms are refractory to treatment, unsuspected nocturnal bladder dysfunction with detrusor overactivity is often the cause.

Desmopressin (DDAVP)

A synthetic analogue of vasopressin. In Australia it is available on Authority Prescription for those who have not responded to or are unsuitable for an alarm. While not curative, it can nonetheless serve a purpose for the short-term (school camps and sleepovers) and medium-term (adolescents who are fed up).

Side effects are uncommon and include nose bleeds, sore throat and abdominal pain. Hyponatremia with convulsions has been reported, particularly with nasal spray DDAVP, and tablets are now the recommended route of administration. It is important to ensure appropriate advice regarding fluid intake is given to minimise this risk. The child should **not** drink for 1 h before and 8 h after the administration of DDAVP.

The oral dose of DDAVP is 200–400 mcg (1–2 tablets) at night. Nasal spray is still available in Australia: the dose is 10–40 mcg/night (1–4 sprays).

Other treatments

Imipramine should no longer be used. It has an unacceptably high relapse rate and there is an ever-present danger of accidental or intentional overdose causing cardiotoxicity. There is no evidence to suggest that fluid restriction or liberalisation influences outcome. There is insufficient evidence to recommend lifting or waking the child, psychotherapy, hypnosis, acupuncture, rewards, chiropractic or bladder training.

Polysymptomatic NE
Treatment plan
- Treat constipation/faecal incontinence first (p. 156) and exclude UTI.
- Use anticholinergics to treat detrusor instability (see below).
- Then use alarm if needed as above.
- Frequent, regular voiding may help.

Anticholinergics
- Oxybutynin (Ditropan). Dose: 2.5–5 mg bd. Dry mouth is common. Less common side effects include rash, mood changes, constipation, headache, epistaxis, blurred vision. Treatment is often needed for many months to years.
- Tolterodine (Detrusitol) is a new bladder-specific anticholinergic. There is currently little experience with use in childhood.

Daytime wetting without NE
Daytime wetting in isolation is not well understood. In a bygone era it was called the 'sham syndrome' as it was (mistakenly) thought to have a psychological or behavioural cause. It affects girls more often than boys and is often difficult to treat. The following classification is useful in determining appropriate investigations and management.

Urge incontinence
Symptoms include urgency, frequency, posturing (squatting) and wetting.

The condition is caused by overactivity in the detrusor muscle during bladder filling. There is an association with recurrent UTI, vulvovaginitis and constipation. Management includes treating any coexistent UTI and constipation, regular voiding, and anticholinergic medication to reduce detrusor spasm.

Dysfunctional voiding
- There is a lack of coordination between detrusor and bladder neck activity with poor relaxation of the external sphincter during voiding.
- The condition is associated with increased intravesical pressure, high residual urine volumes and, at times, upper tract dilatation.
- Management relies on teaching sphincter relaxation (i.e. pelvic floor relaxation) and ensuring optimal voiding techniques.

Neurological and urological pathology
These children do not have jiggling, urgency or frequency and *they may wet at night* Ectopic ureter and fistulae cause constant rather than episodic dribbling. Bladder neck and urethral obstruction and neurogenic bladder may have large or expressible bladders. Examine the back and the neurology of lower limbs for spinal cord anomalies, and inspect the urethral opening.

Investigation
NE alone does not usually require investigation. Children with NE and day-wetting (PNE) should have a urine microscopy, culture and glucose. Where there is diagnostic uncertainty or a poor response to treatment, a renal and bladder ultrasound including an assessment of residual urine volume will exclude major structural pathology. A 2 day voiding volume diary, uroflow (volume/time) measurement and post-void bladder scan can provide information about detrusor overactivity or outflow obstruction and further guide management.

CHAPTER 14

Developmental delay and disability

Catherine Marraffa
Dinah Reddihough

Approximately 3–5% of children have developmental delay of at least mild–moderate severity that may remain undiagnosed unless specific assessment is undertaken. In general, problems affecting motor development and speech present early, but problems affecting receptive language, socialisation and cognition present late. The clinician's role is to ascertain whether a child's development is significantly aberrant for their age and to determine the underlying reasons for this, realising that developmental delay may not have a clearly identifiable medical basis.

Developmental surveillance

Developmental surveillance is a flexible continuous process of skilled observation as part of providing routine health care. It should occur opportunistically whenever a child comes into contact with a health professional.

If a parent is concerned about a child's development it is highly likely that evaluation will confirm developmental delay; however, a lack of concern from parents is no guarantee that the child's development is normal. The PEDS (Parents' Evaluation of Developmental Status) consists of 10 questions based on research of parents' concerns. It aims to systematically elicit parents' concerns and guide referral decisions. It is validated from birth to 8 years. It is simple to administer and can be used in primary care settings.

Informal clinical judgement is unreliable as a method for detecting developmental problems. Milestone checklists (see Table 14.1) serve as an aid to memory by recording what is expected of the average child at each age in several domains of developmental function. Because they record average expectations for each age, it is often difficult to distinguish the child with true developmental delay from the normal child with below-average milestone attainment.

Formal screening tests such as the *Denver II* and the *Australian Developmental Screening Test* allow the objective discrimination of the child who *probably* has a developmental delay from the child who *probably* does not. Results of screening tests are not definitive; a fail on such a test requires referral of the child for formal developmental assessment.

Paediatric Handbook, 8th edition. By Kate Thomson, Dean Tey and Michael Marks. Published 2009 by Blackwell Publishing, ISBN: 978-1-4051-7400-8.

Table 14.1 Developmental milestones

Age*	Gross motor	Fine motor adaptive	Language	Personal–social
1 m	Lifts head momentarily while prone (0–3 w)	Visual following to mid-line (0–5 w)		Watches face (0–4 w)
2 m	Lifts head momentarily to erect position when sitting	Hands predominantly open	Vocalises (0–7 w)	Smiles responsively (0–7 w)
3 m	Lifts head to 90° while prone (0–10 w)	Visual following past mid-line (0–10 w)	Laughs (6–10 w)	
4 m	Head steady when held erect (6–17 w)	Plays with hands together (6–15 w)	Coos and gurgles	Excited by approach of food
5 m	No head lag when pulled to sitting (3–6 m) Rolls over	Grasps rattle (10–18 w) Reaches for object with palmar grasp (3–5½ m)	Squeals (6–18 w)	Smiles spontaneously (6 w–5 m)
6 m	Lifts head forward when pulled to sit (9–19 w)	Passes block hand to hand (4½–7½ m)	Turns to voice (3½–8½ m)	Friendly to all comers
8 m	Maintains sitting position without support		Repetition of syllables (e.g. baba, Dada)	Feeds self biscuit (5–8 m) Tries to get toy out of reach (5–9 m)
10 m	Stands holding on (5–10 m)	Index finger approach	'Mum', 'Dad' without meaning (6–10 m)	Shy with strangers Plays peek-a-boo

(Continued)

Table 14.1 Continued

Age*	Gross motor	Fine motor adaptive	Language	Personal–social
12 m	Walks holding on to furniture (7½–12½ m)	Crude finger–thumb grasp (7–11 m)	Imitates speech sounds (6–11 m)	Gives up a toy
15 m	Walks alone (11½–15 m)	Neat pincer grasp of pellet (9–15 m)	'Mum', 'Dad' with meaning (9–15 m)	Indicates wants (10½–14½ m)
1½ y	Walks well (11½–18 m)	Builds tower of two blocks (12–20 m)	Three words other than 'Mum', 'Dad' (12–20 m)	Drinks from cup (10–17 m)
2 y	Walks up steps without help (14–22 m)	Scribbles (12–24 m)	Points to one named body part (14–23 m)	Feeds self with spoon (12–24 m)
2½ y	Throws ball (15–32 m)	Builds tower of four blocks (15–26 m)	Combines two words (14–27 m)	Helps in house – simple tasks (15–24 m)
3 y	Pedals tricycle (21 m–3 y)	Imitates vertical line (18 m–3 y) Copies circle (2½–3½ y)	Uses three word sentences	Puts on clothes (2–3 y)
4 y	Balances on one foot (2¾–4½ y)	Copies square	Gives first and last name (2–4 y)	Dresses with supervision (2½–3½ y)
5 y	Hops on one foot (3–5 y)	Draws person in three parts (3–5 y)	Knows some colours (3–5 y) Knows age	Dresses without supervision (2½–5 y)

w, weeks; m, months; y, years.

* Age indicates when at least 90% of a normal group of children will achieve the test. Figures in parentheses represent the range from 25th to 90th centiles for achievement.

Formal assessment involves a synthesis of the findings from history, physical and neurological examination, and developmental testing using standardised assessment tools such as the *Bayley Scales of Infant Development* and the *Griffith's Developmental Scales*. The type of testing undertaken depends on the presence or absence of several risk factors for developmental delay (see Table 14.2).

Children with developmental delay or disability, or both, have the same basic needs as all children. They have the potential for further development and the principles of normal development apply.

Specific disabilities in one area may cause secondary disabilities in other areas (e.g. children who have motor disabilities with reduced opportunity for exploration may suffer delayed development of their comprehension abilities).

Transient developmental delay may be associated with:

- Prematurity.
- Physical illness.
- Prolonged hospitalisation.
- Family stress.
- Lack of opportunities to learn.

Causes of *persistent developmental delay (developmental disability)* include

- Language disorders.
- Intellectual disability.
- Cerebral palsy.
- Autism.
- Hearing impairment.
- Visual impairment.
- Degenerative disorders.
- Neuromuscular disorders.

Once suspicion regarding a child's development has been raised, a complete paediatric consultation is required. This should include full details of the family, obstetric, neonatal and developmental histories. Liaison with the GP and a maternal and child health nurse to obtain background information is often helpful. A history of loss of previously attained developmental skills is suggestive of regression rather than delay, and requires more comprehensive investigation to exclude neurodegenerative conditions. Observation of how the child looks, listens, moves, explores, plays, communicates and socialises is essential before the formal examination. Understandably, parents will be anxious and a sensitive approach is essential at all times.

Developmental assessment provides the family with an understanding of the child's development and outlines developmental goals and strategies to reduce any handicapping effects of the disability. Assessment and management may include input from physiotherapists, speech pathologists, teachers, occupational therapists, psychologists and social workers.

Principles of assessment
These include:

Table 14.2 Children at risk of developmental problems

Risk group	Risk factors	Action
High	Developmental regression Abnormal neurology Dysmorphism Chromosomal abnormality Hearing or vision problems	Bypass developmental screening Refer for comprehensive developmental assessment

Moderate	Parents suspect developmental delay
	History of severe pre- or perinatal insult
	Very low birthweight (<1500 g)
	Family history of developmental delay
	Severe socio-economic or family adversity
		Administer a formal screening test
		Pass – reassure that development is
		   within normal range and continue
		   surveillance through a local doctor/
		   maternal and child health nurse
		Questionable – repeat the test 4
		   weeks later
		Fail – refer for comprehensive
		   paediatric consultation and
		   developmental assessment

Low	No parental or professional concerns
	No other risk factors
		Developmental surveillance by a local
		   doctor/maternal and child health
		   nurse is recommended
		Should there be later parental or
		   professional concerns, a formal
		   screening test is recommended
		If there are no further concerns,
		   continue surveillance monitoring

- Utilisation of play as a fundamental assessment tool.
- Promotion of optimal performance of the child.
- Gearing the assessment towards remediation rather than merely producing a profile.
- Involvement of the parents in the assessment process.
- Close linking of the assessment with services offering help and support.

Early intervention

Early intervention includes prevention and early detection of disabilities, as well as health, educational and community services that assist the child, family and community in adapting to the child's developmental needs and disability. Services are based on the principles of inclusion and integration into regular settings.

The aims of early intervention are to minimise the handicapping effects of the child's disability on their development and education, and to support the family in understanding and providing for their child's individual needs. Services include individual teaching and therapy (speech and occupational therapy), family support and counselling, providing resources and support to childcare, preschools and respite care. Services are usually regionally based and are provided by government and non-government agencies. Unfortunately, waiting lists for these Early Childhood Intervention Services (ECIS) can be many months and it is important to provide any other services locally available while awaiting placement. Recently the Australian government has made available five Medicare-funded allied health consultations per person, per year. These are only available by GP referral, and can be used, for example, to obtain private physiotherapy or speech therapy.

Education

There is a range of special educational strategies to optimise learning and development, dependent on the child's abilities and disabilities, with increasing opportunities for integration as resources are moved from special to local schools. A range of special schools is also available. Paediatricians liaise closely with schools to assist with meeting the child's educational needs. Dialogue ensures appropriate support for the child's physical and intellectual function, maximising the child's learning potential and opportunities. This may include applying for government funding for aides, management of physical disability, seizure management and behavioural support.

Family supports

Parents need to be aware of the services that are available to them to assist in the care of their child with a disability. Supports include social security benefits, home help and respite care through foster agencies and community residential units. Consumer organisations can provide parent support, information and advocacy.

Intellectual disability

The definition of intellectual disability comprises three elements:

1 a significantly subaverage general intellectual functioning (i.e. 2 standard deviations below the mean of the intelligence quotient) that exists concurrently with
2 deficits in adaptive behaviour, and
3 manifests itself during the developmental period.

This definition is used by service providers, as well as academics and legislators. The term *developmental disabilities* is used increasingly to reflect the complexity of development.

Up to 2.5% of children have an intellectual disability: approximately 2% mild and 0.5% moderate, severe or profound.

Causes of intellectual disability
Prenatal

- Chromosomal; e.g. trisomy 21, fragile X syndrome and velocardiofacial syndrome (22q11-deletion syndrome).
- Genetic; e.g. tuberous sclerosis and metabolic disorders.
- Major structural anomalies of the brain.
- Syndromes; e.g. Williams, Prader–Willi, Rett.

Development

- Infections; e.g. cytomegalovirus.
- Drugs; e.g. alcohol.

In addition, children of low birthweight are at risk for intellectual disability: the lower the birthweight, the greater the risk.

Perinatal
- Infections.
- Trauma.
- Metabolic abnormalities.

Postnatal
- Head injury.
- Meningitis or encephalitis.
- Poisons.

Presentation
- At birth with a known syndrome or malformation.
- At follow-up in high-risk infants.
- Language delay.
- Global developmental delay.
- Learning difficulties.
- Behaviour problems.
- With associated medical complications (e.g. epilepsy).

A biological cause for moderate, severe and profound intellectual disability can be identified more readily than in those with a mild intellectual disability. In disability requiring extensive support, a cause may be identified in up to 2/3 of cases. In people with mild intellectual disability, the cause is identifiable in <20% of individuals. Where a cause is identified, the majority are caused by problems during the prenatal period with 10% due to perinatal and 5% due to postnatal insults. The three most common identifiable causes of intellectual disability are trisomy 21, fragile X syndrome and velocardiofacial syndrome.

Investigations
It is important to establish aetiology where possible in order to understand prognosis, provide genetic counselling and to ensure that associated problems are detected.
The following investigations should be considered:
- Chromosomes, especially for fragile X, William and Prader–Willi syndromes using DNA probes and FISH for 22q11-deletion.
- MRI of the brain.
- Creatinine phosphokinase in boys (for neuromuscular disorders).
- Plasma amino acids.
- Urinary organic and amino acids.
- Thyroid function tests.
- Mucopolysaccharide screen.

- Investigation for congenital infection: ophthalmological and audiological examination, maternal/infant serology and viral culture (cytomegalovirus).

Despite thorough investigation, the cause is often not identified.

Management

- Support and information for parents.
- Referral to and liaison with other practitioners, early intervention, family support and educational services.
- Child advocacy.
- Regular assessment of vision and hearing.
- Investigation for associated anomalies (e.g. cardiac and thyroid status with trisomy 21).
- Treatment of associated disorders (e.g. epilepsy).
- Monitoring of development.

Cerebral palsy

Cerebral palsy is a persistent, but not unchanging, disorder of movement and posture due to a defect or lesion of the developing brain.

Aetiology

Cerebral palsy is not a single entity but a term used for a diverse group of disorders, which may relate to events in the prenatal, perinatal or postnatal periods. In many children the cause is unknown. Perinatal asphyxia accounts for <10% of cases and postnatal illnesses or injuries for a further 10%. There is a significant association with low birthweight and prematurity, particularly for infants weighing <1500 g at birth. The overall prevalence is approximately 2.0/1000 live births.

Classification

This is according to:

- The type of motor disorder, e.g. spasticity, dyskinesia (includes dystonia and athetosis) and ataxia.
- The distribution, e.g. hemiplegia, diplegia and quadriplegia.
- The severity of the motor disorder, using the Gross Motor Function Classification System.

Spectrum of cerebral palsy and associations

- Children with cerebral palsy are an extremely heterogeneous group and the degree of handicap experienced varies enormously. Approximately 30% are hemiplegic, 25% diplegic and 45% have quadriparesis.
- The most common type of motor disorder is spasticity. This can lead to significant complications if not well managed, the most severe being contractures and hip subluxation.
- Some children have an isolated motor disorder. However, an estimated 70% of children with cerebral palsy have associated disorders including visual problems, hearing impairment, communication disorders, epilepsy, intellectual disability, specific learning disability or perceptual problems.

- Other complications include incontinence and constipation, feeding and nutritional problems, poor dental health and poor salivary control. These are usually multifactorial.

Management
General management
- An accurate diagnosis with genetic counselling.
- Management of the associated disorders, health problems and consequences of the motor impairment.
- An assessment of the child's capabilities and referral to the appropriate services for the child and family. Liaising with the kindergarten, school and GP is important.
- Attention to usual childhood issues of growth, immunisation and dental health.

Management of commonly associated disabilities and health problems
- All children require hearing and visual assessment.
- Careful assessment and management of epilepsy is required.
- Children may benefit from formal cognitive assessment.
- *Nutritional problems*: obesity can occur because of an imbalance between intake and physical activity. Conversely, children may be underweight, particularly in the presence of oromotor problems that may result in major feeding difficulties. Dietary advice is important. The presence of severe slow weight gain, major feeding problems or aspiration, or all of these, may be indications for non-oral feeding by a nasogastric or gastrostomy tube.
- *Gastro-oesophageal reflux* occurs commonly in cerebral palsy.
- *Continence issues.*
- *Undescended testes* occur more frequently in boys with cerebral palsy than in the general population.
- *Constipation* requires dietary and laxative advice.
- *Aspiration and lung disease* may be associated with impaired oromotor control. Chronic cough with wheeze or repeated lower respiratory infections may indicate the presence of chronic lung disease. Videofluoroscopy is a useful test for the detection of aspiration.
- *Osteoporosis* with pathological fractures may occur in cerebral palsy. This is often compounded by vitamin D deficiency and serum levels ought to be monitored, especially in children with limited sun exposure.
- *Psychological and social difficulties* require careful attention.

Management of the consequences of the motor disorder
- *Saliva control* can be improved with techniques employed by speech therapists, or by the use of anticholinergic medication or surgery in a small group of children.
- *Spasticity management* is aimed at improving function, comfort and care and requires a team approach. Options include:
  - Oral medications, e.g. diazepam, baclofen and dantrolene.
  - Inhibitory casts to increase joint range and facilitate improved quality of movement.
  - Botulinum toxin A for localised spasticity.
  - Intrathecal baclofen is suitable for a small number of children with severe spasticity.

   – Selective dorsal rhizotomy – a treatment option for a selected group of children with severe spastic diplegia.

Orthopaedic problems
The orthopaedic management of cerebral palsy requires a team approach. Dynamic spasticity, which interferes with function in young children, is best managed by conservative methods (e.g. orthotics, inhibitory casts or the use of botulinum toxin A). Surgery is mainly undertaken on the lower limb, but is occasionally helpful in the upper limb. Some children also require surgery for scoliosis. Physiotherapy is an essential part of postoperative management. The advice of occupational therapists on strategies and equipment to overcome barriers into and within the home of an immobilised child postoperatively is often of great assistance to families. Gait laboratories are useful in planning the surgical programme for ambulant children. The critical parts of the body to observe are:

- *The hips*: non-walkers and those only partially ambulant are prone to hip subluxation and eventual dislocation. Early detection is important and hip radiographs should be performed at yearly intervals or more frequently if there is concern. Dislocation, which may cause pain and difficulty with perineal hygiene, is extremely difficult to treat once it occurs and prevention by early adductor releases is a better strategy. Hip problems may also occur in mobile children (e.g. those with severe hemiplegia). However, this is rare.
- *The knees*: hamstring surgery may be necessary to improve gait pattern, or the ability to stand for transfers.
- *The ankles*: there may be a range of problems around the foot and ankle. Conservative treatments are used in young children but surgical correction is frequently required later.
- *Multilevel surgery*: sometimes children require surgery at several different levels, e.g. hip, knee and ankle.

Referrals
Referral to and ongoing liaison with allied health professionals is essential to enable children to achieve their optimal physical potential and independence.

- *Physiotherapists* give practical advice to parents and carers on positioning, handling and play to minimise the effects of abnormal muscle tone and encourage the development of movement skills. They also give advice regarding mobility aids, the use of orthoses or special seating. They may provide individual or group treatments or refer to appropriate community services.
- *Occupational therapists* provide parents with advice on developing their child's upper limb and self-care skills, often suggesting suitable toys to encourage skill development. OTs design and make hand splints, and provide advice on equipment and house adaptations for home care.
- *Speech pathologists* provide guidance for those with severe eating and drinking difficulties, and communication and augmentative communication systems for children with limited verbal skills.
- *Orthotists/prosthetists* provide design/fabricate/fit and maintain various orthoses (braces) and prostheses (artificial limbs). Orthoses are used to improve function, support, align, prevent or correct musculoskeletal deformities in different parts of the child's body,

more commonly the lower limbs. As part of the allied health team, orthotists work closely with the referring specialist and other allied health team members to optimise the child's potential.

- *Other professionals* who may be helpful include medical social workers, nurses, psychologists and special education teachers.
- *GPs* play an important role in supporting these children and their families in the community.

Irritability in children with profound disability

Refer to Pain in children and adolescents with disabilities, p. 70.

Irritability in children can present the clinician with diagnostic uncertainty, amplified in those patients with difficulties in communication or complex medical illness. In children with severe cerebral palsy the following differentials should be considered:

- Muscle spasm.
- Seizure.
- Pain:
  - Consider all the usual sites of infection (e.g. otitis media, urinary tract, throat, sinusitis, respiratory tract and skin).
  - Gastro-oesophageal reflux.
  - Dental abscess/caries.
  - Corneal abrasion/foreign body in the eye.
  - Pancreatitis.
  - Renal colic.
  - Surgical – appendicitis, intussusception, torted testes.
  - Severe constipation.
  - Subluxing or dislocated hips.
  - Fractures – accidental or inflicted.
  - Side effects of medication e.g. anticonvulsants.
  - Gynaecological.
  - Sleep deprivation (associated with pain and spasm).
  - Increased intracranial pressure (many children have VP shunts).

Spina bifida (myelomeningocele)

Spina bifida is the most common severe congenital malformation of the nervous system. The degree of impairment from the spinal cord pathology varies. Most children have some element of lower limb dysfunction, sensory loss and a neurogenic bladder and bowel; 80% have progressive hydrocephalus requiring surgery. Many children have specific learning problems.

Prevention

Periconceptional folic acid supplementation (in the month before and in the first 3 months of pregnancy) has been shown to reduce the risk of recurrence in any at-risk family (by ~75%), as well as reduce occurrence in any family. Recommended doses are:

- Low-risk women (no family history of neural tube defects): 0.5 mg daily.
- Women with a previous child with a neural tube defect (or personal, partner or close family history): 4 mg daily (5 mg if 4 mg not available).
- Women with epilepsy on anticonvulsants should also be advised to take the larger dose.

Note: Multivitamin supplements are not recommended because of the potential risks of vitamin overdose to the developing fetus.

Fortification of staple foods with folate has been recommended in many countries and is currently being considered in Australia. Fewer children are now being born with neural tube defects, mainly due to antenatal diagnosis and termination of pregnancy. The effect of folate supplementation on incidence is not yet clear.

Management
Management requires collaboration between health, education and welfare professionals and the child and family. Most children attend regular schools. Families require a great deal of support.

An interdisciplinary team of paediatricians, surgeons, neuropsychologists, physiotherapists, orthotists, occupational therapists, social workers and stomal therapists is required to develop an appropriate developmental and rehabilitation programme, in collaboration with the family, GPs and community agencies (including local primary care service providers).

Initial management
- *Neurosurgical and paediatric assessment* of the newborn infant is undertaken to determine if early surgery to close the spinal defect should be recommended. Clinical and ultrasound observation to detect and monitor the presence of hydrocephalus is important. Insertion of a ventriculoperitoneal shunt may be necessary.
- *Orthopaedic and urological consultations* and investigations are undertaken in the neonatal period to provide baseline information for subsequent management. A small number of infants require early management of talipes or a high-pressure neurogenic bladder.
- The families must be fully informed about the diagnosis, natural history and prognosis, and be reassured that assistance is available.

Specific aspects of management
Medical and therapy staff should monitor children regularly.
- Mobility:
  - Independent mobility is the primary goal of the orthopaedic surgeon, physiotherapist and orthotist.
- Urinary tract:
  - The primary goal is the maintenance of satisfactory renal function and the establishment of urinary continence (dryness) at a developmentally appropriate age.
  - Clean intermittent catheterisation is now the preferred method of treatment, starting in the neonatal period. Additional support may be necessary in the form of medication (e.g. oxybutynin 8–12 hourly), protective clothing and condom drainage.
  - Bladder augmentation may be required, and if it has been performed lifelong surveillance by a urologist is important because of the increased risk of malignant change.

In the past artificial sphincters were used in some patients and long-term urological surveillance is also required for them. The Mitrofanoff procedure (fashioning a conduit from the bladder to the abdominal wall by using the appendix) is being used more frequently to facilitate independence in catheterisation.
- Urinary tract infection is common.
- Neurological functioning:
  - Children with shunts should have neurosurgical assessment regularly (in infancy every 6–9 months; in childhood and adolescence at least every 1–2 years). See also chapter 33, Neurologic conditions, p. 470.
  - Tethering of the spinal cord to surrounding structures occurs in most children. In a small number, traction on the cord causes deterioration in neurological functioning. Surgical de-tethering may be required.
  - Children often have specific cognitive difficulties and a neuropsychological assessment is usually carried out before school entry and repeated before transition to secondary school.
- Miscellaneous medical problems:
  - Constipation is common, and dietary advice, laxatives and enemas may be required. For children with severe continence problems anal plugs can be used following careful assessment by the stomal therapist. The Malone procedure is the fashioning of a non-refluxing appendicocaecostomy so that an antegrade continence enema can be performed to prevent soiling.
  - Scoliosis is a common management problem.
  - Pressure sores occur in all children with spina bifida at some time, most commonly on the feet or the buttocks.
  - Epilepsy occurs in 15% of cases.
  - Latex allergy is much more common in children with spina bifida and has serious implications. Testing is offered to all children.
  - Weight issues can be a problem.
- Adolescent issues:
  - Puberty may be delayed or precocious.
  - Specific adolescent issues including sexuality, relationship difficulties and contraception should be addressed.
  - Mental health should be monitored.
  - Vocational support is important.
  - Transition and transfer to adult services is a major challenge and needs careful planning and support for the young person.

Autism spectrum disorder

Autism is now seen as part of a spectrum of disorders, also known as pervasive developmental disorders. They include autistic disorder, Asperger's syndrome and atypical autism.

Diagnosis requires the presence of three core features by 3 years of age:
- Qualitative impairment of social interaction.
- Qualitative impairment in communication.
- Restricted, repetitive and stereotyped patterns of activities, behaviour and interests.

Prevalence estimates vary with definitions used but autism spectrum disorder is now thought to affect nearly 1% of the population with a sex ratio of 3 males : 1 female.

Aetiology

The aetiology of autism is unknown. Factors involved may include:

- *Genetic*: recurrence rate in families of 2–6%.
- *Syndromal*: there is an association with tuberous sclerosis, fragile X syndrome and congenital rubella. Careful medical assessment to exclude these conditions is important.
- *Structural*: subtle brain abnormalities are described in some children.

Associated disorders

- Intellectual disability (75%).
- Epilepsy (20%).
- Other: ADHD, anxiety disorders and depression, Tourette syndrome.

Clinical features

Parents will often identify that something is different about their child before the second birthday. Early features include *lack of*:

- Pretend play.
- Pointing out objects to another person.
- Social interest.
- Joint attention.
- Social play.

Language development is delayed, with an unusual use of language. Regression of language may be seen.

Diagnosis

There is no single test for autism spectrum disorders. Diagnosis is best made by a multidisciplinary team of a paediatrician/child psychiatrist, speech pathologist and psychologist.

Management

Management is multidisciplinary. It includes:

- Parent support and education.
- Appropriate screening of vision/hearing, investigation for associated disorders/syndromes if suspected.
- Early intervention programmes, including a well-structured and predictable environment with:
  - Behavioural modification.
  - Speech therapy.
  - Special education.
  - Sensorimotor programmes.
- A combination of educational, developmental and behavioural treatments has been shown to improve a child's rate of progress.

Development

- Drug therapy is sometimes used to treat co-morbid psychopathology (e.g. attentional and behavioural problems, anxiety, self injury). It does not affect the core autistic symptoms.
- Advice regarding educational options.
- Support groups.
- Access to respite care.

Families of children with autism spectrum disorder will often seek alternative health care, sometimes at considerable cost. It is important for parents to be aware and informed of what is available and the evidence supporting/refuting such strategies, such that an educated choice can be made.

Asperger's syndrome

Asperger's syndrome is used to describe individuals with:
- Normal intelligence (although it may range from borderline to superior).
- No obvious delay in language development.
- Impaired social and communication skills with an egocentric approach to others.
- Social immaturity.
- A narrow range of obsessional interests (such as knowledge of sporting statistics, astronomy, public transport systems).
- Lack of common sense.

Common co-morbidities
Anxiety disorders
- Obsessive compulsive disorder occurs in about 25% of people with Asperger's syndrome.
- Post-traumatic stress disorder.
- School refusal.
- Selective mutism.
- Social anxiety disorder.

Depression
Up to 1/3 of children and adults with Asperger's syndrome are clinically depressed.

Management
Specific educational, behavioural and supportive psychological and psychotherapeutic treatments are used.

Teaching social skills and friendship skills, emotion education and management, can help young people with Asperger's syndrome deal with their difficulties. Clinicians monitor for the emergence of co-morbidities.

USEFUL RESOURCES
- *www.pedstest.com* – Parent's Evaluation of Developmental Status.

CHAPTER 15

Adolescent health

Susan Sawyer

Adolescence is the transitional period of development between the relative dependence of childhood and the independence of adulthood. Puberty has long been accepted as the starting point of adolescence. Later social transitions such as completion of education, financial independence, marriage and childbearing have generally marked the end of adolescence. In the past such transitions occurred in the late teens and early twenties. As young people now commonly participate longer in education and are marrying and having children later, the end of adolescence has become less distinct. The term 'adolescent' formally refers to those aged between 10 and 19 years while 'youth' refers to those aged 15–24 years. The term 'young person' is commonly used to refer to those aged between 10 and 24 years. These terms are often used interchangeably.

Most adolescents rate their health, including their mental health, as good. Many adolescents describe the period of adolescence as enjoyable and exciting, and a time of satisfaction with the achievement of many milestones such as first relationship, completing school, first job, and learning to drive.

Burden of disease

Changes in the past few decades have led to adolescents experiencing a more complex burden of disease. Increased survival of children with congenital or early-onset diseases (e.g. cystic fibrosis, congenital heart disease) and a true increase in the incidence of other chronic disorders (e.g. asthma, diabetes, cancer) have resulted in a larger proportion of children entering adolescence with chronic disease. Adolescence is recognised as a time of risk for the onset or escalation of various behavioural and mental disorders, such as depression, anxiety, eating disorders, substance use, and attention deficit hyperactivity disorder (ADHD), which have also increased in prevalence. Finally, larger cohorts of young people experience previously uncommon conditions, such as obesity and sexually transmitted infections.

Young people with chronic disease and disability are increasingly recognised to have a higher prevalence of health risk behaviours and mental health problems than healthy young people. They are doubly disadvantaged, as they also have a greater attributable risk from these behaviours (e.g. the effect of smoking is worse in someone with diabetes or asthma than in an otherwise healthy young person).

Paediatric Handbook, 8th edition. By Kate Thomson, Dean Tey and Michael Marks. Published 2009 by Blackwell Publishing, ISBN: 978-1-4051-7400-8.

Social health perspective

Broader social and economic changes appear to have contributed to higher rates of emotional, eating disorders and substance misuse in adolescents. Accompanying changes in lifestyles have led to a rise in sexually transmitted and blood-transmitted diseases. Marginalised young people who are poorly connected to their families and schools are at the greatest risk of these newer psychosocial morbidities. Groups such as young offenders, those in 'out of home care' and the homeless have particularly high levels of these problems.

Adolescent developmental challenges

Engaging adolescents in a productive therapeutic relationship requires the clinician to have a good understanding of both the social context and developmental challenges young people face. The key developmental tasks involve the issues of:

- Autonomy and independence.
- Body self-integrity and personal identity.
- Peer relationships and recreational goals.
- Educational and vocational goals.
- Sexuality.

Health outcomes

Clinicians must have clear therapeutic goals. Management approaches are more likely to be successful when they consider the developmental challenges facing adolescents, the individual behavioural and emotional issues experienced by a young person, and the social context of these issues.

Clinical approach to adolescents

Allowing adequate time is essential to the conduct of a successful consultation. Young people often perceive that they are not listened to or not given adequate time to put their views across, and that their opinions are dismissed. A clinician who listens respectfully and acknowledges a young person's point of view will have made an excellent start in establishing a therapeutic relationship.

Starting the consultation

Greet the young person by name, make eye contact with them and give them your full name. When parents are present, greet the young person first, then introduce yourself to the parents. Remember that the young person is the patient and must be provided with some time alone with the clinician during the consultation.

Confidentiality

In addition to medicolegal requirements, maintenance of confidentiality enhances trust and honesty with adolescents and has been shown to improve health outcomes. Explain the issue of confidentiality at the beginning of the first contact with every adolescent. For example: 'Health consultations are confidential. That means that I cannot talk about anything we discuss today with your parents or anyone else, unless you and I have agreed to do so. However, there are some exceptions. I cannot maintain confidentiality if you are at risk of harm, such as threat of suicide, self-harm, or sexual abuse.'

Young people benefit from reminders about confidentiality when sensitive information is discussed (see Table 15.1).

Psychosocial screening and developmental assessment

Notwithstanding their complex burden of disease, young people are most likely to present for clinical care as a consequence of minor complaints, such as a viral illness or injury. Irrespective of the primary reason for presentation, every consultation should include psychosocial screening.

One approach to taking a psychosocial history and a developmental assessment is to use the HEADSS framework (see Table 15.2). Questions can be asked in any order, although the

Table 15.1 Confidentiality

- Define the term at the start of the interview.
- Consider all information from an adolescent as confidential until discussed or clarified.
- In most states, confidentiality is a legal requirement over 16 years of age.
  Negotiation or compromise may be required for adolescents under 16 years.
- Exceptions to confidentiality are when the adolescent is at risk of significant harm, such as risk of suicide or if they are subject to physical or sexual abuse.

Table 15.2 Adolescent developmental screening: HEADSS*

	Area	Questions
H	Home	Where do you live and who lives there with you?
E	Education and employment	What are you good at in school? What grades do you get?
A	Activities	What do you do for fun? What things do you do with friends?
D	Drugs	Many young people experiment with drugs, alcohol and cigarettes. Have you ever tried them?
S	Sexuality	Most young people become interested in sex at your age. Have you had a sexual relationship with anyone?
S	Suicide risk/Depression Screening	See Table 15.3 (p. 183)

* Goldenring and Cohen, *Contemporary Pediatrics*, July, 1988, pp. 75–80.
From Goldenring JM, Rosen DS. Getting into adolescent heads: An essential update. *Contemporary Pediatrics* 2004; **21**: 64–90.

first three themes generally involve less sensitive questions than the last three. Taking a psychosocial history is a powerful way of engaging a young person and establishing rapport. It also provides an opportunity to assess developmental stage (maturity), identify the balance of health risk and protective factors, and also identify opportunities for early intervention and health promotion.

Physical examination

A thorough physical examination should be conducted whenever appropriate. Protection of the adolescent's modesty and privacy is important. Use reassuring dialogue that explains the reason for the particular examination. Many young people are anxious about many aspects of normal development and benefit from reassurance. Provide feedback on examination findings as much as possible. Monitoring height, weight and pubertal development are essential, and plotting these on to a growth chart and explaining it in the context of the normal range can be very reassuring for the adolescent.

Other health considerations in adolescents

- *Scoliosis*: higher rates in adolescent girls. Screening by clinical examination should be undertaken.
- *Sports injuries*: common as a result of participation in (contact) sports.
- *Immunisation status*: some infectious diseases are known to have incidence peaks in adolescents (e.g. meningococcal disease, measles, HPV). Opportunistic enquiry may lead to better uptake of adolescent immunisations. See chapter 9, Immunisation, p. 117.
- *Sexual health*: respectful inquiry may identify individuals at risk of the physical or emotional sequelae of adolescent sexual relationships. It also offers the opportunity to educate young people about contraceptive options and prevention of sexually transmitted infections. See chapter 28, Gynaecological conditions, p. 357.
- *Substance misuse*: identify those at risk. Taking a non-judgemental, 'harm minimisation' approach leads to preservation of rapport. Over time, important health messages can be conveyed and reasons for using drugs explored. The management of acute intoxication states is presented in chapter 2, Poisoning and envenomation.

Young people with chronic diseases and disabilities

Young people with chronic disease and disability are frequently the most experienced consumers of the health system in the paediatric environment. Clinicians are encouraged to acknowledge and respect the experience and views of these young people and their families.

Conflict of priorities

It is not uncommon for a conflict of priorities to occur between the therapeutic goals of the clinician (focused on disease control and management) and the developmental goals that are frequently the main concern of young people. For example, a young person with persistent asthma who goes on a school camp may be too embarrassed to take their preventer medication while on camp, preferring instead to put up with the unknown consequences (and the unspoken wishful thinking that their asthma will be fine). Negotiating management approaches with the young person is the key to achieving medical goals in ways that the young person is developmentally comfortable with. Providing the young person with a choice of acceptable management options is one useful strategy.

Adherence

Promoting adherence with treatment regimens is a challenge for clinicians, irrespective of the age of the patient. It can be especially difficult with adolescents with chronic disease, as they are generally far less influenced by long-term health goals than adults are. There may be conflict between the young person's (developmentally appropriate) pursuit of increasing autonomy and independence, and the clinician and parents' desire to improve their health. Practical tips include:

- Provide a clear rationale for all treatments.
- Simplify the treatment regimen.
- Focus on developing treatment routines.
- Discuss the acceptability of treatment in relationship to peers and education.
- Use simple language and write down all instructions.
- Don't use threats.
- Work with both parents and young people. Parents may need to be more involved, or encouraged to 'back off' and not be overprotective.

Promoting self-management

As young people with chronic disease mature, they gradually take on increasing responsibility for managing their health. It is important that both clinicians and parents have developmentally appropriate expectations of self-management. It is challenging for both clinicians and parents to educate and empower young people to manage as much of their chronic condition as possible.

Examples of specific elements of self-management include the adolescent being able to:

- Name and explain their condition.
- Explain why each medication is necessary.
- Remember to take their medication.
- Arrange repeat prescriptions before medication runs out.
- Be able to consult with doctors (see the doctor alone, ask and answer questions, arrange and cancel appointments).
- Develop a desire to be independent with health care.
- Prioritise their health over (some) other desires.

Multidisciplinary teams and mixed messages

The value of the multidisciplinary team is well established. However, there is the potential for individual health professionals within the team to give conflicting messages to young people and their families. Excellent communication within the team is crucial to ensure that a mutually agreed set of messages is delivered to the young person and their family.

Working across the sectors

The emotional health and well-being of young people is influenced by many factors, including families, peers and schools. It is valuable to gain information from these other sources, provided young people and their parents consent to the sharing of health information by the clinician with other agencies. Sources may include:

- School and other educational agencies.
- Welfare agencies.
- Recreational programmes.
- Peer support groups.

Transition to adult health care

Transition is the purposeful and planned movement of adolescents with chronic diseases and disability from child-centred to adult-oriented healthcare systems. The term 'transfer' refers to the physical move from one healthcare setting to another. In contrast, 'transition' refers to the process of facilitating developmentally appropriate self-management and generally requires the acquisition of knowledge, attitudes and skills over time. This skill set starts to develop well before transfer to adult health care and continues after any physical move. From the time of diagnosis, anticipation of transfer to an adult setting is one way of ensuring that the physical move is truly part of a broader transition process. Seeing young people alone for at least part of the health consultation from the age of 14–15 years will actively promote self-management skills and facilitate successful transition to adult health care.

A planned and coordinated transfer to adult health care is essential. Community providers, such as GPs, are an important source of continuity of care. When adult tertiary care is indicated, identifying an adult specialist and team that is both interested and capable of providing tertiary care is fundamental. A detailed medical and allied health summary should be compiled and clearly communicated to adult providers.

Adolescents with intellectual or complex disability

The health assessment of adolescents with intellectual and/or complex medical disabilities requires the same diligence and respect as afforded to all patients. The aetiology and treatment of acute distress can be difficult to interpret in adolescents with intellectual or complex disabilities; see chapter 14, Developmental delay and disability, p. 170.

Young people with intellectual disability have variable potential for independent living and self-management. Capability is assessed over the course of childhood and adolescence and it is important to listen to reports from parents, teachers and other community workers who know the patient well. In the long term, GPs often play a central role in the provision of adult medical care for these patients; however, those with complex medical issues often benefit from transfer to specialised clinics.

High-risk young people

High-risk young people include those with significant health risk behaviours (e.g. regular drug use) or mental health problems. A small proportion of young people are considered to be at very high health risk. This includes adolescents who are socially disadvantaged by homelessness, those engaged in multiple health risk behaviours, those with major mental health problems or those within the juvenile justice setting. These young people commonly do not receive appropriate health care. Close consultation and liaison with existing case-managers in the community is a priority and can be more effective than referral to new services. Case managers may be based within a range of community-based facilities, such as general practice, youth mental health services, or protective services. Youth-focused services are preferred to adult specialist services. Young people whose families are chaotic or whose parents have a mental disorder are especially vulnerable.

Adolescent medicine units

Young people who require admission to hospital prefer to be nursed with other people their own age. Adolescent inpatient wards provide developmentally appropriate nursing, recreation and peer support. Specialist adolescent medicine units are increasingly available in Australia. Common reasons for referral include:

- Complex health problems which are relatively unique to the adolescent age group, including eating disorders, deliberate self-harm and suicide attempts, school problems and behaviour disorders.
- Problems occurring at the interface between adolescent general health and adolescent mental health, such as early depression, psychosomatic disorders and chronic fatigue syndrome.
- Complex interactions between young people, disease and disease treatments, including poor adherence.
- Concerns about physical growth, puberty and sexual behaviours.
- Complex problems requiring access to community networks and programmes dealing with young people.

Adolescent mental health

The notion that adolescence is a time of inevitable emotional turmoil, with few implications for future mental health, has given way to a view that the teens and early twenties are critical years for the development of major psychiatric disorders that persist into adulthood (see also chapter 16, Child psychiatry). Major disorders with high rates of first onset in young people include:

- Depression and self-harm.
- Anxiety disorders.
- Obsessional neurosis.
- Schizophrenia and drug-induced psychoses.
- Bipolar affective disorders.
- Substance misuse.
- Personality disorders.
- Anorexia and bulimia nervosa.

The recognition and early diagnosis of adolescent mental health disorders is a clinical challenge. Presenting features may be less well developed than in an adult population.

Development

The mounting evidence that psychological and social treatments are most effective at this early stage of illness underlines the necessity for early diagnosis and referral for treatment.

Adolescent mental health problems commonly arise in the context of interpersonal and social problems. There is an increasing understanding that puberty marks the transition to a phase where new mental disorders commonly begin. During assessment and treatment, consideration should be given to recent stresses arising from grief (e.g. death or illness in the family or among friends), conflict (e.g. victimisation by peers or arguments with parents), relationship breakdowns and problems with school work. Many young people have longer-standing problems with parents, school and a lack of emotional and interpersonal skills to deal with the developmental tasks of adolescence (e.g. difficulties in initiating social contact, dealing with new sexual feelings and negotiating greater independence within the family). It is useful to assess aspects of lifestyle that contribute to good mental health (e.g. regular exercise, sleeping and eating patterns) rather than poor mental health (e.g. substance misuse).

Depression, deliberate self-harm and suicide

After motor vehicle accidents, suicide is the next most common cause of death in 15–25 year olds in Australia. Factors most commonly associated with completed suicide are a history of deliberate self-harm, major depression, substance abuse and antisocial behaviour (see also chapter 16, Child psychiatry).

About 1/200 young people present to emergency departments each year for deliberate acts of self-harm, typically in the form of an overdose. An even greater number do not present for medical care at all. In most instances, deliberate self-harm is not true suicidal behaviour with the intent of causing death; however, most self-harm is associated with a degree of psychiatric disturbance. Key features of assessment of the potentially suicidal adolescent are shown in Table 15.3. Assessment of the act of self-harm should include:

- Attention to suicidal intent.
- Perceived lethality of the act.
- Actual harm incurred.
- Degree of planning.
- Actions taken by the patient after the event.

Assessment should also be made of any associated psychiatric disorders, and the level of social and interpersonal difficulties in a teenager's life. Depression is the most common major psychiatric disorder of young people with symptoms similar to those found in adults. Typical symptoms include:

- Extended periods of low mood.
- Loss of pleasure in activities.
- Irritability.
- Fatigue.
- Somatic complaints.
- Social withdrawal.

Table 15.3 Assessment of suicide risk following an act of self-harm

Act itself	Impulsive or planned?
	Suicidal intent?
	Method and perceived lethality?
	Does life feel worthless or hopeless?
	Any acute precipitant?
	Actions post attempt (e.g. disclosure)?
Background	Stressors (family and peer relationships, school, sexuality)
	Recent suicidal ideation or attempts
Co-morbidity	Depression
	Drug and alcohol use
	Anxiety disorders
	Personality disorders (disturbed past relationships and behaviours)

- Impaired concentration and deteriorating function at school.
- Early and mid insomnia.
- Suicidal ideation.

In most instances, a teenager will give a better account of these symptoms than parents or other informants. Assessment should include the consideration of organic causes (e.g. recent corticosteroid therapy, hypothyroidism, or substance abuse). Adolescents recently commenced on certain anxiolytic drugs may also be at increased risk of suicidality. Mood fluctuations in response to a significant stressor may improve with short-term problem-solving strategies, but persistent low mood lasting longer than a few weeks is likely to require specific treatment. This may include:

- Psychotherapy (cognitive behavioural and inter-personal psychotherapies have been shown to be effective), **and/or**
- Antidepressant medication; selective serotonin re-uptake inhibitors (SSRI) are often used as first line antidepressants as these are usually well tolerated and are safe.

Families provide an important context for adolescent mental health care. Communication with parents about the meaning of a diagnosis of depression as well as the likely time-course and treatment of an episode is usual. Where family conflict is prominent, family therapy may be an important part of the management.

The violent young person and emergency restraint

Physical restraint and emergency sedation should be used only when other reasonable methods of calming the patient down are unsuccessful. **A patient who is acting out and does not need acute medical or psychiatric care should be discharged from**

hospital rather than restrained. Alternative means of calming the patient include prevention of a crisis by anticipating and identifying irritable behaviour (consider the patient's past history), early involvement of mental health services, provision of a safe 'containing' environment, listening and talking, and possibly a plan of collaborative sedation (e.g. patient agreeing to oral medication).

When restraint is required, a coordinated team approach is essential, with roles clearly defined and swift action taken. Unless contraindicated, sedation should usually accompany physical restraint.

Emergency restraint should be considered in any patient who requires urgent medical or psychiatric care, who has aggressive and combative behaviour which is:

- Compromising the provision of urgent medical treatment (physical or psychiatric).
- Placing the patient at risk of self-harm.
- Placing staff at risk.

Contra-indications to physical restraint and emergency sedation include:

- Safe containment possible via alternative means.
- Inadequate personnel/setting/equipment.
- Situation judged as too dangerous, e.g. patient has a weapon (call police if there is concern about the safety of staff or others).
- Known adverse reaction to drugs usually used (e.g. neuroleptic, malignant or other acute brain syndromes related to trauma or infection).

Procedure

1 Establish roles, including defining person in charge (usually attending doctor).
2 Assemble team. Person in charge to assemble team of seven people.
3 Draw up drugs. **Drugs of preference are midazolam 5 mg, and haloperidol 5 mg (draw up together).** Ensure benztropine available.
4 Secure the patient quickly and calmly. At least five people are required – one for the head, and one for each limb (assign roles before approaching the patient). The patient should be prone, with hands and feet held flexed behind back.
5 **Administer midazolam 5 mg (onset rapid) and haloperidol 5 mg (onset 15– 20 min) by intramuscular injection into lateral thigh.** Beware the risk of needle-stick injury. Further titrated doses of 0.1 mg/kg may be required (preferably i.v.).
6 Sedated patients must have continuous oxygen saturation monitoring. They must have a nurse present continuously, with close observation of conscious state, respiration, heart rate, blood pressure and temperature.
7 Explain the procedure to the parents/carers if possible.
8 After restraint the patient must have a complete medical and mental health assessment to guide subsequent management. In some cases certification and transfer to an in-patient mental health facility may be required (Section 9 of the Mental Health Act 1986). Consider the need for ongoing physical restraint and/or for ongoing sedation.
9 Document fully in the patient's unit record.

Complications of emergency sedation include anaphylactic reactions, respiratory depression, hypotension, tachycardia and extrapyramidal reactions. Dystonia may occur with major tranquillisers, particularly as the benzodiazepine is wearing off – treat with benztropine (0.02 mg/kg i.v. or i.m.) or repeated small doses of diazepam.

Eating disorders

Anorexia nervosa and bulimia nervosa typically arise in the early to mid-teens. The most common eating disorders to present clinically are sub-syndromal forms where the mental state is similar but the full picture has not developed. Such disorders may pass spontaneously but should be treated seriously. Where symptoms persist after 3 months, referral for more specific treatment is warranted.

Adolescent dieting is the usual forerunner of an eating disorder. Although most dieters do not go on to develop an eating disorder, preoccupation with dieting that leads to the avoidance of other activities (e.g. not going out with friends because of feeling fat) deserves attention.

Anorexia nervosa

Diagnostic criteria of anorexia nervosa are:
- Refusal to maintain body weight over a minimum normal weight for age and height.
- Intense fear of gaining weight or becoming fat, even though underweight.
- Distorted body image.
- Amenorrhoea.

Severity indices of postpubertal anorexia nervosa include the current weight, rate of weight loss, methods employed (e.g. abstinence, self-induced vomiting, purging, exercise) and any associated depression or other mental health disturbance (e.g. obsessional neuroses). Consideration should be given to the exclusion of other primary psychiatric disorders (e.g. major depression or obsessional neurosis) and physical disorders (thyrotoxicosis and malabsorption). The earlier the onset of the disorder (e.g. peripubertal), the greater the concern for long-term physical complications such as growth retardation and reduced bone mineral density.

Management

- Multidisciplinary outpatient care is the model of care preferred by most specialist centres. They commonly include input from medical, nutritional and mental health professionals.
- Hospital admission is indicated in adolescents where there is evidence of physiological compromise (e.g. bradycardia and hypotension), rather than the extent of weight loss *per se*. Generally, admission is indicated before significant metabolic or physiological complications (e.g. hypokalaemia) are evident. In effect, admission is indicated where outpatient treatments have failed.
- Refeeding is the mainstay of most acute admissions. Nasogastric feeding is commonly used in inpatient settings to achieve physiological stability. Refeeding syndrome (with significant metabolic and physiological consequences) can be fatal. It can follow parenteral, NGT and oral refeeding. Close attention must be paid to electrolyte and cardiovascular status, especially in the first 72 h following refeeding (see chapter 6, Nutrition, p. 99).

Bulimia nervosa

Bulimia nervosa is characterised by frequent loss of control of eating (bingeing), self-induced vomiting and fear of fatness. Intercurrent depression and difficulties with impulse control in other areas (e.g. alcohol use, sexual behaviour and deliberate risk-taking) are common. The psychosocial context in which bulimia arises is often similar to that found in depression, but an antecedent history of dieting is usually evident.

Treatment is usually on an outpatient basis, and focal psychotherapies such as cognitive-behavioural therapy (CBT) are effective both in individual and group treatment settings. Antidepressants such as SSRIs are indicated when severe depressive symptoms are evident, as well as to prevent relapse.

Chronic fatigue syndrome

Chronic fatigue syndrome (CFS) is characterised by unexplained, prolonged (>3 months) and disabling fatigue associated with constitutional and neuropsychological symptoms. It occurs in children, although is more common in adolescents. Most patients have a history of suspected or confirmed viral illness.

Presenting features can include
- Prolonged fatigue.
- Increased need for sleep.
- Pain (headaches, myalgias, abdominal pain).
- Nausea.
- Depressive symptoms.
- Loss of concentration, difficulty with balance.

Examination and investigations (FBE, ESR, U&E, creatinine, LFT, TFT and urinalysis) are usually normal. The diagnosis is a clinical one and differential diagnoses that must be considered include connective tissue disease, inflammatory bowel disease, coeliac disease, gastrointestinal infection and depression.

Management
- Must be developed with patient, family and local doctor in a team approach.
- Individual management plan that is focused on addressing the psychosocial features and impact of their illness.
- Balanced activities and encouragement of social contact and reintegration into normal life.
- Symptomatic management of focal symptoms, e.g. sleep difficulties.

Prognosis
- Most recover with normal function, but it often takes several years (2–5).
- A small number remain more chronically unwell.

CHAPTER 16

Child psychiatry

Maria McCarthy
Chidambaram Prakash

Mental health is defined as a state of emotional and social well-being in which the individual realises their own abilities, can cope with the normal stresses of life, can work productively or fruitfully, and is able to make a contribution to their community.

One in five people will experience mental health problems in their lifetime. The prevalence of mental health problems among children and adolescents in Australia (including subclinical symptoms) is ~14%. Most childhood mental health problems are managed by GPs, paediatricians, schools and community services. Only a small percentage of children and young people are treated by specialist mental health services. As medical practitioners are often well placed to identify mental health problems and facilitate management, it is important that they develop some skills in developmental and mental health assessment. It is important to remember that the family is the most influential force in a child's life.

Key skills required by medical practitioners

- To listen and engage children and young people and their families to discuss emotional and psychological issues in a comfortable manner.
- To manage common and uncomplicated mental health problems either independently or with consultation from mental health professionals.
- To identify when mental health issues are serious, complex and/or chronic and to facilitate appropriate referral.

Approach to mental health problems
Interview and assessment

Each interview of a child and family should lead to an assessment and evaluation of the child (including their strengths and difficulties) and the family's contribution to these difficulties and capacity to help overcome them. Parents are respectful of the clinician who tries to understand their child directly.

- See the child with their parents and siblings.
- Aim to speak with the child directly and engage other family members. This enables a therapeutic relationship to be established with the child.
- Assess the presenting problem, noting the language and narrative used by the child and family.

Paediatric Handbook, 8th edition. By Kate Thomson, Dean Tey and Michael Marks. Published 2009 by Blackwell Publishing, ISBN: 978-1-4051-7400-8.

- Observe the verbal and non-verbal interaction between the child and each parent and siblings if present.
- Aim to make a formulation of the problems based on the initial assessment, decide on an initial management plan and whether to refer for specialist mental health assessment.
- A clinician needs to be able to answer the following questions:
  - What is the problem now?
  - Why is the the child presenting at this stage?
  - What is this child usually like?
  - How does this child's mind work currently?

History

- Presenting problem: duration, severity, exacerbating and relieving factors?
- What is the parent's ideas about this problem?
- Family medical and psychiatric history.
- Perinatal history, including experience of the pregnancy, delivery and the child's early months.
- The child's feeding, sleeping and toileting habits where appropriate.
- Friendships, relationships within the family.
- Possible traumatic events at home and school (directly experienced or witnessed). Consider physical or sexual abuse and ask sensitive questions directly where appropriate.

The child and family should come to feel the problem is taken seriously and understood by the clinician.

Mental state examination
See Table 16.1.

Principles of intervention
At the conclusion of the therapeutic assessment the clinician should form a provisional diagnosis and assess the severity and urgency of the presenting problem.

Options for intervention

- Explain and reassure if the problem is transient or minor. Suggest further contact with GP or community counsellor.
- Further mental health intervention through paediatric or primary care service. Offer follow-up appointment or telephone contact.
- Telephone consultation with regional mental health service or a colleague.

Available mental health interventions

- Brief therapies – family or individual.
- CBT.
- Psychodynamic psychotherapy.
- Family and parent therapy.
- Supportive intervention for the child and family (clinic, school or home based).
- Psychopharmacology.

Table 16.1 Mental state examination

Observe the child's play and behaviour before, during and after the formal consultation. The young child communicates through play. Access to simple toys (e.g. a doll, a ball, or pencil and paper) allows the clinician to assess the child's level of self-organisation as well as their inner world of imagination and thought. Ask the child to draw a person or a house. Interview with the parents.

1. General appearance and behaviour
- Observe the child's appearance, demeanour, gait, motor activity and relationship with examiner.
- What is the child's apparent mood?
- Do they seem sad, happy, fearful, perplexed, angry, agitated?

2. Speech
- How does the child communicate? Consider rate, volume (amount), tone, articulation and reaction time.

3. Affect
- Observe the range, reactivity, communicability, and appropriateness to the context and congruence with the reported mood state.

4. Thought
- Stream: Are there major interruptions to flow of thinking?
- Content: What is the child thinking about?
- Do they seem preoccupied by inner thoughts, obsessional ideas, delusions, fears or have suicidal ideation?

5. Perception
- Are there hallucinations, illusions, imagery in various sensory modalities?

6. Cognition
- Conscious state and orientation: Does the child know where they are, what time it is, who they are and who is around them?
- Concentration: Is the child able to concentrate on developmentally appropriate tasks?
- Memory: How well do they remember things of the recent and more distant past?
- Do they understand questions posed to them and how well do they problem-solve?

7. Insight
- Does the child seem aware of their illness?

8. Judgement
- Personal (as inferred from answers to questions about themselves), social (as inferred from social behaviour) and test situation (answers to specific questions).

Much of this information can be obtained from the child in a non-threatening way by asking them directly in detail about things such as their family, home, school, address, telephone number and their immediate context.

When and how to make a mental health referral

Referral to mental health services should be discussed with families. The manner in which this is done can influence their engagement with these services, their expectations and understanding and even treatment outcome.

- Avoid coercion (unless the patient is at serious risk to themselves or others).
- Ensure an open and honest discussion about why you believe a mental health referral would be helpful.
- Explain what the child and family should expect from an initial mental health consultation in clear and simple language.
- Examine your own responses/feelings about mental health and ensure you do not impose these views on a child or family, e.g. being sceptical about the usefulness of mental health services but referring anyway, or presenting the mental health clinician as the potential cure to all current and future difficulties!
- Where appropriate, continue your involvement and interest in a child and family.

Some children and families accept mental health referral readily, whereas others are wary or even openly opposed to referral. In the latter, referral may be discussed over a period of weeks or months before being made.

Stigma around mental health continues to be a powerful influence. Families may interpret the suggestion of a referral as an indication that you think they are 'mad' or 'crazy'. Such beliefs may not necessarily be overt, and reassurance is helpful.

Talking to children and families in plain language may help them accept mental health involvement. For example,

- Talk about the **stress** they are dealing with, or
- The **worries** they seem to have, or
- How **down** they have been feeling.

Children who are hospitalised or have been subjected to significant medical interventions need to be reassured that the mental health clinician is a talking person (rather than someone who gives needles). Terms such as 'the talking doctor' can be useful. Similarly, talking to parents about mental health 'colleagues' as you would talk about other medical/surgical referrals can help reduce stigma or concerns.

Common childhood problems

This section discusses anxiety and mood disorders, which are common mental health presentations to medical practitioners. More severe problems are also discussed but present less frequently than generalised anxiety disorders and mood disorders.

Anxiety disorders

Fear is a normal response to a frightful stimulus. Anxiety is a fear response that is abnormal in either context or extent. Anxiety is often seen as part of the child's coping with developmental challenges at various stages in life. Common symptoms of anxiety disorders are listed in Table 16.2.

- In infants and toddlers, anxiety often manifests at separation from parents.
- Preschoolers and school-age children may be fearful of the dark or specific situations.

Table 16.2 Common symptoms of anxiety disorders in children

Symptoms
Distress and agitation when separated from parents and home
School refusal
Pervasive worry and fearfulness
Restlessness and irritability
Timidity, shyness, social withdrawal
Terror of an object (e.g. dog)
Associated headache, stomach pain
Restless sleep and nightmares
Poor concentration, distractibility and learning problems
Reliving stressful event in repetitive play

Family factors
Parental anxiety, overprotection, separation difficulties
Parental (maternal) depression and agoraphobia
Family stress: marital conflict, parental illness, child abuse
Family history of anxiety

Reproduced with permission from Tonge B., *Medical Journal of Australia*, 1998; **168**: 241–8.

- Older children and adolescents may exhibit performance anxiety associated with exams, social situations, etc. Anxiety is most commonly experienced at times of transition, e.g. moving house, starting or changing schools.

Anxiety disorders may be characterised by:

- Persistent fears and/or developmentally inappropriate fears.
- Irrational worries or avoidance of specific situations that trigger anxiety.
- Impaired ability to perform normal activities (e.g. inability to attend school).

Generalised anxiety disorder

Generalised anxiety disorder is persistent and pervasive anxiety that is not contextually based. This includes feeling 'on edge' at most times, with bodily symptoms such as tachycardia, palpitations, dizziness, headache and 'butterflies in the tummy'.

School refusal

School refusal is often an indicator of separation difficulties, where the child is frightened to leave their parent or home. Children refusing to attend school often present with somatic complaints such as abdominal pain.

It is important to ascertain the basis of the child's anxiety, which may be related to factors at home, including a parent's physical or mental health, difficulties with parental or peer relationships, school factors such as bullying or academic performance.

Obsessive-compulsive disorder

Obsessive-compulsive disorder (OCD) is one of the more severe forms of childhood anxiety disorders. Although it is relatively rare (1–2% of children and adolescents, more commonly in males), OCD can be associated with childhood anxiety, depressive and pervasive developmental disorders. Symptoms include intrusive thoughts and a variety of compulsive/ritualistic behaviours. Common co-morbid conditions include social anxiety disorder, separation anxiety, agoraphobia (fear of open and public spaces) and generalised anxiety disorder.

Traumatic stress disorders

Post-traumatic stress disorder

Trauma can directly contribute to mental health difficulties in children and young people, and can manifest as post-traumatic stress disorder (PTSD). See Table 16.3 for common symptoms of PTSD in children.

- Children show a variable response to trauma.
- PTSD is **not** an expected outcome of trauma.
- The development of PTSD is not strongly correlated to the severity of the trauma.
- The cluster of symptoms characteristic of PTSD are intrusion, avoidance and arousal.
- PTSD criteria are not particularly sensitive to trauma effects in very young children.
- PTSD is more common in girls than boys.
- Common co-morbid conditions include specific phobia, social phobia and agoraphobia.

Paediatric medical traumatic stress

Children and families may experience traumatic stress response as a result of their experiences associated with pain, injury, serious illness, medical procedures or invasive medical treatment. This cluster of symptoms has been referred to recently as paediatric medical traumatic stress (PMTS). This trauma may be chronic, repetitive, predictable (such as associated with medical procedures) and involve interpersonal interaction. This is referred to as *complex trauma*.

- The child and/or family may experience symptoms of arousal, re-experiencing and avoidance in response to a medical event.
- Symptoms may vary in intensity but may impact on general functioning.
- Symptoms may not reach diagnostic criteria of PTSD or acute stress disorder (ASD) but can occur along a continuum of intensity (from normative stress reactions to persistent and distressing symptoms).
- *Subjective* appraisals of threat rather than *objective* disease/medical factors seem more predictive of stress responses.
- There is debate regarding the need to acknowledge complex trauma experienced by some children as a distinct form of trauma stress disorder.

Depression

Childhood depression is probably underdiagnosed. Symptoms vary according to the age and developmental stage of the child. Infants and younger children may present with irritable mood, failure to gain weight and lack of enjoyment in play and other activities. Children tend to exhibit more symptoms of anxiety (e.g. phobias, separation anxiety), somatic complaints, irritability with temper tantrums and behavioural problems. This is in contrast to adults with depression who are more likely to have delusions and serious suicide attempts. See Table 16.4 for common symptoms of childhood depression.

Depression becomes increasingly common in adolescence (1/4 experience a major depressive episode) and is associated with an increased risk of suicide (see chapter 15, Adolescent health, page 182). Adolescents tend to present with more sleep and appetite disturbance, delusions and impairment of functioning. Compared to adults they tend to have more behavioural problems and fewer neurovegetative symptoms.

Major depressive disorder has a prevalence of 2% in children, and 4–8% in adolescents. There is a male to female ratio of 1 : 1 in childhood and 1 : 2 in adolescents. By 18 years old, the cumulative incidence is 20%. Co-morbidities are common and include anxiety disorder, conduct disorder or attention deficit hyperactivity disorder (ADHD).

Incidence of co-morbidities
- In patients with anxiety disorder, 10–20% have co-morbid depression.
- In patients with depressive disorder, >50% have co-morbid anxiety.
- Average age of onset of co-morbid anxiety and depressive disorders are: anxiety 7.2 years, dysthymia 10.8 years, major depressive disorder 13.8 years.
- In patients with disruptive behaviour disorders, 15–30% have co-morbid anxiety.

Assessment and management of anxiety and mood disorders
General principles
- A thorough history should include details of anxiety symptoms, length of time anxiety has persisted, the degree to which the child is impaired in their day-to-day activities and their relationships.
- Behavioural analysis: how is the problem manifest in the child's behaviour?
- Cognitive analysis: what are the child's thoughts and emotions associated with the problem?
- Family, school and developmental assessment.
- Individual interviews of the child or adolescent to help understand the nature of the symptoms and their impact as age appropriate. This will also help with building a therapeutic rapport with the child or adolescent.
- Structured instruments and questionnaires may be useful. These include the Anxiety Disorder Interview Schedule, Diagnostic Interview Schedule for Children IV, Revised Child Manifest Anxiety Scale, Childhood Depression Inventory, Children's Depression Rate Scale and Yale Brown Obsessive Compulsive Scale.

Specific features
Generalised anxiety/phobias
- If symptoms are mild, explore behavioural and/or family support interventions with the child and family and review.
- Specific fears (e.g. phobias) and more severe or generalised anxiety disorders will require referral to a mental health specialist.

School refusal
- Conduct a physical examination if the child presents with somatic symptoms.
- Assess the source of the anxiety and consider whether further management is required, e.g. family therapy, school-based services such as school counsellor etc.

Table 16.3 Common symptoms of post-traumatic stress disorder in children

Intrusive thoughts and 'Re-experiencing' of the event(s) – may be demonstrated through play, enactment or drawings

Fear of the dark

Nightmares

Difficulties getting to sleep and/or nocturnal waking

Separation anxiety

Generalised anxiety or fears

Developmental regression, e.g. continence, language skills

Social withdrawal

Irritability

Aggressive behaviour

Attention and concentration difficulties

Memory problems

Heightened sensitivity to other traumatic events

Reproduced with permission from Tonge B., *Medical Journal of Australia*, 1998; **168**: 241–8.

Table 16.4 Common symptoms of childhood depression

Symptoms
  Persistent depressed mood, unhappiness and irritability
  Loss of interest in play and friends
  Loss of energy and concentration
  Deterioration in school work
  Loss of appetite and no weight gain
  Disturbed sleep
  Thoughts of worthlessness and suicide (suicide attempts are rare before age 10 years, then increase)
  Somatic complaints (headaches, abdominal pain)
  Co-morbid anxiety, conduct disorder, ADHD, eating disorders or substance abuse

Family factors
  Family stress (ill or deceased parent, family conflict, parental separation)
  Repeated experience of failure or criticism
  Family history of depression

Reproduced with permission from Tonge B., *Medical Journal of Australia*, 1998; **168**: 241–8.

- Return to school is a high priority. If necessary this can be done by gradually increasing the child's time at school over a short period of time.

Obsessive-compulsive disorder

- Provide support and explanation to the patient and family.
- Refer for assessment and management by a mental health specialist.
- Principles of treatment are symptom control, improvement and maintenance of function.
- For children and adolescents with mild symptoms, CBT is the treatment of choice. For adolescents with more severe symptoms a combination of CBT and medication (SSRI, e.g. clomipramine) is indicated.

Post-traumatic stress disorder

Assessment

- PTSD can be diagnosed only when the traumatic event *precedes* the symptoms and symptoms are present for >1 month.
- Co-morbid mental health disorders such as anxiety disorder or depressive disorder can occur. Hence, some presenting symptoms may be indicative of these co-morbid disorders rather than PTSD.
- When symptoms have persisted beyond a period of a few days or weeks, refer to mental health services for further assessment and management.

Management

- Trauma-focused CBT has been shown to be effective. Techniques include graded exposure, cognitive processing, psycho-education, training in stress reduction, relaxation and positive self-talk.
- Medication is not first line treatment (only open-label studies have been conducted), unless co-morbid conditions such as depression are present. In such circumstances, propranolol, clonidine, risperidone and citalopram (an SSRI) can be used.

Paediatric medical traumatic stress

- Healthcare providers are well placed to modify stress experiences of patients and families in the medical context, subsequently reducing the risk of persistent symptoms. This can be done by:
  - Explaining procedures in a developmentally appropriate manner and checking the child's understanding.
  - Teaching parents how to comfort and reassure their children.
  - Looking for opportunities for the child to make decisions in their management, e.g. would they prefer to sit up or lie down, would they like for a parent to hold their hand.
  - Implementing good pain management practice (see chapter 4, Pain management).
  - Screen for persistent symptoms of distress post injury/illness.
- The National Child Traumatic Stress Network in the USA has developed resources for health professionals to enhance 'trauma informed' medical and nursing practice (The Pediatric Medical Traumatic Stress Toolkit for Health Care Providers) and has developed materials for children and families. See their website, *www.nctsnet.org*

Depression

Assessment

- Recognition is important, as untreated childhood depression increases the risk for depression in adulthood.
- Additionally, depression in childhood (and particularly in adolescence) increases the risk of suicide and self-harming behaviours.

Management

- Referral to local mental health services for further management is generally required.
- GPs can play an important role in providing ongoing support and counselling to the child and/or family.

- Psychotherapy is the first line treatment for mild to moderate mood disorder. Effective psychotherapies include CBT and interpersonal therapy for adolescents.
- Antidepressants (generally SSRIs) can be used for non-rapid cycling bipolar disorder, psychotic depression, depression with severe symptoms that prevents effective psychotherapy and poor response to adequate psychotherapy.
- Even when medications are indicated, it is important to address the psychosocial context through psychotherapy.

Suicide risk and self-harm
See chapter 15, Adolescent health, page 182.

Principles of psychotropic medications
- Limited application in early childhood.
- In strictly diagnosed ADHD, methylphenidate or dexamphetamine can enhance concentration and attention and reduce morbidity (see chapter 11, Common behavioural and developmental problems, p. 143).
- In severe depression, SSRIs such as fluoxetine may be helpful on a case-by-case basis with careful monitoring.
- In severe anxiety disorders, imipramine may be helpful.
- Benzodiazepines have no proven role in anxiety or depressive disorders in children, and may produce paradoxical agitation.
- In adolescents with psychosis, early treatment with newer antipsychotics in collaboration with specialised youth psychiatric services are beneficial.

SSRIs and suicidality
A number of studies have indicated that SSRIs are prescribed for a variety of childhood problems including anxiety disorders, major depressive episodes, ADHD and other disorders. Prescribing rates are increasing in Australia, USA and Europe.

There has been some concern regarding increased risk of suicidality and deliberate self-harm associated with SSRI use in children, although the evidence to date is relatively weak. Risk of deliberate self-harm appears to be highest in the first 2–4 weeks of starting an SSRI. The following guidelines should therefore be adhered to:
- Start with a low dose and increase slowly. Side effects are dose-dependent, but efficacy is not. Always use the lowest effective dose.
- Only use as an adjunct to psychotherapy.
- Explain to parents (and child if appropriate) about possible adverse effects of antidepressants. Discuss the issues of deliberate self-harm and suicidality and the need for close monitoring, especially in the first 2–4 weeks.
- Explain the discontinuation syndrome, which occurs when an SSRI is withdrawn abruptly. This can result in irritability, mood lability, insomnia, anxiety, vivid dreams, nausea, vomiting, headache, dizziness, tremor, dystonia, fatigue, myalgia, rhinorrhoea and chills.
- Monitor closely for adverse effects in the first 4 weeks; consider using structured rating instruments.

Psychosomatic problems

Somatic responses to stressful situations are common (e.g. sweating during a job interview, or diarrhoea before taking an exam). Somatic complaints in children are also believed to be relatively common and appear as physical sensations related to affective distress.

Psychosomatic or somatoform disorders refer to the presence of physical symptoms suggesting an underlying medical condition without such a condition being found, or where a medical problem cannot adequately account for the level of functional impairment.

Common symptoms include:

- Headache.
- Abdominal pain.
- Limb pain.
- Fatigue.
- Pain/soreness.
- Disturbance of vision.
- Symptoms suggestive of neurological disorders.

Conversion disorder may present with dramatic symptoms such as:

- Gait disturbance.
- Paraesthesia.
- Paralysis.
- Pseudoseizures.

In this situation the onset of the symptom is closely associated to a psychological stressor. Conversion disorders are generally relatively short-lived. They are often alleviated by identification and management of the stressor(s) and in some instances, symptomatic treatment of the physical problem.

Somatisation disorders may present in children whose families have a history of illnesses or psychosomatic disorders. Such patterns may be evident at a multigenerational level where physical symptoms appear to be the 'currency' by which affective states are communicated. Possible family relationship difficulties (including sexual abuse) should be considered as part of a thorough assessment.

Mental health problems associated with chronic illness

Children and adolescents with chronic illnesses such as asthma and diabetes may present with exacerbations of their physical symptoms that relate to their affective state. Such responses may be related to a precipitating stressor or may reflect the child's changing responses to their illness. Increased understanding of the illness and its implications and developmental changes will influence a child's response to their medical condition.

Children and adolescents may be angry, resent the limitations their condition imposes, and may be particularly sensitive to being different from their peers. Additionally, responses by their parents (e.g. over- or under-protectiveness) may contribute to adjustment problems. Along with somatisation, other difficulties may emerge, such as non-adherence with treatment and family relationship problems.

Management

Management depends on the nature, severity and duration of the problem. Some general principles are:

- It is important to recognise the child's physical symptoms as genuine and distressing.
- Thorough clinical examination, investigation and mental health assessment is usually required. Hospital admission may be required to facilitate this.
- Discussion of mind–body interactions can be useful. Discuss early on the possibility that psychological factors are contributing to symptoms or well-being. This may allow the child and family to begin to discuss possible psychological stressors, reducing resistance to mental health input.
- Symptomatic treatment (e.g. heat packs, relaxation exercises, physiotherapy, mild analgesia) may be appropriate, along with supportive counselling and/or mental health referral.
- Avoid medical over-investigation based on the family's coercion or unwillingness to consider psychological factors.
- It is important that the child and family do not feel they have 'wasted your time' if there is no evident medical problem. Maintain an interest in the child and family with a review appointment or follow-up telephone enquiry as appropriate.

Developmental and family psychiatry
Infant mental health

Infant mental health is an area of clinical work aimed at understanding the psychological and emotional development of infants from birth to 3 years and the particular difficulties that they and their families might face.

Babies come into the world with a range of capacities and vulnerabilities and, together with their parents, negotiate their way through the next months and years. This process of attachment, growth and development may be challenged by a range of experiences that stress or interrupt this course. Examples include traumatic events, developmental concerns, hospitalisation of the infant or parent, prematurity, illness or disability, an experience of loss, changing family circumstances or postnatal depression.

Referral to an appropriate mental health clinician may be considered for:

- Persistent crying, irritability or 'colic'.
- Gaze avoidance.
- Bonding difficulties.
- Slow weight gain.
- Persistent feeding or sleeping difficulties.
- Persistent behavioural symptoms, e.g. tantrums, nightmares, aggression.
- Family relationship problems.
- Infants with chronic ill health.
- Premature babies and their families.

Family relationship difficulties

A family-sensitive approach is crucial to the assessment and management of childhood mental health issues. Behavioural and/or emotional difficulties in a child can occur in the context of chronic family dysfunction. Conversely, such difficulties can arise in the context of well-functioning families where the child's temperament, personality or precipitating stressors may lead to behavioural/emotional difficulties for the child and/or parent–child relationship difficulties. When a child is presenting with behavioural and/or emotional difficulties, assessment should include an understanding of the family situation including:

- Family tree, living arrangements and caregiving roles.
- Quality of family relationships.
- Early attachments/relationships.
- History of significant losses, stressors, precipitating factors.
- Social/family support networks.
- Identifiable 'risk' factors such as poverty, illnesses, absent social supports.

Children can be symptom-bearers for family relationship difficulties. In such instances, treatment of the presenting symptom is unlikely to be successful in the long term without appropriate family and/or couple counselling.

When working with families:

- Conduct at least one family interview when dealing with a child with significant behavioural or emotional difficulties.
- Interview all family members (including siblings, who are often insightful commentators on family life) and provide an empathic response to each member's point of view. In the case of young children, observing and commenting upon play themes is useful.
- Do not assume that different family members agree on what is the presenting problem. It is often useful to ask family members to rank their concerns such as:
  - *What is the problem you are most worried about today?*
  - *What is the number one worry you have at the moment . . . number 2 . . . number 3?*
  - *Who in the family is most worried about this problem? Who is the least worried?*
- If family members are not present, seek further understanding by questions such as:
  - *If your husband were here today, what would he say about this problem?*
  - *Who else in the family has noticed the changes you have described today?*
- Encouraging families to find solutions to their difficulties is more likely to provide long-term change. This may involve helping families identify negative or unhelpful patterns of interaction, helping families identify strengths and resilience and noting small changes/improvements.

Developmental disorders
Mental health problems occur in children with a wide range of developmental disorders. See chapter 11, Common behavioural and developmental problems and chapter 14, Developmental delay and disability.

Oppositional behaviour
See chapter 11, Common behavioural and developmental problems, p. 139.

Grief and loss

Experiences of grief and loss are inevitable. Where losses are severe or traumatic or where a child has pre-existing vulnerabilities, these experiences can contribute to mental health problems or result in complicated grief reactions. Children may believe that they caused a loved one's death or illness. Bereaved children may feel different from other children or have difficulty managing the reactions of their peers.

In most instances, the bereaved child can be supported through family, school, community and religion. Family-based counselling/therapy can be helpful to address the child's grief in the context of other family members' reactions; it may feel less 'blaming' for the child.

Grief and loss experiences for children occur in situations other than bereavement (e.g. chronic illness, refugee status or having a parent with a mental illness). Parental divorce is a common source of grief and loss in children. Grief associated with this situation can be complicated and often remains unacknowledged by significant adults. Children may experience feelings of guilt and self-blame, harbour fantasies of a parental reunion, struggle with divided loyalties and feel anxious about their own future relationships. Feelings of anger, rejection and sadness may lead to behavioural or emotional manifestations of their grief.

Management

- Acknowledge the child's loss in an empathic and appropriate manner; this can be helpful even when a loss is not recent.
- Where a grieving child presents with behavioural or emotional difficulties, gently probe their beliefs about why the loss occurred. This can help the clinican understand the child's predicament. For example:
  - *Sometimes when I see children who have lost their (mum/brother, etc.) they feel like it's their fault that they died or got sick. Does it ever feel like that for you?*
  - *How do you imagine your life would be different if your mum and dad were still together?*
  - *Why do you think people get (cancer, etc.)?*
- Assist the family in gaining access to appropriate support and counselling.
- Seek further specialist mental health services when a child continues to exhibit extreme distress or prolonged behavioural or emotional difficulties.

Eating disorders

See chapter 15, Adolescent health, p. 185.

Psychosis

Psychosis is a general term for states in which mental function is grossly impaired, so that reality testing and insight are lacking, and delusions, hallucinations, incoherence, thought disorder or disorganised behaviour may be apparent.

In the case of 'organic' psychosis there may also be a clouding of consciousness, confusion and disorientation, as well as perceptual disturbances. Short-term memory impairment is common in organic brain syndromes.

Anticholinergics, anticonvulsants, antidepressants, antimalarials and benzodiazepines have been associated with psychotic reactions in young people, as have substances of abuse (amphetamines, cocaine, marijuana, opiates and hallucinogens). Organic brain syndromes may follow even minor head injury.

Adolescents may occasionally present in an acutely psychotic state with no prior history of drug ingestion or head injury. In this case the possibility of a 'functional' psychosis, schizophrenia or bipolar disorder should be considered. The latter often presents with an elated mood, grandiose ideas, increased energy and reduced sleep requirements.

Management
Children presenting with such symptoms require admission for a full psychiatric and medical assessment.

USEFUL RESOURCES
- *www.nctsnet.org* – National Child Traumatic Stress Network. Excellent website containing practical resources for families and healthcare professionals.
- *www.aacap.org* – American Academy of Child & Adolescent Psychiatry. Contains useful practice parameters for doctors and information for families.
- *www.nimh.nih.gov* [Health & Outreach > Topics > Children & Adolescents] – National Institute of Mental Health in USA with parent information.
- *www.zerotothree.org* – Excellent resource for infant mental health in this Washington-based organisation.

CHAPTER 17
Child abuse

Anne Smith
Chris Sanderson

Healthcare providers should consider the possibility of child abuse whenever they evaluate and treat an injured child. Doctors are encouraged to access advice and opinion from local medical professionals with expertise in this area. As the body of knowledge related to child abuse and the demand for expert court testimony increase, there is an additional expectation that doctors will provide evidence and opinion that will withstand the rigours of cross examination in court.

In addition, professionals working with children should remain informed about, and vigilant for, warning signs of children's vulnerability to abuse or harm. Whenever a child's living circumstances suggest the possibility of risk of harm, a comprehensive psychosocial assessment should be carried out. A holistic, ecological view of children's vulnerability to harm promotes effective interventions that alter the trajectory of the child's life for the better.

Mandatory reporting
In most states of Australia, medical practitioners are legally required to notify the relevant statutory authorities about children who have experienced, or are likely to experience, child abuse. The wording of legislation varies between states/territories in Australia but the common theme is a legal requirement to notify local child protection agencies when child abuse is considered. Medical practitioners are encouraged to inform themselves of relevant legislation in their own state or territory.

Definitions
Child abuse
Child abuse is the harming (physically, emotionally or sexually), ill treatment, abuse, neglect, or deprivation of any child or young person.

Child physical abuse
Child physical abuse is physical trauma inflicted on a child. Objective evidence of this violence may include bruising, burns and scalds, head injuries, fractures, intra-abdominal and intrathoracic trauma, suffocation and drowning. Injury can be caused by impact, penetration, heat, a caustic substance, a chemical or a drug, but the definition also includes physical harm sustained as a result of fabricated or induced-illness by carer (Munchausen syndrome by proxy).

Paediatric Handbook, 8th edition. By Kate Thomson, Dean Tey and Michael Marks. Published 2009 by Blackwell Publishing, ISBN: 978-1-4051-7400-8.

Child neglect
Child neglect is the failure of caregivers to adequately provide for and safeguard the health, safety and well-being of the child. It applies to any situation in which the basic needs of a child are not met with respect to nutrition, hygiene, clothing or shelter. It also comprises failure to provide access to adequate medical care, mental health care, dental care, stimulation to promote development, or attendance to a child's moral and spiritual care and education.

Child sexual abuse
Child sexual abuse is the involvement of dependent, developmentally immature children and adolescents in sexual activities that they may not fully comprehend and to which they are unable to give consent.

Psychological maltreatment
Psychological maltreatment of children and young people consists of acts that are judged on the basis of a combination of community standards and professional expertise to be psychologically damaging. Such acts are committed by individuals, singly or collectively, who by their characteristics (e.g. age, status, knowledge and organisational form) are in a position of differential power that renders a child vulnerable. Such acts damage, immediately or ultimately, the behavioural, cognitive, affective or physical functioning of the child. Examples of psychological maltreatment include acts of spurning (hostility, rejecting or degrading), terrorising, isolating, exploiting or corrupting and denying emotional responsiveness.

Signs of neglect and emotional abuse are often non-specific, but suspicion should be raised when infants, preschoolers or school age children behave in the following ways:
- Persistently angry, socially avoidant, defiant, disobedient and overactive.
- Anxiously attached, watchful of, or ambivalent to, their parents.
- Limited ability to enjoy things.
- Low self-esteem, depressed or unresponsive.
- Developmental and emotional retardation, poor social skills and over-inhibition.

Signs of sexual abuse are also usually non-specific, but may include the above and various behavioural problems (phobias, bad dreams, eating and sleeping disorders, depression, school problems or delinquency). There may be overt manifestations of sexual preoccupation, including precocious and inappropriate sexual activity, promiscuity and aggressive sexual behaviour.

Mental health service psychiatric consultation is often useful in conjunction with the involvement of local child protection services.

Child physical abuse
In assessing and treating an injured child, there is a duty to accurately diagnose or exclude child abuse in the differential diagnosis. Most injured children examined have injuries as a result of accidental childhood trauma. If the patterns of injury are familiar and easily recognised as usually being caused by accidental trauma and the injuries are consistent with the

alleged mechanisms of injury, then the child can be investigated and treated without mentioning the possibility of inflicted trauma.

Aims of assessment

- Differentiate accidental from deliberately inflicted trauma.
- State an opinion about the likely cause of the child's injuries.
- Investigate and manage all medical aspects of the child's care.
- Take action to protect the child from additional harm. This usually involves working in partnership with police, protective workers and support agencies.
- Intervene to prevent re-injury to this child or another child in the family.

Staff must discuss all cases of possible child abuse with a senior paediatric fellow or paediatrician. Consider child abuse especially when:

- A child has been severely injured.
- A child has had multiple injuries in the past.
- Any injury has occurred in a child <18 months old.
- History is inconsistent or the mechanism indeterminate.

History

Professionals dealing with injured children must become familiar with the manifestations of accidental and inflicted trauma and take a thorough and detailed history of the alleged mechanism of injury:

- Determine precisely when, where and how the injury occurred.
- Who provided the history and who (if anyone) witnessed the injury.
- Note the child's developmental capabilities.
- What previous injuries, illnesses or emergency department presentations the child has had.

Regardless of whether the injury initially appears to be inflicted or accidental, it is important to obtain details of the child's past medical, social and family history. See Table 17.1 on aspects of history which might alert health professionals to futher investigate.

Examination

A thorough physical examination must be performed. **A parent or legal guardian must give informed consent before the child is physically examined**. Injuries must be described and documented accurately. Record injuries on a body chart and use diagrams whenever possible. Accurate measurements are essential. Include details of the site, size, colour and shape of all injuries and skin lesions (including injuries thought to result from accidental trauma).

Look for:

- Skin injuries such as bruises, petechiae, lacerations abrasions and puncture wounds. Note injuries that may be inflicted by a human hand (finger marks from a slap or fingertip bruising from a firm grip) or an implement.
- Intra-oral injuries such as a torn frenulum, contused gums, dental trauma or petechiae on the soft palate.

Table 17.1 Aspects of history-taking which might alert professionals to the need for further investigation

Alerts on history taking	Examples
Alleged mechanism of injury seems unlikely given the child's developmental level	A parental allegation that a 6 week-old baby rolled from a couch onto the carpet
Alleged mechanism of injury seems implausible or unlikely	A parental suggestion that a 17 month-old sibling could fracture a newborn baby's ribs, skull and femur. Alternative explanations for the infant's injuries are probable
Alleged mechanism of injury is inconsistent over time	A parent gives differing versions of the sequence of events prior to the child's presentation to hospital
Alleged mechanism of injury varies between historians	The child's parents give different versions of their whereabouts for the time prior to the child's presentation to hospital and the disparity in their histories indicates at least one of the parents is offering information that is not factual
The child implicates an adult as the cause of the injuries	A child alleges 'Mummy's smoke burn hot' when you examine skin lesions suggestive of cigarette burns
The injured child's parent seems to be hinting that they and/or their partner have been extremely stressed during recent days. First-time parents with distressed infants are particularly vulnerable. Be sensitive to the needs of a parent with an injured child who might be seeking help to improve their parenting and/or avoid inflicting additional injuries. Ask specifically about shaking and 'rough handling' when assessing injured infants	
Pattern of injury is not one usually associated with accidental trauma	Bruising over the scapula and abdominal wall in a toddler with no history of accidental trauma
Pattern of injury is inconsistent with the explanation offered	A parent suggests that an 18 month-old might have sustained contact burns when he accidentally bumped into a heater but the pattern of injury suggests a contact burn to the palm and dorsum of the hand with sparing of the digits
Pattern of injury suggests deliberately inflicted trauma	The pattern of a large curved bruise on a baby's arm suggests it was caused by a bite mark with indentations from an adult's teeth
A parent alleges that someone else injured their child	

- Nasal trauma such as a nasal septal haematoma.
- Ear trauma: remember to inspect behind the pinnae and examine both tympanic membranes.
- Eye trauma: examine for objective evidence of injury from the lids to the retinae.
- Internal injuries: injuries to internal organs in the thorax and abdomen.
- Genital trauma.

Investigations
- Consider clotting studies and a full-blood examination for children with bruising.
- Radiograph sites of clinically suspected fracture(s).
- Bone scan **and** skeletal survey are recommended in children <3 years of age, to search for occult fractures.

Note: a bone scan is not a sensitive tool for the detection of skull fractures; if suspected, obtain a skull radiograph in addition.
- In older children, bone scans are used if occult or healing fractures are suspected.
- Photography is an important means of documenting injuries. Note the need for a colour wheel and a tape measure/ruler. Also note that photography augments a detailed written description of injuries but should never replace it.

Interviewing parents
- A non-judgemental, sensitive approach is essential.
- Ask open, non-directive questions. Use verbatim quotes whenever possible.

Child neglect
Detail information related to the child's health, growth, nutrition, physical and emotional well-being. Also note the family's access and attendance to services.

Examination includes the nature and appropriateness of a child's clothing, cleanliness of the skin and nails, nutritional status, growth percentiles, evidence of infections, infestations and other medical conditions.

Medical opinion should reflect the doctor's assessment of objective signs of physical neglect, as well as historical evidence of environmental neglect (e.g. if an infant is left unattended in the bath) or medical neglect (medical conditions not treated).

Child sexual abuse
Aim for a single assessment by a suitably trained medical practitioner who has access to facilities for paediatric genital examination and photographic documentation. This doctor should have expertise in assessment, preparation of medical reports and presentation of evidence in court. All other medical practitioners are encouraged to seek advice from regional experts. Doctors must ensure that examination is in accordance with local policies, procedural guidelines and legislation.

These guidelines are for the uncommon situation when the examination cannot be deferred and a clinician with expertise in the assessment of child sexual abuse is not available to conduct the examination, provide supervision or peer review.

Informed consent and the assent of the child are required. Document the time, circumstances and people present.

History

A full paediatric assessment is required. The evaluation should include:

- The nature of the sexual contact (digital, penile, vaginal, rectal, oral or a foreign object).
- The time and circumstances of the alleged abuse, whether ejaculation occurred and whether a condom was used.
- The identity of the alleged perpetrator(s).
- Genital symptoms and concerns (pain, discharge, bleeding or possible injury).

Examination

An examination should be performed as soon as possible after the alleged assault.

- Note signs of injury on general examination.
- Ask the child to indicate the exact sites on their body where there was contact with the offender.
- The external genitalia should be carefully examined for debris from the crime-scene and signs of injury.
- Girls may be examined in the frog-leg position using labial traction or labial separation techniques. Adequate visualisation of the posterior hymenal rim may be achieved with the girl in the knee–chest prone position.
- Boys may be examined in the supine position, flexing the boy's knees to visualise the anus.
- An otoscope provides light and magnification when a colposcope is not available. Many medical examination lights provide a source of magnification and are 'cold' to touch. Ensure the child is comfortable with the procedure and understands the equipment being used.
- Semen may fluoresce under ultraviolet light.
- Speculum examination is not usually required in prepubertal girls or adolescent girls who are not sexually active. Examination under anaesthetic should be considered only if the clinician suspects internal injuries that might require surgical repair.
- Collect the child's clothing (including underwear) for forensic evaluation. Collect forensic specimens. Seek advice if uncertain about what specimens to collect and how to handle the specimens. Forensic swabs should be air-dried, labelled and handed to police. Document the chain of transmission of evidence, i.e. record the name of the person to whom the forensic specimens are handed and the time and date this occurs.
- Swabs and slides for microbiological tests should be performed as clinically indicated. Blood tests for hepatitis B and C, as well as screening tests for syphilis (VDRL) and HIV should be considered when the history raises concern about the transfer of body fluids. Note the need for repeat serology after 3 months. Consider urine polymerase chain reaction (PCR) for identification of *Chlamydia* and gonococcus.

- Consider pregnancy prophylaxis if within 72 h of sexual contact. Arrange for a follow-up pregnancy test (see chapter 28, Gynaecological conditions, p. 359).
- Consider sexually transmitted infection (STI) prophylaxis with azithromycin.
- Arrange for follow-up tests for STI.
- All abused children and their parents should have access to appropriate counselling.

Management

- Multidisciplinary assessment of the child and their family is recommended for all children in whom child abuse is suspected.
- A child with moderate or severe injuries should be admitted to hospital for evaluation.
- Medical staff are expected to attend case conferences with police and protective workers in order to share information and plan intervention.
- Medical reports should be prepared by the senior medical staff responsible for the child's care. The report should use language appropriate for non-medical professionals; it should be clear, concise and informative, including an opinion as to the possible causes of the injuries.
- Before appearing in court, medical staff are strongly advised to consult with senior medical colleagues who are experienced in this field.

Tertiary referral centres

Most major metropolitan paediatric hospitals have established tertiary reference centres for the assessment and treatment of child abuse. Paediatricians and other medical professionals working in these centres provide expert advice in relation to the assessment of injuries and the management of suspected child abuse. Seek advice early.

Report writing

Senior medical staff should write (or supervise the preparation of) the medical report. This report will provide information to non-medical agencies. The report can form the basis of a statement; it will need to be signed and witnessed by the police at a later date. The statement can then form part of the evidence in bringing criminal charges to court. Subsequently, doctors may receive a subpoena (sometimes years later) to give evidence as a witness. It is very useful to have a clear report as a reminder of the case details. Doctors are also required to take the original notes (or hospital record) of the consultation to court and can be cross-examined about the details of this record. Ensure the original notes are clear and non-ambiguous. Use simple medical language in the report.

Providing a medical report involves describing what was observed, which draws on the report writer's experience as a doctor with knowledge of anatomy, physiology, growth and development. However, doctors are not expected to be detectives. For example, medical professionals can offer a description of bruising and may be able to reach a conclusion about the likely mechanism of injury but should refrain from saying who they believe did it and when.

Hints on format for report writing
Heading
Do not use any identifying patient details apart from name and date of birth. Do not include address. Confidentiality cannot be ensured for a report that may pass to legal and welfare systems. Even so, all reports should be headed 'confidential'.

Introduction
Document your credentials clearly. This includes academic qualifications and year of graduation/conferring of degrees, relevant past experience and current position. State who was examined, when and where it took place and who else was present in the room, part or all of the time.

Consent
Record the name of the person giving consent for the medical evaluation and the preparation and release of the report.

Presenting history
- Circumstances: who referred the child, what information they provided, e.g. *Senior Constable Jack Cracklaw requested a medical examination of child A following allegations of attempted digital vaginal penetration by person X, occurring two days prior.*
- History taken from child/adolescent, e.g. *I obtained the following history from child B. Child B told me that 'person X touched . . .'*
- History taken from accompanying person, e.g. *Child B's mother told me that 'I went into child B's bedroom and saw . . .'*

This style of narrative can seem repetitious but provides an unambiguous record and structured report (without winning a literary award). The medical report does not need to contain details of non-relevant medical history, though this should form part of the original history.

Physical examination
- General statement includes whether the child was cooperative, overview of level of function and growth parameters.
- General physical examination should mention relevant positive findings in detail, e.g. *'the following bruises were noted . . .'* A numbered list is useful in avoiding any ambiguity and helps divide those injuries for which there is an explanation from those where the mechanism remains unclear.
- Genital examination should be described separately when this is relevant. It is important to note the position of the child and and any additional lighting and magnification that was used.

Experience is required in the interpretation of abnormal genital signs and genital examination should not be undertaken without full consideration of possible management options, including the need for collection of forensic specimens.

Investigations
Investigations should be noted, with results and interpretation.

Conclusions and opinion
Keep concise. Try to answer the question that is being asked (e.g. the pattern, extent and distribution of bruising observed exceeds that likely to occur as a result of accidental childhood trauma).

Recommendations
Professional recommendations about intervention to improve the child's health, safety, development and well-being.

Court appearances
Few doctors are familiar with the court system. See Table 17.2 for key points to remember when appearing in court. Other important points relevant to the process and giving evidence as a witness are as follows:
- *Swearing in* (the oath).
- *Evidence in chief:* the prosecutor takes the doctor through their statement – non-leading questions.
- *Cross-examination:* to test the evidence and raise doubts about the validity of the basis of the medical opinion – to test whether there are alternative explanations and how firmly the doctor holds their view.
- *Re-examination:* to clarify any remaining points.

Table 17.2 Key points for court appearances

1 Address (and look at) the magistrate or jury rather than the cross-examining counsel
2 Answer the question asked
3 Beware of expressions of absolute certainty. Make concessions if and as required
4 Be dispassionate and not combative or hostile
5 Never try to be an advocate
6 Prepare by talking with experienced colleagues

USEFUL RESOURCES
- *www.rch.org.au/clinicalguide [Child Abuse]* – RCH Clinical Practice Guidelines. Contains useful guidelines for assessment and management of child abuse.
- *www.vfpms.org.au* – Victorian Forensic Paediatric Medical Service. Contains useful relevant literature, educational resources and guidelines.

CHAPTER 18

The death of a child

Peter McDougall
Jenny Hynson
Mary O'Toole

The death of a child causes an intense grieving process in surviving family members that may last for years. For the family's future well-being it is very important that the healthcare team ensures that the processes surrounding death are carried out in a sensitive and caring manner. The purpose of this chapter is to provide some practical guidelines.

Before death

Often the death of a child can be anticipated. Although hospital admission is frequently necessary, most children and families wish to spend as much time as possible at home. With appropriate planning and support, most symptoms can be controlled effectively at home. Domiciliary medical care can be provided by the GP in consultation with hospital staff. Palliative care agencies can provide specialised nursing care and a range of other services. Parents may be reluctant to accept the assistance of such services because they associate the term 'palliative care' with imminent death, 'giving up' and hopelessness. Explaining palliative care as an approach that aims to improve the quality of life for children with life-limiting illness and their families may help overcome some of this resistance. Palliative care can be provided alongside ongoing attempts to modify or even cure disease. Parents do not have to abandon hope in order to receive support from a palliative care service.

Although home care offers many advantages to the family, it is not without difficulties and parents are subject to physical, emotional and financial stress. Re-admission to hospital or hospice should be easily and readily available. A letter detailing the child's condition, plans in case of sudden deterioration and people to contact will facilitate appropriate care in an emergency.

Giving bad news to families: the interview in a hospital setting

The way in which difficult information is communicated sets the stage for the working relationship between staff and family. Staff need to be aware of how their own feelings of anxiety, sadness and impotence may influence this process. Most families appreciate honest information given in an empathic way and tempered with a sense of hope. Realistic hope may be offered in terms of ongoing support, attention to symptoms and help to maximise the child's quality of life.

Paediatric Handbook, 8th edition. By Kate Thomson, Dean Tey and Michael Marks. Published 2009 by Blackwell Publishing, ISBN: 978-1-4051-7400-8.

Psychosocial Problems

Personnel

The consistency of the healthcare team in a child's final illness is essential. Medical interviews with families, in hospital, should be led by a senior doctor together with a junior doctor, nurse, social worker or pastoral care worker. The presence of more than two of these people at an interview may be difficult for the family. Other healthcare team members, especially the family doctor, community nurse and others outside the hospital, must be closely informed.

Comfort

Choose a physically comfortable location where interruptions can be avoided. The open ward or corridor are not the places for interviews. Whenever possible, divert phones and have someone answer pagers. Try to allow plenty of time for the discussion.

Giving clear and simple information

- Begin by asking the family to give their understanding of the situation.
- The prognosis is usually best given first.
- Give an explanation of the disease process.
- Try to determine what it is the family wish to know.
- Avoid the use of unexplained medical jargon.
- Avoid information overload. There is time to deal with complex medical issues at later interviews.
- Avoid ambiguous phrases such as 'we might lose the battle' or 'he's passed away'. The words *death, die* or *dying* should be used.
- Allow expression of emotion.
- Offer to help the parents tell important others such as grandparents and siblings.
- Initial shock may render parents unable to process detailed information, so multiple opportunities for discussion should be provided.

Respect silences

When bad news is delivered it is best to remain silent until the parent responds. This sometimes takes minutes and can be very uncomfortable. These are important moments; they should not be interrupted.

Responsibilities of the accompanying members of the healthcare team

At a medical interview, the accompanying members of the healthcare team need to be sensitive to the parents' needs and to watch for misunderstandings. If they do not understand the medical message, it is unlikely that the parents will. At an appropriate time, the accompanying team member may ask the doctor to clarify some of the explanations given, but it is important not to interrupt a train of conversation or the silences that occur.

The senior doctor should inform the family that all possible reasonable measures will be taken to preserve their child's life. It is not necessary to repeat this message.

When the senior doctor has concluded discussion with the family, other members of the health team may stay with the family for a time in order to offer their support and explore their understanding of the information provided.

Interpreters

The availability of trained interpreters for people with a language other than English is essential. Do not use other family members or friends as interpreters.

Adequate relief of pain and distress of the child

The most common reason for inadequate treatment of physical suffering is the failure to recognise it. It is important to actively ask about symptoms and consider potential contributing factors. For example, fatigue may be an expected part of terminal illness but it may also be due to factors such as anaemia and depression, which may be amenable to treatment.

Many parenteral medications (e.g. morphine, midazolam, and haloperidol) may be successfully administered subcutaneously rather than i.v. and this offers many advantages to children needing palliative care. Community palliative care teams are able to help establish and monitor subcutaneous infusions if the family wishes to be at home. Planning for symptom development and escalation is essential, such that appropriate medications are available for use in a crisis.

Parents and health professionals may be concerned about the use of opioids and benzodiazepines and fear they may hasten the death of the child. These concerns can result in needless suffering. There is no evidence that the appropriate use of medications such as morphine (i.e. when commenced at a conservative dose and titrated to effect, with the intention of relieving physical symptoms such as pain and dyspnoea) alters the timing of death. It is not ethical for a child to suffer as a result of misconceptions about the use of medications. Concerns about the treatment of physical symptoms should be directed to the child's paediatrician, a children's pain specialist or a palliative care specialist.

Communicating with children about death and dying

Parents may feel compelled to protect their children from 'bad news'. Children often know a great deal about their disease and prognosis even when they have not been 'told'. They may not reveal what they know, for fear of upsetting their parents who may (falsely) assume the child knows very little. Attempts to protect the child from accurate information may leave them feeling anxious and isolated as they sense distress in those around them and generate incorrect explanations for this such as '*I have been bad*' or '*Mummy and Daddy are angry with me*'. In general, it is best to encourage parents to be honest with children, but information needs to be provided in a manner appropriate to their cognitive ability and developmental level. It may be helpful to anticipate questions and work with the family in planning responses.

It is important to listen to what the child is asking. The child who asks '*Am I going to die?*' may actually not be concerned about dying as such but more about who will look after their parents, what their friends will think, or whether they will be in pain. A response such as '*What makes you ask me that?*' will provide further information upon which to base an answer. Children may not wish to express themselves verbally or directly. Stories, artwork, music and play allow expression, build trust and facilitate communication.

Concepts of death

The child's concept of death becomes more complete with development and life experience. A number of variables influence this process, so statistical averages serve as a guide only. Preschoolers typically view death as a reversible phenomenon (e.g. Snow White) and do not yet appreciate that people die as a consequence of age, illness or trauma. Magical thinking may lead them to believe they have caused death through bad behaviour or thoughts. By 7 years of age most children understand the concepts of irreversibility, causality, universality and cessation of bodily functions. Most 8 year olds also understand that dead people cannot feel pain or fear.

Siblings

Siblings of children with life-threatening conditions suffer not only the distress of having a brother or sister who is sick and dying, but the isolation of having parents who are frequently either physically or psychologically unavailable to them. They may feel guilty that they do not have the condition, or may fear for their own health. They may resent the attention given to the sick child. They may feel they have somehow caused the illness. Siblings often don't want to burden their parents with their concerns and may express distress through developmental regression, school failure and physical symptoms.

Siblings benefit from inclusion in visits to the hospital and where possible, the care of the child. Staff can help by dedicating special time to children in which they may be given information and allowed to ask questions. Specific reassurance that the illness is not their fault may be needed, especially for siblings who have donated organs.

Preparations for death

Time and space

The healthcare team must not overwhelm families. Parents need to spend time alone together and with their child, either in the hospital ward, a quiet room, at home, or at a children's hospice.

Arrangements

These may need to be made for baptism, religious advice, photographs, videos and other memories of the child.

Permission

Many families have specific needs and sometimes they are unsure whether these are permissible. If these issues can be anticipated and discussed, the family's wishes may be facilitated.

The child

The preparation for death is largely dependent on the age and particular illness of the child. The older child with a chronic illness is often aware of impending death and the healthcare team needs to be sensitive to the family's and child's wishes in the delivery of information.

The place of death

Decisions need to be made about where the child will die. This largely depends on the family, but it may be at home, in a hospice or the hospital. When appropriate, the child may be included in this planning.

Taking the deceased child's body home

Some families wish to take their child home after death. This may be for a brief period or several days. This allows family and friends to say goodbye and can be very helpful in facilitating the grieving process. The funeral may then commence from home, or the family may be happy to allow an undertaker to remove the deceased body earlier. Families should be advised to consult with a funeral director before taking the child home. In most cases parents can transport their child's body from hospital to home, but it is important for the medical team to provide them with a brief document explaining the situation.

Sudden unexpected death

The sudden death of a child from a wide variety of causes may occur in the community, the emergency department, or a hospital ward. Sudden infant death syndrome (SIDS – see p. 219) is particularly traumatic because it is the unexpected and unexplained death of a previously well infant. Although most of the preceding guidelines are applicable, there are some additional considerations regarding sudden death.

Resuscitation

This is frequently attempted either at home or in hospital. Some parents may wish to be present and they should not be excluded, but an experienced health professional needs to be available to provide them with support.

When it becomes clear that further resuscitative attempts are futile, it is the responsibility of the senior hospital doctor, GP or senior ambulance officer to:

- Introduce themselves and explain their role in the child's care.
- Explain to the family what happened and what treatments were attempted (this may need to be repeated).
- Listen to the family's account of the events.
- Allow the family to express their emotions.
- Provide a non-judgemental understanding for any pre-existing difficult family relationships.
- Provide access to telephones for the notification of relatives.
- Facilitate the attendance of siblings and other important family members at the hospital.
- Encourage the family to see the child's body, say their farewells and take as much time as required.
- Ensure the family can reach home safely.

The family response

The immediate responses to sudden death vary from emotional withdrawal to outbursts of profound grief. Unexpected reactions commonly occur; for example, anger towards healthcare providers who have done their best. Any response is appropriate, provided it does not threaten harm to self or other people.

Brain death

Brain death is defined as the irreversible cessation of all brain function including that of the brain stem. There are strict clinical criteria for the determination of brain death. Occasionally it becomes clear that a child who is dependent on mechanical ventilation is brain dead. In such a situation:

- The senior doctor needs to explain the meaning of brain death. Avoid using confusing words. The unambiguous message that death has occurred, together with the distinction between brain death and coma, needs to be clearly explained.
- It can be helpful to say that, although the child's body is still alive, the brain is dead and therefore the person is dead.
- It frequently helps parents to understand that their child has died by encouraging them to witness some or all of the brain death tests.
- The request for organ donation generally requires a separate interview, made in a positive manner, without coercion and with the clear acknowledgement of the family's vulnerability. Issues related to organ donation need to be discussed in order to receive an informed consent.

After death
The moment of death
Although usually anticipated, the moment of death is an important event and needs medical confirmation.

Mementos
Offer to create the family mementos for the family such as photographs, locks of hair, hand-and footprints together with personal belongings. Families will vary in what mementos they would like and how involved they want to be in the process of creating these. Remember that:

- Black and white photographs of the dead child produce better-looking pictures.
- Some families may not want to take mementos with them on the day of the child's death but may like to collect them at a later time.

Viewing the body
This can be valuable for family members. It may eliminate the disbelief that death really occurred or, in the case of stillbirth, that the child was profoundly abnormal.

- A private and comfortable area should be provided where the family can spend uninterrupted time with their child.
- Families should feel able to spend as long as they need with their child.
- Families should be offered the opportunity to wash and dress their child as a last act of love and care.

Autopsy
There has been a large amount of adverse publicity regarding the previous practice of organ retention without parental informed consent for autopsy procedures. Clear and accurate explanations need to be provided to families regarding the autopsy procedure and its purpose. Parents need to understand that the purpose of the autopsy is to seek full information regarding the cause of the child's death, the nature of the illness and the risk of recurrence

of the illness in other family members or future children. If you are concerned about your ability to do this, seek support and assistance from senior colleagues.

The autopsy may be limited to a system or area or be designated as a full autopsy. In particular, details need to be given regarding the removal, careful study and microscopic examination of tissues and organs, and that some organs such as the heart and brain may need to be retained for a period of time before a proper examination can be performed. Informed consent is essential if removed organs are to be disposed of or retained for teaching purposes.

The parents should be informed that the autopsy will be performed on the next working day after the child's death and may interfere with the funeral arrangements. The full results of the autopsy are usually not available until approximately 6 weeks after the autopsy procedure and this needs to be made clear to the family. Written consent forms need to be completed before the autopsy can proceed.

Many parents decide against an autopsy. They need to be reassured that a hospital autopsy will not be performed without their consent. However, there are occasions where a death needs to be reported to the Coroner for further investigation and a Coroner's autopsy can be performed without their consent.

Coroner's cases
A doctor must report a death to the Coroner as soon as possible if:
- The cause of death is unable to be determined.
- The death appears to have been unexpected, unnatural or violent.
- The death appears to have resulted, directly or indirectly, from accident or injury.
- The death occurred during an anaesthetic and is not due to natural cause.
- The deceased person was held in care immediately before death.
- The deceased person's identity is unknown.

The Coroner then decides whether or not an autopsy needs to be performed. Parents can request (on a special form) that the Coroner does not direct that an autopsy be performed. In many cases where the cause of death is not in doubt (e.g. severe head injury), the Coroner will respect the wish of the family.

Reviewable deaths
The second or subsequent death of a child with the same parent(s) must also be reported to the Coroner's Court. The ensuing investigation may be limited to a review of medical files and contact with medical staff and family members or in some cases an autopsy.

Funeral options
These need to be discussed and the family assisted to make their own arrangements in their own time with a funeral director and religious personnel as appropriate. Encouragement is given to the family to involve siblings in this important ritual.

Sedation
Unless a parent has a well-defined psychiatric illness, sedation should be avoided for the acute stages of grief as it interferes with and suppresses the normal mourning process.

Breast-feeding

In the case of neonatal death or the death of an infant, advice needs to be given to the breast-feeding mother regarding suppression of lactation. Consultation with a specialist is recommended.

Surviving siblings

Children react in their own way to a sibling's death. They may blame themselves and may fear their own death or that of others close to them. This fear is often unspoken. At times children may not appear to be grieving the death of their sibling as they often grieve in short bursts. Distress may be expressed by regression to an earlier stage, difficulties at school, acting out or in other ways. Parents often need help and support to understand the responses of their surviving children who may need repeated reassurance. Opportunities to talk as a family about the death, their feelings and their day-to-day challenges and achievements are important. A return to family routines can help them to feel more secure.

Availability of the healthcare team

The healthcare team should be available to the family after death and follow-up arranged. It is usually important to both families and team members that farewells are made.

Notification of other professionals

Notify the health professionals who have been and who will continue to be involved with the family following the child's death, including the referring doctor or institution, the family's GP and the maternal and child health nurse. This must be done as soon as possible.

Other families

The death of a child often affects the parents of other children in the hospital ward or local community. The acknowledgement of a child's death with these families is very important.

Follow-up
Medical interview

Whether an autopsy is performed or not, it is essential that an appointment be made for the parents to see the child's treating doctor. Some parents are reluctant to attend, but most see the interview as a 'final farewell'. The discussion should include the autopsy results, the child's period of illness, future childbearing and issues related to bereavement. If a family is reluctant to attend this important interview, alternative interviews with other healthcare providers should be arranged.

If the child has died in hospital, the child's doctor should see the family for one or more follow-up visits, although they may not be the best person to conduct ongoing bereavement counselling. Families are more likely to attend if they receive both a written and a verbal invitation, and social workers may be helpful in both facilitating attendance and offering support during the visit. Parents may find it helpful to discuss the reactions of siblings and ways in which to support them. It is important the family be given information regarding potential sources of support and ongoing counselling if required.

Condolences

Communication such as a letter or card from the medical practitioner/team involved with the care of the child can be important.

Ongoing support

The course of parental grief following the death of a child may vary greatly. Many families manage their grief with the support of family and friends and may not utilise more formal supports. The grieving process changes over time, often intensifying after the initial period of shock, around important dates and sometimes unexpected triggers. Over time (usually years, not months) parents develop ways of living with their loss and are able to regain some sense of purpose and happiness in their lives. The death of a child is considered a risk factor for a more complicated and prolonged grieving process. Information needs to be provided to all families about the support groups that are available both at the hospital and in the community. Other factors to consider when assessing the risk of a more complicated grieving process include the preparedness of the family for their child's death, their view of pre-death care, their perception of available supports, their own physical and mental health, substance use or addiction issues and life stressors. If someone is struggling more than expected, formal referral for psychotherapy should be considered. Medication is not a solution for grief.

Sudden infant death syndrome

Sudden unexpected death in infancy (SUDI) is a term used to describe all infants under the age of 1 year who die unexpectedly after they are placed to sleep. Any unexpected death of an infant should be reported to the Coroner.

The causes of death for SUDI include:
- Sudden infant death syndrome (SIDS).
- Other sudden death, cause unknown (autopsy carried out).
- Other ill defined and unspecified causes of mortality (no autopsy).
- Suffocation while sleeping (including asphyxiation by bedclothes and overlaying).
- Explained: child abuse/homicide, infection, metabolic disorders, genetic disorders, other causes.

SIDS is only one of the causes of SUDI. The definition of SIDS was refined by Krous et al. (2004) as the sudden death of any infant or young child that is unexplained by history and in which a thorough post-mortem evaluation fails to demonstrate an adequate cause of death.

Key features include age <1 year, onset of the fatal episode apparently occurring during sleep, and the death remains unexplained after a thorough investigation, including a complete autopsy, review of the circumstances of death and the clinical history.

This definition has four main categories:
- Category IA SIDS: classic features of SIDS present and completely documented.
- Category IB SIDS: classic features of SIDS present but incompletely documented.
- Category II SIDS: infants meeting category I except for ≥1 factor(s).
- Unclassified sudden infant death.

Epidemiology

Until 1990, about 550 babies a year died of SIDS in Australia, approximately 140 of these in Victoria, which correlated with the national and international average of 2 SIDS cases per 1000 live births. Following the 'Reducing the Risks' campaign initiated in 1990 by the Sudden Infant Death Research Foundation (now SIDS and Kids), the number of infants dying from SIDS in Victoria has steadily fallen to 15 in 2005 (Consultative Council on Obstetric and Paediatric Morbidity and Mortality 2005). A drop in incidence has also been observed in Europe and New Zealand, where similar campaigns have been promoted.

The decline in SIDS rates is due to changing babies' sleeping position from lying on their front to lying on their back.

SIDS is rare in the first 2 weeks of life and among babies over the age of 12 months. See Table 18.1 for further epidemiological features of SIDS.

The SIDS and Kids 'Safe Sleeping Campaign' recommends:

- Place baby on back to sleep from birth (not on side or face down).
- Baby should sleep with head uncovered.
- Avoid exposing baby to tobacco smoke before birth and afterwards.
- Place baby to sleep in a safe cot, safe mattress, safe bedding and safe sleeping environment.

Additional risk factors are discussed in Table 18.2. Further information on the campaign can be obtained from the appropriate SIDS organisations.

Apparent life-threatening episode

An apparent life-threatening episode (ALTE) is an event that is frightening to the observer, characterised by a combination of apnoea, colour change, marked change of muscle tone, choking or gagging. The terms 'near-miss SIDS' or 'aborted cot death' should not be used as they imply a close association between ALTE and SIDS.

- Up to 13% of infants who die from SIDS have a preceding history of an ALTE.
- No cause for the ALTE is found in over 50% of cases presenting under the age of 6 months.

Table 18.1 Epidemiological features of SIDS

Parents of SIDS infants	Infants who die from SIDS
1 Younger mothers and fathers	1. Male (63%)
2. Single and unsupported mothers	2. Lower birthweight
3. Higher maternal parity	3. Lower gestation
4. Lower family income	4. Lower Apgar score
5. Previous stillbirths	5. Admitted to a special care unit
6. Previous SIDS infant (~1.6 times higher risk)	6. Congenital abnormalities

Data from the United Kingdom Confidential Enquiry for Stillbirths and Deaths in Infancy (CESDI) study into sudden unexpected deaths in infancy (SUDI) (Fleming et al. 2000).

Table 18.2 Risk factors for SIDS

Risk factors for SIDS	Items that were *not confirmed* as risk or protective factors for SIDS
1. **Sleeping positions** – face down or on the side.	1. **Breast-feeding** – no independent factor found in the reduction of SIDS.
2. **Tobacco smoke** – daily exposure of infant to smoke from either father, mother or other household members, is highly significant and dose related.	2. **Dummies** (pacifiers) – no increased risk.
	3. **Aeroplane flights** – no evidence of risk.
	4. **Bed sharing** – no apparent increased risk in the absence of cigarette smoke, alcohol or drug abuse.
3. The **cot environment** – infants dying from SIDS were found wrapped more warmly, wore hats, used quilts or 'dooners', had covers over their heads or were wrapped loosely.	5. **Cot bumpers** no increased risk or benefits.
	6. **Apnoea monitors** – no evidence of protection.
	7. **Mattress type or age** – no relationship.
4. **Room sharing** – evidence suggests that sharing a room with the baby in the first 6 months may be beneficial.	
5. **Bed sharing** – when either parent has been smoking, drinking alcohol or using illegal drugs has been shown to be a risk factor.	
6. **Sofa sharing** – with an adult conveys a higher risk of SIDS.	
7. **Illness recognition** – parents should be taught to recognise significant features of illness in babies.	
8. **Immunisation** – infants who are fully immunised are at lower risk of SIDS than those who are not immunised.	

The United Kingdom Confidential Enquiry for Stillbirths and Deaths in Infancy (CESDI) study into sudden unexpected deaths in infancy (SUDI).
Reference: 'Sudden unexpected deaths in infancy: the CESDI SUDI Studies'.
Editors: Peter Fleming, Pete Blair, Chris Bacon, Jem Berry.

Associations that have been found with ALTE are:
- *Gastro-oesophageal reflux:* a small number of infants with this common condition experience coughing and choking episodes and occasionally apnoea. These episodes occur most frequently when the infant is awake and are often recurrent. Most resolve within a month of onset but some persist for several weeks. The chest radiograph of these infants rarely shows signs of aspiration.
- *Respiratory syncytial virus:* can cause apnoea. Other upper airway viruses and pertussis can also be associated with apnoea.

- *Upper airway obstruction:* due to Pierre Robin syndrome, midnasal narrowing or adenoidal hypertrophy. It is usually suspected by a history of inspiratory stridor, snoring and sleep disturbance.
- *Epilepsy:* usually suggested by a good history. Investigations of ALTE by electroencephalogram (EEG) are usually fruitless unless there is clinical suspicion of a seizure disorder.
- *Cardiac arrhythmia:* this is an uncommon cause but should be suspected in recurrent episodes. Obtain an electrocardiogram (ECG).

Most infants with ALTE need minimal resuscitation; however, some need cardiopulmonary resuscitation. These infants have at least a 10% chance of further episodes, which almost always occur in the first month after the previous episode.

A cause will often be found in infants presenting with ALTE over the age of 6 months. If no cause is found in this age group and the episodes are recurrent, formal investigation including sleep polysomnography should be done. Munchausen's syndrome by proxy should be considered as a possibility, but this diagnosis is rare and in >50% no cause is found.

All infants presenting with ALTE should be admitted to hospital for monitoring, investigation and counselling of the parents. However minor the episode may appear to healthcare professionals, the parents usually believe that their infant's life was endangered at the time.

Home apnoea monitoring

No study has demonstrated that home apnoea monitoring programmes reduce the incidence of SIDS.

Home apnoea monitoring is not routinely recommended; however, there is a community awareness of its availability. Many baby goods stores sell monitors over the counter without any back-up or counselling. Advice regarding home monitoring should concentrate on the lack of its proven efficacy together with the positive message about the falling incidence of SIDS. Families may be given inaccurate advice regarding frequency of false alarms. Consider home apnoea monitoring in:

- Infants with a history of SIDS in the family.
- ALTE – particularly if cardiopulmonary resuscitation has been used.

There are families who demand monitors and in this situation they are best used under medical supervision after appropriate counselling. Some examples of these are:

- Siblings of a previous SIDS victim.
- Extremely low birthweight infants.
- Infants with minor ALTE.
- Previous family bereavement.
- Extreme family anxiety about apnoea and SIDS.

Counselling and instruction in cardiopulmonary resuscitation, together with complete medical and device back-up are essential to a home monitoring programme.

USEFUL RESOURCES
- *www.rch.org.au/rch_palliative* – Victorian Paediatric Palliative Care Program.
- *www.vifm.org* – Victorian Institute of Forensic Medicine.
- *www.nalagvic.org.au* – National Association for Loss and Grief (NALAG).
- *www.vsk.org.au* – Very Special Kids.
- *www.sidsandkids.org* – SIDS and Kids (1800 240 400 – 24 h consult). Usually for those affected by the sudden and unexpected death of a child ≤6 years old, but some rural area services take referrals for children up to 18 years old.
- *www.sandsvic.org.au* – Sudden and Neonatal Death Support (SANDS) Victoria.
- *www.health.vic.gov.au/perinatal* – Consultative Council on Obstetric and Paediatric Mortality and Morbidity. Annual Report for the Year 2005, incorporating the 44th Survey of Perinatal Deaths in Victoria. Melbourne, 2007.
- Fleming P, Blair P, Bacon C, Berry J. *Sudden unexpected deaths in infancy: the CESDI SUDI studies 1993–1996.* The Stationery Office, London, 2000.
- Krous HF, Beckwith JB, Byard RW. Sudden infant death syndrome and unclassified sudden infant deaths: a definitional and diagnostic approach. *Pediatrics* 2004; 114(1); 234–238.

CHAPTER 19

Allergy and immunology

Mimi Tang
Joanne Smart

Allergic diseases

Allergic disease is an increasingly common problem in the community, affecting up to 40% of children. The allergic conditions include asthma, eczema, allergic rhinitis and allergies to food, insects or drugs. Children who have allergic diseases are often atopic; that is, they produce IgE antibodies to common allergens such as house dust mite, animal dander, pollens and foods. The presence of IgE antibodies (i.e. sensitisation) to these allergens does not necessarily cause disease; however, exposure to an allergen to which a patient is sensitised may exacerbate or precipitate symptoms (e.g. inhalant, food, insect or drug allergy).

Allergy tests include skin-prick tests (SPT) and radioallergosorbent tests (RAST). Both detect specific IgE antibodies against allergens. SPT and RAST are available for numerous allergens. Testing should be individualised for each clinical situation and is used to *confirm* suspected allergy. Testing to 'routine' allergen panels is not recommended.

Skin-prick tests

- Preferred because they are highly sensitive, inexpensive, simple and rapid.
- Age is not a contraindication to skin-prick testing. Skin-prick testing can be done from early infancy, but a negative skin test in infancy does not preclude the later development of sensitisation.

Limitations

- SPTs have a poor positive predictive value (<50%) for the presence of clinical allergy in the absence of a previous clinical reaction. The finding of a positive SPT to a food in this context does **not** necessarily indicate presence of clinical allergy.
- May be affected by medications. Antihistamines should be withheld for 2–4 days. Inhaled β_2-agonists, oral theophylline and corticosteroids do not interfere with SPTs.
- Dermatographism may complicate the interpretation of SPTs. Saline and histamine controls must be done.

Paediatric Handbook, 8th edition. By Kate Thomson, Dean Tey and Michael Marks. Published 2009 by Blackwell Publishing, ISBN: 978-1-4051-7400-8.

Indications

- Evaluation of suspected IgE-mediated food reactions. A negative SPT almost eliminates the possibility that a food will induce an IgE-mediated immediate reaction. A positive SPT must be correlated with the history. When there is a clear history of reaction to a specific food, a positive SPT confirms food allergy. If the history is uncertain, a positive test only indicates the possibility of food allergy and a cautious supervised inpatient food challenge in a specialist centre is required to confirm the presence or absence of allergy. SPT should not be routinely used to screen for the presence of food allergy. If there is a high suspicion of food allergy, refer the child to a specialist.
- Skin-prick testing to the relevant environmental allergens can identify major allergic factors that may exacerbate or contribute to symptoms and can guide the application of appropriate environmental modification. Consider performing in:
  - Patients with asthma or rhinitis who require maintenance steroid therapy to control symptoms, including patients with frequent episodic asthma.
  - Patients with moderate or severe eczema despite appropriate medical therapy.

Radioallergosorbent tests

- Have reduced sensitivity, are more expensive and have a slower turnaround time.
- Are useful alternatives to SPTs if there is dermatographism, widespread skin disease, or if antihistamines cannot be discontinued.
- May be useful in the primary care setting as initial **limited** investigation to confirm a suspected, **simple** allergy (e.g. confirmation of IgE-mediated food allergy to cow's milk, egg or peanut; or assessment for HDM, pet dander or pollen sensitisation in asthma or allergic rhinitis).

Interpretation of SPT and RAST

- A positive SPT or RAST only identifies the presence of specific IgE against an allergen (i.e. sensitisation).
- **A positive test does not prove that an allergic disease exists, nor does it necessarily predict that the patient will develop symptoms on exposure to that substance**. For example, only 50% of individuals with a positive SPT to a food allergen will develop symptoms when exposed to that food.
- In general, the larger the SPT and/or the higher the RAST result, the greater the likelihood of clinical allergy.

In vivo challenges

- _In vivo_ challenges are primarily used for diagnosis of food allergy and the evaluation of antibiotic reactions.
- They may also be used to assess the development of tolerance to foods.
- They are highly specialised procedures that should only be done in specialist centres with facilities for the early identification and management of allergic reactions.
- They are usually not done if there is a clear history of food allergy or anaphylaxis and the trigger has been identified.

- Cautious inpatient challenge is used to test the clinical relevance of a positive SPT where the history is unclear.
- In these circumstances, less than half of the patients with a positive SPT to a food will react to the food during a challenge. In general the larger the SPT size the greater the likelihood of clinical allergy. However, the size of a SPT does not correlate with the severity of reaction.
- Diagnosis of delayed non-IgE-mediated reaction to foods requires a formal food challenge, as there are no skin-prick or blood tests for this type of food reaction.

Allergic rhinitis

Allergic rhinitis refers to nasal symptoms of paroxysmal sneezing, itching, congestion and rhinorrhoea caused by sensitivity to environmental allergens. It can have a major impact on the quality of life and school performance, and appropriate recognition and treatment is important. This condition is commonly unrecognised.

Traditionally, allergic rhinitis has been classified as perennial (symptoms throughout the year, commonly due to HDM sensitisation), seasonal (symptoms occurring in a particular season, i.e. seasonal rhinitis/hay fever) or related to a specific allergen (e.g. cats or horses). More recently an alternative classification has been proposed which describes symptoms as 'persistent' (symptoms for >4 days a week **and** >4 weeks a year) or 'intermittent' (symptoms <4 days a week or <4 weeks a year), and as mild, moderate or severe (Fig. 19.1). Both classification systems may be used in combination.

Diagnosis requires the demonstration of an allergic basis for symptoms. Other causes of rhinitis should be considered: nonallergic rhinitis with eosinophilia syndrome (NARES), infective rhinitis, vasomotor rhinitis, hormonal rhinitis or rhinitis medicamentosa (rhinitis induced by excessive use of topical decongestants).

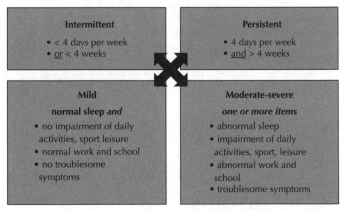

Fig. 19.1 Classification of allergic rhinitis. (Reproduced with permission from ARIA Workshop Executive Summary. (2002) *Allergy*. **57**; 2002: 841–855.)

Perennial allergic rhinitis

- Can occur at any age and is more common than seasonal rhinitis in preschool and primary school children.
- Sneezing and congestion are prominent especially on waking in the morning. There may be significant nasal obstruction and snoring at night.
- House dust mite is the major allergen involved but concurrent sensitivity to pollens is also common.
- Consider the possibility of perennial allergic rhinitis in any atopic child – this diagnosis is frequently missed.
- Any patient with allergic rhinitis and significant obstructive symptoms is at risk of obstructive sleep apnoea.

Seasonal allergic rhinitis

- More frequent in teenagers and young adults.
- Seasonal sneezing, itching and rhinorrhoea are prominent. Nasal symptoms are frequently associated with symptoms of itchy, red and watery eyes.
- Symptoms occur in the relevant pollen season.
- In general, trees pollinate in early spring, grasses in the late spring and summer, and weeds in the summer and autumn, although there is some overlap. Rye grass is the commonest provoking antigen in Australia, but multiple sensitivities to tree, grass and weed pollens are also seen.

Examination

No examination is complete until you have looked in the nose!

- Assess the nasal mucosa and nasal airflow.
- Pale oedematous mucosa and swollen turbinates indicate ongoing rhinitis. In seasonal rhinitis, examination may be normal outside the relevant pollen season.

Management

- Topical corticosteroid nasal sprays are the treatment of choice for both allergic and non-allergic rhinitis. The presence of congestion, nasal drainage or persistent symptoms (>4 days a week and >4 weeks per year) warrants treatment with topical corticosteroid nasal sprays. In general, full strength (prescription requiring) forms of nasal corticosteroid are recommended where there is significant rhinitis. Refer to Table 19.1.
- Continuous topical corticosteroid therapy for allergic rhinitis has not been shown to cause suppression of the hypothalamic–pituitary–adrenal axis. In seasonal rhinitis, commence treatment 1 month prior to the relevant pollen season and continue over the symptomatic period.
- Topical sodium cromoglicate is generally not effective.
- Topical anti-inflammatory treatment must be taken regularly for benefit. Improvement may not be apparent for 3–4 weeks and an initial course of treatment should last for 2–3 months.
- Allergen avoidance measures should be considered for patients using topical anti-inflammatory therapy. These are most feasible with certain allergen triggers (e.g. pets in animal dander sensitivity, house dust mite allergen in perennial rhinitis with dust mite

sensitivity). Dust mite reduction involves washing bedding in hot water weekly, removing soft toys and soft furnishings from the bedroom, vacuuming carpet and damp-dusting hard surfaces (including hard flooring) weekly and using allergen-impermeable covers for the mattress, pillow and doona or duvet. Avoidance of grass pollens is generally not possible.

- Antihistamines are not helpful in relieving nasal obstruction and are not indicated as first line treatment for significant rhinitis. Antihistamines may be used for intermittent symptoms (<4 days per week or <4 weeks a year) in the absence of congestion or significant rhinorrhoea (see Table 19.2). They may also be useful for control of break-through sneezing, itching or rhinorrhoea while on topical corticosteroid therapy or prophylactically before allergen exposure in allergen-specific rhinoconjunctivitis (e.g. cats or horses). Second-generation less-sedating antihistamines (loratadine and cetirizine) are well tolerated. Terfenadine and astemizole should be avoided as they may cause cardiac arrhythmia when taken with other medications.

Table 19.1 Nasal corticosteroids

Nasal corticosteroid type	Brand name	Dose
Prescription only		
Budesonide	Rhinocort	64 mcg
Mometasone	Nasonex	50 mcg
Over-the-counter		
Budesonide	Rhinocort aqueous	32 mcg
Fluticasone propionate	Beconase Allergy & Hayfever 24	50 mcg

Table 19.2 Antihistamines

Antihistamine type	Brand name	Doses
Less sedating		
Loratadine	Claratyne (10 mg tablet, 1 mg/mL syrup)	1–2 years: 2.5 mg/dose once daily
		3–6 years: 5 mg/dose once daily
	Lorastyne (10 mg tablet)	>6 years & adults: 30 mg/dose once daily
Fexofenadine	Telfast (30 mg, 60 mg, 120 mg, 180 mg tablets)	>6 years: 30 mg/dose twice a day
		Adults: 60 mg/dose twice a day
Cetirizine	Zyrtec (10 mg tablet, 1 mg/mL syrup, 10 mg/mL drops = 0.5 mg/drop)	>1 years: 0.125 mg/kg/dose twice a daily
		2–5 years: 2.5–5 mg/day in 2 doses
		6–12 years: 5–10 mg/day in 1–2 doses
		Adults: 10–20 mg/day in 1–2 doses
Sedating antihistamine		
Trimeprazine	Vallergan (1.5 mg/mL syrup)	>2 years (allergy): 0.1–0.25 mg/kg/dose 6-hourly
	Vallergan Forte (6 mg/mL syrup)	(Sedation) dose: 1–2 mg/kg nocte
		Adults: 10 mg/dose 3 times a day (max 100 mg/day)

Allergic conjunctivitis

Allergic conjunctivitis is commonly associated with allergic rhinitis.

- Occasionally eye symptoms occur in isolation.
- Red, watery, itchy eyes.
- May be persistent or intermittent.

Management

- Eye toilet with normal saline to flush out allergen, cool compresses.
- Oral antihistamine may be adequate.
- Topical therapies, i.e. eye drops such as antihistamine, combination antihistamine/mast cell stabilisers (e.g. Patanol).
- Occasionally symptoms may be severe and warrant topical corticosteroid therapy, but this should only be prescribed with caution and in consultation with an allergy specialist or ophthalmologist.

Food allergy

Food allergy is commonest in infancy; affecting 6–8% of children. More than 90% of food allergy reactions are caused by eight food groups – milk, egg, wheat, soy, peanut, tree nuts, fish and shellfish. Most food allergies resolve by 5 years of age. The exceptions are peanut, tree nut and shellfish allergies, which frequently persist and account for most food allergies in adults (affecting ~2% of the adult population).

Allergic reactions to foods fall into two broad groups: IgE-mediated and non-IgE-mediated reactions.

IgE-mediated food reactions

- Are common.
- Occur within 30–60 min of food ingestion.
- Typically occur in young infants and frequently resolve by the age of 3–5 years.
- Are most commonly triggered by milk, eggs and peanuts.
- Common symptoms are angioedema (usually facial), urticaria and vomiting immediately after the ingestion of the food.
- More severe reactions (anaphylaxis) involve the respiratory tract (stridor, wheezing, hoarse voice) and/or the cardiovascular system (hypotension, collapse). See chapter 1, Medical emergencies, p. 6.

Management

History

- Take a detailed history including details of the reaction, time after ingestion, treatment required, prior and subsequent exposures and co-existence of other atopic disease.
- Clarify whether there are symptoms of allergy to any other foods: 30% of children with food allergy will be allergic to more than one food. The finding that a food is being taken in the diet in significant quantities (i.e. whole egg rather than small amounts of

egg contained within cakes or biscuits) without reaction effectively excludes the presence of clinical allergy to that food and SPT and RAST to that food is **not** indicated.
- Patients are instructed to avoid the food that caused the allergic reaction. This requires careful reading of ingredient labels. Current Australian food labelling laws require that the common food allergens are listed as an ingredient if they are used in the preparation of a food.
- In IgE-mediated cow's milk allergy, cow's milk products should be eliminated. In infants and young children, a soy-based milk can be used if the child is not also allergic to soy. Where a child is also allergic to soy, a formula in which the milk proteins are broken down into hypoallergenic fragments (protein hydrolysate) should be used. Examples in Australia include Alfaré and Pepti-Junior. Occasionally, children may react to the hydrolysed milk proteins in these formulas and in such cases an elemental amino acid formula is indicated (e.g. Neocate or Elecare). Some clinicians advise that infants <6 months proceed directly to a protein hydrosylate formula (without trial of soy), because of the theoretical adverse effects of phytoestrogens in soy products, although this is not universal.

Allergy and anaphylaxis plans
- All patients with IgE-mediated food allergy must be provided with a written management plan in the event of an accidental exposure to the offending food allergen.
- Mild–moderate allergy:
  - Avoid causative food.
  - Give Allergy Action Plan (without an EpiPen) which is available from *www.allergy. org.au*
- Anaphylaxis:
  - Avoid causative food.
  - Refer for specialist allergy advice.
  - In the interim period, consultation with a clinical immunologist, allergist, paediatrician or emergency physician should be sought to determine the need for an EpiPen.
  - Prescription of an EpiPen must be accompanied by education on its use and provision of an Anaphylaxis Action Plan (available at *www.allergy.org.au*).
  - Dose for EpiPen:
    Child >20 kg, EpiPen 300 mcg.
    Child 10–20 kg, EpiPen Jr 150 mcg.
    Child <10 kg, not usually recommended (discuss with specialist).

Note: This is different to current product information dosage guidelines, where Epipen 300 mcg is recommended for children >30 kg.

Investigation
- Confirm the presence of mild–moderate IgE-mediated reaction (not anaphylaxis) to the suspected food if it is one of the common food allergens (e.g. milk, egg, peanut) with a

SPT or RAST to that food. A negative SPT or RAST almost eliminates the possibility of an immediate IgE-mediated reaction to that food. A positive SPT or RAST **confirms** food allergy if there is a convincing history. If the history is uncertain, further evaluation by formal challenge is required. Parents should not challenge children with a suspected food at home as severe reactions and even death have occurred.

- Performing SPT or RAST to other common food allergens (egg, milk, wheat, soy, peanut, shellfish, fish) to which the child has not yet been exposed may be indicated.

Refer to paediatric allergy specialist

- Children with anaphylaxis.
- Children suspected of having multiple food allergies, including children with confirmed allergy to one food and not yet exposed to one or more of the other common food allergens.
- Children with an unclear history or those who are likely to require retesting or challenge.
- Children with multiple atopic diseases.

Non-IgE-mediated and mixed IgE/non-IgE mediated food reactions

- Non-IgE-mediated food reactions are much less common.
- Generally these are delayed reactions occurring 24–48 h after food ingestion, although some infants may have immediate non-IgE-mediated food reactions that occur within 1–2 h of food ingestion.
- Typically, gastrointestinal symptoms are prominent with vomiting, diarrhoea and abdominal cramps. Occasionally there may be malabsorption, weight loss or slow weight gain. Worsening of eczema may also occur.
- In severe cases (e.g. food protein induced enterocolitis syndrome, FPIES) there may be cardiovascular collapse.
- Cow's milk and soy proteins are the most common foods implicated.
- Diagnosis requires elimination of the suspected food followed by formal food challenge.
- Skin-prick testing is usually negative, but may be positive if there is a mixed aetiology, which includes some IgE-mediated reaction.
- Treatment is with avoidance of the offending food. Specialist consultation is recommended.
- Infants with non-IgE-mediated cow's milk allergy should be given an extensively hydrolysed protein formula.
- 50% of cases resolve within 1–2 years.

Food-protein-induced enterocolitis syndrome (FPIES)

- A form of non-IgE mediated food allergy seen in young infants usually <6 months.
- Usually due to cow's milk, soy or cereals (e.g. rice).
- Can be seen in exclusively breast-fed infants.
- Can be seen in older children with other foods (e.g. egg).
- Typically delayed onset (>1–2 h) of projectile vomiting (that may become bilious) and protracted diarrhoea.
- May be associated with hypotension in 15% of cases (significant pallor and lethargy) that may be misdiagnosed as sepsis.

- Stool: occult blood, polymorphonuclear cells (PMNs), eosinophils, reducing substances.
- Symptoms resolve within 72 h of substance elimination.

Food-protein-induced enteropathy

- A spectrum of disorders that present with protracted diarrhoea, vomiting in 2/3 and slow weight gain.
- Cow's milk is the most frequent cause. Others include soy, egg, wheat, rice, chicken and fish.
- It has been suggested that coeliac disease represents the most severe form.
- Endoscopy/biopsy shows patchy villous atrophy with cellular infiltrates.
- Symptoms resolve after 6–12 weeks of elimination of the responsible food allergen. Improvement in appetite, vomiting, and diarrhoea may occur within 2–4 weeks; however, weight gain may take 8–12 weeks.

Food-protein-induced colitis

- First weeks to months of life.
- Usually cow's milk or soy, but 50% of infants with this condition are breast-fed.
- Present with isolated bloody stool (gross or occult).
- Otherwise clinically well.
- Endoscopy shows mucosal oedema, ulceration, erosions that are restricted to distal bowel.
- Symptoms resolve within 72 h of elimination of the offending food.

Eosinophilic oesophagitis

- May be a cause of gastroesophageal reflux (GOR).
- Up to 40% of GOR in infants <1 year that is unresponsive to medical therapy may be due to cow's milk allergy.
- May present as infantile colic.
- Infants often have other allergic disease, elevated IgE, peripheral blood eosinophilia and positive SPT to foods.
- Can occur in older children and adults, where it commonly presents as dysphagia.
- Endoscopy shows eosinophilic infiltrates in the oesophagus.
- Symptoms resolve within 72 h of elimination of the offending food.

Eosinophilic enteritis

- Presents with postprandial symptoms of nausea, vomiting, abdominal pain and diarrhoea.
- Other presentations include slow weight gain in infants, iron deficiency anaemia, hypoalbuminaemia and steatorrhoea in adults.
- Endoscopy shows eosinophilic infiltrates in the stomach and/or duodenum.
- Symptoms resolve within 72 h of elimination of the offending food.

Allergic factors in atopic dermatitis (eczema)

See also chapter 23, Dermatologic conditions, p. 277.

Atopic dermatitis has a major impact on the lives of patients and their families. Allergic and infective factors may play an important role in the exacerbation of eczema and this should always be considered in moderate or severe disease. Avoiding the relevant allergic factors can improve symptom control in the context of optimal medical management.

- *Staphylococcus aureus* infection can have several clinical presentations including folliculitis (often punctuate), impetigo (crusting) and discoid lesions. Treatment of acute staphylococcal infection and reduction of staphylococcal loads on the skin can provide significant improvement of eczema control. Staphylococcal infection and/or colonisation must be controlled before the benefits of other allergen-avoidance measures can be assessed.
- House dust mite sensitivity is another important exacerbating factor in atopic dermatitis. Dust mite allergen is ubiquitous in the home environment, particularly in the bedroom where a child spends up to 10 h each day. In patients with sensitivity to house dust mite allergen, instituting the appropriate avoidance measures may be beneficial (see Allergic rhinitis, p. 228).
- Immediate food hypersensitivity reactions can also act as exacerbating factors, particularly in young children with severe atopic dermatitis and generalised erythema. Patients requiring investigation for possible food triggers should be referred for specialist allergy advice.
- In a small number of severe cases, there may be delayed reactions to foods. There are no skin or blood tests that can reliably identify whether delayed reaction to a food is occurring. The implementation of a restricted diet followed by systematic reintroduction of suspected foods is used to assess this. These dietary manipulations are often complex and difficult to interpret. Specialist advice from a paediatric allergist and dietician is required. Appropriate case selection is important. Dietary restrictions should not be instituted in children with mild atopic dermatitis that can be readily controlled with the appropriate topical medication.

Allergic factors in asthma

See also chapter 36, Respiratory conditions, p. 505.

Allergic factors may contribute to the symptoms of asthma, particularly in cases of chronic persistent asthma. Investigation for allergens to which a patient is sensitised should be pursued in any patient requiring maintenance anti-inflammatory corticosteroid therapy, particularly those with interval symptoms. The avoidance of relevant allergic factors represents a simple, inexpensive and non-pharmacological approach to anti-inflammatory therapy. However, allergen avoidance represents only one component of the overall management of asthma. Patients should understand that allergic factors are not the sole cause of asthma.

- The major allergens implicated are the indoor inhalants (house dust mite, cat and dog dander). Pollens may also contribute to seasonal exacerbations of asthma, especially if the patient also suffers from seasonal allergic rhinitis. Moulds may trigger asthma symptoms in arid climates.
- Allergic rhinitis can exacerbate asthma and untreated persistent rhinitis may be one of the reasons for a failed response to standard anti-asthma therapy. Co-existent allergic rhinitis should be considered in all patients with asthma – it is common and treatable.
- Foods generally do not induce asthma symptoms in isolation. They may cause asthma symptoms as part of an immediate allergic reaction (i.e. anaphylaxis) when cutaneous eruptions are usually also observed.

- In some patients with chronic asthma, the preservative metabisulfite can provoke an acute exacerbation. Confirmation of this requires specialist consultation.
- NSAIDs (e.g. aspirin) may exacerbate asthma symptoms in some patients with chronic asthma. Specialist consultation is required to confirm this.

Urticaria and angio-oedema
Urticarial rashes
Also known as hives, urticarial rashes are raised areas of erythema and oedema, which are usually itchy and move over the body over several hours. They are classified as acute (<6 weeks' duration) or chronic (>6 weeks' duration).

Acute urticaria
- Often only lasts a few days.
- In the vast majority of cases, no precipitating factor is identified.
- The most important step is to take a careful history to look for possible exposure to drugs (especially antibiotics) or foods that may have induced an immediate hypersensitivity reaction. If a precipitating factor cannot be identified on history, SPT and RAST will generally not provide additional information and are **not** indicated.
- Some cases follow viral or streptococcal infections.

Chronic urticaria
- Can persist or occur intermittently for months or years.
- The possibility of a physical urticaria (e.g. heat, cold or cholinergic) should be considered.
- In protracted cases, it is important to consider the possibility of an underlying connective tissue or autoimmune disorder that may (rarely) present as chronic urticaria. In these cases, there are usually other suggestive features such as arthritis or vasculitis. Biopsy of lesions for histologic analysis may be helpful in identifying vasculitis.
- Chronic urticaria is rarely caused by specific allergic factors and therefore investigation with SPT and RAST is not helpful.

Angio-oedema
- Swelling of the deeper tissues that is not necessarily itchy. It often involves areas of low tension, such as the eyelids, lips and scrotum.

Treatment of both acute and chronic urticaria
- Symptomatic: treat with second-generation antihistamines. Cetirizine is particularly effective (for doses see Table 19.2).
- Manipulation of the diet is generally not helpful and is not indicated in children. A small number of subjects may respond to a preservative and colouring-free diet; however, this should only be considered if symptoms are particularly troublesome.
- In resistant cases, the combined use of an H_2 antihistamine (cimetidine) with standard H_1 antihistamines may be considered but success is limited.

Hereditary angio-oedema

- Rare autosomal dominant condition in which C1 esterase inhibitor levels are reduced (HAE type I) or poorly functional (HAE type II), resulting in uninhibited activation of the complement, kinin and fibrinolytic cascade.
- This results in recurrent episodes of angio-oedema involving limbs, upper respiratory or gastrointestinal tract. Hence patients present with:
  - Angio-oedema **without** pruritis or urticaria.
  - Abdominal pain ± nausea/vomiting (due to intestinal oedema).
  - Laryngeal oedema.
- Diagnosed by the finding of low C1 esterase inhibitor level or function. C4 level is also low during episodes of angio-oedema.

Management

Refer to the Clinical Practice Guideline *www.rch.org.au/clinical guide* [C1 Esterase Inhibitor Deficiency].

- Adrenaline, antihistamines and corticosteroids have **no** role in the management.
- Tranexamic acid may be considered in mild episodes to shorten the duration of symptoms.
- Severe angio-oedema episodes can be fatal. I.v. C1 esterase inhibitor concentrate should be administered.
- Children undergoing surgery: preoperative discussions with the anaesthetist, immunologist and intensive care unit are recommended. Consider the use of danazol for 5–10 days before surgery.

Antibiotic allergy

Reported allergy to antibiotics in children is common; however, many patients are incorrectly labelled as 'antibiotic allergic'. Careful history is required to identify those patients who are likely to have experienced true antibiotic reactions. This includes details of the reaction and its timing in relation to drug dose; prior and subsequent drug exposure; concurrent illness; and other concurrent new food or drug ingestion.

Reactions may be IgE mediated or non-IgE mediated. The most common presentation is a cutaneous eruption, either urticarial or maculopapular. More severe reactions are anaphylaxis with angio-oedema and bronchospasm or laryngeal oedema, exfoliative dermatitis, Stevens–Johnson syndrome, or serum sickness with arthralgia. Multiple antibiotic allergies where a child is reported to react to a significant number of antibiotics are not uncommon.

The most common reactions are to the penicillin family. Allergy to penicillin or its derivatives is associated with a 10% risk of reaction (through cross-reactivity) to the first- and second-generation cephalosporins. This does not extend to third-generation cephalosporins, as reactions to these are usually directed to side chains.

Management

- No completely adequate *in vitro* or *in vivo* tests diagnose drug allergy.
- The detection of IgE antibodies by RAST or SPT may be helpful in the evaluation of penicillin or amoxycillin reactions.

- Skin-prick testing regimens have been established for the penicillin metabolites; however, neither positive nor negative tests accurately predict actual reaction to drug administered. Skin testing for other antibiotics is even less helpful.
- In most cases, an oral challenge initiated under observation and then continued on an outpatient basis is required to confirm or exclude allergy.
- An assessment should be made of the severity of the reaction. Each case must be judged on its merits.
- If there has been anaphylaxis with cardiovascular and/or respiratory problems, the patient should **not** be challenged with the drug again except in exceptional circumstances and after appropriate evaluation.
- Other contraindications to challenge include severe mucocutaneous reactions such as Stevens–Johnson syndrome or exfoliative dermatitis and serum sickness. In these instances, an alternative class of antibiotic should be selected. In deciding whether to proceed with a challenge, a judgement should also be made regarding the importance of the antibiotic in question.
- In the vast majority of cases with the question of multiple antibiotic allergies, a challenge is carried out with a single antibiotic selected as being appropriate for future use and the challenge is completed without reaction.

Latex allergy

Latex products contain two types of compounds that can cause reactions: chemical additives that cause dermatitis and natural proteins that induce immediate allergic reactions. Most reactions to latex in the hospital setting involve disposable gloves; however, other items including catheters, dressings and bandages, i.v. tubing, stethoscopes and airways may contain latex. Common latex products used in the community include balloons, baby-bottle teats and dummies, elastic bands and condoms. Reactions to latex products may be irritant or immune mediated.

Irritant dermatitis

Irritant dermatitis is the most common problem encountered with the use of latex gloves. This is a non-allergic skin rash characterised by erythema, dryness, scaling and cracking. It is caused by sweating and irritation from the glove or its powder or by irritation as a result of frequent washing with soap and detergents.

Immediate allergy to latex

Type I hypersensitivity reactions to latex are the most serious as they are potentially life threatening. They are caused by IgE antibodies to latex proteins. Reactions may occur after contact with latex (e.g. gloves and catheters) or the inhalation of airborne powder particles containing allergenic latex proteins.

- Sensitisation may occur following direct exposure of mucosal surfaces to latex (e.g. catheterisation).

- The severity of the reaction may vary widely, ranging from isolated allergic rhinoconjunctivitis, urticaria or asthma, to anaphylaxis and death.
- Certain populations are at high risk for developing latex allergy: children with spina bifida or other urogenital anomalies and individuals undergoing multiple surgical procedures, particularly if they are atopic.
- SPTs and/or RASTs are useful in confirming suspected sensitisation. SPTs are more reliable than RAST; however, well-standardised SPT extracts are not widely available.
- There is no cure for latex allergy. The best approach is to avoid exposure.
- There may be cross-reactivity between latex and certain foods, in particular avocado, kiwi fruit and banana. Latex-allergic individuals who experience discomfort in the mouth or throat while eating these foods should avoid them.

Contact dermatitis

This is a delayed type IV hypersensitivity to chemical additives used in processing latex. Reactions are limited to the site of contact. Use of rubber gloves results in eczematous lesions on the dorsum of the hands. The skin may become dry, crusted and thickened. Oral reactions caused by dental appliances or balloons, and genital reactions caused by condoms have been described. The use of cotton lining gloves inside latex gloves or a change to gloves that do not contain the chemicals contained in latex gloves usually reduces the problem. Patients with irritant and contact dermatitis are at an increased risk of developing immediate hypersensitivity to latex and exposure to latex should be minimised.

Management

- Patients at high risk for latex sensitivity should be referred to a paediatric allergist/immunologist for further evaluation.
- Patients who have a confirmed latex allergy (either immediate or delayed) should undertake strict latex avoidance including having latex-free precautions during surgery.

Immunotherapy

There are relatively few indications for specific injection immunotherapy in paediatric practice.

Immunotherapy has traditionally been administered by subcutaneous injections. In general, injections are given weekly, in increasing dosage until the maintenance dose has been achieved. This is done under close supervision by practitioners trained in the early identification and management of allergic reactions and anaphylaxis. Once maintenance doses have been achieved, injections are continued monthly, often by a GP, for a period of 3–5 years. Immunotherapy is not undertaken lightly. It requires a long-term commitment to therapy and may be associated with severe reactions (anaphylaxis). Consideration of pain management and psychological support is essential, especially in young children or those who are frightened of needles.

Bee venom anaphylaxis

- Immunotherapy with purified bee venom is indicated for life-threatening anaphylactic reactions to bee stings in children. Referral should be made to a paediatric allergist/immunologist for allergy testing and further management.
- Severe local reactions to bee stings are **not** an indication for immunotherapy and do not require further investigation with skin-prick testing.
- SPTs and RASTs to bee venom are not predictive of systemic reactions and in general are not indicated except to confirm the presence of bee venom sensitisation before initiation of bee venom immunotherapy in those with previous bee sting anaphylaxis.

Allergic rhinitis

- Immunotherapy may be an option in severe seasonal allergic rhinitis if the symptoms are not controlled with allergen avoidance and maximal medical therapy (topical anti-inflammatories and antihistamines), particularly if a limited number of allergens can be identified.
- Extreme caution is required in administering immunotherapy to unstable asthmatic patients, as deaths have resulted.

Note: Sublingual administration of allergen for immunotherapy (to environmental allergen) is used widely in Europe and is being used increasingly in Australia. Evidence of efficacy in children is currently lacking. Further studies are required before routine use can be recommended, but it may offer an alternative approach in the future.

Guidelines for the investigation and treatment of immunodeficiency
When to suspect immunodeficiency

Immunocompetent children average 5–10 viral upper respiratory tract infections per year in the first few years of life (even more if the child attends childcare or has older siblings). Recurrent viral infections in a well, thriving child do not suggest immunodeficiency. Immune deficiency should be suspected when there is a history of severe, recurrent or unusual infections.

- Recurrent or chronic bacterial infections (e.g. persistently discharging ears or purulent respiratory secretions) or more than one severe pyogenic infection may indicate antibody deficiency.
- Severe or disseminated viral infections, persistent mucocutaneous candidiasis, chronic infectious diarrhoea and/or failure to thrive in infants suggest a severe T-cell deficiency. These children should be investigated for severe combined immune deficiency (SCID). SCID should be managed as a paediatric emergency.
- The presence of autoimmune cytopenias, together with recurrent sinopulmonary infections, raises the possibility of less severe forms of combined immune deficiency.
- Recurrent pyogenic infections affecting lymph nodes, skin, lung and bones suggest a neutrophil defect.
- Recurrent or severe meningococcal disease suggests a late component complement deficiency.

- Early component complement deficiencies may present with clinical features that are similar to antibody defects or with autoimmune disease.

Which tests to order

Basic immunodeficiency screen

- An FBE with differential and immunoglobulin levels (IgG, IgA and IgM) will identify the vast majority of treatable primary immunodeficiencies (e.g. agammaglobulinaemia, common variable immune deficiency, selective IgA deficiency and SCID). IgG subclass levels should **not** be done as part of a basic immunological screen, as isolated IgG subclass deficiency is of uncertain clinical significance.
- Note that immunoglobulin levels vary with age and are lower in infancy and early childhood. It is therefore important that the relevant age-related reference ranges are used (see Table 19.3).
- If these tests are normal and the clinical suspicion of immune deficiency persists, referral to a clinical immunologist for further evaluation is indicated.

Specific antibody responses

- Only consider when there is evidence of persistent or recurrent suppurative upper and/or lower respiratory tract infection and hypogammaglobulinaemia has been excluded.
- Ask the question: 'If an antibody defect is found, does this clinical condition warrant regular gammaglobulin therapy?'
- The most important question is whether appropriate antibodies can be made to specific protein and polysaccharide antigens. Abnormal IgG subclass levels may be a clue to an evolving antibody deficiency. However, isolated abnormalities of IgG subclasses with normal specific antibody responses rarely result in clinical problems. In general, regular gammaglobulin therapy is only indicated for severe recurrent infections when a specific antibody defect has been identified.

T-lymphocyte numbers and function

- Consider a chest radiograph to look for absent thymic shadow when a T-lymphocyte defect is suspected.
- Specialised T-lymphocyte function tests are used to help in the diagnosis of SCID and Di George syndrome (absent thymus, hypocalcaemia and cardiovascular anomalies). Referral to an immunologist is recommended if these conditions are suspected.

Neutrophil function tests

- Specific defects of neutrophil function (e.g. chronic granulomatous disease and leucocyte adhesion deficiency 1) are very rare. They are almost always associated with gingivitis and careful examination of the mouth is important when considering abnormalities of neutrophil function.
- Markedly elevated circulating neutrophil counts and delayed separation of the umbilical cord (>4 weeks) suggest the possibility of a leucocyte adhesion deficiency.
- Suspected cases of defective neutrophil function should be referred to an immunologist for further evaluation.

Table 19.3 Immunoglobulin normal ranges (5th to 95th percentile)

Age	IgG (g/L)	IgA (g/L)	IgM (g/L)
0–1 month	2.5–12.0	<0.07–0.94	0.19–1.93
1–2 months	2.5–12.0	<0.07–1.31	0.19–1.93
2–3 months	2.5–12.0	<0.07–1.31	0.21–1.92
3–4 months	2.86–16.8	<0.07–1.31	0.21–1.92
4–12 months	2.86–16.8	0.1–1.29	0.21–1.92
1–2 years	2.86–16.8	0.19–1.75	0.43–1.63
2–3 years	3.41–19.6	0.22–2.20	0.43–1.63
3–4 years	3.41–19.6	0.48–3.45	0.43–1.63
4–5 years	5.28–21.9	0.61–3.45	0.48–2.26
5–6 years	5.28–21.9	0.43–2.53	0.48–2.26
6–7 years	5.28–21.9	0.41–2.97	0.48–2.26
7–10 years	5.28–21.9	0.51–2.97	0.48–2.26
10–13 years	5.28–21.9	0.44–3.95	0.48–2.26
13–19 years	5.28–21.9	0.44–4.41	0.48–2.26

Source: Davis *et al.* IFCC-standardised pediatric reference intervals for 10 serum proteins using the Beckman Array 360 system. *Clin Biochem*, Oct 1996; **29(5)**: 489–92.

Complement studies
- Deficiencies of complement are rare.
- The best screening test for congenital deficiency is a CH50, which measures the function of the classical complement pathway.

HIV tests
HIV testing should be considered in the setting of recurrent, severe or unusual infections, particularly if there is hypergammaglobulinaemia. Testing requires informed consent and appropriate counselling. This specialised immune function testing is best undertaken in consultation with a clinical immunologist.

Immunodeficiency treatment
Immunisation
See also chapter 9, Immunisation.

- As a general rule, all live viral vaccines should be avoided in immunodeficiency unless advised by a specialist.
- Patients with a T-cell defect and their immediate family should receive the killed injectable polio (Salk) vaccine, not live oral polio vaccine. This is now the standard form of polio vaccine in Australia.
- In certain circumstances, measles immunisation may be given to patients with a T-cell defect (e.g. Di George syndrome or paediatric HIV infection) as the risks of wild-type measles infection are considerable, but adverse reactions to the vaccine are largely theoretical.
- In cases of antibody deficiency, T-cell deficiency and combined immunodeficiency, immunisation with killed vaccines will not promote a significant antibody response.
- If the patient is on immunoglobulin replacement therapy, passively acquired antibody will prevent viral infections such as measles and chickenpox. See also chapter 9, Immunisation.
- Patients of any age with asplenia should be immunised with Hib, pneumococcal and meningococcal vaccines.

Immunoglobulin therapy

- Immunoglobulin therapy (400–600 mg/kg i.v. monthly) is given when a significant deficiency of antibody production is demonstrated in a patient with clinically significant infections (usually sinopulmonary).
- In hypogammaglobulinaemia, immunoglobulin therapy is generally lifelong.
- In patients with combined immunodeficiency, immunoglobulin treatment may be discontinued once normal B-cell function can be demonstrated following bone marrow transplantation.
- In patients with IgG subclass deficiency, immunoglobulin therapy is indicated only if a significant functional antibody deficit is demonstrated and the patient has significant symptoms. In this instance, a trial of immunoglobulin therapy may be used for a restricted period of time to determine if there is clinical benefit. This should only be instituted in conjunction with a clinical immunologist.
- The finding of a low immunoglobulin subclass level alone is not a sufficient indication for immunoglobulin therapy. Immunoglobulin therapy is not indicated for isolated IgA deficiency. These patients should be referred to a specialist for further evaluation and/or follow up.
- Three forms of immunoglobulin are currently available for i.v. administration in Australia: Intragam P (produced from Australian plasma), Octagam and Sandoglobulin (imported products).
  - IgG concentrations and rates of administration differ in the different products and need to be taken into account when these products are administered.
- The subcutaneous route for administration of immunoglobulin for replacement purposes is being used widely overseas and increasingly in Australia. Potential benefits include ease of administration in patients where venous access is limited and capacity for home immunoglobulin delivery. A more concentrated immunoglobulin product is used for these purposes.

Antibiotics
- As immunoglobulin therapy does not provide significant levels of IgA antibody (the mucosal surface antibody), aggressive treatment of respiratory infections in patients with antibody deficiency is important in order to prevent bronchiectasis and permanent damage to the lungs.
- In severe cases, prophylactic rotating antibiotics are used to prevent recurrent severe sinopulmonary infections.
- Antibiotic prophylaxis with cotrimoxazole 2.5/12.5 mg/kg (max. 80/400) p.o. b.d. 3 days per week is indicated in patients with T-cell or combined immune deficiency to prevent infection with pneumocystis.

Use of blood products
- If it is suspected or known that the patient has a significant T-cell deficiency, blood products that contain cells (e.g. whole blood, packed red cells or platelets) should be irradiated to prevent graft versus host disease.
- In infants with SCID or any significant T-cell deficiency, attempts should be made to provide cytomegalovirus (CMV) antibody-negative blood, as CMV infection can be a significant problem in such patients. If this is not possible, the blood product should be filtered to remove contaminating white blood cells as it is delivered to the patient. If possible, Epstein–Barr virus (EBV) antibody-negative blood should also be given, as EBV can induce lymphoproliferative states in severely immunodeficient subjects.
- Patients with IgA deficiency may develop IgE antibodies to IgA and have an anaphylactic reaction to blood products containing IgA (i.v. immunoglobulin, packed red cells, platelets). Immunoglobulin preparations that are depleted of IgA should be used and packed cells or platelets should be washed four times in physiological saline before infusion.

Bone marrow transplantation
- Bone marrow transplantation is the definitive treatment for SCID. It may also be useful for the treatment of other immune deficiencies (e.g. chronic granulomatous disease, hyper IgM syndrome).
- The cure rate can be of the order of 80% if the transplant is from a matched sibling or a parent.
- Survival is less, in the order of 50%, if the transplant is only partially matched and from an unrelated donor.

USEFUL RESOURCES
- *www.allergy.org.au* – The Australian Society of Clinical Allergy and Immunology. Contains excellent information for patients and health care professionals. Includes anaphylaxis action plans.
- *www.primaryimmune.org* – Immune Deficiency Foundation. Patient organisation website containing excellent handouts for primary immune deficiencies.
- *www.esid.org* – Eurpean Society for Immunodeficiencies. Contains a useful clinical section which details diagnostic criteria of various primary immunodeficiencies.

CHAPTER 20

Burns

Russell Taylor

Treatment aims
- Prevent and treat burn shock.
- Provide adequate analgesia.
- Prevent infection.
- Obtain early skin cover.
- Prevent hypertrophic scar formation.
- Restore function and correct cosmetic defect.
- Prevent recurrence of injury and promote accident prevention.

Assessment
Age
The younger the child, the more likely shock will occur for a given extent of burn.

Estimating the surface area burned
The usual adult formula (rule of nines) is not applicable to children. In infancy, the head is relatively large and contributes proportionately more to the total surface area. As the child grows, the lower limbs contribute more to the total surface area. The burned areas should be plotted accurately on the body chart and the area calculated with the aid of the Lund–Browder chart (see Fig. 20.1). The extent of the burn is commonly overestimated, leading to excessive fluid administration.

Assessment of the depth of burn
In most burns, there are varying grades of injury (see Table 20.1).

First aid
- Remove clothing or smother the flame immediately.
- In minor burns, apply cold water from a bowl or by compressing for up to 30 min.
- In major burns, bathe for 20 min whilst awaiting transportation to hospital. Never use ice or ice slush.

Paediatric Handbook, 8th edition. By Kate Thomson, Dean Tey and Michael Marks. Published 2009 by Blackwell Publishing, ISBN: 978-1-4051-7400-8.

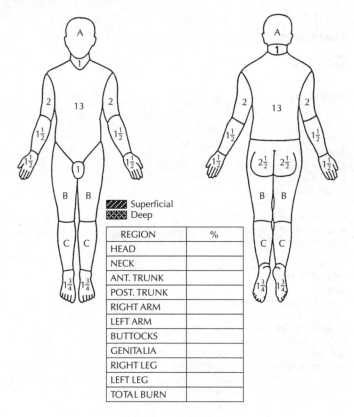

REGION	%
HEAD	
NECK	
ANT. TRUNK	
POST. TRUNK	
RIGHT ARM	
LEFT ARM	
BUTTOCKS	
GENITALIA	
RIGHT LEG	
LEFT LEG	
TOTAL BURN	

Superficial
Deep

Relative percentage of areas affected by growth

Age (years)	0	1	5	10	15	Adult
A—$\frac{1}{2}$ of head	$9\frac{1}{2}$	$8\frac{1}{2}$	$6\frac{1}{2}$	$5\frac{1}{2}$	$4\frac{1}{2}$	$3\frac{1}{2}$
B—$\frac{1}{2}$ of one thigh	$2\frac{3}{4}$	$3\frac{1}{4}$	4	$4\frac{1}{4}$	$4\frac{1}{2}$	$4\frac{3}{4}$
C—$\frac{1}{2}$ of one leg	$2\frac{1}{2}$	$2\frac{1}{2}$	$2\frac{3}{4}$	3	$3\frac{1}{4}$	$3\frac{1}{2}$

Fig 20.1 Lund–Browder chart

Table 20.1 Assessment of burn depth

Depth	Cause	Surface/colour	Pain	Treatment
Superficial (partial loss of skin)	Sun, flash, minor scald	Dry, minor blisters, erythema	Painful	Expose Non-adherent dressing
Superficial partial	Scald	Moist, reddened with broken blisters	Painful	Nanocrystalline silver dressing, e.g. Acticoat
Deep partial	Scald, minor flame contact	Moist, white slough, red mottled	Painless	Nanocrystalline silver dressing, e.g. Acticoat
Deep (complete loss of skin)	Flame, severe scald or contact	Dry, white, charred	Painless	Nanocrystalline silver dressing, e.g. Acticoat or SSD cream until split skin graft

- Cover to guard against hypothermia or cold injury with special foam transport dressing (if available) or plastic cling wrap, with a blanket for warmth. Give i.v. fluid, oxygen and morphine.
- Chemical and eye burns should be irrigated with copious volumes of cold water.
- Check tetanus immunisation status and boost with tetanus toxoid ± tetanus immunoglobulin as appropriate (see chapter 3, Procedures, p. 51).

Pain relief
- Paracetamol (oral), 20–30 mg/kg.
- Codeine (oral), 0.5–1 mg/kg.
- Morphine (i.v.), 0.1 mg/kg given in titrated boluses.
- Morphine (i.m.), 0.2 mg/kg (useful if only a single dose is anticipated).

Minor burns
Superficial burns <5% of the body surface area (BSA) are suitable for outpatient treatment, unless they occur on the face, neck, hands, feet or perineum. Infants <12 months are more likely to require admission.

Initial management
- Blisters should be left intact.
- Gently cleanse and remove loose skin.

- If burns are definitely superficial, dress with tulle gras and an absorbent dressing (e.g. gauze). Do not use Hypafix-type dressing directly on the burn.
- Immobilise with a crepe bandage, plaster slab or sling, if indicated.
- In partial thickness burns of indeterminate depth, the use of nanocrystalline dressing is recommended e.g. Acticoat. These dressings should be left in place for 3 or 7 days depending on the product used.

Subsequent management
- Leave the initial dressing for 5–8 days. If the dressing is soaked by exudate, redress without disturbing the adherent tulle.
- If the healing process is not complete by the end of the second week, grafting may be required. Deep, second-degree burns should be grafted by 5–10 days.
- Pain, fever and soiled or offensive dressings indicate that the dressing should be changed and the child assessed and treated for infection if necessary.

Major burns
Superficial burns >5% of the BSA and deep burns require admission to hospital. **For any child with burns >10% of the BSA, consider transfer to a specialist paediatric burns centre**. Older children with more extensive superficial burns, such as sunburn, may be managed as outpatients (see Table 20.1).

General
- Document the time, causative agent, circumstances of the burn, therapy initiated and the child's general health. If the history is inconsistent with the injury, consider child abuse.
- Carefully chart the extent and depth of the burn.
- Weigh the patient if possible.
- In burns >10% of BSA, insert an i.v. line. If a central venous line is needed, a specialist burn centre should be involved. Plan i.v. therapy (see below) and commence treatment with Hartmann's solution.
- Draw blood for baseline laboratory studies, including haemoglobin, haematocrit and serum electrolytes. In severe burns include blood group and a cross-match.
- In burns >15% of BSA, insert a silastic urethral catheter for hourly urine volume.
- Analgesia or sedation should be administered as necessary (see chapter 4, Pain management).
- Prevent infection. Care should be taken in ward management to guard against cross-infection. Antibiotics should not be prescribed routinely.
- Observations of general condition, pulse, respiration rate, temperature, BP and fluid balance (including hourly urine output estimations) are necessary.

Respiratory management
- With severe burns to the face, consider early endotracheal intubation. As the face swells, airway obstruction may occur, making intubation difficult.

- Smoke inhalation may lead to acute respiratory distress syndrome (ARDS) where ventilation perfusion defects result in hypoxemia, alveolar collapse, shunting and decreased lung compliance.
- Carboxyhaemoglobin (COHb) and cyanide concentration should be measured in all burn/smoke inhalation patients. Symptoms of hypoxemia manifest at levels >30% COHb. Treatment is oxygen therapy, as CO binding to Hb is reversible.

Fluid management
Fluid resuscitation
See Figure 20.2.
- **Fluid volume** = 3 mL/kg body weight/% burn surface area (BSA) in the first 24 h.
- In less severe burns, fluid volume = 2 mL/kg body weight/% BSA may be sufficient.
- **Type of fluid** = 4% normal serum albumin solution (NSAS) and Hartmann's solution (use 50% of each solution concurrently).

Fluid maintenance
- 5% dextrose with 0.9% saline (to calculate maintenance fluid rate see chapter 5, Fluids, p. 73).

Burns surface area (BSA) .. ... % Date ......
Weight (kg) ...... Time i.v. commenced (24 h clock) ......
Urinary output expected (0.75 mL/kg per h) = ... mL/hr Time of burn (24 h clock) ......

	1st 24 h (volume)	1st 8 h (volume)	2nd 8 h (volume)	3rd 8 h (volume)
(A) Burn resuscitation *3 × kg × % = ... mL Type of infusion: concurrently use 50% of each of **4% normal serum albumin solution (NSAS) ***Remainder as Hartmann's solution	_____ mL _____ mL	1/2 of 24 h vol _____ mL _____ mL	1/4 of 24 h vol _____ mL _____ mL	1/4 of 24 h vol _____ mL _____ mL
(B) Maintenance fluid (see oral fluids information p248) 5% dextrose with 0.9% saline (estimated volume on bodyweight in kg)	_____ mL	1/3 of 24 h vol _____ mL	1/3 of 24 h vol _____ mL	1/3 of 24 h vol _____ mL
(C) Total A & B burn (burn resuscitation & maintenance fluid)	_____ **mL**	_____ **mL**	_____ **mL**	_____ **mL**

* In less severe burns, 2 mL × kg × 1% in the first 24 h may be sufficient.

** Normal serum albumin solution (NSAS) is interspersed and not given as one bolus.

*** If no Hartmann's available, use normal saline.

Figure 20.2 Resuscitation of a burnt child during the first 24 hours

Rate of infusion (first 24 h)
- First 8 h: 1/2 resuscitation fluid plus 1/3 maintenance fluid.
- Second 8 h: 1/4 resuscitation fluid plus 1/3 maintenance fluid.
- Third 8 h: 1/4 resuscitation fluid plus 1/3 maintenance fluid.

For example, in a 16 kg child with 5% burns:
- Total resuscitation fluid = 3 × 16 kg × 5% = 240 mL (use 120 mL NSAS + 120 mL Hartmann's).
- Total maintenance fluid = 1300 mL.
- First 8 h = 120 mL (1/2 total resus fluid) + 433 mL (1/3 total maintenance fluid) = 553 mL (69 mL/h).
- Second 8 h = 60 mL (1/4 total resus fluid) + 433 mL (1/3 total maintenance fluid) = 493 mL (62 mL/h).
- Third 8 h = 60 mL (1/4 total resus fluid) + 433 mL (1/3 total maintenance fluid) = 493 mL (62 mL/h).

The 24 h period commences from the time of burning, not from the time of admission.

Adjustments are made according to the hourly urine output, which is the best guide to the adequacy of fluid replacement. Expected flow is 0.75 mL/kg per hour in children; in infants and toddlers, a urine output of up to 1 mL/kg per hour is required. Record the urine specific gravity, serum and urine osmolality if renal function is poor.

Continue monitoring haemoglobin, haematocrit and electrolytes, more frequently in severe injury. Restlessness may indicate inadequate fluid replacement.

Rate of infusion (second 24 h and onwards)
After the initial 24 h of fluid replacement, the type of fluid replacement will depend on urinary output, serum electrolytes and haemoglobin.
- The volume of burn resuscitation fluid is approximately 1/2 of that given for the first 24 h.
- Total volume is given at an even rate over 24 h.
- The volume and type of fluid given are adjusted according to urine flow and electrolyte estimations, and then decreased as the shock diminishes over the succeeding days. Diuresis occurs 2–3 days post-burn.

Oral fluids
Most children will tolerate small amounts of feeds (30–60 mL/h) after 4–8 h. If this is tolerated, increase the quantity to 4 hourly. In minor burns, oral fluids may be commenced earlier. If vomiting secondary to gastric dilatation occurs, a nasogastric tube should be inserted. **If oral fluids are not tolerated see (B) in Figure 20.2.**

After 48 h, most fluid intake is usually oral. Children who refuse to drink, or who have burns to the face and mouth, may require nasogastric feeding.

Blood
Whole blood is not required initially except in severe, deep burns, and then usually only 24 h post-burn, when the haemoglobin concentration is falling.

Local wound care

Minimal debridement of loose skin is done initially and management continued by exposed or closed methods.

Escharotomies should be considered if the peripheral circulation to a limb is jeopardised. Before commencing this procedure contact a paediatric burns unit.

Respiratory difficulties require particular attention; intensive care or escharotomy to the trunk may be required.

Exposed

- *Indications:* for burns on the face, perineum, or one surface of the trunk.
- *Treatment:* apply Solugel if superficial; Acticoat dressing or topical silver sulfadiazine (SSD) cream should be used depending on the extent of the burn.

Closed

- *Indications:* for small children and burns on extremities. Except for burns to the face or perineum, nearly all children are ultimately nursed with closed dressings.
- *Treatment:* an antiseptic tulle gras and gauze for superficial burns, or Acticoat dressing for deep burns. Fingers and toes are separated and wrapped together (not separately). Acticoat dressings can be left intact for 3 or 7 days.

Fever in patients with burns and antibiotic choice

- On admission, swabs should be taken of the burn area, nose, throat and rectum. The burn area should be re-swabbed twice weekly. In major burns, multiple 3 ml punch biopsy specimens are the most reliable method of detecting infection.
- Antibiotics are usually only given for proven infection and on the basis of sensitivity tests.
- If septicaemia is suspected clinically, blood culture should be performed and empiric antibiotics commenced. First line antibiotics are flucloxacillin and gentamicin, with change to timentin and gentamicin to cover *Pseudomonas* if there is no clinical improvement.

Nutrition

- All children with burns should receive a high-calorie diet containing adequate protein, vitamin and iron supplements.
- In severe burns there is a marked increase in metabolic rate and gastric tube feeding with a complete fluid diet (e.g. Isocal or Ensure) should be instituted early and adjusted to maintain or increase body weight. The involvement of a dietician is recommended.

Room temperature

It is desirable that this is in the range of 22–26 °C. If a child is partly exposed and nursed in a cool environment, metabolic requirements will increase.

Special therapy

Physiotherapy and occupational therapy should be commenced early and continue throughout the course of burn care. Splints and pressure dressings are necessary to control hypertrophic scar formation. The play therapist also has an important role.

Social rehabilitation is important, as many burned children come from disadvantaged homes. **Maltreated children constitute approximately 6% of admissions to the burns unit**. Psychological and psychiatric consultation is often required. The hospital teacher should also liaise with the child's schoolteachers.

Follow-up

Healed burns and grafts are kept soft with emollient (e.g. Sorbolene cream). Pressure therapy and supervision of splints should be continued by a physiotherapist and occupational therapist. Parents and children need continuing support. Further operations are sometimes necessary to correct contractures and relieve cosmetic defects.

USEFUL RESOURCES
* *www.sagediagram.com* – Fantastic resource from Oregon Burn Center which allows users to draw on areas of partial and full thickness burns, print out diagrams, calculate burn areas and fluid resuscitation.

CHAPTER 21

Cardiac conditions

Paul Brooks
Dan Penny

When to investigate a murmur
Background
At least 50% of school-age children have a systolic cardiac murmur with no structural or physiological cardiac problem. Chest radiograph (CXR) and electrocardiogram (ECG) are specific but not sensitive tests for cardiac disease.

Features of a physiological, functional or 'innocent' murmur
History
- Benign family history.
- Asymptomatic.
- Normal growth.

Examination
- Normal general physical examination.

Murmur characteristics
- Continuous murmur, which varies with posture.
- Soft, systolic murmur with:
  - Normal second heart sound.
  - Separate, audible heart sounds.
  - A musical, vibratory quality.

When to refer
A cardiac murmur associated with any of the following requires clinical assessment by a specialist:

History
- Family history of cardiomyopathy or sudden unexplained death.
- Chromosomal disorder.
- Congenital malformation of other organs.
- Maternal diabetes.

Paediatric Handbook, 8th edition. By Kate Thomson, Dean Tey and Michael Marks. Published 2009 by Blackwell Publishing, ISBN: 978-1-4051-7400-8.

- Exertional syncope or unexplained collapse.
- Palpitations.
- Symptoms of cardiac failure.

Examination
- Cyanosis.
- Breathlessness.
- Failure to thrive not clearly due to other causes.
- Unequal pulses.
- Thrill associated with murmur.

Murmur characteristics
- Diastolic murmur.
- Continuous murmur with no postural variation.
- Pan-systolic murmur.
- Loud murmur (amplitude grade 3/6 or greater).
- Murmur harsh or high pitched.
- Murmur heard best at left upper sternal border.
- Abnormal second heart sound.
- Early or mid-systolic click.

Worrying CXR
- Enlarged heart.
- Abnormal cardiac contour.
- Pulmonary plethora.
- ↓ Pulmonary vascular markings.

Worrying ECG
- Abnormal QRS axis.
- Increased voltages.
- Abnormal intervals.
- ST/T wave changes.

The neonate with symptomatic congenital heart disease
Background
- The greatest mortality risk for a neonate with symptomatic congenital heart disease (CHD) is before diagnosis.
- Critically obstructed systemic circulation (e.g. critical aortic stenosis, coarctation and hypo-plastic left heart syndrome) can be indistinguishable from shock due to sepsis.
- CHD should be considered as a differential diagnosis in any unwell neonate, and prosta-glandin may be life-saving in duct-dependent lesions.

Clinical syndromes

Clinical syndromes of presentation with symptomatic CHD include:
- Shock due to low cardiac output, often with poor peripheral pulses and acidosis.
- Persistent cyanosis.
- Congestive cardiac failure with respiratory distress and hepatomegaly.

Management

Use of prostaglandin (PGE₁)

- There are no congenital cardiac lesions for which PGE_1 is absolutely contraindicated.
- Initial dose PGE_1 10 ng/kg per min i.v. (= 0.01 mcg/kg per min) then increase to 20–100 ng/kg per min depending on response.
  - Aim for saturations in the 80s and improving systemic perfusion if compromised.
- Hypotension and apnoea are the major side effects at higher doses, intubation and ventilation may be required.
- The risk–benefit is in favour of PGE_1 infusion if:
  - Patient is *in extremis*.
  - Patient is cyanotic with a murmur.
  - Patient has poor peripheral pulses.

Seek early advice from a specialist centre for support to arrange timely transfer for assessment.

Neonatal cyanosis

Cyanosis in any neonate must be investigated. Consider structural CHD, parenchymal lung disease and persistent pulmonary hypertension (PPHN).

Clinical syndromes

- Cyanotic CHD is often more likely if there is persistent cyanosis with no respiratory distress and normal CO_2 clearance. The presence of a murmur increases the likelihood of a prostaglandin sensitive lesion.
- Parenchymal lung disease is likely if the infant has respiratory distress, elevated P_{CO_2}, lung field changes on CXR and a likely cause (e.g. meconium aspiration).
- PPHN is difficult to distinguish clinically from cyanotic CHD.

Initial assessment

- Examination: respiratory effort, abnormal pulses and presence of murmur.
- CXR: look at cardiac silhouette, pulmonary vascularity and parenchymal lung disease.
- Arterial blood gases: look for acidosis, P_{CO_2}.
- 12-lead ECG: look at axis, rhythm, presence of sinus P waves, QRS complexes.
- Echocardiography: remains the diagnostic test of choice.
- Hyperoxia test:
  After 10 min breathing 100% O_2, take a right arm, preductal (radial artery) arterial blood gas.

- A Pa_{O_2} <70 mmHg will occur with most major cyanotic defects.
- A Pa_{O_2} >150 mmHg suggests cyanosis is **not** due to structural heart disease.
• Trial of prostaglandin (PGE_1).
  - Will generally result in considerable improvement with duct-dependent CHD.

Seek early advice from a specialist centre.

Heart failure after the neonatal period
Main causes
• Congenital heart defects with pressure or volume overload (±cyanosis).
• Myocardial dysfunction after repair or palliation of heart defects.
• Cardiomyopathies: genetically determined metabolic and muscle disorders, infectious or anthracycline medications.
• Tachyarrhythmias.
• Rheumatic heart disease.

Clinical syndromes
• Infants and young children have non-specific symptoms and signs:
  - Dyspnoea, fatigue, feeding difficulties, increased sweating.
  - Failure to thrive, poor exercise tolerance.
  - Gallop rhythm, hepatomegaly, cardiomegaly.
• Older children may have signs more like those in adults:
  - Breathlessness, fatigue, poor exercise tolerance, orthopnoea.
  - Nocturnal dyspnoea, venous distension, peripheral oedema.

Management principles
• Seek early advice from a specialist centre.
• Arrange urgent echocardiography for an anatomical and functional diagnosis.
• Oxygen for hypoxia related to pulmonary congestion or respiratory infection.
• Diminish pulmonary and systemic venous congestion:
  - Frusemide: 1 mg/kg per dose (8, 12 or 24 hourly).
  - Spironolactone (dose by weight): 0–10 kg 6.25 mg/dose oral (12 or 24 hourly), 11–20 kg 12.5 mg/dose oral (12 or 24 hourly) and 21–40 kg 25 mg/dose oral (12 or 24 hourly).
• Decrease loading conditions:
  - Captopril: 0.1–1 mg/kg per dose (max 50 mg) oral 8 hourly.
  - Commence ACE inhibitor in hospital to monitor blood pressure.
  - Monitor serum potassium if using spironolactone.
• Inotropes for acute, low-output cardiac failure:
  - Dobutamine: initially 5 mcg/kg per min i.v.
  - Dopamine: initially 5 mcg/kg per min i.v.
  - Milrinone: 50 mcg/kg over 10 min i.v. then 0.375–0.75 mcg/kg per min.

- Positive pressure ventilation.
- Treat complications:
  - Infection.
  - Anaemia.
  - Arrhythmia.
  - Malnutrition.

Hypercyanotic spells ('tetralogy spells')

Severe cyanotic spells are a characteristic feature of tetralogy of fallot (TOF) but may occasionally occur with other cyanotic lesions. The TOF consists of (1) right ventricular hypertrophy, (2) right ventricular outflow tract obstruction, (3) ventricular septal defect, with (4) over-riding aorta.

Clinical presentation and background

- Severe cyanosis with agitation and breathlessness.
- Often precipitated by exertion, feeding or crying, but can be spontaneous.
- Mechanism probably involves increased right ventricular outflow tract contractility, peripheral vasodilatation and hyperventilation.
- The right ventricular outflow tract murmur becomes softer and may become inaudible.
- Most episodes are self-limiting, lasting 15–30 min, but can be prolonged or result in loss of consciousness.

Management

Initial

- Avoid exacerbating distress.
- Try to console the child by cradling, soothing or nursing in a knee–chest position.
- Give high-flow oxygen via mask or head box.
- Morphine 0.2 mg/kg i.m. may help in severe cases.
- Continuous ECG and oxygen saturation monitoring, frequent BP monitoring.
- Correct any underlying cause, e.g. arrhythmia, hypothermia, hypoglycaemia.

If prolonged

- I.v. fluids: 0.9% normal saline 10 mL/kg bolus followed by maintenance fluids.
- Correct acidosis: sodium bicarbonate 1–2 mmol/kg i.v.
- Beta-blocking drugs: i.v. esmolol 0.5 mg/kg over 1 min, then 50–200 mcg/kg per min for up to 48 h.
- Intubation and positive pressure ventilation may be required in extreme cases.

Longer term

- In most cases, hypercyanotic spells are an indication for palliative or corrective surgery.
- Oral propranolol may be given prophylactically to prevent spells in a child awaiting surgery.

Supraventricular tachycardia (SVT)

Seek urgent specialist advice if any tachycardia is broad complex or irregular, or fails to respond to the management.

Definition

Supraventricular tachycardia is usually a regular, narrow complex tachycardia, with heart rate 160–300 beats/min.

Differential diagnosis

Sinus tachycardia up to 230 beats/min may occur in the neonate with:

- Hypovolaemia.
- Hypoventilation.
- Pain.
- Fever.
- Pulmonary hypertension.

Note: Ventricular tachycardia in the neonate can have a relatively narrow QRS complex.

Clinical features

- *In utero:* may cause hydrops.
- Infancy: irritability, pallor, poor feeding and dyspnoea secondary to congestive cardiac failure.
- Older children: palpitations, chest discomfort.
- Hypotension may be present at any age.

Initial management

- Physical examination:
  - Pulse, BP, murmur.
  - Signs of cardiac failure (tachypnoea, increased work of breathing, hepatomegaly).
- 12-lead ECG to confirm a narrow-complex tachycardia.

Patient normotensive and well perfused

Vagal manoeuvres

- Infant or young child:
  - Ice water in bag or icepack to face for a few seconds only.
  - Oropharyngeal suctioning.
  - Gag with spatula.
- Older child:
  - Valsalva manoeuvre (e.g. forced blow through a blocked straw).

I.v. adenosine

- Full resuscitation facilities should be available.
- I.v. access in a large, proximal vein.
- Record a continuous ECG rhythm strip throughout administration, to monitor the pattern of reversal.

- Begin with adenosine 0.1 mg/kg as an initial bolus (max 6 mg):
  - Repeat doses can be given at 2 min intervals increasing by 0.05 mg/kg each dose to maximum 0.3 mg/kg (18 mg).
- Dilute small doses of adenosine with saline to allow rapid infusion.
- Give adenosine quickly, followed immediately by a 5 mL normal saline flush.
- Check patient's vital signs.
  - Rapid re-initiation of the tachycardia may occur due to premature atrial contractions, a repeated and often **lower** dose may be successful in this case.
- Side effects of adenosine: facial flush, chest pain, bronchospasm.

Patient shocked (hypotensive, poor perfusion, impaired mental state)
- Ensure child is given oxygen and has i.v. access.
- The airway should be managed by experienced staff.
- Administer midazolam 0.2 mg/kg (max 10 mg) i.v. to minimise awareness and fentanyl 1–2 mcg/kg (max 50–100 mcg) if rapidly available for analgesia.
- D/C revert using a **synchronised** shock of 1 J/kg.

Subsequent management
After stabilisation of SVT, specialist review is required for:
- 12 lead ECG in sinus rhythm (pre-excitation and other abnormality).
- Echocardiogram (structural associations of atrioventricular re-entry SVT, e.g. Ebstein's anomaly, cardiomyopathy).
- 24 h Holter monitor (intermittent pre-excitation and initiating triggers such as premature atrial contractions).
- Decisions regarding prophylaxis, electrophysiological study.

Infective endocarditis
For infective endocarditis to develop, two independent events are normally required: a damaged area of endothelium and a bacteraemia.

Presentation
- Usually insidious and non-specific presentation.
- Often suggestive of intercurrent viral illness.
- Fever, anorexia, myalgia, arthralgia, headache, general malaise.
  - Splenomegaly, splinter haemorrhages, petechiae and other peripheral stigmata are rarely seen in children but do occur. Careful repeated examination for these signs is necessary as they may not develop until several days into the illness.

Diagnosis
- Suspect endocarditis in any patient with a structural cardiac anomaly and prolonged fever, or who develops fever and a new murmur.
- Multiple blood cultures (at least three) from separate sites and at different times, before antibiotic administration.

- Full blood count.
- ESR and CRP.
- Echocardiogram.
  - Transoesophageal echo may be more sensitive than transthoracic echo but is often non-contributory in young children with good imaging through a relatively thin chest wall.
  - The sensitivity and specificity of echo for endocarditis are limited, thus **a normal echocardiogram does not exclude endocarditis**.

Management
- Admission to hospital.
- Commence empiric antibiotics which should be chosen to cover endocarditis as well as other potentially serious causes for the presenting illness.
  - Native valve/homograft: benzylpenicillin 60 mg/kg (max. 2 g) i.v. 6 hourly **plus** flucloxacillin 50 mg/kg (max. 2 g) i.v. 6 hourly **plus** gentamicin 2.5 mg/kg (max. 240 mg, synergistic dose) i.v. 8 hourly.
  - Prosthetic valve: vancomycin 15 mg/kg (max. 500 mg) i.v. 6 hourly **plus** gentamicin 2.5 mg/kg (max. 240 mg, synergistic dose) i.v. 8 hourly.
- Prolonged antibiotic therapy is required. Specialist consultation is recommended to tailor the antibiotic regimen to individual patients and pathogens.
- Close monitoring of clinical and cardiovascular status including serial echo, blood cultures and inflammatory markers.
- Close monitoring for evidence of other embolic phenomena.

Endocarditis prophylaxis
- Children at risk should establish and maintain the best possible oral health to reduce potential sources of bacteraemia.
- Single dose antibiotic prophylaxis is recommended for children at risk, undergoing procedures likely to cause a bacteraemia (see Table 21.1).
- Recommended prophylaxis is with amoxicillin 50 mg/kg oral 1 h preoperatively (max. 2 g).
- If unable to take oral medication, give amoxicillin 50 mg/kg i.v. at induction (max. 2 g).
- For penicillin-allergic patients, see Antimicrobial guidelines, page 603.

Basic ECG interpretation
ECG interpretation should include a systematic assessment of rate, rhythm, axis, P waves, QRS, ST segments, T waves and intervals; PR, QT and QTc.

A normal ECG should have an appropriate rate for age and a P-wave, which should be upright in leads I and aVF, preceding each QRS complex (see Fig. 21.1).

Table 21.1 Indications for antibiotic prophylaxis for endocarditis

High-risk cardiac conditions	High-risk procedures	Children not at risk
• Cyanotic defects • Prosthetic valves • Conduits/shunts • Previous endocarditis	• Dental procedures (involving manipulation of gingival tissues, periapical region of teeth or perforation of oral mucosa) • Invasive procedure of respiratory tract (involving breach of respiratory mucosa) • Procedures on infected skin, skin structures or musculoskeletal tissue • Genitourinary or gastrointestinal procedures	• Confirmed 'innocent' or physiologic murmurs • Non-structural problems (e.g. arrhythmia) • Previous Kawasaki disease without valvular dysfunction

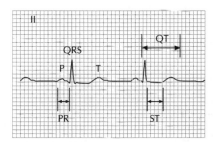

Fig. 21.1 Normal ECG

There are age-related normal values for axis, P waves, QRS complexes and all intervals on the 12 lead ECG (see Table 21.2). For children >12 years, adult normals can be used as a guide.

Rate

Calculate as 300/(number of big squares). At a normal paper speed of 25 mm/s, each small square represents 0.04 s, and each big square 0.20 s.

Rhythm

Sinus rhythm is present when there is a P wave with normal axis followed by a QRS complex. Alternatives include:
• Ectopic atrial rhythms; P wave with abnormal axis followed by QRS complex.
• AV nodal or junctional rhythm; narrow QRS complexes unrelated to P waves.
• Ventricular rhythms; broad often bizarre QRS complexes unrelated to P waves.

Table 21.2 Age-related ECG normal values

	Neonate	Young child (1–2 years)	Older child (3–12 years)
Heart rate (per min)	107–182	89–151	62–130
QRS axis (°)	+65 to +161	+7 to +101	+9 to +114
PR (s)	0.07–0.14	0.08–0.15	0.09–0.17
QRS (s)	0.03–0.08	0.04–0.08	0.04–0.09
R V_1 (mm)	3–21	2.5–17	0–12
S V_1 (mm)	0–11	0.5–21	0.3–25
R V_6 (mm)	2.5–16.5	6–22.5	9–25.5
S V_6 (mm)	0–10	0–6.5	0–4
Q V_6 (mm = 98th centile)	3	3	3

QRS axis

Normal QRS axis values are listed in Table 21.2. An abnormal QRS axis can indicate ventricular hypertrophy (or hypoplasia with the larger ventricle contributing to relatively greater voltages) or be associated with anatomically abnormal conduction pathways in complex lesions.

P waves

A normal axis sinus P wave is upright in leads I and aVF. Other appearances may result from ectopic atrial foci or structural congenital heart lesions. Tall P waves reflect RA enlargement (p pulmonale), broad P waves LA enlargement (p mitrale). A prolonged PR interval occurs in first-degree heart block.

QRS complexes and T waves

The neonatal ECG shows right-sided dominance with large R waves and upright T waves in leads V1, V2, aVR and V4R. The T waves should have inverted by 1 week of age in the normal child. Persistence beyond this time indicates RVH.

The T waves become upright in right-sided leads again in later childhood and the ECG takes on the adult appearance of dominant left-sided forces with small Q waves and large R waves in the lateral leads I, II, aVL, V5 and V6.

ST segments

Normal adolescents and young adults may have sloping elevation of the ST segment due to early repolarisation. Elevation or depression of >1 mm in limb leads and 2 mm in precordial leads is abnormal and occurs in pericarditis, ischaemia or infarction and with digoxin treatment.

Corrected QT interval

The QT interval can be corrected for heart rate by measuring the QT occurring after the shortest RR in sinus rhythm and applying Bazett's formula (all measurements in seconds). The QT is measured to the point where a tangent to its slope crosses the baseline (see Fig. 21.2).

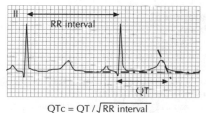

$$QTc = QT / \sqrt{RR\ interval}$$

Fig. 21.2 Bazett's formula for calculating corrected QT interval (QTc)

USEFUL RESOURCES
- *www.rch.org.au/cardiology/defects.cfm* – RCH Cardiology Website. Excellent website with pictures and parent handouts regarding the major structural abnormalities.
- *www.heartkids.org.au* – Parent support organisation.

CHAPTER 22
Dental conditions

Nicky Kilpatrick

Dental development
Primary dentition

Teeth start to form from the 5th week *in utero* and may continue until the late teens or early twenties. The first teeth to erupt are usually the lower central primary incisors at around 7 months of age. Table 22.1 summarises the eruption dates for primary teeth.

An infant who shows no sign of any primary teeth by the age of 18 months should be referred to a paediatric dentist.

By the age of 2.5 years most children will have a complete primary dentition consisting of 20 teeth: 8 incisors, 4 canines, 8 molars. In most cases all primary or deciduous teeth are ultimately replaced, but some individuals are missing permanent teeth and primary teeth may be retained into adulthood.

Permanent dentition

At around the age of 6 years the primary incisors become mobile and fall out. The tooth fairy then comes to visit. The permanent dentition begins to develop, starting with the eruption of the lower first permanent molars (Table 22.2). Permanent teeth are much larger than the primary predecessors and often look more yellow or cream in colour. The period that follows, referred to as the mixed dentition phase, is highly variable. Some second primary molar teeth are replaced by the second premolars as late as 14 years of age.

The simultaneous presence of primary and permanent teeth in the same site during the mixed dentition stage is common and is not a cause for concern.

Dental caries

Dental caries (or decay) remains one of the most common childhood diseases. In Australia just over 60% of 5 year olds and 55% of 12 year olds are decay free; 80% of all decay is experienced by 20% of children. It is therefore important to identify children at high decay risk and specifically target them for prevention (Table 22.3).

Dental decay can occur as soon as teeth erupt. Early childhood caries (ECC) is a particular form of dental decay that is seen in infants as young as 18 months of age. It affects >6% of Australian infants and has a characteristic appearance in which the upper front teeth are affected on their labial (or lip) surfaces. The cariogenic bacteria causing ECC are transmitted from primary caregiver to child, and decay is closely associated with infant feeding habits.

Paediatric Handbook, 8th edition. By Kate Thomson, Dean Tey and Michael Marks. Published 2009 by Blackwell Publishing, ISBN: 978-1-4051-7400-8.

Table 22.1 Eruption sequence of primary dentition (months after birth)

Central incisors	Lateral incisors	Canines	First molars	Second molars
6–12	9–16	16–23	13–19	23–33

Table 22.2 Eruption sequence of permanent dentition (years of age)

Central incisors	Lateral incisors	Canines	First premolars	Second premolars	First molars	Second molars	Third molars
6–8	6.5–8.5	9–13	9.5–11.5	10–13	5.5–7.0	11–13	17+

Table 22.3 Dental caries: common risk factors assessable by medical practitioners

Risk factor	Influence
Sugar exposure	Infant feeding habits are very important with frequency of exposure being most relevant. High risk associated with prolonged on-demand night-time feeds and daytime grazing patterns
Family oral health history	Poor parental oral health places child at risk of decay as cariogenic bacteria are transmitted from the primary caregiver
Fluoride exposure	Exposure to fluoridated water source and the regular use of fluoridated toothpaste are two key factors that reduce caries risk
Social and family practices	Low socio-economic status, ethnic and migrant groups have higher levels of dental disease
Medical illness	Medically compromised children are more at risk of dental decay and are less likely to receive appropriate treatment

Prevention

The prevention of dental decay should start as soon as the first tooth erupts. There are four aspects to preventing decay:

Diet

- Minimise the total amount and frequency of intake of sugary foods and drinks.
- Limit sugary snacks to meal times when salivary flow is optimal.
- Minimise intake of drinks with high acidity (e.g. carbonated, fruit and sports drinks), as they cause erosion of the teeth.
- Increase water intake.
- Encourage drinking from feeder cup from the age of 12 months.
- Avoid demand feeding at night time.

Oral hygiene
- Tooth cleaning should commence within 6 months of the eruption of the first tooth.
- Parents should supervise toothbrushing until around 8 years of age.
- Use a toothbrush with a small head for infants and use only a 'smear' of toothpaste.
- Under 5 year olds should use a low-fluoride (junior) toothpaste unless they are at increased risk of developing dental caries.

Fluoride
- Fluoride enhances the ability of teeth to resist demineralisation caused by sugar acids.
- Apart from systemic water fluoridation, the most common source of fluoride is toothpaste.
- Most adult toothpastes contain around 1000 ppm.
- Junior toothpastes contain a lower concentrations of fluoride, ~400 ppm.
- Fluoride supplements in the form of tablets or drops to be chewed and/or swallowed should no longer be used (new guideline, 2006).

Regular dental check-ups
- A child should see a dental professional within 6 months of the eruption of the first tooth.
- The first visit is a 'well baby' visit and aimed at providing 'anticipatory guidance'.
- A child should have a dental check-up at least annually.
- The frequency of dental attendance will vary according to disease risk assessment.

Dental emergencies
Toothache
- Assess level and nature of pain (e.g. intermittent pain on eating or in response to hot/cold or spontaneous pain at night).
- Provide analgesia (paracetamol should be adequate).
- Refer to dentist for assessment and treatment of the affected tooth.

Dental abscess
Presentation
- History of spontaneous pain, particularly at night; pain may be constant.
- May have recently had fillings.
- Swelling evident intra-orally near teeth.
- Red swollen face, unilateral and often spreading up under the orbit or under the mandible.
- Limited mouth opening.
- Elevated temperature, enlarged lymph nodes and a generally unwell child.
- Tender teeth on side of the swelling.

Investigations
- Orthopantogram (OPG): will show dental pathology, usually decay.

Management

- Consider oral amoxicillin for early infection.
- Admit to hospital if red swollen face, fever and generally unwell.
- I.v. antibiotics (benzylpenicillin in the first instance) and i.v. fluids.
- Extraction of the tooth is almost always indicated.
- Occasionally additional soft tissue drainage is required; however, dental abscesses in young children usually manifest with cellulitis rather than a collection of frank pus.

Dental trauma

Traumatic injuries to the facial region can affect the teeth, soft tissues and jaw bones.

History

Consider:

- How did the injury occur?
- Were there any other injuries?
- Time of the injury?
- Where are the teeth or fragments of teeth?
- How much of the tooth is broken off, or how far is the tooth displaced?
- Can the patient bite their teeth together or does the displaced tooth get in the way?
- Are there associated soft tissue (mucosal) injuries?
- Is the avulsed tooth stored in milk?

Locate all teeth or tooth fragments because:

- Most permanent teeth and tooth fragments can be replaced/re-cemented.
- 'Missing' teeth may have been intruded (pushed in) rather than knocked out.
- Never replant a primary tooth.
- Injury (particularly intrusion) to a primary incisor can damage the permanent successor, therefore dental review for all injuries is important.
- Associated mucosal injuries may require suturing. Refer to a dentist.

Permanent teeth

Whenever possible an OPG is useful as it allows a full review of the jaws, jaw joints and teeth. A chest radiograph is useful if the tooth or fragments cannot be located. Many injuries can be managed under local anaesthesia, depending on the cooperation of the child and the presence of associated soft tissue or other bony injuries.

- An avulsed permanent tooth is a genuine emergency and should be triaged as such. The longer the tooth is out of the mouth, the worse the prognosis.
- The long-term psychosocial and economical impact on a young person of losing a front tooth should not be underestimated. Appropriate emergency management can make a significant difference to the prognosis of any injured tooth.

Mucosal lacerations

- Check carefully intraorally for degloving injuries (where the gum tissue around the teeth is stripped away from the underlying bone). Unless the lips are retracted, this injury is easily missed. These injuries need suturing under general anaesthesia.

Table 22.4 Dental trauma – primary dentition

Injury	Management
No tooth displacement	Non-urgent referral to dentist for review
Intrusion – tooth upwards and inwards	Needs dental review within 24 h to accurately locate the tooth. Likely course is re-eruption, otherwise extraction will be required
Luxation – tooth palatal or sideways	Needs dental review within 12 h
Avulsion – knocked out completely	Extraction is required sooner rather than later **Do not** replant primary teeth Needs dental review within 24 h

Table 22.5 Dental trauma – permanent dentition

Injury	Management
Fractures <1/3 crown >1/3 crown	Non-urgent referral to dentist Locate fragments, store in milk Needs dental review within 24 h Some fragments can be reattached to broken teeth
Mobile but not displaced	Soft diet and analgesia Needs dental review within 12 h May need dental splint
Displacements Intrusions (tooth upwards and inwards) Luxations (tooth palatal or sideways) Avulsions* (knocked out completely)	All such injuries should be referred to a paediatric dentist within 12 h Locate teeth, using radiographs Tooth may re-erupt or require surgical/orthodontic repositioning Use gentle finger pressure to reposition teeth, if in doubt leave alone Loose splinting can be achieved using tin foil until patient sees dentist Urgent referral to dentist Urgent referral to dentist Replace tooth in socket if possible If not, store in milk at all times

* An avulsed permanent tooth is a genuine emergency.

- Many tongue and intraoral lip lacerations do not need suturing and heal well when left.
- Extraoral lacerations, particularly those crossing the vermilion border on to the skin, should be referred to a plastic surgeon.
- **In all cases of dental trauma, lift the lips and look in!**

Fractures to the jaw bones

- Whenever a jaw fracture is suspected, a maxillofacial surgeon should be called. If teeth are also obviously displaced or lost, a paediatric dentist should also be called.
- An OPG, lateral cephalometric view and/or a variety of occipitomental/anteroposterior radiographic views can be useful in inspecting the facial complex for fractures.
- Tetanus prophylaxis should be considered in any compound fractures opening to mouth or skin, and antibiotics commenced.

Bleeding from the mouth

- Clean the mouth with cold water or saline and remove any debris, blood, tissue etc.
- Identify source of bleeding – usually an extraction socket.
- If child has been bleeding for some time, assess haemodynamic status.
- Bleeding socket:
    - Compress the sides of the socket together using finger pressure.
    - If child is co-operative place a slightly damp gauze pack over the socket and have child bite down on to it for 20 min. Parents may be asked to assist. Do not pack anything into socket.
    - Refer to dentist.

USEFUL RESOURCES
- Spencer AJ. The use of fluorides in Australia: guidelines. *Australian Dental Journal* 2006; 51(2): 195–199.
- *www.aapd.org/pediatricinformation* – American Academy of Pediatric Dentistry includes links to Parent Education Brochures and Clinical Guidelines.
- *www.ada.org/public/topics/tooth_eruption.asp* – The American Dental Association website includes eruption charts and animations.

CHAPTER 23
Dermatologic conditions

Rod Phillips
David Orchard

The key to accurate diagnosis and hence to appropriate management of skin disorders in children is a careful history and astute observation of rashes, particularly focusing on their appearance, site and pattern of development. During the examination consider a few key questions (see also Fig. 23.1).

- Are there any vesicles, i.e. fluid-filled lesions? Finding these greatly narrows the range of possible diagnoses. Small circular erosions may be the only signs of an underlying vesicular process.
- Is the rash raised (papular) or flat (macular)?
- Is the rash red? Redness is from haemoglobin. Most red rashes blanch, i.e. the redness disappears with pressure. If not, the haemoglobin is outside the blood vessels (purpura).
- Is the rash scaly? If so, the epidermis may be broken (eczematous) to give weeping, crusting or bleeding, or it may be intact (papulosquamous).

Vesiculobullous rashes
Vesicles are usually caused by infections (herpes simplex virus (HSV), varicella zoster virus (VZV), enterovirus, tinea, scabies or impetigo) or contact dermatitis. Also, consider drug reactions and erythema multiforme. Larger blisters may be from staphylococcal infections, tinea, Stevens–Johnson syndrome, arthropod bites, contact dermatitis, burns or trauma.

Impetigo (school sores)
Cause
Staphylococcus aureus or *Streptococcus pyogenes* (impetigo but not bullous lesions), or both.

Clinical features
Impetigo presents as areas of ooze and honey-coloured crusts on the face, trunk or limbs. Occasionally, the primary lesions are bullous. Lesions are rounded and well demarcated and are most often grouped and asymmetrical but may be solitary and widespread. Their onset and spread may be rapid or occur over days. In more chronic cases, there may be central healing with peripheral spread to give annular lesions.

Paediatric Handbook, 8th edition. By Kate Thomson, Dean Tey and Michael Marks. Published 2009 by Blackwell Publishing, ISBN: 978-1-4051-7400-8.

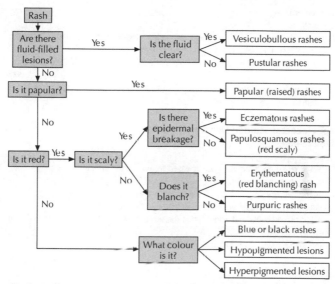

Vesiculobullous rashes
- Impetigo (school sores)
- Eczema herpeticum
- Erythema multiforme
- Single blisters
- Stevens–Johnson syndrome/toxic epidermal necrolysis

Pustular rashes
- Acne

Papular (raised) rashes
- Scabies
- Urticaria/serum sickness
- Papular urticaria
- Keratosis pilaris
- Papular acrodermatitis
- Molluscum
- Warts

Eczematous rashes
- Atopic eczema

Red scaly rashes (papulosquamous)
- Seborrhoeic dermatitis
- Psoriasis
- Tinea corporis
- Pityriasis rosea

Red blanching rashes (erythematous)
- Fever and exanthem
- Erythema infectiosum

Red blanching rashes (erythematous)
- Roseola infantum
- Kawasaki disease

Purpuric rashes
- Enteroviral infection
- Septicaemia
- Leukaemia
- Henoch–Schoenlein purpura
- Child abuse
- Idiopathic thrombocytopenic purpura (ITP)
- Trauma and vasomotor straining

Blue or black rashes
- Vascular malformations
- Haemangiomas
- Mongolian spots

Hypopigmented lesions
- Tinea versicolor
- Pityriasis alba
- Vitiligo
- Post-inflammatory hypo- and hyperpigmentation

Hyperpigmented lesions
- Congenital pigmented naevi
- Acquired pigmented naevi

Fig 23.1 Classification of skin disorders in children

Management
- Bathe off crusts.
- Apply topical mupirocin 2% ointment 8 hourly if localised, or cephalexin 25 mg/kg (maximum 500 mg) orally, 12 hourly if severe or extensive.
- Isolate the child from other children or from sick adults unless all lesions are covered or treated.
- Treat any underlying condition such as scabies (a common cause of widespread impetigo) or eczema.

Staphylococcal scalded skin syndrome
Clinical features
- Usually seen in younger children.
- Mediated by an epidermolytic toxin released from an often insignificant staphylococcal focus (e.g. eyes, nose or skin).
- Fever and tender erythematous skin are early features.
- Exudation and crusting develops, especially around the mouth.
- Wrinkling, flaccid bullae and exfoliation of the skin are seen – Nikolsky sign ('normal' skin separates if rubbed).
- Blisters are very superficial and heal without scarring.

Management
- Flucloxacillin 50 mg/kg (max 2 g) i.v. 6 hourly if there is evidence of sepsis or systemic involvement.
- Look for a focus of infection. Drain foci of pus if present.
- Monitor temperature, fluids and electrolytes if large areas are involved. Increased fluids will aid renal excretion of toxin.
- Handle skin carefully and use an emollient ointment.

Erythema multiforme
Clinical features
This is a specific hypersensitivity syndrome that occurs at any age. Lesions are usually symmetric and appear most commonly on the hands, feet and often the face. They can be found anywhere, including mucous membranes.

Typical target lesions have an inner zone of epidermal injury (purpura, necrosis or vesicle), an outer zone of erythema and sometimes a middle zone of pale oedema. They are not migratory. Most cases are caused by herpes simplex, some by other infections. Drugs are an uncommon cause.

Management
- Fluid maintenance.
- Apply emollient ointment to the lips, if needed.
- If the condition is recurrent, it is highly likely to be related to HSV. Prophylactic aciclovir should be considered if recurrences are frequent and affecting the quality of life.

Stevens–Johnson syndrome/toxic epidermal necrolysis
Clinical features

Stevens–Johnson syndrome and toxic epidermal necrolysis are believed by many to be variants of the same condition.

- They are characterised by widespread blisters on an erythematous or purpuric macular background, often with extensive mucous membrane haemorrhagic crusting.
- There may be tender erythematous areas with a positive Nikolsky sign ('normal' skin separates if rubbed).
- Conjunctivitis, corneal ulceration and blindness can occur. Some degree of permanent scarring around the conjunctivae is common even if eye symptoms are not severe.
- Anogenital lesions can lead to urinary retention.
- Fever, myalgia, arthralgia and other organ involvement can occur.
- Drugs are the most common cause, occasionally *Mycoplasma*.

Management

- Cease any drug that may be the cause.
- Fluid maintenance. Monitor temperature, fluids and electrolytes.
- Apply emollient ointment to the skin, lips and anogenital areas – this may be required many times a day. Careful attention to emollients and/or dressing of the glans and undersurface of the foreskin may prevent secondary scarring, adhesions and phimosis.
- A regular eye examination with a specialist review for topical steroid drops if any eye involvement is noted.
- Good pain management is essential. Occasional or regular brief inhalational general anaesthetics may be necessary to facilitate dressings, eye care, etc., which **must** not be compromised.
- I.v. gammaglobulin is seen by many as standard therapy for cases threatening to become severe.
- Cyclosporin (5–6 mg/kg per day for a few days, then taper to 3–5 mg/kg per day for 2–3 weeks) commenced at diagnosis may prevent worsening. Immunosuppression is controversial (beware sepsis).

Note: Stevens–Johnson syndrome is not severe erythema multiforme (EM). They are distinct conditions with different aetiologies. Permanent sequelae are rarely seen in severe EM and concurrent drug use is unlikely to be the cause. Skin lesion morphology is the best discriminating factor. Classic target lesions are not seen in Stevens–Johnson syndrome. Mucous membrane involvement can be seen in both conditions but is usually localised in EM, often confluent in Stevens–Johnson syndrome.

Eczema herpeticum
Clinical features

HSV infection in children with eczema is common, but many cases are misdiagnosed as either an exacerbation of the eczema or bacterial infection. Grouped vesicles may be prominent, but more often vesicles are rudimentary or absent and the infection presents as a group of shallow 2–4 mm ulcers on an inflamed base. The infected area may not be painful or itchy and does not respond to standard eczema therapy. If untreated, resolution usually occurs in 1–4 weeks, but dissemination may occur. Recurrences may occur at different sites.

Management

- Collect epithelial cells from the base and roof of the vesicles for herpes immunofluorescence and culture.
- Local disease in an otherwise well child requires regular observation but does not need antiviral therapy.
- A child with fever or multiple sites of cutaneous herpes infection may need admission to hospital and treatment with i.v. aciclovir 20 mg/kg per dose (2–12 weeks), 250 mg/m^2 per dose (12 weeks–12 years), 5 mg/kg per dose (>12 years) 8 hourly i.v. over 1 h.
- Milder cases demonstrating progression or facial involvement can be managed with oral aciclovir.
- Eye involvement should be managed with topical or systemic aciclovir, or both, **and** urgent review by an ophthalmologist.
- The underlying eczema can be treated with moisturisers, topical steroids and wet dressings.

Single blisters

When a child presents with a single blister as an isolated finding, consider impetigo, tinea, mastocytoma, insect bite, cigarette burn, friction or spider bite. The latter can grow over days to become a non-tender blister with a diameter of many centimetres.

Pustular rashes

Consider acne, folliculitis, scabies, perioral dermatitis, acute generalised exanthematous pustulosis and rarely psoriasis.

Acne
Clinical features

Acne mainly affects the forehead and face but can involve other sebaceous gland areas (neck, shoulders and upper trunk). Early lesions include blackheads, whiteheads and papules. In more severe cases there may be pustules or inflammatory cysts that can lead to permanent scarring. Undertreated acne is a cause of significant morbidity in adolescents and may be a factor in teenage suicide. Consider underlying endocrine disorders if acne begins before puberty.

Management

- Acne is treatable. No person with acne should just be told it is an inevitable part of adolescence. Effective acne therapies are now available and should be used to control the disease.
- For mild disease, use topical benzoyl peroxide 2.5–5%. Other topical agents include antibiotics (clindamycin, erythromycin or tetracycline), isotretinoin (not in pregnancy) or azelaic acid. These can be used singly or in combination. Improvement occurs over 1–2 months,

not within days. All of these topical agents have side effects with which practitioners must be familiar.

- Treatment of moderate acne often involves the addition of oral antibiotic therapy (e.g. tetracycline 500 mg twice daily, erythromycin 500 mg twice daily, doxycycline 50–200 mg per day) for 3–6 months.
- Oral hormone therapy can help female patients.

If antibiotics and topical treatment have not resulted in considerable improvement in 3 months, oral isotretinoin (Roaccutane®) is indicated. Provided pregnancy is avoided, this is safe and highly effective. Isotretinoin is also indicated if there is scarring, cyst formation, or significant depression. Treatment of severe acne with isotretinoin may decrease the risk of suicide. Assessment and treatment of any depression is also required.

Papular (raised) rashes

If the child is itchy, consider scabies, urticaria, serum sickness, papular urticaria or molluscum. If not, consider urticaria, molluscum, warts, melanocytic naevi, keratosis pilaris and papular acrodermatitis. For vascular swellings, consider pyogenic granuloma.

Scabies
Clinical features

An intensely itchy papular eruption develops 2–6 weeks after first exposure to the *Sarcoptes scabiei* mite or 1–4 days after subsequent reinfestation. The characteristic lesion is the burrow that is several millimetres in length. Burrows are best seen on the hands, especially between the fingers, and on the feet. Early burrows may be vesicular. A clue to the diagnosis of scabies is the distribution of papules and pruritus. Involvement of the palms, soles, axilla, umbilicus, groin and genitalia is common and the head is usually spared. Excoriations and secondary impetigo may be present. There is currently a worldwide pandemic of this contagious disease affecting both adults and children.

Management

- Treatment is expensive and upsetting. If diagnosis is unclear, confirm by scraping to find a mite, or refer before treating.
- Use permethrin 5% cream. An alternative for pregnant women or neonates is sulfur 2% in yellow soft paraffin.

Note: The following are **not recommended:** lindane 1% (contra-indicated in infants or women who are pregnant or breast-feeding) or benzyl benzoate 25% (too irritating for children and ineffective if diluted).

- Treat all family members and any other people who have close skin contact with the affected individuals.
- Apply to dry skin (not after a bath) from the neck down to all skin surfaces. For infants, apply to the scalp as well (not face). Use mittens if necessary to prevent finger sucking.

- Leave the cream on for at least 8 h.
- Wash the cream off. Wash clothing, pyjamas and bed linen at this time.
- The itch takes a week or two to settle and can be treated with potent topical steroids.
- Reinfestation is common. The family should notify all social contacts (e.g. crèche, school or close friends) to ensure that all those infected receive treatment.

Urticaria/serum sickness
See also chapter 19, Allergy and immunology.

Clinical features
Urticaria is characterised by the rapid appearance and disappearance of multiple raised red wheals on any part of the body. Individual lesions are often itchy and clear within 1 day. There may be central clearing to give ring lesions (these are not the so-called target lesions of EM that persist for several days). The child is usually well. Urticarial episodes usually resolve over days or weeks and rarely last longer than 6 months. In most cases of short duration, the trigger is either a transient viral infection, allergic reaction or cannot be determined.

Some children develop fever and arthralgias in association with urticarial lesions that are more fixed and may bruise or be tender (serum sickness). In Australia, serum sickness is usually idiopathic or following a course of cefaclor.

Management
- Urticaria may be the first sign of anaphylaxis. If there is associated angio-oedema (prominent subcutaneous swelling) or wheeze, continued observation and appropriate treatment is required (see chapter 1, Medical emergencies).
- Investigation is usually not required.
- Ask about medications; new foods and environmental allergens.
- Treat the itch with oral antihistamine (see chapter 19, Allergy and immunology, p. 228). Oral prednisolone (1 mg/kg per day, max. 50 mg) for 2–5 days is beneficial in serum sickness and is warranted in urticaria when pruritus is severe.
- Urticaria can become chronic, and in the vast majority of cases no underlying ongoing trigger is found. Consider mast cell degranulating drugs, foods, animals, parasitic infections, heat, cold and physical pressure. Consider investigating with a throat swab (for streptococcal carriage), full blood examination (for eosinophilia and anaemia), antinuclear antibodies, urine culture for bacteriuria, nocturnal check for threadworms and a possible challenge with any suspected agent. Adding cimetidine (10 mg/kg (max 200 mg) p.o. 6 hourly) to the antihistamine may help.
- If individual lesions last >2 days or are tender or purpuric, consider investigation for cutaneous vasculitis.

Papular urticaria
Clinical features
This is a clinical hypersensitivity to insect bites. New bites appear as groups of small red papules, usually in warmer weather. Older bites appear as 1–5 mm papules, sometimes with surface scale or crust, or with surrounding urticaria. Vesicles or pustules may form. Individual

lesions may resolve in a week or last for months and may repeatedly flare up after fresh bites elsewhere. The itch is often intense and secondary ulceration or infection is common.

Management
- Prevent bites (e.g. adequate clothing, modifying behaviour that leads to exposure, occasional repellent and the treatment of pets and house for fleas if necessary).
- Treat the itch with an agent such as aluminium sulfate 20% (Stingose), liquor picis carbonis 2% in calamine lotion, potent steroid ointment or antihistamines (see chapter 19, Allergy and immunology, p. 228). Protective dressings (e.g. Duoderm) can speed the healing of lesions.
- Treat secondary infection with topical mupirocin ointment 2% or oral antibiotics.

Keratosis pilaris
Clinical features
This is a rough, somewhat spiky papular rash on the upper outer arms, thighs, cheeks, or all three areas, with variable erythema. It is common at all ages.

Management
- Reassure the patient that this is rarely a problem. Soap avoidance and moisturisers can improve the feel. Steroids don't help.
- Older children may get some benefit from topical keratolytics (e.g. Dermadrate, Calmurid).
- Older children with troublesome facial redness can be treated with vascular laser (V beam).

Papular acrodermatitis
Clinical features
This is characterised by the acute onset of monomorphic red or skin-coloured papules mainly on the arms, legs and face. It is usually asymptomatic. It can be caused by coxsackie virus, echovirus, mycoplasma, EBV, adenovirus and others.

Management
Reassure and advise that clearing can take several weeks.

Molluscum
Clinical features
Uncomplicated molluscum lesions are easily recognised as firm, pearly, dome-shaped papules with central umbilication; however, presentation to a doctor is often prompted by the development of eczema in surrounding skin. In such cases, recognition can be difficult as eczematous changes can obliterate the primary lesions. A careful history of the initial lesions is usually diagnostic.

Management
Education – molluscum is caused by a virus and is very common. A child may develop a few, or a great many lesions and individual lesions may last for months. Complete resolution will not happen until an immune response develops, which may take from 3 months to 3 years.

Children with molluscum should not share towels but should not be restricted in their activities.

The treatment depends on the age of the child, the location of the lesions and any secondary changes. Things to note include:

- Treatment of the surrounding eczema may be all that is required.
- Uncomplicated lesions not causing problems and not spreading can be left alone.
- Isolated or troublesome lesions (e.g. on the face) can be physically treated. One method is gentle cryotherapy.
- Rarely, children warrant curettage under topical anaesthesia. This is well tolerated and usually curative but can potentially scar. Alternatively, the stimulation of an immune response can be attempted with cantharidin, aluminium acetate solution (Burow's solution 1:30) for large areas, or benzoyl peroxide 5% daily to small areas and covered with the adhesive part of a dressing.
- Inflamed lesions do not require antibiotic treatment but if true cellulitis or abscess formation occurs, treat with antibiotics and/or drainage.

Warts

Many serotypes of the papilloma virus can cause warts. Different serotypes have a predilection for different areas of the skin. No treatment is necessary unless the warts are causing a problem to the child (e.g. social embarrassment, or pain from a plantar wart). Avoid painful procedures unless chosen by older children. Resistant warts on the limbs often respond to contact sensitisation (e.g. Diphenylcyclopropenone (DCP) 0.1% cream after sensitisation with 2% solution). Diphenylcyclopropenone use requires caution, supervision and possible dose adjustment, as there is a wide variation in individual responses.

- *Ordinary warts*: if tolerated by the child, paring every 2–3 days with a razor blade or nail file will remove the surface horn. Apply a proprietary keratolytic agent that contains salicylic or lactic acid, or both, each day or two as directed.
- *Plantar warts*: these can be painful and can appear flat. Pare as for ordinary warts. Apply a proprietary keratolytic agent that contains salicylic or lactic acid, or both, each day or two. Alternatively, place a small pad of cotton wool soaked in 3% formalin in a saucer on the floor. Rest the wart-affected sole on the pad/saucer for 30 min each night. Cryotherapy and surgery are often ineffective and can lead to painful keloid scarring.
- *Plane (flat) warts*: these are smooth, flat or slightly elevated, skin-coloured or pigmented lesions. They may occur in lines or coalesce to form plaque-like lesions. If treatment is needed for plane warts on the hands, apply a formalin solution as for ordinary warts. Lesions on the face are often subtle and may not need treatment. Treatment may cause complications such as pigmentary changes and requires considerable caution.
- *Anogenital warts*: these are soft, fleshy warts that occur at the mucocutaneous junctions, especially around the anus. They may be isolated flesh-coloured nodules or may coalesce into large cauliflower-like masses. Management options include awaiting resolution, topical podophyllotoxin, imiquimod, curettage and diathermy and carbon dioxide laser.

Note: the presence of genital warts in a young child is not an indication for mandatory reporting to government protective services. Genital warts in children should lead to consideration of sexual abuse, but transmission is usually by normal close parent–child contact.

Eczematous rashes

Consider atopic eczema, allergic contact dermatitis, irritant contact dermatitis, photosensitivity eruptions, molluscum, tinea corporis and scabies.

Atopic eczema

See also chapter 19, Allergy and immunology.

Clinical features

Eczema usually begins in infancy. It commonly involves the face and often the trunk and limbs as well. In older children the rash may be widespread or may be localised to flexures. Erythema, weeping, excoriation and rarely vesicles may be seen in acute lesions. Chronic lesions may show scale and lichenification. In some children the lesions are more clearly defined, thickened discoid areas that may intermittently be itchy. There is usually a cyclical pattern of improvement and exacerbation. Weeping and yellow-crusted areas that do not respond to therapy may indicate secondary bacterial or herpetic infection.

Management

- *Education*: parents need to know the triggers and that treatments are effective in controlling the disease.
- *Avoid irritants* which may worsen eczema: soaps, bubble baths, prickly clothing, seams and labels on clothing, car seat covers, sand, carpets, overheating or contact with pets. Smooth cotton clothing is preferred.
- *Keep the skin moist*: use a moisturiser such as paraffin ointment (50:50 white soft paraffin/liquid paraffin) as often as several times a day if necessary.
- *Treat inflammation*: in mild or moderate cases, steroid creams can be used intermittently with good effect. Hydrocortisone 1% is usually adequate. If not, moderate potency (e.g. beta-methasone valerate 0.02%) or potent (e.g. mometasone 0.1% or methylprednisolone 0.1%) ointment can be used for exacerbations in areas other than the face or nappy area. Prolonged regular use of moderate-potency steroids to the skin of young children can cause atrophy and adrenal suppression. Oral steroids are rarely indicated in eczema. For chronic eczema on the limbs, zinc and tar combinations are alternatives to steroids.
- *Control itch*: advise parents to avoid saying 'Stop scratching' all the time, and to distract the child instead. Avoid overheating, particularly at night. Wet bandaging is very helpful if warranted. Antihistamines are often unhelpful but may be tried if the itch is not controlled by other measures (see chapter 19, Allergy and immunology). *Note:* Terfenadine (Teldane) and astemizole (Hismanal) should not be used because of occasional fatal interactions if erythromycin is also taken.
- *Treat infection*: take cultures and treat with simple wet dressings and oral antibiotics (e.g. erythromycin, cephalexin or flucloxacillin). Consider if herpes simplex is present (see p. 271). For recurrent bacterial infection, use antiseptic wash or bath oil (e.g. triclosan).
- *Diet*: a normal diet is usually indicated. If a child has immediate urticarial reactions to a particular food, that food should be avoided. Environmental and food allergens may contribute to the exacerbation of symptoms in some patients. Allergen avoidance in these children may be of some benefit. In difficult cases, consider a more formal allergy assessment.

- *Hospitalisation*: if a child is missing school because of eczema, they should generally be in hospital for intensive treatment.

Red scaly rashes (papulosquamous)

Consider seborrhoeic dermatitis (infants), psoriasis, tinea corporis, pityriasis rosea, pityriasis versicolor and atopic eczema. Ichthyosis vulgaris is a common cause of generalised scale without itch or redness.

Seborrhoeic dermatitis

Clinical features

- This condition presents in the first months of life, partly due to the activity of commensal yeasts.
- Red or yellow/brown scaly areas will commonly affect the scalp and forehead. (The 'seborrhoeic' rash in infants affecting areas without sebaceous glands (e.g. axillae, napkin area) is probably best considered as a form of psoriasis.) The folds behind the ears and around the neck, axillae, groin and gluteal clefts are also affected.
- Resolution by the age of 1 year is usual.

Management

- Paraffin or olive oil applied to scalp to loosen scale.
- Imidazole creams with hydrocortisone 1% cream or with a mixture of salicylic acid (1%) and sulfur (1%) ointment, twice daily.
- Anti-yeast shampoos (e.g. selenium sulfide – Selsun) can be helpful. Use carefully to avoid irritation or toxicity.

Psoriasis

Clinical features

Psoriasis can occur at any age. Lesions begin as small red papules that develop into circular, sharply demarcated erythematous patches with prominent silvery scale. Common presentations include plaques on extensor surfaces, generalised guttate (small) lesions, red scaly scalp lesions or moist red anogenital rashes. Itch can be a variable feature. Nail changes are often seen in childhood.

Management

The treatment depends on the site and extent of disease and the age of the child. Adolescents are less tolerant of tar creams.

- Treat isolated skin plaques with either topical steroids (e.g. intermittent mometasone with clinical monitoring) or tar-based creams (e.g. liquor picis carbonis 3%, salicylic acid 2% in sorbolene cream). Generally avoid tars on the face, flexures and genitalia.
- Use hydrocortisone 1% ointment on the face and anogenital region. Topical steroids are not used for large areas in childhood psoriasis because of the possible development of rebound pustular disease.

- Thick scalp plaques can be softened overnight with a similar tar cream and removed with a tar shampoo.
- Topical calcipotriol can be used in conjunction with steroid creams.
- Widespread psoriasis may need treatment with one or more of dithranol, etretinate, methotrexate, cyclosporin or ultraviolet therapy, all of which are effective.

Tinea corporis
Clinical features
The typical lesion is a slow-growing erythematous ring with a clear or scaly centre; however, tinea corporis can present in a wide variety of ways, particularly if previously treated with steroid ointments. It can be pustular, vesicular or bullous, or spread to many sites within days. Tinea should be considered in any red scaly rash where the diagnosis is unclear.

Management
- If in doubt about the diagnosis, confirm by scraping the scale for microscopy and culture.
- Lesions are treated with terbinafine cream (twice daily for 1 week) or an imidazole cream (e.g. clotrimazole, miconazole or econazole 2–4 times daily, for 4 weeks).
- Oral griseofulvin (20 mg/kg per day in divided doses) is required for tinea capitis or for widespread lesions.

Pityriasis rosea
Clinical features
The condition is common between the ages of 1 and 10 years. Initially, a pink scaly patch appears, followed a few days later by many pink/red scaly oval macules mainly on the trunk. It is usually asymptomatic but can be itchy.

Management
Reassure the patient. The condition can persist for weeks.

Red blanching rashes (erythematous)
Macular erythematous lesions are most commonly caused by viral infections (e.g. coxsackie, echovirus, Epstein–Barr virus, adenovirus, parainfluenza, influenza, parvovirus B19, human herpes virus 6, rubella and measles) or drug reactions. Consider also septicaemia, scarlet fever, Kawasaki disease (see chapter 30, Infectious diseases) and *Mycoplasma* infection.

Fever and exanthem
The onset of fever and exanthem is usually due to a viral illness, often enterovirus. Some infections have specific clinical features that aid diagnosis; for example measles and erythema infectiosum. However, in most instances a diagnosis cannot be made with certainty. To manage such a child, consider:
- Is the child sick? Is the child lethargic, cold peripherally or young? Consider meningococcal disease, other bacterial sepsis and Kawasaki disease. Investigate and treat.

- Are they taking any medication? Consider ceasing medication.
- Are there other people at risk? If relatives are immunosuppressed or pregnant, consider serology, stool viral culture and advising the at-risk person to consult their doctor.
- Is the rash papular? Consider papular acrodermatitis.

If the answer to all the above is 'no', reassurance and review is probably appropriate.

Erythema infectiosum and Kawasaki disease
See chapter 30, Infectious diseases.

Roseola infantum
This condition is seen every day in paediatric emergency departments. Typically, an infant has had a high fever for 2–4 days and has often been put on antibiotics. The fever then goes but a widespread erythematous rash appears. The family need reassurance that the rash is not a drug reaction. See chapter 30, Infectious diseases.

Purpuric rashes
Consider viral infections, meningococcal sepsis, platelet disorders, vasculitis, drug reactions and trauma.

Septicaemia
Suspect septicaemia (usually meningococcal) in a child with recent onset of fever and lethargy. Skin lesions may be erythematous macules progressing to extensive purple purpura. Even if there is doubt, take blood cultures, give antibiotics and arrange admission (see also chapter 1, Medical emergencies).

Enteroviral infection
Scattered petechiae are common in children who have fever from enteroviral infections. These children are usually well. If in doubt, or if the child appears unwell, investigate (full blood examination, blood cultures) and consider treatment for septicaemia. See Approach to the febrile child, p. 381.

Leukaemia
Suspect leukaemia in a child with generalised petechiae or purpura in the absence of trauma. Look for tiredness or pallor. Obtain an urgent full blood examination (see chapter 29, Haematologic conditions and oncology).

Henoch–Schönlein purpura
See detailed summary including Investigations and Management in chapter 37, Rheumatologic conditions.

Non-itchy, painless macules, papules or urticarial lesions with purpuric centres occur in a symmetrical distribution mainly on the buttocks and ankles, occasionally on the legs, arms and elsewhere. There may be associated abdominal pain, arthralgia, arthritis or haematuria. Renal involvement leading to chronic renal failure is rare, but can occur irrespective of the severity of the rash and other symptoms and may be delayed until weeks or months after the onset of the illness.

Idiopathic thrombocytopenic purpura

See also chapter 29, Haematologic conditions and oncology.

Bruises, petechiae or purpuric lesions appear over a period of days or weeks, mainly in sites of frequent mild trauma. The child is otherwise well. Full blood examination will show a low platelet count.

Child abuse

See chapter 17, Child abuse.

Twisting, compression, pinching and hitting can all cause petechial or purpuric lesions. Look for bruises of bizarre shapes and different ages, evidence of bony fractures and an abnormal affect.

Trauma and vasomotor straining

In some ethnic groups it is common to treat a febrile or unwell child by rubbing or suctioning the skin with a variety of implements. This produces bizarre circular and linear patterns of petechiae that can alarm the unwary.

Petechiae can appear around the head and neck in normal children after coughing or vomiting. Restraining a small child for a procedure such as a lumbar puncture or venepuncture can also lead to the development of petechiae on the upper body.

Blue or black rashes

Consider vascular malformations, haemangiomas, Mongolian spots, blue naevi and melanoma.

Vascular malformations

- These can be blue, red, purple or skin coloured. They are developmental defects and do not resolve.
- Such malformations can involve any mix of capillaries (e.g. portwine stain), veins, arteries (e.g. arteriovenous malformation) and lymphatics (e.g. cystic hygroma).
- Extensive malformations can be associated with pain, soft tissue or bony hypertrophy, bone erosion, haemorrhage, infection and platelet trapping.
- Management requires a multidisciplinary approach using expertise from surgical, paediatric, dermatological and radiological fields.

Haemangiomas
Clinical features

Superficial haemangiomas begin as macular erythematous lesions in the first weeks of life and become soft, partly compressible, sharply defined, red or purple swellings that can occur anywhere on the body. Deeper houraemangiomas may appear as blue or skin-coloured swellings. Most haemangiomas are not present at birth; they grow for several months and resolve fully over several years.

Management

Parents need reassurance about the inherently benign nature of these lesions. Most haemangiomas are best left alone and allowed to involute spontaneously. In some sites, however, haemangiomas can rapidly lead to problems such as ulceration, blindness, destruction of cartilage, respiratory obstruction or death.

Urgent assessment by an experienced clinician is needed if any developing haemangioma:

- Is ulcerating and potentially disfiguring.
- Is on the eyelid or adjacent to the globe of the eye.
- Deforms structures such as the lip, ear cartilage or nasal cartilage.
- Begins as an extensive macule that grows thicker.
- Is associated with stridor, thrombocytopenia or multiple lesions.

Corticosteroids are usually used, occasionally with vascular laser, surgery or interferon.

Hypopigmented lesions

In hypopigmented lesions, look for a fine scale. If it is scaly, consider pityriasis versicolor or pityriasis alba. If it is not scaly, consider pityriasis versicolor, post-inflammatory loss of pigment, halo naevi or vitiligo.

Pityriasis versicolor

- This is common in adolescents and is caused by an increased activity of commensal yeasts.
- Multiple oval macules, usually covered with fine scale, appear on the trunk or upper arms. The lesions may appear paler or darker than the surrounding skin.
- Treatment with anti-yeast shampoos is effective. For example, apply selenium sulfide 2% (Selsun shampoo). Leave on for 5–10 min, rinse and treat weekly for 4 weeks and then monthly. The pigmentation takes weeks to resolve and relapses are common without ongoing maintenance.

Pityriasis alba

This condition is common in prepubertal children and represents post-inflammatory hypopigmentation secondary to mild eczema. Single or multiple, poorly demarcated hypopigmented 1–2 cm macules are seen on the face or upper body. Lesions are not itchy but often have a fine scale. Reassure and treat with hydrocortisone 1% to active lesions and educate regarding skin care for eczema. Resolution of the discolouration takes weeks.

Vitiligo

This condition is characterised by sharply demarcated, often symmetrical areas of complete pigment loss. Eventual repigmentation in childhood vitiligo is common and is helped by topical steroids. In troublesome cases refer to a specialist for advice regarding treatment (e.g. corrective cosmetics or psoralen therapy).

Post-inflammatory pigmentation changes

This condition occurs particularly in dark-skinned people. Many inflammatory skin disorders may heal leaving diffuse, hypo- or hyperpigmented macules that can persist for months or years. No treatment is satisfactory.

Hyperpigmented lesions

If they are flat, consider junctional melanocytic naevi, café-au-lait spots, naevus spilus, pityriasis versicolor and post-inflammatory hyperpigmentation. If raised, consider compound melanocytic naevi, Spitz naevi and warts.

Congenital pigmented naevi

Congenital melanocytic naevi that cover large areas or are likely to cause significant cosmetic concern need very early assessment by a skin specialist and plastic surgeon, preferably in the first week of life, for diagnosis, surgery, laser treatment and/or long-term follow up. Small congenital melanocytic naevi have no increased risk for the development of melanoma over other moles.

Acquired pigmented naevi

During childhood, most children develop multiple pigmented lesions, which may be freckles, lentigines, naevus spilus, acquired melanocytic naevi or very rarely, melanoma.

Immune-suppressed children and those who have had chemotherapy are at greater risk of skin malignancy.

Anogenital rashes

Most anogenital rashes seen in infants who wear nappies are primarily caused by reaction with urine or faeces (irritant napkin dermatitis) or by seborrhoeic dermatitis. Soaps, detergents and secondary yeast infection may contribute. In older children, threadworms (*Enterobius vermicularis*) are a common cause of an itchy anogenital rash. Look for the worms at night and treat with mebendazole 50 mg (<10 kg), 100 mg (>10 kg) (not in pregnancy or <6 months) or pyrantel 10 mg/kg (max 500 mg) once oral. A repeat dose 2 weeks later helps reduce the high rate of reinfestation.

Consider also less common causes such as malabsorption syndromes (diarrhoea, erosive dermatitis and failure to thrive), zinc deficiency (a sharply defined anogenital rash with associated perioral, hand and foot 'eczema'), Langerhans' cell histiocytosis, psoriasis and Crohn's disease.

Irritant napkin dermatitis
Clinical features

This is the most common cause of napkin dermatitis in infants and typically presents as confluent erythema that typically, but not always, spares the groin folds. Variant presentations include multiple erosions and ulcers, scaly or glazed erythema and satellite lesions at the periphery. Satellite lesions are suggestive of *Candida* infection.

Management
- Keep the area clean and dry. Leave the nappy off whenever possible.
- Gel-based disposable nappies or a non-wettable under-napkin can be helpful. Cloth nappies should be thoroughly washed and rinsed.
- Use topical zinc cream or paste for mild eruptions.
- Add hydrocortisone 1% cream if inflamed. Do not use stronger steroids.
- Consider mupirocin 2% cream if not settling. Antifungal therapy is often not needed, even if *Candida* is present.

Candida napkin dermatitis
This occurs secondary to irritant napkin dermatitis and antibiotic use. Swab to confirm and treat the underlying cause as above and use topical imidazole cream.

Perianal streptococcal dermatitis
Streptococcus pyogenes infection.

Clinical features
- A localised, well-demarcated erythema that covers a circular area of 1–2 cm radius around the anus.
- Tenderness and painful defecation are typical.
- If not treated, it may persist for months.
- May have fissures and constipation.

Management
- Take perianal and throat cultures to confirm the presence of *Streptococcus pyogenes*.
- Apply paraffin ointment three times daily to the perianal area for symptomatic relief. Treat with oral antibiotics (phenoxymethylpenicillin 15 mg/kg (max 500 mg) 6 hourly) for a minimum of 2 weeks. Several weeks of therapy may be required. Intramuscular penicillin can be used if there are concerns about compliance.
- Keep stools soft with oral liquid paraffin for several weeks.

Lichen sclerosis
This condition presents as an area of atrophy with white shiny skin, purpura or telangiectasia in the perivulval region of girls aged 3 years or older. It may be itchy. Cases have been mis-diagnosed as sexual abuse. Management is with moisturisers and brief courses of moderately potent steroid ointment. About 50% of cases resolve spontaneously.

Hair problems
Consider alopecia areata, traumatic alopecia, tinea capitis, kerion and head lice.

Alopecia areata
Clinical features

Typically one or more oval patches of hair loss develop over a few days. Some hairs may remain within the patches but usually there is complete alopecia in the affected areas. Occasionally, the hair loss is diffuse. The scalp appears normal and does not show scaling, erythema or scarring. Most cases in childhood resolve spontaneously but progression to total scalp or body hair loss or recurrent alopecia can occur. Regrowth can occur decades later.

Management
- For isolated small patches present for weeks without further progression, no treatment is needed.
- For recent or progressive hair loss, treatment with intralesional steroids for a few weeks is beneficial. In difficult cases, other therapies including contact sensitisation, irritant agents and pulsed corticosteroids need to be considered.

Traumatic alopecia
Clinical features

This condition is usually caused by rubbing (as on the occiput of many babies), cosmetic practices (e.g. tight braiding) or hair pulling as a habit (trichotillomania). Trichotillomania may be largely nocturnal and parents are often unaware of it. The affected areas are usually angular and on the anterior or lateral scalp. The areas contain hairs of different lengths and are never completely bald, unlike alopecia areata.

Management
- Recognition of the problem and a careful explanation to the family is often sufficient.
- Trichotillomania in younger children does not usually indicate that significant psychological problems are present. It is a habit similar to thumb sucking or nail biting, and a low-key approach similar to that used in those conditions is appropriate.

Tinea capitis
Clinical features

In Australia, tinea capitis is usually caused by *Microsporum canis* contracted from cats or dogs. It is characterised by patches of hair loss with some short, lustreless, bent hairs a few millimetres in length. Redness and scaling are present in the patch. Hair loss without any of these features is not likely to be fungal.

Management
- Confirm the diagnosis, if possible, by greenish fluorescence of the hair shafts with Wood's light (not present with some fungi) or by microscopy and culture of hair and scale.
- Treatment usually comprises griseofulvin orally 15–20 mg/kg (max. 1 g) daily for 4–6 weeks or until non-fluorescent. Pulse therapy (1 week treatment, 3 weeks off, then repeat) with newer antifungals (terbinafine, itraconazole) is also effective.
- Children may attend school provided that they are being treated.

Kerion (inflammatory ringworm)

This represents an inflammatory scarring immune response to tinea. It is an erythematous, tender, boggy swelling that discharges pus from multiple points. The swellings appear fluctuant but skin incision should be avoided. Treatment is with oral antifungals, often with antibiotics for secondary infection, and a brief course of oral steroids to suppress the immune response. Other inflammatory granulomas can mimic kerions.

Head lice
Clinical features

Infestation of the scalp with *Pediculus capitis* is associated with itching. Eggs (nits) can be seen attached to the hairs just above the scalp surface. Epidemics of head lice regularly sweep through primary schools in all areas.

Management

- Suitable treatments include pyrethrin 0.165% (e.g. Pyrifoam), maldison 0.5% and permethrin 1% (e.g. Nix and Lyclear cream rinse), although resistance to all of these therapies has been reported.
- Wash the hair with soap and water. Thoroughly moisten the hair with the treatment and leave for 10 min. Rinse well and comb out with a fine-toothed comb. Reapply 1 week later to kill any eggs that have subsequently hatched.
- Reinfestation is common. A regular physical inspection, use of conditioner and combing of the hair are as important as chemical treatment.

Nail problems

Congenitally abnormal nails are usually atrophic and can be the presenting feature of rare inherited conditions such as ectodermal dysplasias, dyskeratosis congenita, pachyonychia congenita, congenital malalignment of the great toenails and the nail–patella syndrome.

Acquired nail disease is usually a result of fungal infection, psoriasis, ingrown toenails or 20-nail dystrophy. It may also be seen in association with diseases such as alopecia areata and lichen planus. Nail biting and picking can lead to marked deformity of involved nails.

Tinea unguium (onychomycosis)
Clinical features

- Dermatophyte infection may affect one or more nails.
- White or yellow patches develop at the distal and lateral nail edges. The rest of the nail may become discoloured, friable and deformed with accumulation of subungual debris.
- Tinea is often also present on the adjacent skin, particularly in between the toes.

Management

- Always confirm the diagnosis by microscopy and culture of nail clippings.
- Oral terbinafine is the therapy of choice, taken daily for 12 weeks (<20 kg 62.5 mg, 20–40 kg 125 mg, >40 kg 250 mg).

USEFUL RESOURCES
- *www.dermnet.org.nz* – An excellent website with online courses (including pictures, investigations and management) and patient information.

CHAPTER 24

Ear, nose and throat conditions

Robert Berkowitz
Michael Marks

Upper respiratory tract infections

The average child has 4–12 upper respiratory tract infections (URTIs) a year, the peak incidence being between 1 and 6 years. Risk factors include exposure to other young children (either at home, childcare or school) and passive exposure to tobacco smoke.

Causes

Viruses are responsible for at least 90% of upper respiratory tract infections. Bacterial causes include Group A streptococcus and *Mycoplasma pneumoniae*.

Local symptoms include coryza, cough, sore throat and ears. There may be fever, lethargy and decreased feeding. Infants and young children with an URTI may appear quite unwell. It is important to exclude serious bacterial infections in children who have severe constitutional symptoms.

Management

Symptomatic if necessary.
- Ensure adequate fluid intake.
- Give paracetamol if the child is distressed.
- The following may be administered for temporary relief of nasal congestion interfering with feeding or sleeping: saline nasal drops/spray, eucalyptus inhalant (e.g. chest rub), or ephedrine nose drops (maximum duration of therapy is 48 h).

Note: Antihistamines are not indicated in URTIs unless co-existent allergic rhinitis is suspected. Refer to chapter 19, Allergy and immunology. Antihistamines, especially sedating varieties, should be avoided in children <12–24 months of age.

Otitis media

This term covers a spectrum of conditions, which are characterised by the presence of fluid in the middle ear. Fluid may be recognised by tympanic membrane appearance or by assessment of tympanic membrane mobility. Otitis media may be classified according to clinical presentation as either:

Paediatric Handbook, 8th edition. By Kate Thomson, Dean Tey and Michael Marks. Published 2009 by Blackwell Publishing, ISBN: 978-1-4051-7400-8.

- Acute suppurative otitis media (ASOM).
- Otitis media with effusion (OME).

Acute suppurative otitis media

This condition is characterised by both:
- Middle ear effusion:
  - Otoscopic features include loss of the normal tympanic membrane translucency, loss of the light reflex and yellowish discolouration rather than the usual grey colour of the tympanic membrane
  - Reduced tympanic membrane motility – as assessed by pneumatic otoscopy and/or tympanometry

and
- Clinical features of inflammation, that are either:
  - Localised (e.g. ear pain) **or**
  - Generalised (e.g. fever, irritability), provided there is no other cause apparent to explain these symptoms.

Note: **Be wary of accepting ASOM as the sole diagnosis in an unwell infant with a fever. There may be a coexistent serious bacterial infection. Consider a septic work-up or careful observation.**

ASOM is very often preceded by a viral upper respiratory tract infection. The causative bacteria are usually:
- *Streptococcus pneumoniae.*
- Non-typeable *Haemophilus influenzae.*
- *Moraxella catarrhalis.*

Management
Initial management
- Adequate analgesia:
  - Paracetamol – 15 mg/kg p.o. 4–6 hourly (max. 90 mg/kg per day) as required.
- Consider antibiotics:
  - Acute symptoms resolve without antibiotics within 24 h in most cases.
  - Withhold in children >12 months who are only mildly unwell.
  - Commence if child is unwell or distress continues beyond 24–48 h; amoxicillin 15 mg/kg (max 500 mg) p.o. 8 hourly for 5 days **or** roxithromycin 2.5–4 mg/kg (max. 150 mg) p.o. 12 hourly for 5 days if allergic to penicillin.

Note: Antibiotics do not reduce the incidence of recurrent ASOM or OME (see below).

Follow-up
The key features of ASOM, clinical inflammation and middle-ear effusion, need to be considered separately.

Clinical inflammation

Review in 48 h. If the inflammation has not resolved, consider these possible explanations:
- Wrong diagnosis (e.g. viral URTI, serious bacterial infection).
- Failure to take the medication (antibiotics not given or vomited).
- Inappropriate antibiotic was prescribed (i.e. bacterial resistance: switch to amoxicillin with clavulanic acid 15 mg/kg (max 500 mg) orally, 8 hourly).
- Antibiotic reaction.
- Uncommonly, a suppurative complication of ASOM may have developed (e.g. mastoiditis, facial paralysis, labyrinthitis, intracranial infection).

If the medical treatment has been unsuccessful and the child remains symptomatically unwell, early drainage of the ear (myringotomy) with or without insertion of a tympanostomy tube may need to be considered. Refer to an otolaryngologist.

Middle ear effusion

A middle ear effusion is present for a variable period of time following ASOM and may be associated with noticeable hearing loss, particularly if bilateral. A middle ear effusion will be present in approximately:
- 80% of cases at 2 weeks following ASOM.
- 40% at 1 month.
- 20% at 2 months.
- 10% at 3 months.

Review at 3 months is recommended, particularly if symptomatic hearing loss is present. Management – see below (otitis media with effusion).

Recurrent ASOM

ASOM is common in the first 3 years of life and is generally a seasonal condition with a peak incidence in winter and early spring, paralleling the incidence of viral URTI. Prevention of recurrent ASOM may need to be considered during this period, depending on the frequency, severity and duration of infections. Prophylactic measures include:
- Limiting exposure to viral URTI (e.g. by avoiding excessive attendance at large childcare groups).
- Long-term prophylactic antibiotics (e.g. co-trimoxazole for 6 weeks).
- Insertion of tympanostomy tubes, which should be considered particularly if infections are associated with morbidity and are thought likely to persist for a significant period of time.

Mastoiditis

This is a severe complication of ASOM. Children are unwell; presenting with features of ASOM associated with more severe systemic symptoms and postauricular inflammation (ranging from cellulitis to subperiosteal abscess). Management involves referral to otolaryngologist and i.v. antibiotics. Unless mild, children will require insertion of tympanostomy tubes and drainage of the subperiosteal abscess. Mastoidectomy is performed where cholesteatoma is suspected or in the presence of an additional suppurative complication.

Otitis media with effusion (OME)

A persistent middle ear effusion (which has been present for a variable period of time) can be associated with varying degrees of hearing loss, behavioural, language and educational difficulties. OME usually resolves spontaneously over time. Factors contributing to persistence include recurrent upper respiratory tract infection, recurrent ASOM, poor eustachian tube function and exposure to tobacco smoke.

Management

Medical

- Antibiotics: for symptomatic cases that have not resolved in 3 months, a prolonged course of antibiotics (amoxicillin 15 mg/kg (max. 500 mg) 8 hourly for 3 weeks) will usually result in resolution.
- No other medical treatment has proven benefit (except for steroids, which are not recommended in the treatment of OME).
- Eustachian tube exercises (auto-inflation) are of limited value because of the difficulty of adherence in children.

Tympanostomy tubes

Tympanostomy tubes provide good short-term benefit, but their long-term value is widely debated. It does not cure the underlying eustachian tube dysfunction responsible for OME, but temporarily removes the symptoms by providing an alternative means for middle ear ventilation. Adenoidectomy may be beneficial (by removing a reservoir of infection from the nasopharynx), particularly in children requiring recurrent tympanostomy tube insertion. The long-term impact of tympanostomy tube insertion on language, literacy and cognitive function is the subject of ongoing research.

Consider insertion of tympanostomy tubes **only** if:

- Middle ear effusion present for **at least 3 months** and appears likely to persist long term, **and**
- significant symptoms are present: either recurrent ASOM or functionally significant hearing loss (e.g. speech delay, behavioural disturbance or poor school performance).

OME and ASOM are commonly related to URTI and are therefore more common in winter and early spring. Inserting tubes towards the end of this period should be avoided, in the expectation that there may be resolution with the onset of warmer weather.

The benefits of temporary alleviation of symptoms by tympanostomy tube insertion need to be balanced against the disadvantages:

- Need for general anaesthesia and surgery.
- Tubes usually remain *in situ* for only 6–9 months (although longer-stay tubes are available) and the reinsertion rate of tubes is ~25%.
- Tympanic membrane perforation occurs at a rate of approximately 1% per year that tubes remain *in situ*. A range of other tympanic membrane and middle ear complications are associated with tubes.
- Otorrhoea occurs in up to 25% of cases. It is often associated with an URTI, and may also occur because of external contamination (e.g. swimming or bathing without ear protection).

Management of discharging ears in children with tympanostomy tubes
- Ear toilet; gentle removal of excess discharge and debris from the outer external canal using cotton wool.
- Topical antibiotics, e.g. ciprofloxacin.
- For refractory discharge:
  - Ear swab.
  - 1.5% hydrogen peroxide ear washes.
  - Refer to an otolaryngologist.
  - Consider possibility of underlying immunodeficiency or cholesteatoma.

Hearing loss
Children with impaired hearing (Table 24.1) are at risk of speech and language delay, which may contribute to learning, behavioural and social problems (see chapter 11). Hearing level is measured in decibels (dB).

Screening
Infant screening is carried out in some centres and is associated with earlier diagnosis, which may improve developmental outcomes. All infants admitted to a neonatal intensive care or special care nursery are now routinely screened.

Formal audiological testing
Hearing can be assessed behaviourally in children from 9 months of age, but younger children require electrophysiologic testing by ABR (auditory brainstem response audiometry). Audiology assessment should be carried out in the following 'at risk' children:
- Prematurity or other significant neonatal condition.
- Developmental delay or other disability.
- Family history of hearing loss.
- Bacterial meningitis.
- Strong parental concern about hearing (e.g. the child who shouts, can't follow instructions).

Table 24.1 Levels of hearing impairment

No impairment	Can hear <15 dB	
Mild	Can't hear <26–40 dB	Soft speech
Moderate	Can't hear <41–65 dB	Ordinary speech
Severe	Can't hear <66–95 dB	Shout
Profound	Can't hear <95 dB	

Hearing impairment may be conductive, sensorineural or mixed and may be unilateral or bilateral. The more severe and prolonged the hearing loss, the greater the chance of developmental impairment. However, some children may be affected by even mild levels of impairment (e.g. difficulty learning in a noisy classroom). Associated disabilities may magnify the risks of hearing impairment.

Sensorineural impairment may be due to a range of congenital or acquired problems in the cochlear and/or central auditory pathways (Table 24.2). Specialist referral is suggested for children with significant impairment to consider genetic testing and imaging studies.

Management options for hearing-impaired children

These will be considered by otolaryngologist, audiologist and family. Some causes will be amenable to surgical interventions but most permanent causes of hearing impairment require optimisation of communication potential by other means. For example:

- Amplification (with hearing aids).
- Cochlear implant.
- Sign language.

The impact of hearing impairment and the optimisation therapies listed above on patients and their families is significant. Family support is available through a variety of organisations, for example Hearing Australia (*www.hearing.com.au*).

Otitis externa
Clinical features

Commonly occurs due to water contamination following swimming or in children with dermatitis of the external auditory canal. It is characterised by pain (often severe) **and**:

- Inflammation of the ear canal, which may include the tympanic membrane (mobility of the tympanic membrane on pneumatic otoscopy excludes otitis media).
- Pre-auricular tenderness.

Table 24.2 Commonest causes of hearing impairment in children

Conductive	Sensorineural
Recurrent ASOM/OME	Congenital: Genetic or chromosomal Syndromic Temporal bone malformations Infections (TORCH organisms)
Chronic otitis media: Non-suppurative, e.g. tympanic membrane perforation Suppurative	Acquired: Prematurity Meningitis Drug-related, e.g. aminoglycosides Postviral (measles, mumps)

Management
- Ear toilet.
- Topical antibiotics combined with steroids (e.g. ciprofloxacin HC).
- An ear wick should be inserted when the ear canal is very oedematous (to maintain patency of the ear canal and allow topical antibiotics to enter the ear canal) and moistened frequently with topical antibiotics.
- Hospital admission for administration of (antipseudomonal) i.v. antibiotics may be necessary when ear pain is severe and not relieved by regular analgesics, or where cellulitis has extended beyond the ear canal. See Antimicrobial guidelines, Appendix 3.

Acute pharyngitis/tonsillitis

The combination of fever and sore throat is a common presenting problem in children. Determining the aetiology and deciding whether to treat with antibiotics can be difficult.

Background

Most sore throats are due to a viral infection (almost all in children <4 years of age). The only clinically important bacterial pathogen is group A β-haemolytic streptococcus (GABHS), *Streptococcus pyogenes*.
- GABHS is found in around 20–30% of older children presenting with an acute sore throat.
- GABHS colonises the throat in some normal children (up to 20%).
- Distinguishing colonisation from acute infection is a major problem. A child with a sore throat may be colonised with GABHS and therefore have a positive throat swab (or a positive antigen test), yet the cause of the episode may be a viral infection.
- GABHS is more likely if the child is 4 years of age or older, has tenderness and enlargement of the tonsillar cervical lymph nodes, inflammation of the tonsils and pharynx (pharyngotonsillitis), unilateral signs or a generalised erythematous (scarlatiniform) rash.
- The presence of tonsillar exudate is not helpful in distinguishing viral infection from GABHS.
- GABHS is less likely if the child has associated coryza, cough, generalised lymphadenopathy or splenomegaly.
- Streptococcal serology (ASOT, antiDNase-B titre) can only be used to make a retrospective diagnosis (rise in titre between baseline and 3 weeks later).
- Penicillin reduces the duration of symptoms, possibly by up to a day or more. Penicillin reduces the incidence of uncommon suppurative complications (e.g. quinsy) and acute rheumatic fever. However, penicillin to prevent acute rheumatic fever is of questionable use as this is now rare except in some indigenous communities and developing countries.

Practical management

Children who probably **do not** need antibiotics are those aged <4 years and/or those with associated cough or coryza, unless they are unwell enough to require hospitalisation.

Children who might benefit from antibiotics are those aged >4 with marked pharyngotonsillitis, tender tonsillar cervical nodes, and without cough and coryza.

- Send a throat swab for culture and give oral phenoxymethylpenicillin 250 mg (500 mg if >10 years) 12 hourly.
- Erythromycin 15 mg/kg (max. 500 mg) 8 hourly or roxithromycin 2.5 mg/kg (max. 150 mg) 12 hourly may be used for children with true penicillin allergy.
- If the throat swab does not grow a GABHS (the result is normally available 48–72 h later) the antibiotics can be stopped. If GABHS is grown, continue antibiotics for a total of 10 days.

In populations with high rates of acute rheumatic fever (e.g. Aboriginal Australians in remote/rural settings), all sore throats should be treated with antibiotics and throat swabs are not needed.

Infectious mononucleosis is a relatively common cause of acute pharyngitis in older children. The diagnosis often becomes apparent when there is no response to penicillin, other characteristic features develop (e.g. generalised lymphadenopathy, splenomegaly, mild jaundice and rashes) and the illness follows a more prolonged course.

Quinsy (peritonsillar abscess)

Infection can extend beyond the tonsil as cellulitis (peritonsillar cellulitis) or as a peritonsillar abscess (quinsy). In addition to features of severe tonsillitis, quinsy presents with drooling, a 'hot potato' voice, and trismus. Inflammation of the hemipalate adjacent to the tonsil is evident and an area of fluctuance (perceived as a softening) can be palpated. In the earlier cellulitic stage, the condition will settle with i.v. antibiotics, but where an abscess is present, drainage is necessary. Refer to an otolaryngologist.

Recurrent acute pharyngitis/tonsillitis

Recurrent sore throats are a normal part of growing up for many children. Many of these children have recurrent viral pharyngitis. True recurrent GABHS pharyngotonsillitis is much less common but often over-diagnosed.

A variety of strategies have been used to reduce recurrences of GABHS pharyngotonsillitis. None of these is universally effective in preventing recurrent episodes and each has its own disadvantages.

- Use of another antibiotic to attempt eradication of GABHS (e.g. amoxicillin/clavulanic acid).
- Use of low-dose prophylactic penicillin.
- Treatment of culture-positive family members.
- Tonsillectomy. Tonsillectomy (with or without adenoidectomy) probably works by removing a reservoir of GABHS infection. It should be considered if the pattern of infection (i.e. frequency, severity and duration of infections) is such that significant morbidity is expected to continue for a prolonged and unacceptable period of time. The presence of associated airway obstruction may influence treatment choice.

Children with suspected recurrent GABHS pharyngotonsillitis should have a throat swab taken during an acute episode to aid in treatment decisions. Streptococcal serology may also be of value.

Obstructive adenotonsillar hypertrophy

See chapter 12, Sleep, p. 152).

Epistaxis

This is usually due to bleeding from the anterior nasoseptal vessels, often in association with nasal crusting or nose picking. Acute bleeding usually settles with local pressure to the lower nasal septum, but occasionally the application of a cottonwool pledget soaked with a topical decongestant (e.g. ephedrine) is necessary.

Recurrent bleeding can be treated by the application of an antibiotic ointment if significant nasal crusting is present, or by cautery if enlarged blood vessels are seen (use a silver nitrate stick following the application of a topical anaesthetic and decongestant, e.g. co-phenylcaine spray – lignocaine (lidocaine)/phenylephrine). Epistaxis in children is very unlikely to be due to a nasal tumour or a previously undiagnosed coagulopathy.

Trauma

Nasal trauma

Treatment is required for either cosmesis or drainage of septal haematoma.

Cosmesis

A nasal deformity due to a displaced nasal fracture should be reduced within 7–10 days of injury. The presence of a bony deformity due to a nasal fracture is best determined at about 5 days following the injury, once the soft tissue swelling has resolved. The decision to reduce the nasal fracture is based on clinical grounds and radiology is unhelpful.

Septal haematoma

- This can occur after nasal trauma, regardless of whether a fracture is present or not. It invariably leads to septal abscess formation with cartilage destruction and nasal collapse.
- It presents with nasal obstruction and pain associated with a bulge of the septum that can be confirmed by palpating with an instrument (e.g. wax curette) following application of a topical anaesthetic. Treatment involves incision and drainage, nasal packing to prevent recurrence and antistaphylococcal antibiotics.

Oral/oropharyngeal trauma

This invariably occurs after a fall with a stick or similar object in the mouth and may sometimes be associated with a significant injury.

Admit and evaluate if:
- Unable to feed.
- Upper airway obstruction.
- Significant laceration, requiring debridement, closure or both.
- Significant retropharyngeal injury.

- Suspicion of injury to the internal carotid artery. The internal carotid artery lies posterolateral to the tonsil. An injury to this region may be associated with injury to the internal carotid artery whether the trauma is blunt or sharp. Internal carotid artery injuries are rare; they are usually due to blunt trauma causing intimal disruption and progressive thrombosis and they typically present with neurological signs over a period of 24 h.

Involvement of the retropharynx may not be obvious by oral examination, particularly for injuries that penetrate the soft palate. Investigate by:
- Lateral cervical spine radiograph (look for widened retropharynx, evidence of cervical spine injury, or presence of foreign material).
- Flexible nasopharyngoscopy.

Consider involvement of the teeth in cases of oral trauma; see chapter 22, Dental conditions, p. 265.

Aural trauma

Trauma to the external auditory canal is usually associated with bleeding, but it is an insignificant injury and requires no treatment. The tympanic membrane can be perforated by direct trauma or a pressure wave (e.g. a slap across the ear or diving). Acute tympanic membrane perforations usually heal within weeks and do not require acute intervention. Topical antibiotics are recommended for water-related injuries. Direct trauma may rarely cause ossicular disruption, facial paralysis or inner ear damage (with complete deafness and vertigo). Follow-up at around 4 weeks after injury is required to ensure perforations have healed.

Foreign bodies

The first attempt at foreign body removal is always the easiest and should be undertaken by an experienced clinician with the appropriate instruments and good illumination. Take into account the child's developmental stage and their level of anxiety in planning this procedure. Failure of the initial removal may lead to an otherwise unnecessary general anaesthetic.

Ear

Foreign bodies in the external auditory canal are best removed with a hook-shaped instrument, which is passed behind the foreign body and then used to pull it out. Grasping instruments, such as forceps, invariably lead to the foreign body being displaced further medially. Suction may also be useful.

Nose

The technique for the removal of nasal foreign bodies is the same as for foreign bodies in the external auditory canal. A topical anaesthetic (e.g. co-phenylcaine) should be applied before the attempted removal. The risk of inhalation of a nasal foreign body is minimal and therefore acute removal should be deferred until appropriate personnel and equipment are available.

Fish bone in pharynx

A fish bone usually lodges in the tonsil or at the base of the tongue and therefore can be seen on oral examination and removed after the application of a topical anaesthetic. If the fish bone cannot be seen during the oral examination, a more thorough examination by nasopharyngoscopy is required. Fish bones rarely reach the oesophagus and so oesophageal evaluation is usually unnecessary. Where a fish bone is not found, despite a suggestive history, the child should be reviewed until symptoms resolve and an examination under general anaesthetic considered. Although fish bones are radiolucent, radiology (particularly CT) may be helpful to detect the presence of complications when symptoms persist.

Oesophagus

The vast majority of swallowed foreign bodies pass without difficulty. If a foreign body becomes lodged in the oesophagus, it usually does so in the upper oesophagus, at the level of the cricopharyngeus. Lower oesophageal foreign bodies suggest the presence of underlying oesophageal pathology (e.g. stricture).

If a swallowed object reaches the stomach it will almost always pass without incident. Two types of object, however, may cause problems:

- Long, thin objects (e.g. hairpins and locker keys) may impact at the duodenojejunal flexure.
- Button batteries, if held up at any point in the alimentary canal, may release alkali, causing local necrosis and perforation. Their removal is a matter of urgency.

Radiographs (including neck, chest and abdomen) should be taken if there are symptoms suggestive of oesophageal impaction (e.g. drooling and dysphagia), or if long, thin objects or button batteries have been swallowed. Oesophageal foreign bodies impact in the coronal plane, whereas tracheal lodgement occurs in the sagittal plane. Radiolucent foreign bodies may be imaged by barium swallow. If an object is impacted in the oesophagus, endoscopic removal is required.

Tracheobronchus

See chapter 36, Respiratory conditions.

USEFUL RESOURCES
- *www.hearing.com.au* – Hearing Australia
- *www.entnet.org* – American Academy of Otolaryngology and Head and Neck Surgeons. Links to websites and case scenario teaching.
- *www.tracheostomy.com* – Aaron's tracheostomy page. An excellent site regarding tracheostomy management, run by an American parent and nurse.

CHAPTER 25

Endocrine conditions

Margaret Zacharin
Garry Warne
Fergus Cameron
George Werther

Type 1 diabetes mellitus
Diagnosis
Diagnosis is made by either:
- Random blood glucose >11 mmol/L, or
- Fasting blood glucose >7 mmol/L.

Note: There is no need for oral glucose tolerance testing.

Clinical features
- Typical symptoms are polyuria, polydipsia or weight loss. Glycosuria and ketonuria are often present.
- Children presenting with diabetes may range from being mildly unwell to severely unwell in diabetic ketoacidosis. Management varies according to presentation.

Differential diagnosis
Transient hyperglycaemia
Transient elevation of blood glucose and glycosuria (and possibly ketonuria) may occur in children with an intercurrent illness or with therapy such as glucocorticoids. The risk of later developing diabetes mellitus is about 3%, but it is approximately 30% if these findings are picked up in an otherwise well child. Check HbA1c and diabetes-related autoimmune markers (antibodies against insulin, glutamic acid decarboxylase (GAD) and islet cells) and discuss with a specialist.

Type 2 diabetes mellitus
This form of diabetes was rare in children. It is being seen increasingly in children who are overweight, those with a family history of type 2 diabetes mellitus and in some specific ethnic groups.

Paediatric Handbook, 8th edition. By Kate Thomson, Dean Tey and Michael Marks. Published 2009 by Blackwell Publishing, ISBN: 978-1-4051-7400-8.

New presentation, mildly unwell
Assessment
Less than 3% dehydration, no acidosis and not vomiting.

Management
Initial treatment
- 0.25 units/kg of quick-acting insulin s.c. stat. Halve dose if <4 years old.
- If within 2 h of a meal give mealtime dose only (see below). Halve dose if <4 years old.
- Before breakfast and lunch give 0.25 units/kg of rapid-acting insulin. Before the evening meal give 0.25 units/kg rapid-acting insulin and 0.25 units/kg of intermediate-acting insulin. If this is the first insulin dose give 0.25 units/kg rapid-acting insulin only, then a further 0.25 units/kg rapid-acting insulin at midnight followed by a snack. Continue until normoglycaemia and negative ketonuria are achieved.
- Encourage fluid intake with sugar-free fluid and a normal diet according to appetite, but exclude foods with quick-acting sugars.

Ongoing treatment
- Once normoglycaemia is achieved and ketonuria disappears, change insulin to twice-daily mixtures of short and intermediate insulins. Several regimes and insulin types with varying profiles are available.
- The usual initial total dose is 1 unit/kg/day. This is given as:
  - 2/3 in morning and 1/3 at night.
  - 2/3 of each dose intermediate-acting and 1/3 as rapid-acting.
- Older adolescents often go on to a basal bolus regimen: 30–40% intermediate acting insu-lin given at 2200 h, remainder given as quick-acting insulin in three equal doses before meals.
- Other treatment modalities now include insulin pump therapy; see p. 307.

Hyperglycaemia, mildly unwell (known diabetic)
Usually advised to take 10% of total daily dose as rapid acting insulin every 2 h until nor-moglycaemic (in addition to normal insulin). Consult with a specialist if uncertain.

Diabetic ketoacidosis
This is the mode of presentation in >30% of newly diagnosed diabetes in childhood and adolescence. Diabetic ketoacidosis (DKA) may occur in any child or adolescent with established type 1 diabetes. Rapid onset is more likely in patients with poor underlying control or in patients on an insulin pump.

Definition
- Hyperglycaemia >14 mmol/L.
- Metabolic acidosis (pH <7.3 or bicarbonate <15 mmol/L).
- Hyperketonaemia or moderate to severe ketonuria.

Causes
- Delayed diagnosis of insulin-dependent diabetes mellitus (IDDM).
- Omission of insulin (especially in adolescents with recurrent DKA).

- Acute stress (infection, trauma, psychological).
- Poor management of intercurrent illness.

History
- Polyuria, polydipsia, loss of weight and lethargy. These symptoms are usually of 1–3 weeks' duration in newly diagnosed patients. Symptoms are either absent or of shorter duration in patients with established diabetes.
- There may be a family history of diabetes or other autoimmune disease.

Examination
- Degree of dehydration (often overestimated):
  - Mild/nil (<4%): no clinical signs.
  - Moderate (4–7%): easily detectable dehydration (e.g. tachycardia, reduced skin turgor, poor capillary return).
  - Severe (>7%) poor perfusion, rapid pulse, reduced blood pressure, i.e. shock.
- Altered level of consciousness.
- Body temperature – hypothermia is common.
- Presence of a precipitating cause (e.g. infection).

Investigations
- Blood glucose, urea and electrolytes.
- Arterial or capillary acid/base.
- Urine – ketones, culture.
- Check for precipitating cause e.g. infection (urine, FBE, blood cultures; consider chest radiograph).
- In all newly diagnosed patients: islet cell antibodies, insulin antibodies, GAD antibodies, total IgA, antiendomyseal IgA gliadin and transglutaminase antibodies and thyroid function tests.
- Calculate:
  - Serum osmolality = $2Na^+$ + glucose + urea.
  - Adjusted Na^+ = plasma Na^+ + 0.3(plasma glucose – 5.5).

Management
Initial fluid requirements
- If hypoperfusion is present, give normal saline at 10 mL/kg stat.
- Repeat until perfusion is re-established (warm, pink extremities with rapid capillary refill).
- Commence rehydration with normal saline (see Table 25.1).
- Keep nil by mouth (except ice to suck) until alert and stable.
- Insert a nasogastric tube if patient is comatose or has recurrent vomiting; leave on free drainage.
- Rehydration may be completed orally after the first 24–36 h if the patient is metabolically stable.

Table 25.1 Diabetic ketoacidosis fluid rates (mL/h) including deficit and maintenance fluid requirements, to be given evenly over 48 h

Weight (kg)	Mild/Nil	Moderate
5	24	27
7	33	38
8	38	43
10	48	54
12	53	60
14	58	67
16	64	74
18	70	80
20	75	87
22	78	91
24	80	95
26	83	100
28	86	104
30	89	108
32	92	112
34	95	116
36	98	120
38	101	125
40	104	129
42	107	133
44	110	137
46	113	141
48	116	146
50	119	150
52	122	154
54	124	158
56	127	162
58	130	167
60	133	171
62	136	175
64	139	179
66	142	183
68	145	187
70	148	191

Note: Include fluids given as a bolus and deduct these from ongoing rate.

Fluids once insulin is commenced
- **Aim for maximum rate of fall of blood sugar of <5 mmol/L per hour**. If the blood sugar falls more rapidly than this, very quickly, i.e. within the first few hours, change to normal saline (0.9%) with 5% dextrose.
- When the blood sugar reaches 12–15 mmol/L, use 0.45% NaCl with 5% dextrose. Aim to keep the blood sugar at 10–12 mmol/L.
- If the blood glucose falls below 10–12 mmol/L and the patient is still sick and acidotic, increase the dextrose in the infusate to 7.5–10%.
- Do not turn down insulin infusion.

Insulin
- Commence after treatment of shock.
- Add 50 units of clear/rapid-acting insulin (Actrapid or Humulin R) to 49.5 mL 0.9% NaCl (1 unit/mL solution).
- Ensure that the insulin is clearly labelled.
- Start at 0.1 unit/kg per hour in newly diagnosed children >2 years and those already on insulin who have glucose levels >15 mmol/L.
- Children who have had their usual insulin and whose blood sugars are <15 mmol/L and those <2 years of age should receive 0.05 units/kg per hour.
- Adjust the concentration of dextrose to keep blood glucose 10–12 mmol/L.
- Adequate insulin must be continued to clear acidosis (ketonaemia).
- Insulin infusion can be discontinued when the child is alert and metabolically stable (blood glucose <10–12 mmol/L, pH >7.30 and HCO_3 >15 mmol/L). The best time to change to s.c. insulin is just before meal time.
- The insulin infusion should only be stopped 30 min after the first s.c. injection of insulin.

Potassium
- Add potassium chloride (KCl) to the i.v. fluid at the time of starting the insulin infusion.
- Start KCl at a concentration of 40 mmol/L if body weight <30 kg, or 60 mmol/L if ≥30 kg.
- Measure levels 2 h after starting therapy and 2–4 hourly thereafter.
- Specimens should be arterial or venous. Do not give K^+ if the serum level is >5.5 mmol/L or if the patient is anuric.

Bicarbonate
- This is usually not necessary if shock has been adequately corrected. Continuing acidosis usually means insufficient resuscitation.
- In extremely sick children (with pH <7.0 ± HCO_3 <5 mmol/L), small amounts may be given. Liaison with paediatric intensive care unit is advisable.
- The HCO_3 dose (mmol) = 0.3 × body weight (kg) × base deficit. **Infuse half** over 30 mins with cardiac monitoring. Reassess acid–base status. Remember risk of hypokalaemia.

Monitoring
Clinical
- Strict fluid balance.
- Check all urine for ketones.
- Hourly observations: pulse, BP, respiratory rate and neurological observations.
- Hourly glucose (glucometer) while on insulin infusion.
- 4 hourly temperature.

Note: Any headache or altered behaviour may indicate impending cerebral oedema.

Biochemical
- 2–4 hourly laboratory blood glucose levels (with hourly bedside glucometer readings).
- Serum sodium (adjusted for hyperglycaemia), potassium, chloride.
- pH.
- Serum osmolality: should not fall >0.5 mmol/kg per hour.

Note: Beware of falling adjusted sodium levels as glucose declines – hyponatraemia may herald cerebral oedema. If the sodium level falls, consider decreasing the rate of fluid administration to replace over 72–96 h; see Hypernatraemia section below.

Other instructions
- Intensive care is required if age <2 years, coma, cardiovascular compromise or seizures.
- Patient should remain nil orally until alert and stable.
- Nurse the patient in a head-up position and in good light.

Complications of diabetic ketosis
Hypernatraemia
Measured serum sodium is depressed by the dilutional effect of the hyperglycaemia. If Na is >160 mmol/L, discuss with a specialist. Sodium should rise as the glucose falls during treatment. If this does not happen or if **hyponatraemia** develops, it usually indicates overzealous volume correction and insufficient electrolyte replacement. This may place the patient at risk of cerebral oedema.

Hypoglycaemia
If blood glucose <2.2 mmol/L give i.v. 25% dextrose 2 mL/kg over 3 min or 10% dextrose 5 mL/kg. Do not discontinue the insulin infusion. Continue with a 10% dextrose infusion until stable. Where hypoglycaemia is recurrent, increase concentration of dextrose in i.v. fluids (e.g. to 12.5% or 15%).
Note: 15% infusions require central access.

Hypokalaemia
Monitor frequently and adjust potassium concentration in the infusate. Children at particular risk of this complication are those who are very acidotic or have low potassium levels at presentation.

Cerebral oedema

This is an uncommon (0.5–3.0%) but extremely serious complication of diabetic ketoacidosis in children, usually occurring 6–12 h after commencement of therapy. This condition is often fatal. If the patient survives there may be profound neurological impairment.

Prevention

Slow correction of fluid and biochemical abnormalities. Optimally, the rate of fall of blood glucose and serum osmolality should not exceed 5 mmol/L per hour, but in children there is often a quicker initial fall in glucose. Patients should be nursed head up.

Risk factors

- Newly diagnosed diabetes, young age, poorly controlled diabetes.
- Excessive fluid rehydration, particularly with hypotonic fluids.
- Severe initial acidosis.
- Hyponatraemia or hypernatraemia and negative sodium trend during the therapy.

Note: With appropriate therapy the serum sodium should remain stable or rise slightly as blood glucose falls. If the adjusted serum sodium falls during resuscitation, this may be a sign of excess fluid administration and may be associated with the development of cerebral oedema. If this occurs, decrease the rate of fluid administration to replace over 72–96 h.

Signs

- Early: negative sodium trend, headache, behaviour change (sudden irritability, depression of conscious state) and incontinence.
- Late: bradycardia, elevated blood pressure and depressed respiration.

Treatment

Cerebral oedema is a medical emergency.

- Administer 20% mannitol i.v. as a bolus dose at 0.25–0.5 g/kg (1.25–2.5 mL/kg of 20%). This can be repeated if the response is inadequate.
- Nurse the patient in a head-up position, maintain the airway.
- Severely restrict fluids.
- Transfer to an intensive care unit for intubation, intermittent positive pressure ventilation and further management.
- Do not delay treatment for radiological confirmation – diagnosis is clinical.

Hypoglycaemia in children with diabetes

Common causes

- Missed meal/snack.
- Vigorous exercise (can be during exercise or hours afterwards).
- Alcohol.
- Too much insulin.

Management
See Table 25.2

Sick day management during intercurrent illness in the child with diabetes
Principles
- Frequent testing of blood sugar and urine ketones (Table 25.3).
- The meal plan may temporarily be dropped – replace with fluids and easily digested carbohydrates.
- Ensure good fluid intake – alternate sugar and non-sugar-containing fluids depending on blood sugar levels (water is best if high).
- Insulin doses usually need to be increased; never omit insulin.
- Keep in touch with medical staff.

Management of children with diabetes undergoing surgery
The main aims are to prevent hypoglycaemia before, during and after surgery and to provide sufficient insulin to prevent the development of ketoacidosis. Factors that must be considered are:
- Time of surgery.
- Duration of surgery.
- Urgency of surgery.

Minor elective morning surgery
- Admit the child on the evening before surgery.
- Aim for the patient to be first on the operating list.
- Administer normal food and insulin until midnight on the night before surgery.
- At 0600 h check blood glucose. If blood glucose is <10 mmol/L give lemonade or sugar-containing clear fluid at 5–10 mL/kg (max = 200 mL) and inform the anaesthetist.
- Monitor blood glucose every 2 h and immediately before surgery. If blood glucose is <6 mmol/L insert i.v. line and give i.v. glucose.
- Give rapid-acting insulin equal to 1/10 of the total daily insulin dose (rapid- and intermediate-acting) at the usual time.
- An i.v. line with glucose will be inserted in the operating theatre (if not required preoperatively).
- Perform regular blood glucose every 2–4 h postoperatively, and adjust the i.v. glucose infusion as necessary. Give extra insulin 0.25 units/kg every 4–6 h to keep glucose between 5 and 10 mmol/L.
- When the patient can tolerate oral fluids stop the i.v. infusion and resume the normal insulin regimen.

Table 25.2 Management of hypoglycaemia in children with diabetes

Awake	Sugar, e.g. 1 cup lemonade, orange or apple juice; jelly beans; honey (1 tbs); condensed milk in tube Repeat in 5–10 min if no improvement, follow with 'sustaining serve', e.g. bread, milk
Drowsy/uncooperative/unconscious/fitting (at home)	Glucagon* i.m. injection 1 mg (1 ampoule) if >25 kg or >8 years old (0.5 mg if <25 kg or <8 years) Blood sugar rises in 5–10 min. Give sips of sugar-containing fluid when awake
Uncooperative/unconscious/fitting (in hospital)	Glucose 2 mL/kg of 25% dextrose i.v. over 2 min, then infuse 3–5 mg/kg per min until awake and able to eat/drink

* Note: As glucagon can cause headache/vomiting, mini-glucagon rescue is preferred. It is used when vomiting is associated with hypoglycaemia or for persistently low blood glucose levels resistant to oral therapy. The doses vary with age: ≤2 years 0.02 mg; 2–15 years 0.01 mg/year of age; >15 years 0.15 mg.

Table 25.3 Sick day management

Group BSL Urine ketones Vomiting	1 high 0–trace ±	2 high > 1 + none or occasional	3 normal/low 0–trace ±
Danger	Progress to group 2	DKA	Hypoglycaemia
Fluids	Ensure good intake (to thirst)	Increase intake ++	Ensure good intake
Meals	Normal meal plan	Can drop meal plan. Replace with fluids and easily digested carbohydrates	Normal to ↑ meal plan
Insulin	Increase normal dose by 10%	Give rapid acting insulin at 10–20% total daily dose. Repeat 4 hourly (2 hourly if 3+ ketones or mild vomiting)	Reduce normal insulin by 10–25%. May drop intermediate insulin if giving rapid insulin 4–6 hourly
Monitor	4–6 hourly BSL and urine ketones	2–4 hourly	2–4 hourly
Further action	If ketones increasing move to group 2	If not improving admit	If BSL low, manage as hypoglycaemia If BSL high move to group 2.

Minor elective afternoon surgery

- Continue normal food and insulin until midnight on the night before surgery.
- Provide a light breakfast at the usual time.
- Give rapid-acting insulin equal to 1/10 of the total daily insulin dose, half an hour before breakfast.
- Monitor blood glucose every 2 h (commence i.v. glucose if BSL is <6 mmol/L, otherwise i.v. glucose can be commenced in theatre).
- Give additional insulin at the same dose at 1200 h.
- Adopt same regimen as above postoperatively.

Minor surgery/short anaesthetic

I.v. glucose may not be necessary, provided that the oral intake can be resumed soon after surgery and that the pre-operative blood glucose concentration does not fall below 6 mmol/L. If in doubt, it is safer to follow the routines outlined above.

Emergency and major surgery

- Urgent clinical and biochemical assessment as for diabetic ketoacidosis.
- Rehydrate and start i.v. insulin as required.
- Maintain i.v. 0.45% saline with 5% dextrose and insulin infusion at 0.05–0.1 units/kg per hour pre- and postoperatively until the patient is able to resume oral feeding.

Continuous subcutaneous insulin infusion use in children and adolescents

Continuous subcutaneous insulin infusion (CSII), or insulin pump therapy, is gaining increasing use in the treatment of type 1 diabetes in children and adolescents. It relies on the continuous delivery of rapid-acting insulin into the subcutaneous tissues by an insulin pump, which is worn on the belt or in a bra, or carried in a pocket. The insulin pump is connected to a subcutaneous cannula by a dual-lumen flexible catheter. The subcutaneous cannula is re-sited and the pump reloaded with insulin every 3 days. Insulin pumps can be disconnected for 1–2 h at a time for bathing, swimming or contact sports.

Indications

- CSII can be used at any age but is currently most common in adolescent patients.
- Although it offers benefits in terms of reduction of hypoglycaemia, improved glycaemic stability and improved quality of life, it is not suitable for all patients.
- At a minimum, patients must do 4–6 finger-prick blood glucose measures per day, be able to carbohydrate count accurately and be cognitively able to cope with the challenges of operating the insulin pump.

Calculating dose

Insulin is delivered in two ways:

- A continuous background delivery (*basal delivery*). Basal delivery is pre-programmed and automatic.

- An intermittent meal or correction-based insulin delivery (*bolus delivery*). Bolus delivery is manually undertaken by the patient at the time of meals or when blood glucose levels are to be corrected.

Total daily insulin dose (TDD) on CSII is derived from pre-existing insulin requirements or based on weight.

- 40–50% of the TDD is given as basal insulin and the remainder given as bolus insulin.
- Patients may have multiple basal rates at varying times of the day and according to the varying levels of activity.
- Bolus insulin doses are calculated using the '500' rule (500 ÷ TDD = the number of grams of carbohydrate covered by 1 unit of bolus insulin). Correct calculation of the amount of bolus insulin requires that the patient is able to accurately 'carb count' their meals.
- The amount of insulin given to correct a high blood glucose level (correction factor) is calculated using the '100' rule (100 ÷ TDD = the number of mmols drop in blood glucose that will result from a correction bolus of 1 unit of insulin).
- Most modern insulin pumps will automatically calculate bolus doses after they have been configured and a blood glucose level has been entered into the pump software.

Note: Infants and toddlers will usually require lower insulin bolus doses than are indicated by the '500' and '100' rules.

Complications
Diabetic ketoacidosis is the most concerning acute complication of CSII use (Table 25.4). These patients are at higher risk of DKA because they do not use any long- or intermediate-acting insulin.

If CSII therapy is discontinued it is critical that these patients have ongoing, regular and frequent review due to the risk of rapid onset of ketosis.

Short stature
Stature must be assessed in the context of parental heights and pubertal status. Growth velocity must be compared with age-matched peers and assessed with regard to the child's pubertal status. Consider: is a growth spurt occurring at an expected time for this child?

Stature
Measure the child and, wherever possible, both biological parents. Plot all three heights on appropriate height percentile charts, and compare the percentiles (see Appendix 1). For girls, adjust father's height by subtracting 12.5 cm; for boys, adjust mother's height by adding 12.5 cm. The child's height percentile should approximate the mean of the parents' percentiles.

Table 25.4 Complications of CSII use

Complication	Causes	Management
Diabetic ketoacidosis	When insulin delivery is disrupted or when requirement increases. Ketosis ensues within 2–3 hours. • Cannula dislodgement • Tube kinks • Pump malfunction • Infected insertion site • Intercurrent illness	All patients receiving CSII therapy should also carry a back-up insulin pen containing rapid-acting insulin. • Hyperglycaemia – give correction bolus with pump • Recheck blood glucose in 1–2 h • Glucose remains high and/or ketones in urine – disconnect pump and give insulin bolus using insulin pen • CSII therapy can be recommenced once glycaemic stability and a lack of ketosis has been re-established
Hypoglycaemia	• Excessive basal rate • Increased physical activity	• Temporarily cease pump therapy and give 'hypo' food • CSII should be recommenced as soon as normoglycaemia is re-established • Hypoglycaemia causing altered conscious state should be treated with glucagon as per the protocol (in addition to temporary cessation of CSII)

Questions to consider:
- Is the child short in relation to other children the same age (i.e. below the third percentile)?
- Is the child unexpectedly short for the family?

Growth rate
Ask for any previous height measurements and plot them on the percentile chart. If no previous measurements are available, review at 3 month intervals; after 6 months, calculate the height velocity and check this against a growth velocity (GV) chart. Growth velocity can only be reliably calculated from measurements taken over 6–12 months. In most children, GV tends to fluctuate and only a consistently low GV will lead to a falling-off in height percentile. The criterion for further investigation in a short child is a GV below the 25th percentile.

Questions to consider:
- Is the child growing slowly?
- If the child's growth really is slow, what is the reason?
- Is the child growing at the rate expected for pubertal status? A growth spurt should always accompany puberty.

Causes
Physiological
Constitutional delay in maturation
This is a common (and often familial) normal variant. Characteristically, growth slows at about 2 years of age, producing a fall in the height percentile. Thereafter, growth is parallel to the 3rd percentile, but the prepubertal decline in growth is exaggerated and the onset of the growth spurt is later than average. Bone age is delayed. The final height is likely to be in keeping with that of other family members.

Familial short stature
- Several adult family members are short. Skeletal proportions and GV are normal. Bone age is equivalent to the chronological age.
- Some children from short families also have constitutional delay in maturation. Parents who have suffered protein–calorie malnutrition as children may not have achieved their own genetic potential and may be on a lower percentile than their children.

Organic
Organic causes of short stature are classified in Table 25.5. Clues to the diagnosis may emerge from the history and the child's general appearance. Some serious medical conditions (e.g. chronic renal failure, coeliac disease, inflammatory bowel disease, craniopharyngioma) may present with slow growth as the only abnormal sign. Important clues include:
- Dysmorphic features (e.g. Turner syndrome).
- Cutaneous changes (e.g. café au lait markings).
- Hand changes (e.g. short 4th/5th metacarpals, narrow deep-set nails).
- Fundal changes (e.g. optic atrophy).

Measure the skeletal proportions (arm span/height and upper/lower segment ratios).
- The lower segment should be >1/2 the height beyond the age of 8 years.
- The arm span should be within a few centimetres of height at all ages.

Investigations
Check the bone age initially. If the GV is <25th percentile for bone age then tests are indicated.
- Thyroid function tests – thyroid stimulating hormone (TSH) is the usual screening test, check free T_4 (FT_4) if central dysfunction is considered.
- Haemoglobin and erythrocyte sedimentation rate (ESR) (inflammatory bowel disease).
- Renal function and urine MC&S.
- Serum calcium, phosphate and alkaline phosphatase.
- Consider testing for coeliac disease.
- Chromosomes (all short girls; lack of dysmorphism does not exclude Turner syndrome).
- Skeletal survey (if disproportionate).
- Consider growth hormone (GH) studies as a second step (always done fasting):

Table 25.5 Organic causes of short stature

	Examples	Clues to diagnosis
Intrauterine	Russell–Silver syndrome	Birth length <3rd centile for gestational age
Skeletal	Bone dysplasia (e.g. achondroplasia) Spinal irradiation	Skeletal disproportion (short limbs) Low upper:lower segment ratio
Nutritional	Rickets	History of poor nutrition or limited sunlight/dark skin
	Protein–calorie malnutrition (world no.1)	Low weight-for-height (if not chronic)
	Malabsorption (e.g. coeliac disease)	Abdominal distension
	Chronic illness (e.g. renal failure, Crohn's disease)	Anaemia, high ESR
Iatrogenic	Corticosteroid therapy	Cushingoid features
Chromosomal/genetic	Turner, Down, Prader–Willi, Noonan, Cornelia de Lange, Rubinstein–Taybi syndromes	Specific dysmorphic features
	Inborn errors of metabolism: storage disorders (MPS, Gaucher)	Particular odour
	Organic/amino acidopathies (e.g. MMA, MSUD)	Metabolic acidosis
Endocrine	Hypothyroidism, Cushing disease, growth hormone deficiency, pubertal arrest, parathyroid disorders, AHO	Height centile < weight centile (i.e. short and plump) and associated examination findings

AHO, Albright hereditary osteodystrophy; MMA, methylmalonic aciduria; MPS, mucopolysaccharidosis; MSUD, maple syrup urine disease.

- Exercise.
- Glucagon stimulation (the current definitive test for GH deficiency).

Note: Basal GH is a useless test and does not define GH deficiency.

Interventions
Growth hormone therapy
Recombinant human GH is government-controlled in Australia; it costs an average of $20 000–$30 000 per year per child. To qualify, children must meet certain criteria:

- Height is below the 1st percentile.
- GV is below the 25th percentile for bone age.

- Bone age is <13.5 years for girls, or <15.5 years for boys.
- Must be free of any condition known not to respond to GH (e.g. high-dose steroid therapy or thalassaemia) or that could be worsened by GH therapy (e.g. insulin-dependent diabetes mellitus (IDDM), Fanconi anaemia or active malignancy).

Children with GH deficiency or Turner syndrome respond to growth hormone with an increase in final height. Use of growth hormone for other conditions without biochemical GH deficiency will increase growth velocity in the short term but usually does not result in significant increase in final height.

Note: These criteria differ if a child has GH deficiency following intracranial pathology or treatment including cranial radiation. Specialist assessment is required.

The dose of growth hormone is 14–22 units/m^2 per week divided into 6–7 doses/week.

Tall stature
Causes
- Familial.
- Precocious puberty.
- Hyperthyroidism.
- Syndromes: Marfan, Klinefelter, triple X, homocystinuria and Sotos.
- Pituitary gigantism (juvenile acromegaly).

Assessment
Height must be considered in the context of midparental expectation and pubertal status, e.g. if puberty is 2–3 years earlier than average, the child may appear to be very tall for chronological age but have a perfectly normal final height expectation for the family.

Investigations
Consider:
- Thyroid function.
- Karyotype.
- Urine metabolic screen/antithrombin III/coagulation/lipids (homocystinuria).
- 3 h oral glucose tolerance test for GH/IGF1.

Management
Management of any underlying disorder, for example, precocious puberty. High-dose oestrogen is very seldom used in very tall girls, to hasten epiphyseal closure. Tall boys may be similarly treated with testosterone. Treatment is managed by a paediatric endocrinologist.

Hypothyroidism
Hypothyroidism may be congenital or acquired.

Congenital hypothyroidism

Incidence is 1 : 3200 births.

Causes

- Absent thyroid 40–45%.
- Thyroid arrested in line of normal descent (lingual) 40–45%.
- Abnormal function (dyshormonogenesis) 10–15%.
- Thyroid hypolasia or hemithyroid (may be part of a genetic syndrome).
- Maternal iodine deficiency.

Clinical

- Unusually sleepy baby.
- Jaundice.
- Large anterior fontanelle, persistent posterior fontanelle.
- Coarse features.
- Dry skin.
- Periorbital oedema.
- Umbilical hernia.
- Harsh or hoarse cry.
- Slow feeding.
- Distal femoral epiphysis that is not ossified.

Investigations

- Most cases are detected by neonatal screening (high thyroid stimulating hormone (TSH)).
- Confirmation of the diagnosis on whole blood thyroid function tests (TFT) is essential.
- Technetium (Tch) scanning for position, function, size (presence of goitre, Tch uptake).

Management

Thyroxine therapy (8–12 mcg/kg per day) must be started as early as possible – before 2 weeks. Evidence suggests better outcome if treatment started at 10 days and T_4 in upper range. Aim for:

- FT_4 at the upper limit of normal range for age or just above.
- Normalisation of TSH.

Acquired hypothyroidism

Acquired hypothyroidism is called primary when the thyroid gland itself is abnormal (e.g. ectopic thyroid dysgenesis, autoimmune chronic lymphocytic thyroiditis and dyshormonogenesis) and secondary when the abnormality is a deficiency in pituitary TSH.

Clinical features

Hypothyroidism is often very difficult to detect clinically in children. Growth retardation may be the only sign, often with a relatively excess weight for height. The classical signs are usually absent when the cause is hypothalamic–pituitary.

- Growth retardation.
- Weight gain.
- Lethargy.
- Constipation.
- Cold intolerance.
- Goitre.
- Dry cool skin, dry hair.
- Prolonged ankle-jerk relaxation time.

Investigations
- TSH as screening test.
- FT_4 for degree of deficit and for primary diagnosis when cause is central.
- Thyroid autoantibodies.
- Urinary iodine (early morning).
- Technetium thyroid scan.
- Thyroid ultrasound where indicated (for assessment of gland structure).

Note: Referral to a specialist is important for the management of hypothyroidism.

Hyperthyroidism

Hyperthyroidism is usually due to Graves' disease in children and adolescents (different spectrum from that of adults). Six times as many girls are affected as boys, most commonly during puberty. A family history of thyroid disease (hyper- or hypothyroidism) is common. A family history should be sought for IDDM, vitiligo, pernicious anaemia, Addison disease or premature gonadal failure, as part of the spectrum of autoimmune polyglandular syndrome types I and II. Other causes to consider are:
- Toxic phase of Hashimoto thyroiditis (usually 4–6 weeks' duration and usually not detected clinically).
- Thyroid adenoma (rare in childhood).
- Factitious (thyroxine consumption for weight loss).

Clinical features
- Goitre (nearly all), diffuse, with bruit.
- Weight loss, heat intolerance, tiredness.
- Warm sweaty hands, tremor, tachycardia.
- Irritability and restlessness.
- Proximal muscle weakness and wasting, accelerated ankle-jerk relaxation time.
- Lid lag; exophthalmos, peri-orbital oedema, extraocular muscle trapping causing diplopia on upward and lateral gaze.
- Accelerated growth velocity.

Investigations
- FT_4, FT_3. TSH should be suppressed to undetectable (<0.01 mU/L).
- TSH receptor antibodies.

- Bone age (usually advanced).
- Technetium thyroid scan – expect diffuse increased uptake.
- Thyroid ultrasound if adenoma suspected.

Management
Antithyroid drugs are used for long-term treatment in childhood and adolescence. The long-term remission rate in this age group is 40%. Management by a specialist is necessary.

Antithyroid drugs
- Carbimazole: 0.2 mg/kg (max 30–60 mg/day depending on age, size), oral 8–12 hourly, for 2 weeks. Then reduce dose to 0.1 mg/kg (max. 5 mg) oral 8–24 hourly for at least 18–24 months, until remission is achieved. Short courses of treatment result in low remission rates.
- Propylthiouracil (PTU): 5–7 mg/kg per day in three divided doses oral 8 hourly with similar reduction in dose after 2 weeks. Propylthiouracil prevents conversion of T_4 to T_3 and is the preferred treatment in severe toxicity.

Idiosyncratic reactions may occur to either drug with urticaria and/or neutropaenia. This can occur at any time during treatment but is more common with high doses early in treatment. There is approximately 40% crossover intolerance.

Surgery
Used for:
- Non-compliance.
- Allergy to drugs.
- Large goitre, increasing in size.
- Long-term patient choice.

Radioactive iodine
The use of radioactive iodine in children and young adolescents is controversial and is not advocated. WHO considers it safe after the age of 17 years. It is the treatment of choice for adults.

Thyroid storm
Thyroid storm is a rare complication of untreated primary hyperthyroidism or non-compliance with thyroid medication. It is characterised by tremor, anxiety, tachycardia, fever and confusion. It requires treatment (usually in ICU), with i.v. beta blockade, sedation, Lugol's iodine and propylthiouracil.

Delayed puberty
Delayed puberty is defined as the absence of pubertal changes by 13–14 years for girls and by 15 years for boys. There is no absolute age for diagnosis; later than average and inappropriately late in a family being common reasons for referral (see Appendix 1 for pubertal stages charts/diagrams).

Causes

With normal or low serum gonadotrophins

- Constitutional delay (usually familial) is the most common cause. It is associated with slow growth and a delayed bone age in an otherwise healthy child.
- Chronic illness/poor nutrition (e.g. inflammatory bowel disease, anorexia nervosa, cystic fibrosis).
- Endocrine causes:
  - Hypopituitarism (gonadotrophin and possibly GH and other hormonal deficiencies).
  - Kallmann syndrome (isolated gonadotrophin deficiency with anosmia).
  - Hyperprolactinaemia (prolactinoma, secondary to medication (e.g. antipsychotics), functional (e.g. postcranial irradiation)).

With elevated serum gonadotrophins

This signifies primary gonadal failure, which may be due to:

- A genetic abnormality associated with gonadal dysgenesis (e.g. Turner, Klinefelter and Noonan syndromes).
- Anorchia.
- Gonadal destruction secondary to vascular damage, irradiation, infection, torsion or auto-immune disease.

Investigations

- Serum follicle-stimulating hormone (FSH), luteinising hormone (LH), testosterone or oestradiol; serum prolactin; other pituitary function tests (e.g. GH studies), as indicated by growth.
- Full blood examination, ESR.
- Urea, creatinine, serum proteins.
- Thyroid function test.
- Chromosomes.
- Bone age.

Management

Referral to a specialist is advised. Testosterone may be used in boys and oestradiol in girls; however, excess or too early use of sex hormones for pubertal management will result in rapid advancement of bone age, epiphyseal fusion and stunting of final height in both sexes. Growth hormone therapy may be offered to girls with Turner's syndrome (see Short stature, pp. 309–312).

Precocious puberty

Precocious puberty is defined as the onset of pubertal changes under 8 years in girls and under 9.5 years in boys. For pubertal staging, see Appendix 1.

Cause
Gonadotrophin dependent ('central' or 'true' precocious puberty)
- True precocious puberty is 20 times more common in girls than boys.
- Girls are less likely to have an underlying pathological cause than boys.
- Girls with this disorder have accelerated growth, with development of both pubic hair and breasts, and the vaginal mucosa has a pale, shell-pink colour with increased mucus secretion due to the effects of oestrogen.
- Boys with true precocious puberty have enlargement of both testes, as well as accelerated linear and genital growth.
- The commonest pathological cause is hypothalamic hamartoma. Practically all intracranial pathologies (malformation, trauma, tumour, infection and haemorrhage) are associated with an increased prevalence of precocious puberty. After cranial irradiation, puberty occurs on average 2 years earlier than usual, in both boys and girls.
- Investigations are designed to demonstrate the premature activity in the hypothalamic–pituitary–gonadal axis and to exclude intracranial pathology.

Gonadotrophin independent ('pseudo' precocious puberty)
- Congenital adrenal hyperplasia.
- Adrenal, testicular or ovarian neoplasms.
- Tumours that secrete non-pituitary gonadotrophin such as chorionic gonadotrophin (hCG).
- McCune–Albright syndrome.
- Familial male precocious puberty.

Investigation of precocious puberty (both types)
- Serum FSH and LH.
- Gonadal steroid (testosterone or oestradiol).
- βHCG where indicated.
- Bone age.
- MRI of the head
  - If increased FSH or LH is found.
  - All boys with central precocious puberty must have an MRI scan.
  - In girls with central precocious puberty MRI is less likely to yield an intracranial organic lesion. It is not commonly done if puberty occurs at >5 years, unless there is a specific clinical indication (e.g. headache, visual change).
- Pelvic ultrasound in girls for ovarian cyst or tumour.
- Testicular ultrasound if indicated.

Management
Refer to a specialist, who may use medroxyprogesterone acetate, cyproterone acetate or a luteinising hormone releasing hormone superagonist (LHRH agonist). Not all cases require treatment.

Conditions resembling precocious puberty
Premature thelarche
- Isolated breast development is common in girls <2 years of age (8–10%) and can be expected to regress spontaneously in most cases.
- Simple observation is usually sufficient but if the condition is associated with rapid growth velocity, consider true oestrogen excess of any cause and investigate (as above).

Premature adrenarche
- The isolated appearance of pubic hair (usually in a girl) under the age of 8 years may occur as a normal variant, but it may also signify non-classical congenital adrenal hyperplasia.
- Appropriate investigations are bone age, basal serum dehydroepiandrosterone sulfate (DHEA-S), androstenedione, testosterone and 17-hydroxyprogesterone (17-OHP). The measurement of 17-OHP at 30 and 60 min after intramuscular Synacthen (synthetic adrenocorticotrophic hormone (ACTH)) is recommended to diagnose non-classical congenital adrenal hyperplasia.

Note: Referral to a specialist is recommended.

Pubertal gynaecomastia
- In true gynaecomastia there will be a palpable disc of breast tissue; this is to be distinguished from adiposity of the breast area.
- Breast development occurs transiently in many boys midway through puberty and is usually physiological.
- If associated with testicular volumes <6 mL, Klinefelter syndrome must be excluded by a chromosomal analysis (boys with Klinefelter syndrome are usually tall (>50th percentile), but this is not universal).
- Adrenal and gonadal tumours can cause gynaecomastia, but this is rare.
- Prolactinoma must be considered, particularly if gynaecomastia is associated with galactorrhoea.
- Many drugs, notably cimetidine, digoxin, spironolactone and i.m. testosterone can induce breast development, as can heavy use of marijuana.
- Prepubertal gynaecomastia also occurs, but in most cases no cause can be found.

Assessment
Most require no investigation, refer if concerned about diagnosis. Baseline FSH, LH, LFTs, prolactin, oestrogen can be helpful.

Management
90% of gynaecomastia disappears spontaneously within 2 years of onset. Refer boys with significant breast enlargement to a plastic or general surgeon for subareolar mastectomy. Tamoxifen is contraindicated in the young male as it inhibits oestrogen action and may delay epiphyseal fusion.

Table 25.6 Endocrine causes of obesity

Cause	Clinical features	Screening investigation
Cushing disease	Growth retardation, hypertension, hirsutism, striae, typical facial changes, bruising	24 h urinary free cortisol
Hypothyroidism	Growth retardation, tiredness, constipation, cold intolerance, dry skin	Thyroid function tests (TSH)
Growth hormone (GH) deficiency	Growth retardation	GH studies
Prader–Willi syndrome	Neonatal hypotonia, growth retardation, developmental delay, hyperphagia, hypogonadism, typical facial appearance, small hands and feet	Specific DNA FISH test

Obesity

See chapter 8, Obesity, and Table 25.6.

Nutritional obesity is associated with growth acceleration and advancement of bone age. Endocrine obesity is associated with growth retardation and a delay in bone age.

Ambiguous genitalia

An underlying endocrine or genetic cause should be sought in:
- Any infant with ambiguous genitalia.
- Boys with perineal hypospadias.
- Boys with any combination of the following: micropenis, hypospadias, short stature, dysmorphic features or undescended testis.
- Girls with inguinal herniae containing gonads.

Note: Clitoral enlargement of any degree is abnormal.

Causes

In decreasing order of frequency:
- Gonadal dysgenesis.
- Congenital adrenal hyperplasia.
- Androgen insensitivity syndrome.
- Testosterone biosynthetic defects.

Investigations

- Electrolytes, urea and blood glucose.
- Serum 17-hydroxyprogesterone and 24 h urine steroid profile.
- Chromosomes.
- Pelvic ultrasound.

Management

- Refer urgently to an experienced paediatric endocrinologist and surgeon.
- Inform the parents about the problem and show them the genitalia; tell them that the infant appears otherwise healthy and that the true sex will be ascertained within a few days. Do not attempt to predict the child's sex.
- Offer emotional support (refer to a social worker or an experienced mental health professional).
- Transfer the baby to a tertiary referral centre without delay.
- Call a meeting of all nursery staff and discuss policy about communication with the parents about the baby. Keep detailed notes about communication with the parents.

Adrenal hypofunction

Primary adrenal insufficiency

This is rare in childhood and adolescence. It should be considered in the presence of vomiting, weight loss, pigmentation, chronic tiredness, low serum sodium and high serum potassium of unknown cause.

X-linked adrenoleukodystrophy

This is the commonest cause of primary adrenal insufficiency in school-age boys.

- Clinical hyperpigmentation of the skin (ACTH-mediated), tiredness, nausea, anorexia and weight loss.
- Adrenal features are usually but not always preceded by the development of a neurological disability (e.g. memory loss, sleep disturbance or ataxia).
- Test blood and skin fibroblasts for very-long-chain fatty acids.
- Dietary modification and bone marrow transplantation may be helpful in cases with normal MRI.

Autoimmune destruction (Addison disease)

- *Autoimmune:* This is usually part of the autoimmune polyglandular syndrome (in combination with either chronic mucocutaneous candidiasis, primary hypoparathyroidism, or both). Presenting in later childhood or adolescence, it may also be associated with thyrotoxicosis, diabetes mellitus, Hashimoto's thyroiditis, coeliac disease, Graves disease, Sjögren syndrome, rheumatoid arthritis and less commonly with T or B cell deficiency.
- *Infective:* Worldwide, the commonest cause of Addison's disease is TB, followed by HIV infection.

Congenital adrenal hyperplasia

- 21-Hydroxylase deficiency.
- Other rare types.
- Signs of androgen excess are usually obvious, with ambiguous genitalia and precocious sexual development.

Investigations
- Serum electrolytes (low sodium and high potassium).
- Simultaneous serum cortisol and plasma ACTH.
- Specific investigations if congenital adrenal hyperplasia (CAH) is suspected; 17-OH progesterone, urine steroid profile.

Management
- Hydrocortisone 12–20 mg/m^2 BSA per day in divided doses.
- Fludrocortisone 0.05–0.2 mg daily, orally.
- Steroid cover for stress (see below).

'Secondary' adrenal insufficiency (due to ACTH deficiency)
Causes
Hypothalamic pituitary failure due to tumour, trauma, post surgery, cranial irradiation (where it may be subtle) or Langerhan's histiocytosis.

Clinical
- Not usually associated with salt-wasting.
- No hyperpigmentation of the skin.
- Treat with hydrocortisone alone; fludrocortisone is unnecessary.

Steroid cover for stress (primary and secondary adrenal insufficiency)
- **All patients with adrenal insufficiency of any cause are at risk for adrenal crisis during periods of severe stress.**
- **All need extra steroid cover.**
- In cases of acute medical illness (e.g. gastroenteritis, influenza), any surgery requiring general anaesthetic and any major fracture:
  - Hydrocortisone 0.2 mg–0.3 mg/kg (usually 25–100 mg) i.m./i.v. stat.
  - Repeat every 4–6 h until recovery.
  - Follow by triple the usual daily doses of hydrocortisone for 2 days, then double for 3 days.

Adrenal hyperfunction
Adrenocortical tumours
- This may manifest as Cushing syndrome, virilisation, hypertension, abdominal mass or pain.
- These tumours are very rare.

Adrenocortical hyperplasia
- This is usually secondary to a pituitary adenoma secreting ACTH (Cushing disease).
- The primary micronodular form (genetic cause) is rarely seen.

Cortisol excess is more difficult to detect clinically in children than in adults. It is characterised by poor growth velocity and excessive weight gain. The child usually looks obese but the clinical features of moon face, thin limbs and striae may be absent.

Investigation
- 24 h urinary free cortisol. Plasma cortisol is often abnormal in obesity and may give a spurious result.
- Overnight dexamethasone suppression (1 mg dexamethasone given at 2400 h and a plasma cortisol at 0800 h the following day) will differentiate Cushing syndrome from obesity.

Further investigation for origin and type of cortisol excess is by a specialist. Treatment is surgical.

Adrenal medullary tumours
- Neuroblastoma usually occurs in very young children, but may present in adolescence.
- Phaeochromocytoma in older children (leading to hypertension).

Note: Phaeochromocytoma may be associated with various genetic conditions – MEN, neurofibromatosis, von Hippel Lindau, SDH mutations.

Disorders of calcium metabolism
Hypocalcaemia
For causes, see Table 25.7.

Clinical features
- Rachitic changes in long bones (swollen wrists, etc.), rachitic rosary.
- Tetany (may be demonstrated using sphygmomanometer cuff above systolic pressure for up to 2 min).
- Laryngeal stridor.
- Fitting.
- Weakness, tiredness, irritability.
- Even extreme hypocalcaemia may be asymptomatic in an infant.

Investigations
- 25-OH vitamin D.
- Renal function, lipase, albumin.
- Magnesium, phosphate.
- Alkaline phosphatase.
- Parathyroid hormone (PTH).
- Total and ionised calcium.
- 1,25-diOH-vitamin D if hypophosphataemic rickets is suspected.
- Radiographs of wrist, knee (metaphyseal splaying).
- Malabsorption studies.
- ECG (prolonged QT interval).

Treatment
Emergency
- I.v. calcium chloride 10% (infusion 1 mmol/kg per 24 h in 5% dextrose), monitor calcium levels 6 hourly.
- Occasionally i.v. calcium chloride 10%, 0.2 mL/kg stat may be required for severe tetany.

Table 25.7 Causes of hypocalcaemia

Neonatal presentation	Infant/childhood presentation
Prematurity/IUGR/ birth asphyxia Hypoparathyroidism ± Di George syndrome Phosphate load (high phosphate milk) Low magnesium Maternal gestational diabetes	Vitamin D deficiency. Groups at risk: • Families where covering clothing is worn at all times, especially breast-fed infants in such families • dark skin colour • Indoor lifestyle • Anticonvulsants (alter vitamin D metabolism/calcium absorption) • Chronic immobilisation • Malabsorption, liver disease
	Hypoparathyroidism • Association with autoimmune polyglandular syndrome. Look for mucocutaneous candidiasis and/or Addison disease in a young child
	Pseudohypoparathyroidism • Albright hereditary osteodystrophy
	Chronic renal failure Pancreatitis Organic acidaemia Critical illness 1-α-hydroxylase deficiency (rare) Vitamin D resistant rickets

- Correct magnesium if low.
- ECG monitor.
- 25-OH-vitamin D if nutritional rickets is suspected: 4000 IU/day for 2 weeks then maintenance (see below).
- 1,25-diOH-vitamin D if parathyroid disorders suspected: 0.01–0.02 mcg/kg per day starting dose may need to be increased.
- Treatment of underlying condition.

Note: In the first days to weeks after treatment is begun for rickets, bones are 'hungry' – large doses of calcium supplement may be required to maintain normocalcaemia and prevent carpopedal spasm once vitamin D is started.

Maintenance
- Adequate calcium intake, preferably as dairy products, 600–1500 mg/day depending on age.
- 500 IU/day 25-OH-vitamin D for months–years depending on cause (for infant rickets, usually treat to age 4).

- Stoss therapy is alternative method, using 100 000–150 000 units 25-OH-vitamin D every 3–6 months as required. Monitoring is required.
- 1,25-diOH-vitamin D (Rocaltrol) for vitamin D resistant rickets, hypoparathyroidism, patients on anticonvulsants.
- 1,25-diOH-vitamin D and phosphate for hypophosphataemic rickets (high dose).

Hypercalcaemia
For causes, see Table 25.8.

Clinical features
- Polyuria, polydipsia.
- Vomiting, dehydration.
- Failure to thrive.
- Abdominal pain (constipation, renal stones, pancreatitis).
- Confusion, apathy (if severe).

Investigation
- Total and ionised calcium, phosphate.
- Magnesium, albumin.
- Alkaline phosphatase.
- 25-OH-vitamin D ± 1,25-diOH-vitamin D.
- Thyroid function.
- Chest radiograph ± skeletal survey.
- Parathyroid imaging.
- Renal ultrasound (nephrocalcinosis).
- ECG (short QT interval).

Table 25.8 Causes of hypercalcaemia

Neonatal	Infant/childhood
Hyperparathyroidism (rare) Iatrogenic	Primary hyperparathyroidism
	Familial hypocalciuric hypercalcaemia
Subcutaneous fat necrosis	Vitamin D 1,25-diOH-D excess (nutritional, inflammatory disease e.g. sarcoidosis, leukaemia)
Familial hypocalciuric hypercalcaemia – severe form	Neoplasia (lytic bone lesions or humoral hypercalcaemia PTHrP)
Hypophosphatasia	Immobilisation e.g. burns (severe), quadriplegia – can be very severe and cause renal calculi, pancreatitis
Bartter syndrome	Drugs (lithium, thiazides)
William syndrome (with elfin face, supravalvular aortic stenosis)	Endocrine disorders: Hyperthyroidism (mild, usually asymptomatic), phaeochromocytoma, adrenal insufficiency

Management of severe hypercalcaemia

- Rehydration with 0.9% saline/5% dextrose. For infants <2 years use 0.45% saline/5% dextrose.
- Diuretics (thiazide) are used in two situations:
  - Acute hypercalcaemia: frusemide is given to reduce fluid overload while the patient is aggressively rehydrated.
  - Chronic hypercalcaemia with hypercalciuria (or normocalcaemia with hypercalciuria): thiazides are given to reduce oedema and prevent nephrocalcinosis (by decreasing urinary calcium excretion).
- Bisphosphonates, particularly for increased bone resorption (e.g. immobilisation).
- Steroids for vitamin D excess (prednisolone 2 mg/kg per day, reducing).
- Low-calcium diet.
- Surgery if indicated, treatment of underlying condition.

USEFUL RESOURCES
- *www.apeg.org.au* – Australian Paediatric Endocrine Group includes downloadable booklets for patients.
- *www.rch.org.au/chas/pubs* – Complete Androgen Insensitivity Syndrome by Garry Warne.
- *www.magicfoundation.org* – Major Aspects of Growth in Children, a USA-based organisation supporting families and children with conditions affecting growth.

CHAPTER 26

Eye conditions

James Elder
Peter Barnett

Important principles

- Eye examination:
  - Always test and record vision as the first part of any eye examination.
  - In infants, observe following and other visual behaviour and listen to the parents' impressions of their child's vision.
- Instilling eye drops:
  - Do not use local steroid drops unless corneal ulceration has been excluded by fluorescein staining. Only use steroids for short periods (2 days or less), unless an ophthalmologist directs otherwise.
  - Instilling eye drops/ointment in a young child: carer sits on the floor with legs extended; lay child between carer's legs with child's arms under the carer's thighs and the child's feet near the carer's feet. This leaves the child's head secured and the carer with both hands free to hold open the child's eyelids and instil eye medication.
- Padding eyes:
  - Never pad a discharging eye.
  - Pad an eye or keep the child indoors if local anaesthetic has been instilled, until the effect of the local anaesthetic has worn off (10–20 min).
- Referral to an ophthalmologist:
  - Transient malalignment of the eyes is common up to 6 months of age. However, a child with a transient squint after 6 months or a constant squint at any age should be referred promptly to an ophthalmologist. True squints rarely improve spontaneously.
  - All children with a white red-reflex or white masses in the retina must be referred immediately to an ophthalmologist to exclude retinoblastoma.
  - In cases of photophobia or watery eyes with no significant discharge in the first year of life, consider congenital glaucoma.

Trauma

Trauma to the eye can take many forms. Physical trauma to the eye and surrounding structures may be blunt or sharp. Trauma can also result from radiation (thermal and electromagnetic) and chemical agents.

Paediatric Handbook, 8th edition. By Kate Thomson, Dean Tey and Michael Marks. Published 2009 by Blackwell Publishing, ISBN: 978-1-4051-7400-8.

Foreign bodies

Foreign bodies on the surface present with a painful, watery eye. If a foreign body or corneal ulcer is suspected, instil 1 drop of local anaesthetic to ease the pain and facilitate examination. Suitable local anaesthetics are proxymetacaine 0.5%, amethocaine 0.5 or 1%, or benoxinate 0.4%. **Do not use local anaesthetics for the continuing treatment of ocular pain under any circumstance**.

Conjunctival foreign bodies are common and often found on the posterior surface of the upper lid. Therefore, eversion of the lid is essential. Most foreign bodies are easily removed with a moist cotton wool swab. If they are embedded and/or difficult to remove, refer the child to an ophthalmologist. Beware of an iris naevus (small pigmented lesion on the iris that can be mistaken for a corneal foreign body) or iris prolapse through a perforating injury of the cornea mimicking a corneal foreign body.

Intraocular foreign bodies are generally the result of high-velocity fragments. Suspect them if the history involves an explosion, metal(s) striking on metal, or any other situation that involves high-speed objects (e.g. power tools or a lawn mower). If the history is at all suggestive, even in the absence of local signs, radiography of the orbit (AP and lateral) is necessary. If an intraocular foreign body is demonstrated or suspected, immediate referral to an ophthalmologist is mandatory.

Eyelid injuries

All eyelid lacerations except the most minor should be repaired under general anaesthesia. Refer to an ophthalmologist if lacerations involve the lid margin or the medial aspect of the eyelids (canalicular injury is likely).

Hyphaema (blood in the anterior chamber)

This is the result of blunt trauma to the eye and all cases require referral to an ophthalmologist. The potential complications include other eye injuries, secondary haemorrhage and vision loss. Minor hyphaemas can be managed as an outpatient. More significant hyphaemas require admission and bed rest.

Fracture of the orbital bones

A blowout fracture through the wall of the orbit is suspected if ≥1 of the following three cardinal signs are present:
- Restricted movement of the eye, particularly in a vertical plane, with double vision.
- Infra-orbital nerve anaesthesia.
- Enophthalmos – this may be difficult to assess initially because of eyelid haematoma.

Diagnosis is usually clinical. Refer to an ophthalmologist before organising a CT scan. A CT scan is used to demonstrate the fracture of the orbital wall and entrapped orbital tissue (the classic sign is a tear-drop 'polyp' hanging from the roof of the maxillary antrum).

Penetrating injury (including intraocular foreign body)

This should always be considered in patients with lacerations involving the eyelids, particularly after motor vehicle accidents. Clinical clues include distortion of the pupil, prolapse of the iris through the cornea, or presence of pigmented tissue over the sclera. If suspected, protect the eye with a cone or shield that does not place pressure on the eyelids or eye and admit. Prevent vomiting with an antiemetic, as this may cause extrusion of eye contents. Refer to an ophthalmologist immediately.

Chemical burns
Irrigate the eye with saline or water copiously for 15 min using an i.v. giving set under local anaesthesia. Continue this until the fluid is neutral on pH testing. Refer all chemical burns to an ophthalmologist.

Thermal burns
The ocular surface is rarely involved. Check for ulceration with fluorescein staining. Butesin picrate ointment is suitable for use on lid burns. Secondary lid swelling may result in corneal exposure and should be treated with ocular lubricants.

Non-accidental injury
The presence of retinal haemorrhages in cases of unexplained head injury raises the possibility of non-accidental injury. Appropriate investigation of the circumstances of the injury should be initiated. The retinal haemorrhages must be assessed by an ophthalmologist (refer to chapter 17, Child abuse)

Acute red eye
Common causes of the acute red eye are conjunctivitis, corneal ulceration, corneal or conjunctival foreign bodies (see above). Less common causes are preseptal and orbital cellulitis. Table 26.1 gives a brief outline of the presenting features of red, sticky and watery eyes, which have a large number of causes and whose clinical presentations may overlap.

Conjunctivitis
Aetiology
- Bacterial: generally pus is present.
- Viral: generally there is watery discharge.
- Allergic: history of atopy and 'itchy eyes'.

Neonatal conjunctivitis (ophthalmia neonatorum)
Neisseria gonorrhoeae
- *Clinical.* Presents within a few days of birth with acute, severe, purulent discharge associated with marked conjunctival and lid oedema ('pus under pressure').
- *Diagnosis.* Urgent Gram stain for Gram-negative intracellular diplococci and direct culture to appropriate culture media.
- *Treatment.* **This is an ocular emergency because of the risk of corneal perforation.** Admit and give i.v. cefotaxime 50 mg/kg 8 hourly for 7 days (dose may need adjustment according to age and birthweight). Penicillin (same duration) is an alternative if the

Table 26.1 The causes of red, watery and sticky eyes

Problem	Pain	Itch	Epiphora	Discharge	Erythema	Photophobia	Reduced Eye Movements	Other
Neonatal conjunctivitis (ophthalmia neonatorum)	+++		++	+++	++ to +++			
Congenital nasolacrimal duct obstruction			+ to ++	+ to +++				
Infantile glaucoma	++		++		–	++		Enlarged & cloudy cornea
Viral conjunctivitis	++		++	+	+ to ++			
Bacterial conjunctivitis	++ to +++		++	+++	++ to +++			
Allergic conjunctivitis		++ to +++	++ to +++	Stringy	+			
Chemical conjunctivitis	+++		+++	+	++ to +++			
Corneal abrasion	+++		++		Variable			
Foreign body	+++		++		Variable			Variable fluorescein staining
Preseptal cellulitis	++		+	Variable	+++ Swelling of eyelids			Conjunctiva not inflamed
Septal cellulitis	+++		–	Variable	+++ Swelling of eyelids		+ to +++	Eye is often inflamed and proptosed

organism is known to be susceptible. In all cases local measures such as ocular lavage and topical antibiotics (chloramphenicol) may be helpful.
- Investigate and treat the mother and partner.

Chlamydia
- Usually occurs at 10–14 days of age. Fails to respond to routine topical antibiotics. If left untreated, there is a risk of pneumonitis.
- *Diagnosis.* Giemsa stain of conjunctival scraping for intranuclear inclusions. Also antibodies in tears and immunofluorescent stains of conjunctival scrapes. Use a *Chlamydia* kit, ensuring conjunctival cells are collected.
- *Treatment.* Erythromycin 10 mg/kg oral 8 hourly for 21 days and eye toilet.
- Investigate and treat the mother and partner.

Other bacteria
- Other causes of conjunctivitis are *Staphylococcus*, *Streptococcus* or diphtheroids. Culture and treat with chloramphenicol eye drops/ointment. A rapid clinical response is anticipated.
- Occasionally *Neisseria meningitidis* can cause conjunctivitis and should be treated as for invasive infection (see chapter 30, Infectious diseases).

Blocked nasolacrimal duct
Presents with mucopurulent discharge with a watery eye. On waking the discharge is worse and conjunctiva is not inflamed (see Watering eyes, p. 332).

Conjunctivitis in older children
Bacterial
- *Severe:* Chloramphenicol eye drops: 2 hourly by day and ointment at night.
- *Less severe:* Chloramphenicol eye drops or ointment three times a day.

Viral
- This condition usually clears spontaneously.
- If it is unclear whether the infection is viral or bacterial, chloramphenicol eye drops may be given.

Herpes simplex conjunctivitis
- Suspect if the child has eyelid vesicles.
- Check for corneal ulceration and treat with 4 hourly aciclovir ointment if ulceration is present.
- Refer to an ophthalmologist.

Allergic
- In mild cases use an astringent (phenylephrine 0.12% or naphazoline 0.1%).
- In moderate cases use a topical antihistamine (antazoline 0.5%).
- In severe cases refer to an ophthalmologist. Topical steroid or sodium cromoglicate should only be given under the supervision of an ophthalmologist.

Corneal ulceration

Ulceration causes pain, photophobia, lacrimation and blepharospasm. It is diagnosed by eye examination – fluorescein stain after the instillation of a local anaesthetic.

For causes and management, see Table 26.2.

Periorbital and orbital cellulitis

Both periorbital and orbital cellulitis present with erythematous, swollen lids in a febrile child. Orbital cellulitis is differentiated by the presence of proptosis and ophthalmoplegia. Hence the lids **must** be separated (a Desmarres lid retractor may be used) to enable a thorough examination.

Periorbital (preseptal) cellulitis

Periorbital (preseptal) cellulitis refers to infection in the soft tissues of the eyelids. This may arise from purulent conjunctivitis, dacryocystitis, or gain entry via local trauma or insect bite.

- Distinguish this from a *periorbital allergic reaction*. A well child, who has eyelid swelling with minimal or no erythema, fever, tenderness nor local warmth, is quite likely to have an allergic reaction to an allergen that has been blown or rubbed into the eye, or secondary to an insect bite. In this case no specific radiological imaging is required. An oral antihistamine may be used. The child should be reviewed if the swelling does not settle in the next 24 h or if signs of inflammation develop (fever, pain or unwell child).

Recommended antibiotics

In children who are systemically unwell, use both cefotaxime and flucloxacillin initially (Table 26.3). Any child in whom there is a reasonable suspicion of primary skin infection, or who is not improving on flucloxacillin alone should have cefotaxime added. Failure to respond in 24–48 h may indicate orbital cellulitis or underlying sinus disease – treat as for orbital cellulitis.

Orbital (septal) cellulitis

Orbital (septal) cellulitis occurs when infection is present around and behind the globe of the eye, and is usually due to spread from sinus infection (especially the ethmoid sinuses). It usually

Table 26.2 Causes and management of corneal ulceration

Cause	Management
Trauma (with or without a foreign body)	Chloramphenicol ointment (1%) and pad if possible Review in 24 h. If not healed in 48 h, refer to an ophthalmologist When ulcer has healed, continue chloramphenicol ointment twice daily for 1 week
Herpes simplex (dendritic ulcer)	Aciclovir eye ointment (1 cm inside the lower conjunctival sac) 5 times a day for 14 days and refer to an ophthalmologist

Table 26.3 Recommended antibiotics in periorbital cellulitides

Mild	Amoxicillin/clavulanate (400/57 mg per 5 mL) 12.5–22.5 mg/kg per dose p.o. 12 hourly
Moderate	Flucloxacillin 50 mg/kg (2 g) i.v. 6 hourly
Severe **OR** under 5 years of age and non-Hib immunised (treat as for orbital cellulitis)	Flucloxacillin 50 mg/kg (2 g) i.v. 6 hourly and cefotaxime 50 mg/kg (2 g) i.v. 6 hourly

occurs in children >2 years. **Orbital cellulitis is a medical emergency and should be treated with the same level of urgency as meningitis or a brain abscess**. The potential for loss of vision and suppurative intracranial complications is significant.

Orbital cellulitis is differentiated from periorbital cellulitis by the presence of:

- Chemosis.
- Proptosis.
- Ophthalmoplegia.
- Systemic symptoms.

If the features of orbital cellulitis are present, a CT scan is required to determine if the sinusitis is complicated by abscess formation. This is most commonly a subperiosteal abscess on the medial wall of the orbit adjacent to the ethmoid sinus, which requires surgical drainage (usually by an external ethmoidectomy approach). If no abscess is present, treatment is by i.v. antibiotics alone; however, CT scanning may need to be repeated if there is clinical deterioration, or if there is lack of improvement with medical treatment.

Recommended antibiotics

Flucloxacillin 50 mg/kg (max. 2 g) 4–6 hourly and cefotaxime 50 mg/kg (max. 2 g) 6 hourly. See also Antimicrobial guidelines.

AND Urgent ENT and ophthalmology consultation are required in suspected orbital cellulitis.

Watering eyes

Watery eyes are common in children and are the result of either poor tear drainage or overproduction. The latter is usually the result of eye irritation and causes include foreign bodies (see p. 327), corneal ulcer (see p. 331), conjunctivitis (see p. 328) and infantile glaucoma (see p. 334).

Nasolacrimal duct obstruction is the most common cause of watery eyes and discharge that persist after the first 2 weeks of life. The discharge is worse on waking and the conjunctiva is not inflamed. It usually resolves spontaneously, due to an opening of the lower end of the nasolacrimal duct. Local eye cleaning is usually the only treatment indicated. If the eye is red and inflamed, topical framycetin sulfate eye drops may be given (avoid repeated courses of chloramphenicol). If the discharge and watering have not settled by 12 months of age, refer to an ophthalmologist for probing.

Strabismus or squint (turned eye)

Refer all children with squint or suspected squint to an ophthalmologist. This will allow early detection (and possibly prevention) of amblyopia and detection of any underlying pathology such as retinoblastoma or cataract. Examine the red reflex of all children suspected to have a squint; if the reflex is abnormal (very dull or white) urgent referral to an ophthalmologist is required to exclude cataract or retinoblastoma.

A child does not 'grow out of' a squint. However, in the first few months of life, babies may have an intermittent squint, especially when feeding. A child of any age with a constant large-angle squint or a child over 6 months with any squint (constant or intermittent) should be referred to an ophthalmologist. All children with a first-degree relative with a squint should be seen by an ophthalmologist at about 3–3.5 years of age, even if there is no squint, as they may have a refractive error alone.

A pseudo-strabismus (pseudo-squint) is due to a broad nasal bridge or epicanthic folds, or both. This results in the appearance of a squint, but corneal light reflexes are central and there is no movement on cover testing (see Figs 26.1 and 26.2). Only make the diagnosis of pseudo-strabismus if absolutely certain. Refer doubtful cases to an ophthalmologist.

Eyelid lumps and ptosis

- *Styes* are acute bacterial infections of an eyelash follicle. They occur at the eyelid margin and are red and tender. Removing the lash directly related to the stye will often result in discharge of pus and hasten its resolution. Local antibiotics are sometimes indicated. Systemic antibiotics are rarely needed.
- A *chalazion* is an obstructed tarsal (or meibomian) gland. These glands are situated within the substance of the eyelid and thus a chalazion will present as a lump within the eyelid. There may be no associated symptoms. Redness associated with a chalazion is

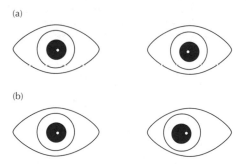

(a)

(b)

Fig. 26.1 Corneal light reflex. Shine a light at the child's eyes and observe the reflection. (a) Eyes are straight and the corneal light reflex is symmetrical. (*Note*: It is displaced slightly to the nasal side of the centre in each eye.) (b) Left convergent strabismus. The reflection from the deviated eye is displaced laterally

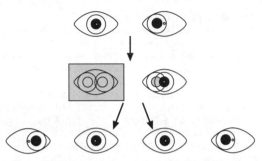

Fig. 26.2 The cover test. The child's attention is attracted with a toy. The eye that appears not to be deviating is covered. The uncovered eye is then observed for movement. If there is a convergent squint, the eye will move outwards (top and middle). The uncovered eye should also be observed when the cover is removed from the fellow eye. In an alternating squint there will be no movement of the uncovered eye and the previously covered eye will now be deviated (bottom left). In non-alternating or constant squint (vision is usually reduced in the deviating eye), there will be a rapid return to the original situation (bottom right). If no movement is detected, the test should be repeated but cover the other eye first

usually the result of sterile inflammation due to leakage of the contents, rather than a bacterial infection. Thus local or systemic antibiotics seldom influence the natural history of these lesions. Warm compresses may hasten resolution. If the chalazion is persistent (>6 months), large or causes discomfort, incision and drainage under general anaesthesia may be indicated.

- *Ptosis* is a droopy or lowered upper eyelid. In children it is usually the result of a minor and isolated anomaly in the development of the levator muscle. It may be unilateral or bilateral, and is sometimes inherited in a dominant manner. If the lowered eyelid obstructs the pupil in a young child, visual loss will occur secondary to amblyopia. Urgent referral to an ophthalmologist is appropriate in such cases. In more minor degrees of ptosis, surgical intervention is for cosmesis and is less urgent.

Rare but important eye conditions
Iritis
Acute iritis is very rare in children and presents with an acute red eye similar to the symptoms for a corneal ulcer. The pupil is small and does not react well to light. Refer to an ophthalmologist. Consider iritis in children with juvenile chronic arthritis (JCA). This form of iritis is chronic and painless.

Infantile glaucoma
The presenting features are:
- A hazy cornea.
- An enlarged cornea.

- Watery eyes.
- Photophobia.

This is a rare condition, but early recognition is vital. Prompt surgery offers a chance of cure and preservation of vision. All infants with suspected glaucoma require urgent referral to an ophthalmologist for examination under anaesthesia to measure corneal diameter, optic disc cupping and intraocular pressure.

Congenital cataracts

Congenital cataracts are rare, but early detection and removal with subsequent optical correction (contact lenses or spectacles) offers a good chance of visual preservation. All newborn infants should have their red reflexes examined before discharge from hospital. Check the red reflexes and fundi in any infant with poor visual performance (fixation and following). Nystagmus is a late sign of congenital cataracts. A unilateral cataract will often present as a squint. Any child suspected of having a congenital cataract must be referred urgently.

Retinoblastoma

This is a rare childhood cancer of the retina and presents with squint, a white pupil (cat's eye reflex), poor vision or a family history of the tumour. Prompt recognition is vital to maximise the possibility of preserving vision. Untreated this is a fatal disorder. If suspected refer urgently to an ophthalmologist.

USEFUL RESOURCES
- *cim.ucdavis.edu/eyes/version1/eyesim.htm* – A brilliant simulation program addressing eye movements and associated defects in muscles or cranial nerves.
- *www.aapos.org/* – American Association for Pediatric Ophthalmology and Strabismus™. Covers information on most major topics in paediatric ophthalmology.
- *www.eyesite.ca/7modules/index_e.html* – Self-directed learning modules in ophthalmology with excellent slides, from the Canadian Ophthalmological Society.

CHAPTER 27

Gastrointestinal conditions

George Alex
Lionel Lubitz

Acute infectious gastroenteritis

The most common cause is rotavirus infection, with the seasonal peak period during autumn and winter in Australia. It is responsible for 40–50% of cases requiring hospital admission, while adenovirus infection causes between 7–17% of cases. Bacterial gastroenteritis is less common, causing 5–10% of all cases; causes include *Salmonella* spp., *Campylobacter jejuni*, *Yersinia enterocolitica* and *Escherichia coli*. Parasites, such as *Cryptosporidium*, are also a known cause of acute gastroenteritis.

The two most important issues in the management of acute infectious diarrhoea are:
- Exclusion of other important causes of vomiting and diarrhoea.
- Adequate assessment and treatment of dehydration.

Differential diagnoses of vomiting and diarrhoea
- Appendicitis.
- Urinary tract infection.
- Other sepsis (including meningitis).
- Other surgical conditions including intussusception, enterocolitis associated with Hirschsprung disease and malrotation of the bowel.
- Haemolytic uraemic syndrome.

Clinical features

Presenting symptoms include poor feeding, vomiting and fever, followed by diarrhoea. Stools are frequent and watery in consistency. Bacterial gastroenteritis is suggested by a history of frequent small-volume stools with passage of blood and mucus, and abdominal pain. Be wary of diagnosing gastroenteritis in the child with vomiting alone who is dehydrated or unwell.

It is essential that all children with acute onset of vomiting, diarrhoea and fever are **re-evaluated regularly** so as to confirm the diagnosis of acute gastroenteritis and adequacy of rehydration therapy.

Paediatric Handbook, 8th edition. By Kate Thomson, Dean Tey and Michael Marks. Published 2009 by Blackwell Publishing, ISBN: 978-1-4051-7400-8.

Assessment of dehydration (see Table 27.1)

- Risk of dehydration is increased with younger age, as infants (<6 months) have an increased surface area:body volume ratio resulting in increased insensible fluid losses.
- Recent change in body weight provides the most accurate indication of fluid depletion. Starvation produces no more than 1% body weight loss per day.
- Decreased skin turgor and peripheral perfusion accompanied by deep (acidotic) breathing are the only signs proven to discriminate between dehydration and hydration.
- Actual degree of dehydration may be underestimated with obesity and overestimated with wasting or sepsis.

> <5% body weight loss represents no or mild dehydration
> 5–9% body weight loss represents moderate dehydration
> >9% body weight loss represents severe dehydration.
> *Note*: These percentages are approximate and given only as a guide.

Table 27.1 Guidelines to assessment and management of dehydration

Assessment of dehydration	Management
Mild: ≤5% body weight loss dry mucous membrane* thirsty, alert and restless	Rehydrate over 6 h with ORS/water ORS only is preferred in high-risk patients (infants <6 months)
Moderate: 5–9% body weight loss all of the above signs (mild group) PLUS rapid pulse decreased peripheral perfusion* sunken eyes and fontanelle deep acidotic breathing* pinched skin retracts slowly (1–2 s)*	May require rehydration via the nasogastric route Re-assessment (including body weight and clinical examination) is required at 6 h If fluid replete, maintenance age-appropriate fluids can then be used Weigh inpatients every 6 h during the first 24 h of admission Introduce food intake after rehydration, if dehydration has been corrected
Severe: >9% body weight loss all of above signs (mild–moderate groups) PLUS *in infants* – drowsy, limp, cold, sweaty, cyanotic limbs and altered conscious level *in children* – apprehension, cold, sweaty, cyanotic limbs, rapid feeble pulse and low blood pressure	If shock is present, give normal saline 20 mL/kg i.v. (repeated fluid boluses may be required until organ perfusion is restored) Can start ORS once initial resuscitation is completed – give over 6 h Following rehydration, the same general principles as those for mild–moderate group apply

* These are the only signs proven to discriminate between hydration and dehydration (4% or greater).

Guidelines to management of acute gastroenteritis
Hydration
- For children/infants with dehydration, rapid enteral rehydration over 4–6 h is now suggested (see Table 27.1). Past regimens aimed at gradual rehydration over 24 h were not evidence based. The exceptions are children with significant neurological or biochemical disturbance (see sections on hyper- and hyponatraemic dehydration below).
- Most children/infants with dehydration can be safely and adequately rehydrated using oral rehydration solutions (ORS) (Table 27.2). If these are not tolerated by the oral route, nasogastric administration is an alternative. Vomiting is not a contraindication to a nasogastric tube.
- Oral rehydration solutions use the principle of glucose-facilitated sodium transport in the small intestine. The solutions currently used in Australia are outlined in Table 27.3.
- Parent education is vital, especially in the outpatient management of children. The important message is the need to drink more fluid more often, which is best given in small volumes and frequently (see Table 27.4). It should be emphasised that home-made solutions and ORS should be carefully prepared according to instructions provided, as they can be potentially dangerous if made up incorrectly.

Nutritional management
Early re-feeding (after rehydration) has been shown to enhance mucosal recovery in children/infants with acute gastroenteritis and reduces the duration of diarrhoea.
- Breast-feeding should continue through rehydration and maintenance phases of treatment.
- Formula-fed infants and children should re-start oral age appropriate formula or food intake after completion of rehydration.
- Children can have complex carbohydrates (e.g. rice, wheat, bread and cereals), yoghurt, fruit and vegetables once rehydration is complete.

Transient lactase deficiency with acute gastroenteritis may occur but is not common in infants <6 months. Lactose-free diets are infrequently required after acute gastroenteritis. If there is persistent diarrhoea after re-introduction of feeds, evidence for lactose intolerance should be sought (stool pH <5 and ≥0.75% reducing substances). A lactose-free formula can be used if the patient is lactose intolerant.

Admission to hospital
- Infants/children who have moderate or severe dehydration.
- Patients at high risk of dehydration on the basis of young age (<6 months) with a high frequency of diarrhoea (8 per 24 h) and vomiting (>4 per 24 h) should be observed for 4–6 h to ensure adequate maintenance of hydration.
- High-risk infants/children (e.g. ileostomy, short gut, cyanotic heart disease, chronic renal disease, metabolic disorders and malnutrition).
- Infants/children whose parents and carers are thought to be unable to manage the child's condition at home.
- If the diagnosis is in doubt.

Table 27.2 Recommended hourly oral or nasogastric rehydration rate for children

Weight (kg)	Maintenance (per h)	Moderate dehydration (4–6%) (mL/h)		Severe dehydration (≥7%) (mL/h)	
		1st 6 h	Next 18 h	1st 6 h	Next 18 h
5	20	45	35	70	35
10	35	85	55	135	55
15	50	125	70	200	70
20	60	140	80	220	80
30	70	190	95	300	95
40	80	250	110	400	110
50	90	300	120	500	120

The daily fluid requirement is relatively high in neonates (150 mL/kg per day), reducing to 100 mL/kg per day in older infants and 80 mL/kg per day between 1 and 5 years.

Table 27.3 Oral rehydration preparations available for use in Australia (concentrations are expressed as mmol/L of made-up solution)

	Na	K	Cl	Citrate	Glucose
Gastrolyte	60	20	60	10	90
Repalyte	60	20	60	10	90
Hydralyte	45	20	35	30	80

Table 27.4 Suitable fluids for non-dehydrated children

Solution	Dilution
Sucrose (table sugar)	1 teaspoon in 200 mL boiled water
Fruit juice	1 in 6 with tap water
Cordials	1 part in 16 parts water
Lemonade	1 part in 6 parts water

Do not use undiluted or low-calorie lemonade or fruit juice.

Biochemical investigations

Glucose, electrolyte and acid–base studies are required in children with:
- A history of prolonged diarrhoea with severe dehydration.
- Altered conscious state.
- Convulsions.
- Short-bowel syndrome, ileostomy, chronic cardiac, renal and metabolic disorders.
- Infants <6 months of age who are judged as being dehydrated.

Pharmacotherapy

- Infants and children should not be treated with antidiarrhoeal agents, as there is no substantial clinical evidence to suggest that this treatment alters symptoms.
- Most bacterial infections do not require antibiotics.
- *Salmonella* or *Campylobacter* gastroenteritis may require antibiotic treatment (see chapter 30, Infectious diseases).
- *Shigella* dysentery requires antibiotic treatment.

Complications

Hypernatraemic dehydration (sodium >150 mmol/L)
- Results from severe water and sodium depletion with greater loss of water. This can lead to severe neurological sequelae if rehydration is not carried out appropriately.
- Oral rehydration therapy is preferred to i.v. rehydration. If the patient is in shock, give a bolus of normal saline 20 mL/kg i.v., repeat until organ perfusion is restored.
- Following this, 'slow ORT' aiming to complete rehydration over 12 h is required, followed by maintenance fluids.
- Serum electrolytes should be monitored on a 4 hourly basis. As a guideline, **serum sodium should not fall by >0.5 mmol/L per hour.**
- Consultation with an intensive care unit is recommended for these patients.

Hyponatraemic dehydration (serum sodium <130 mmol/L)
- Can cause seizures and coma, and requires consultation with an intensive care unit.
- Be aware of iatrogenic hyponatraemia due to fluid (hypotonic) overload.

Sugar intolerance
Lactose intolerance

Following infectious diarrhoea, infants may have temporary lactose intolerance. This sequela of acute gastroenteritis used to be prominent in infants <6 months of age, but it is now uncommon. This may be due in part to early oral feeding which aids mucosal recovery. Clinical features of sugar intolerance include:
- Persistently fluid stool.
- Excessive flatus.
- Excoriation of the buttocks.
- Typically, these infants appear well.

Diagnosis

Collect the fluid stool in napkins lined with plastic. Dilute 5 drops of stool with 10 drops of water. Add a Clinitest tablet. A colour reaction corresponding to ≥0.75% or more reducing substance indicates that sugar intolerance is present.

Management

- Breast-feeding should continue unless there are persistent symptoms with buttock excoriation and failure to gain adequate weight.
- Formula-fed infants should be placed on a lactose-free formula for 3–4 weeks.

Note: A clinical response after change to soy formula may indicate either post-infectious lactose intolerance or allergy to cow's milk protein, as soy formulae available in Australia are lactose-free.

Monosaccharide intolerance

Infrequently, infants with severe bowel damage secondary to gastroenteritis may be unable to absorb normal amounts of monosaccharide such as glucose or fructose. Diarrhoea will continue even with a lactose-free formula. Monosaccharide intolerance requires specialist consultation.

Chronic diarrhoea

An increase in stool frequency or fluid content is often of concern to parents, but does not necessarily imply significant organic disease, although this needs to be excluded. In every child who presents with chronic diarrhoea, the decision must be made as to whether further investigation is required. The algorithm in Fig. 27.1 outlines an approach to the child with chronic diarrhoea.

Toddler diarrhoea

This is a clinical syndrome characterised by chronic diarrhoea often with undigested food in the stools of a child who is otherwise well, gaining weight and growing satisfactorily. Stools may contain mucus and are passed 3–6 times a day; they are often looser towards the end of the day.

- Onset is usually between 8 and 20 months of age.
- Often there is a family history of functional bowel disease, such as irritable bowel syndrome.
- The treatment consists of reassurance and explanation. No specific drug or dietary therapy has been shown to be of value in toddler diarrhoea. Some toddlers on a high-fructose intake may have ('apple-juice') diarrhoea that responds to dietary change.

Coeliac disease

Coeliac disease is an autoimmune enteropathy triggered by the ingestion of gluten in genetically susceptible individuals. The prevalence of this disorder amongst first-degree relatives is

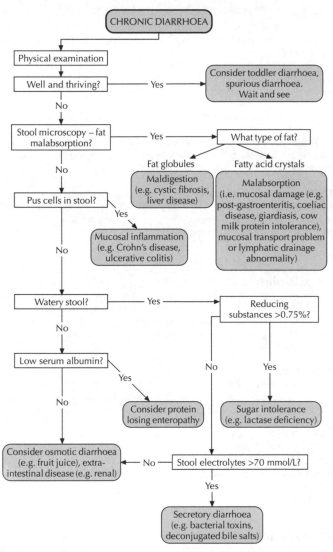

Fig. 27.1 Investigation of chronic diarrhoea

Table 27.5 Presentations of coeliac disease

Classical presentation	First 2 years of life poor weight gain Chronic diarrhoea Anorexia, apathy and abdominal distension
Atypical presentation	Growth retardation/pubertal delay only Amenorrhoea Arthritis Recurrent spontaneous foetal loss Peripheral neuropathy Cerebellar atrophy Hepatitis Recurrent mouth ulcers
Associated disorders	Insulin dependent diabetes mellitus Addison disease Down syndrome Selective IgA deficiency

approximately 10%. The clinical expression of this disorder is more heterogeneous than previously thought (Table 27.5) and onset may be at any time, after years without symptoms.

Serological screening tests
- An IgA antibody to tissue transglutaminase (result of enterocyte damage) which is 98% specific and sensitive, has replaced the anti-endomysial antibody test in many hospitals. False-negative results can occur in IgA-deficient patients, hence all patients will require total IgA levels measured to interpret the results appropriately.
- Previously, three tests were commonly used: antigliadin IgG (high sensitivity) and antigliadin IgA antibodies (high specificity) which can both be falsely positive in other gut conditions including cow's milk protein intolerance, Crohn's disease and post-infectious gastroenteritis; and anti-endomysial antibody test, which is more specific and sensitive than the antigliadin tests. It can be falsely negative if the patient is IgA deficient.

Diagnosis
- Small-bowel biopsy remains the gold standard.
- The need for subsequent biopsies to confirm or refute the diagnosis is dependent upon the clinical response of the patient to a gluten-free diet or if the patient is <2 years of age.

Management
A gluten-free diet excluding wheat, barley, rye and oats.

Non-IgE mediated cow's milk protein allergy
Allergic responses to cow's milk protein may result in a rapid (IgE) or delayed (non-IgE or mixed IgE/non-IgE) onset of symptoms. IgE-mediated allergy is characterised by sudden

onset vomiting, angio-oedema, urticaria and rarely anaphylaxis (cardiovascular–respiratory involvement).

Non-IgE mediated allergy may be more difficult to diagnose and present with diarrhoea, malabsorption or failure to thrive, as well as intermittent intestinal loss of protein or blood in a well child. Non-IgE cow's milk protein allergy predominantly affects young infants; prospective studies suggest a prevalence of 2% in this group (see chapter 19, Allergy and immunology).

- Cow's milk protein intolerance can only be diagnosed with a complete and thorough history, and with unequivocal reproducible reactions to elimination and challenge.
- Blood tests (i.e. RAST) and skin prick testing are generally unhelpful, as the underlying immunological mechanism is usually non-IgE mediated.
- After a definitive diagnosis is established, cow's milk protein should be removed from the diet and replaced with an extensively-hydrolysed (e.g. Alfare™ or Pepti-junior™) or elemental formula (e.g. Neocate™ or Elecare™). A full soy formula is not recommended in young infants with severe enteropathy, as co-existent soy allergy occurs in 15–20% of such patients.
- Most food allergies in infants improve or resolve with increasing age.

Note: Hydrolysed and elemental milk formulas are expensive and should only be prescribed following specialist review.

Rectal bleeding

See Fig. 27.2.

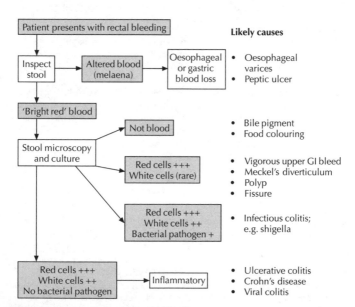

Fig. 27.2 Assessment of lower gastrointestinal blood loss

Inflammatory bowel disease

The incidence of Crohn's disease has increased dramatically in Australian children since the 1970s. In contrast, ulcerative colitis shows an annual fluctuation without an upward trend.

- *Crohn's disease* can present in several ways including recurrent abdominal pain, weight loss, chronic diarrhoea, mouth ulcers and perianal disease. It may also present with isolated growth failure without any gastrointestinal symptoms.
- *Ulcerative colitis* is associated with bloody diarrhoea, which extends beyond the time frame of infective colitis.
- Extra-intestinal manifestations can occur in both disorders and include arthritis, erythema nodosum, hepatitis and ophthalmological complications (uveitis, episcleritis and conjunctivitis).
- Initial laboratory investigations should include a full blood count (anaemia and thrombocytosis), ESR (often raised) and albumin level (low with active disease). Stool cultures for bacterial pathogens and *Clostridium difficile* and toxin should be collected.
- Evaluation and management, including pain management, should occur under specialist guidance.

Gastro-oesophageal reflux

Oesophageal reflux of gastric contents occurs normally and is more frequent after meals. It is regarded as pathological if associated with frequent regurgitation, or if it results in clinically significant adverse sequelae. The number of reflux episodes is normally greater in infants than in older children.

Reflux of gastric acid with heartburn may result in episodic irritability, but this is usually associated with obvious regurgitation and is rarely 'silent'. Although gastro-oesophageal reflux may cause infant distress, it is important to consider other possible causes. Both infant distress and frequent regurgitation are common in the first 6 months of life. Co-existence does not prove cause and effect. Investigations such as 24 h oesophageal pH monitoring can be useful to correlate any episodes of reflux with irritability.

It is important to recognise that vomiting in infants may result from other causes, such as urinary tract infection, metabolic disturbances, bowel obstruction and increased intracranial pressure. These need to be excluded on the basis of history, physical examination and further tests (if clinically indicated).

Complications

- *Peptic oesophagitis:* this is usually correlated with an increase in the number and duration of reflux episodes. Blood-flecked vomitus and anaemia may result.
- *Peptic strictures:* these are well recognised in childhood and present with dysphagia and failure to thrive.
- *Failure to thrive:* severe cases of gastro-oesophageal reflux may cause the loss of calories and anorexia.
- *Pulmonary complications:* recurrent or persistent cough and wheeze may be present and can occur without marked vomiting. These symptoms may result from aspiration of

refluxed material (inhalation pneumonia) or through reflex bronchospasm. This mode of presentation requires a high degree of clinical suspicion to make the diagnosis.

Specialist advice should be sought if complications are present.

Management
Regurgitation of gastric contents is common in infancy. In most cases this 'possetting' does not result in any adverse sequelae and the most appropriate therapy is parental reassurance. 'Physiological' gastro-oesophageal reflux with regurgitation usually resolves by the age of 9–15 months.

Simple measures
In the absence of signs of significant oesophagitis, aspiration or growth failure, the following should be suggested:
- Avoid excessive handling.
- Posture after feeds: the infant should be placed in a cot in the head-up position at or near 30°.
- Thicken feeds: use a proprietary thickening agent or a prethickened formula if formula-fed.

Medication
Note: Medications are not indicated in otherwise healthy, thriving infants with frequent regurgitation.
- Mylanta may offer relief from symptoms of heartburn (0.5–1.0 mL/kg per dose given 3–4 times a day). There are some concerns about its long-term use because of its mineral content.
- H_2 receptor antagonists such as ranitidine (2–3 mg/kg per dose given 2–3 times a day before meals) will reduce gastric acidity. There may be a role for a brief empirical trial of anti-reflux therapy in infants in whom it is thought reflux is the cause of their distressed behaviour. However, these agents are not without risk and should not be prescribed for prolonged periods without evidence to substantiate the severity of reflux.
- Proton pump inhibitors are prescribed to infants and children with severe oesophagitis that is unresponsive to an H_2 receptor antagonist.

Surgery
Fundoplication is indicated for reflux with complications when medical therapy has failed or is inappropriate. This is rarely indicated, but if needed, can now be done laparoscopically.

Recurrent abdominal pain
Recurrent abdominal pain affects about 10% of school-age children. There is usually no specific identifiable cause, though it has been speculated that this condition may be a result of dysmotility of the bowel. Occasionally it can result from a significant emotional problem.

Recent evidence suggests there may be a subgroup with migrainous abdominal pain (associated with pallor and family history). Emotional factors, lifestyle and temperamental characteristics can modulate the child's response to pain, irrespective of its cause.

Assessment

- It is essential to take a careful history, including psychosocial details. It may be helpful to interview the parents alone, the child alone and the family together. Onset of pain after the consumption of dairy products in older children and young adolescents should be sought, as lactase deficiency can present in this manner. Constipation needs to be excluded. 'Red flags' in the evaluation of chronic abdominal pain include pain localised away from the umbilicus, accompanying vomiting, diarrhoea, poor weight gain or linear growth, and pain awakening the patient from sleep.
- A thorough physical examination is essential.
- Urine microscopy and culture is an appropriate baseline investigation.

Management

The two major causes in childhood are constipation and functional pain.

- The treatment of underlying *constipation* is essential and management of non-organic issues may be required.
- *Functional pain* may be related to variation in the perception of visceral sensation in the absence of an identifiable organic cause. A detailed explanation to the child and reassurance is often all that is required.
- The diagnosis of psychogenic recurrent abdominal pain cannot be made simply in the absence of positive findings for an organic disorder. Positive evidence of emotional maladjustment is required separately. If present, referral to a general paediatrician or mental health service is appropriate.

Pancreatitis

Acute pancreatitis has a variable presentation in children (Fig. 26.3) and symptoms may range from mild abdominal pain to severe systemic involvement with accompanying metabolic disturbances and shock.

- The pain is commonly in the epigastrium but may also be in the right and left upper quadrant.
- Back pain is an uncommon feature in children, unlike in adults.
- Diagnosis is based on clinical symptoms and signs, accompanied by a threefold increase above the normal range, in either amylase or lipase. – serum lipase having the greater sensitivity and specificity of the two.
- Other accompanying features may include vomiting, anorexia and nausea.
- Pancreatitis should be considered in children with complex disability, presenting with irritability.
- On examination the child may appear unwell and features of an acute abdomen may be present.

Management

Is primarily supportive and aims at limiting exocrine pancreatic secretion and managing pain. Most mild to moderate cases will settle with bowel rest, i.v. fluids and analgesia for 3–5

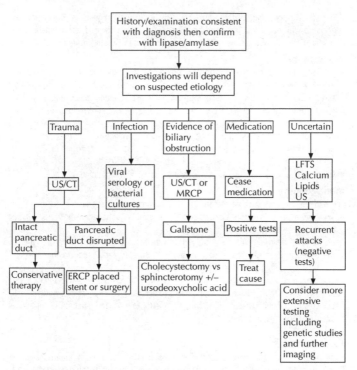

Fig. 27.3 Diagnstic algorithm for acute/recurrent pancreatitis.
CT, computed tomography; ERCP, endoscopic retrograde cholangiopancreatography; LFT, liver function tests; MRCP, magnetic resonance cholangiopancreatography; US, ultrasound. (Reproduced with permission from Nydegger et al. *Journal of Gastroenterology and Hepatology* 21;2006:499–509)

days. In children with recurrent attacks and/or a complicated course, specialist input is recommended.

Liver disease
For causes, see Table 27.6.

Infants
Infants (1–3 months of life) may present with:
- Jaundice (usually conjugated hyperbilirubinaemia). See also page 439.
- Passage of pale grey or white stools and dark tea-coloured urine.
- Hepatosplenomegaly.

Table 27.6 Causes of liver disease in children

Infection:	Viral (hepatitis A, B, C, D; CMV; EBV), bacterial sepsis
Inflammatory:	Autoimmune hepatitis, sclerosing cholangitis
Metabolic:	Galactosaemia, tyrosinaemia, fructose intolerance, Wilson disease, α1 antitrypsin deficiency
Drugs	Particularly paracetamol
Structural	Gallstones, choledochal cyst
Malignancy	Histiocytosis x, leukaemia, lymphoma
Others	Cystic fibrosis

- Failure to thrive.
- Bleeding diathesis.
- Hypoglycaemia.

Biliary atresia is the most common cause of obstructive jaundice in young infants. Infants with this condition will present with jaundice in the first 4–6 weeks of life. They appear well on clinical examination, with conservation of growth. The degree of jaundice may be variable, but onset is usually from birth. They consistently pass acholic (pale white) stool. If untreated, the outcome is fatal. However, the natural history of this condition can be modified by early surgery, which must be done before 70 days of age for success.

Apart from this condition there are several other causes of early-onset liver disease, many of which may have dire consequences if not recognised or treated adequately, including galactosaemia, tyrosinaemia, fructosaemia and other metabolic conditions. Therefore, prompt referral of infants with liver disease to a specialist is essential.

Children
May present acutely with a sudden onset of jaundice, cholestasis (dark urine and pale stools), pruritus, irritability and vomiting. Signs of chronic liver disease should be sought and include poor growth, delayed puberty, dilated abdominal veins and palmar erythema. In general, prompt specialist consultation for acute and chronic liver disorders is required, as both forms of liver disease require urgent investigation and treatment.

USEFUL RESOURCES
- *www.naspghan.org* – The North American Society for Pediatric Gastroenterology, Hepatology and Nutrition. Site includes pdf factsheets for parents, online continuing medical education and publications.
- *www.aafp.org/afp/990401ap/1823.html* – Excellent article from the American Academy of Family Physicians on chronic abdominal pain.

CHAPTER 28
Gynaecological conditions

Sonia Grover

Prepubescent problems
Vaginal discharge
Most newborn girls have some mucoid white vaginal discharge. This is normal and disappears by about 3 months of age.

Vulvovaginitis
This is the most common gynaecologic problem in childhood, usually occurring in girls aged between 2 years and the start of puberty. The vaginal skin in childhood is thin and atrophic. Overgrowth of mixed bowel flora occurs in this environment and the resultant discharge can be an irritant to the vulval area, which is also atrophic. The moist environment between the opposed skin surfaces may also be exacerbated by urine dribbling, particularly in an obese young girl.

Presentation
- Erythema/irritation of the labia and perineal skin.
- Itch and dysuria may also be present.
- ± offensive vaginal discharge.

Management
Investigations are usually not required. If urinary symptoms are present, check the urine to exclude urinary tract infection (UTI).
- Explanation and reassurance.
- Vinegar (1 cup white vinegar in a shallow bath).
- Simple soothing, barrier cream to the labial area (e.g. zinc–castor oil or nappy rash cream).
- Toileting/hygiene advice: avoid potential irritants such as soaps and bubble bath.

Rarely, if the problem persists, further action may be required. The natural history is for recurrences to occur up until the age when oestrogenisation begins.
- If a heavy discharge persists or marked skin inflammation beyond labial contact surfaces is present, take swabs from the perineum in case of an overgrowth of one organism

Paediatric Handbook, 8th edition. By Kate Thomson, Dean Tey and Michael Marks. Published 2009 by Blackwell Publishing, ISBN: 978-1-4051-7400-8.

(e.g. group A *Streptococcus*) and treat it with the appropriate antibiotics (usual culture findings are mixed coliforms).
- Do not take vaginal swabs, as it is painful and distressing. If swabs for culture are required, introital area swabs are adequate.
- If itch/irritation is the main complaint, consider pinworms.
- If eczema occurs elsewhere on the body, this can be superimposed on the irritated skin. Combined treatment of the vulvovaginitis (as above) and hydrocortisone may be indicated.
- Foreign bodies are a potential cause for a persistent, unresolving, often blood-stained discharge. An examination under anaesthesia with vaginoscopy is required to exclude this.
- Although it is rare, consider sexual abuse if other indicators are present.

Thrush is rare in prepubertal girls unless there has been significant antibiotic use. Thrush thrives in an oestrogenised environment, not in the atrophic setting.
Note: Vaginal pessaries should never be prescribed to prepubertal girls.

Vaginal bleeding
Many girls will have some vaginal bleeding in the first week of life, caused by the withdrawal of maternal oestrogens. This is normal. In older girls bloodstained discharge may indicate:
- Vulvovaginitis: associated with atrophic changes (see vulvovaginitis).
- A foreign body: particularly if it is persistent despite management of vulvovaginitis.
- Trauma (including straddle injuries and sexual abuse).
- Excoriation secondary to threadworms or eczema.
- Haematuria.
- Urethral prolapse.

Urogenital tract tumors are rare, and usually a mass is also present at time of presentation.

Labial adhesions
- Labial adhesions are seen in infancy and usually resolve by about 8 years. They may occasionally persist through to puberty but will resolve around the time of menarche.
- The adhesion is not congenital, but acquired from a secondary adherence of the atrophic surfaces of the labia minora, presumably as a result of irritation.
- **Uncomplicated labial adhesions in girls do not need division.** Refer to a specialist if the child has difficulty voiding or recurrent UTIs. Treat vulvovaginitis or nappy rash if present. Parents should be reassured that the labia will separate when oestrogenisation occurs as the child grows. Although it is possible to divide the adhesions with lateral traction this is frequently distressing for the child and the parents and recurrence is common.
- The use of topical oestrogen cream is unnecessary and is associated with significant rates of failure and recurrence.

Menstrual problems
Dysmenorrhoea
Clinical features

- Cramping lower abdominal pain, lower back pain and pain radiating to the anterior aspects of the thighs with menses (symptoms may begin a few days before menstruation).
- Associated symptoms such as nausea, vomiting, change in bowel actions (usually softer bowel actions or diarrhoea, but occasionally constipation), headaches and general lethargy may occur. These symptoms should be looked for as they support the diagnosis of a prostaglandin-induced dysmenorrhoea. Occasionally these symptoms may begin intermittently a few months before menarche.
- Stress will often precipitate more severe episodes of dysmenorrhoea.
- Vaginal examination is not done if the young woman is not sexually active, and even then only with careful consent. Occasionally, vaginal examination in young women who are using tampons may be possible, but alternatives such as a transabdominal pelvic ultrasound examination will usually provide all the required information (e.g. obstructive congenital anomalies and ovarian cysts).

Management

- General measures: assess and manage other adolescent issues (see chapter 15, Adolescent health) and encourage exercise.
- Antiprostaglandins (e.g. mefenamic acid, naproxen, ibuprofen; see Pharmacopoeia) should ideally be commenced before the onset of symptoms. Failure to respond to one type of antiprostaglandin warrants the trial of an alternative type.
- Hormonal treatment can be used to regulate the menstrual cycle if it is too irregular for prophylactic antiprostaglandins. The oral contraceptive pill (OCP) can also be used for dysmenorrhoea. This may be the first line treatment, particularly in a sexually active teenager.
- Non-responsive or worsening dysmenorrhoea will require investigation. Pelvic ultrasound can usually identify an obstructive congenital anomaly and detect significant endometriosis (e.g. an endometrioma).
- Diagnostic laparoscopy may identify mild endometriosis. However, the value of treating this with specific hormonal therapy or operative laser diathermy is unclear from both the short-term and long-term perspective. Therefore, this invasive investigation should be withheld until optimal management with antiprostaglandin therapy or OCP, or both, has been tried, and other adolescent issues explored.

Amenorrhoea
Primary
See chapter 25, Endocrine conditions, Delayed puberty, p. 316.

Secondary
Consider the following diagnoses:
- Pregnancy.
- Weight loss/anorexia nervosa.
- Strenuous exercise.

- Stress (e.g. exams, social/family or travel).
- Polycystic ovaries.

Polycystic ovary syndrome (PCOS)

- Irregular menses with multiple follicles found on pelvic ultrasound **and**
- Signs of excess androgen (severe acne and/or hirsutism).
- Obesity is a common association.

Care needs to be taken, as many teenagers who have multiple follicles found on pelvic ultrasound are inappropriately told they have PCOS. Without the associated features, multiple follicles (10–20) are completely normal. These patients often have irregular, infrequent periods rather than amenorrhoea.

Investigations can help confirm the diagnosis (e.g. follicle-stimulating hormone, luteinising hormone and pelvic ultrasound).

Management

- *Addressing obesity* (see chapter 8, Obesity) can significantly improve the other features of PCOS.
- *Amenorrhoea* itself does not need treatment, but associated problems may require intervention.
- *Hirsutism* responds to OCP containing cyproterone acetate (an antiandrogen). This initiates withdrawal bleeds, which are lighter and more regular.
- *Infertility:* irregular ovulation may impede fertility. Specialist advice is recommended when planning conception.
- *Osteopenia:* prolonged amenorrhoea associated with low oestrogen levels potentially leads to a negative effect on bone mineral density. The addition of hormonal treatment may then be indicated.

Metrostaxis (severe heavy loss)

See also chapter 29, Haematologic conditions and oncology.

Investigations

- Check haemoglobin (Hb).
- Check clotting profiles: APPT, INR, vWF, collagen-binding assay (CBA), platelet function (platelet function assay, PFA-100) or platelet aggregometry.
- Exclude pregnancy.

Management

- *Tranexamic acid (TEA):* antifibrinolytics work via non-hormonal pathways to reduce the degree of blood loss. It can be used in combination with hormonal treatment.
- *Oestrogen therapy* is usually required for a young woman having her first or second period (Fig. 28.1).
- *Progestogen therapy* is more appropriate for a young woman who has been menstruating for some time (Fig. 28.2)

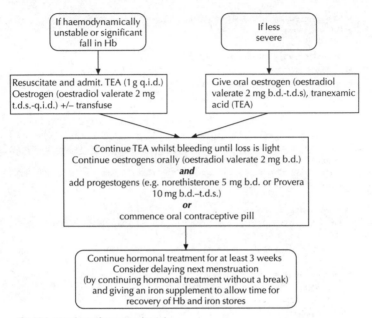

Fig. 28.1 Heavy loss at first or second period

Ongoing management – see menorrhagia section
If a transfusion is required, treatment should be continued for at least 3–6 months before a trial without hormonal therapy is considered.

Menorrhagia
- Menstrual history.
- FBE, iron studies.
- Clotting screen if good history for heavy loss (changing soaked pads <3 hourly), ask for other bleeding history – epistaxis, bruising, family history, post tonsillectomy/postoperative bleeding).
- βHCG (β-human chorionic gonadotrophin) if sexually active and delayed menses (possible threatened abortion or ectopic pregnancy).

Management
Non-hormonal
- If anaemic, use iron supplements.
- NSAIDs can reduce flow by 30% if taken regularly (see dysmenorrhoea section (p. 352) and Pharmacopoeia).

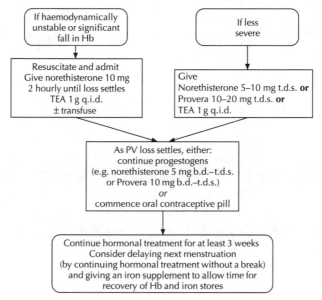

Fig. 28.2 Heavy loss in the young woman who has been menstruating for some time

- Antifibrinolytic agents (tranexamic acid 500 mg 2 tablets q.i.d.) can reduce flow by 50%.

Hormonal
The alternatives are:
- Cyclical progesterones (Primolut = norethisterone 5 mg, or Provera = medroxyprogesterone acetate 10 mg daily or twice daily for 14 or 21 days/month).
- Combined oral contraceptive pill (can reduce flow by 50%).
- Depo-Provera (75% amenorrhoea after 1 year use).

Pelvic pain: gynaecological causes
See Fig. 28.3.

Midcycle pain (Mittelschmerz)
This occurs midcycle, so it can often be diagnosed on history.

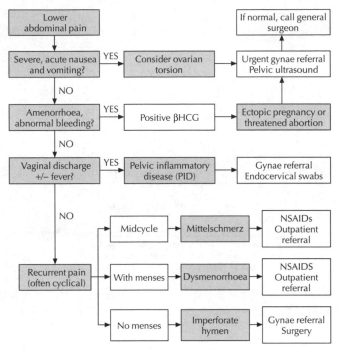

Assess menstrual history, sexual activity, associated symptoms and consider performing βHCG in all patients. Always consider urinary or gastrointestinal causes.

Fig. 28.3 Adolescent gynaecology – Assessment of lower abdominal pain

Ovarian cysts

Most ovarian cysts detected on an ultrasound scan are normal follicles, hence reassurance that these are physiological and represent healthy functioning ovaries is important. Presume that all cysts <6 cm are physiological unless specific features are present to suggest otherwise. Repeating a scan 6 weeks later to prove the resolution of cysts <6 cm can prevent operative intervention.

Torsion of the ovary is uncommon, but it occurs in the presence of an enlarged ovary or ovarian cyst. It presents with the sudden onset of severe pain, with associated nausea, vomiting and dizziness. A diagnostic laparoscopy is the best way of excluding ovarian torsion, although the appearance of normal ovaries on an emergency ultrasound makes the diagnosis most unlikely. Detection of blood flow to the ovary at the time of ultrasound does not exclude a diagnosis of ovarian torsion.

Pelvic inflammatory disease
- This occurs only in females who have been sexually active.
- A history of dyspareunia, discharge and fever may be associated with the pelvic pain.
- Chlamydial pelvic inflammatory disease (PID) may cause endometritis with intermenstrual bleeding, menorrhagia or metrostaxis.
- Other common causative organisms include *Neisseria gonorrhoea,* coliforms, *Gardnerella vaginalis, Haemophilus influenza,* group B *Streptococcus* and *Bacteroides* species.
- As these young females are sexually active it is appropriate that cervical swabs be taken, including specific swabs for *Chlamydia* culture. PCR testing for *Chlamydia* on cervical swabs and urine should also be requested.

Management
- If febrile (severe infection) admit for i.v. antibiotics:
  - Doxycycline 100 mg orally 12 hourly
  - **plus** metronidazole 500 mg i.v. 12 hourly
  - **plus either** ceftriaxone 1 g i.v. daily or cefotaxime 1 g i.v. 8 hourly.
- For mild to moderate infection:
  - Azithromycin 1 g orally as a single dose
  - **plus** ceftriaxone 250 mg (in 1% lidocaine), i.m. as a single dose (for gonorrhoea)
  - **plus** doxycycline 100 mg orally, 12 hourly for 14 days
  - **plus** metronidazole 400 mg orally, 12 hourly, for 14 days or tinidazole 500 mg orally daily for 14 days.
- Papanicolaou (PAP) smears:
  - Remember that all sexually active teenagers should have a PAP smear taken every 2 years, commencing approximately 2 years after intercourse began.
- Discuss contraception and sexually transmitted infections (STIs):
  - If PID is suspected it generally implies that condoms are not being used.
  - Discuss the benefits of condoms for protection against STI and pregnancy.
  - Consider screening for other STIs including hepatitis B and HIV1/2 (this will need informed consent and may need to be discussed with the paediatrician).
  - Ask about immunisation status for HPV (Gardasil introduced to Australia in 2007). See chapter 9, Immunisation, p. 121.

Ectopic pregnancy
- A recent 'period' does not exclude this diagnosis.
- The use of contraception does not exclude this diagnosis.
- Perform a pregnancy test and organise a pelvic ultrasound unless the clinical situation (i.e. shock) necessitates immediate resuscitation and surgical intervention.
- Contraception, PAP smear and STIs will need to be discussed, see above.

Congenital obstructive anomalies
- May cause acute-onset pain, progressive dysmenorrhoea (if there is unilateral obstruction) or progressive pelvic pain without menstruation (if there is complete obstruction; most commonly this is due to an imperforate hymen).
- Pelvic mass may be palpable. Perineal examination may reveal an imperforate hymen. Gentle pressure on the lower abdomen will enhance bulging of the hymen.
- Pelvic ultrasound or other imaging techniques will help clarify the anatomy.
- Associated renal agenesis on the side of an obstructed double genital tract may occur.

Breast problems
- Asymmetrical development of the breast bud may lead to presentation with a 'breast lump'. Biopsy at this early stage is not indicated. Reassure during the time of breast growth and development. Growth that is initially asymmetric may correct itself.
- Persistent unequal breast size can cause considerable embarrassment and distress to the teenager, and referral to a specialist (usually a plastic surgeon with an interest in breast surgery) may be appropriate. Eventually, surgical correction may be required, but this would not usually be undertaken until growth has ceased.
- Breast cysts can occur and may present acutely with inflammation, presumably due to leakage of cyst contents. Breast ultrasound can be used to confirm the presence of the cyst. Anti-inflammatories are useful.

See chapter 25, Endocrine conditons, Premature thelarche, p. 318.

Contraception: best options for young women
Other issues pertinent to adolescence and health risk behaviours must be explored (see chapter 15, Adolescent health, HEADSS approach, p. 177).

Condoms
Condoms offer the advantage of protection from STIs, as well as fairly good contraception. They may not be a reliable form of contraception if alcohol and drug-taking are issues.

Oral contraceptive pill
Contraindications
- Thromboembolic disease.
- Liver disease.
- Oestrogen-dependent tumours.
- Migraines with neurological signs.

Note: Migraines can be oestrogen-induced (onset with commencement of OCP) or secondary to oestrogen withdrawal (onset with menses).

Short-term side effects
- Nausea.
- Breakthrough bleeding (this should resolve with continuing usage or change of pill type).

Types
- *Constant dose* (e.g. Microgynon 30ED and Nordette): for the patient who suffers erratic, heavy periods, premenstrual moodiness or irregular lifestyle routines (there is a slightly greater leeway in the time of taking such pills).
- *Higher oestrogen content*. if using anticonvulsants (which increases hepatic metabolism of OCP) or if there is persistent breakthrough bleeding.

Other forms of contraception
- *Implanon*: Hormonal implant inserted under the skin in the upper arm. Very effective contraception that lasts 3 years. Often associated with a reduction in menstrual loss, although irregular periods occur in up to 30% of young women. Amenorrhoea can also occur.
- *Depo-Provera*: a 150 mg, 3-monthly injection. This often causes irregular bleeding initially but amenorrhoea after 6–9 months. This is a very reliable form of contraception. Long-term usage in teenagers may have some impact on bone density although this now appears to be reversible.

The following options are generally not appropriate for young women:
- Intrauterine contraceptive devices (IUDs) and diaphragms.
- Progesterone-only pill: less reliable than combined OCP and must be taken at the same time every day to be effective.

Emergency contraception: the morning-after pill
- Can be used up to 72 h after unprotected intercourse.
- Some evidence for its use up to 5–7 days, although with reduced efficacy.

Postinor 2 (levonorgestrel 75 mcg, 2 tablets).
- Taken 12 h apart or both tablets may be taken at once, as soon as possible after intercourse.
- Available over the counter.

- These treatments are >90% effective, but do not provide continuing contraception.
- It is essential to plan ongoing contraception, STI prevention, PAP smears and follow-up strategies to ensure that the emergency treatment has worked.

CHAPTER 29

Haematologic conditions and oncology

John Heath
Paul Monagle

Anaemia
Anaemia is defined as having a haemoglobin (Hb) less than the lower limit of the reference range for age (Table 29.1).

Clinical features suggestive of anaemia
- Pallor.
- Poor growth.
- Pale conjunctivae.
- Signs of cardiac failure.
- Flow murmur.
- Listlessness.
- Lethargy.
- Shortness of breath.

Investigation
If anaemia is suspected, begin with a full blood examination (FBE), blood film, ferritin and reticulocyte count. The initial classification is based on the mean corpuscular volume (MCV) (see Fig. 29.1).

Iron deficiency
Iron deficiency is common among Australian children, but it is often subclinical. Anaemia only occurs in those with more severe deficiency. Iron deficiency may be present in 10–30% of children in high-risk groups. Iron deficiency (see Table 29.1) may lead to impaired cognitive and psychomotor performance, even in the absence of anaemia.

Most cases of iron-deficiency anaemia in young children are due to inadequate dietary intake, although faecal blood loss may be provoked by cow's milk protein. In adolescent girls, blood is lost through menstruation (Table 29.2).

In iron-deficiency anaemia, the ferritin, Hb, mean corpuscular volume (MCV) and mean corpuscular Hb concentration (MCHC) are low. In mild iron deficiency, the FBE is normal but the ferritin is reduced, which demonstrates low iron stores. Ferritin is an acutephase

Paediatric Handbook, 8th edition. By Kate Thomson, Dean Tey and Michael Marks. Published 2009 by Blackwell Publishing, ISBN: 978-1-4051-7400-8.

Table 29.1 Haemoglobin reference ranges for age

Age	Lower limit of normal range of Hb (g/L)	
2 months	90	
2–6 months	95	
6–24 months	105	
2–11 years	115	
>12 years	girls – 120	boys – 130

reactant and may be misleadingly normal/high during an acute febrile illness. In such circumstances, a repeat measurement a month later or an empiric trial of iron therapy are alternative strategies.

Iron studies are frequently requested, but in otherwise well, community-based children, results other than **ferritin** contribute little to the diagnosis. Serum iron concentration, total iron binding capacity (TIBC), serum transferrin and transferring saturation are not clinically useful. Serum iron concentration varies considerably throughout the day and week in normal individuals, is low in chronic disease and as an acute phase response.

Remember that iron-deficiency anaemia secondary to a poor diet may be associated with other macro- and micronutrient deficiencies.

Prevention of iron deficiency
- Introduce iron-containing solids from 4–6 months.
- Avoid cow's milk in the first 12 months of life (apart from small amounts in custards and cereals).
- Cow's milk should only form a small part of the diet up to 2 years of age.
- Ensure that formulas (if used) and cereals are iron fortified.
- Consider supplementation in high-risk groups (see Table 29.2).

Good sources of iron for children
See also chapter 6, Nutrition.
- Infant milk formulas.
- Fortified breakfast cereals.
- Meat (including red meat, chicken and fish).
- Green vegetables (especially legumes, e.g. peas and beans).
- Dried beans and fruit.
- Egg yolk.

Note: Iron absorption from non-meat sources is increased when taken with foods high in vitamin C (citrus fruit, strawberries, cauliflower and broccoli).

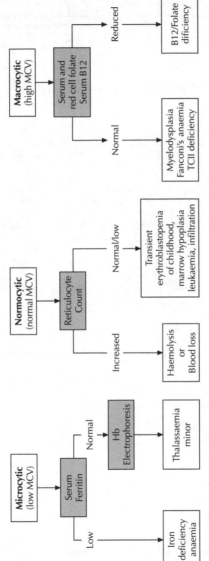

Fig 29.1 Classification of anaemia

* TCII, transcobalamin II deficiency

Table 29.2 Children at high risk for iron-deficiency anaemia

Group	Additional risk factors	Mechanisms
<6 months of age	Prematurity Low birth weight Multiple births Maternal iron deficiency	Inadequate stores

6–24 months of age	Exclusive breast-feeding after 6 months
	Delayed introduction of iron-containing
	    solids
	Excessive cow's milk
		Inadequate intake
		Cow's milk may cause
		  microscopic gut blood
		  loss

Adolescents	Females Poor diet	Menstruation Rapid growth spurt
Aborigines Migrant families Socially disadvantaged Vegetarian/fad diets	Poor diet Excessive cow's milk	Inadequate intake

Management

- Dietary advice should be given in all cases. This includes increasing the amount of iron containing foods and limiting the intake of cow's milk. Parents often need considerable support to manage behavioural issues around the diet, especially in the toddler age group.
- Supplemental iron should be recommended for any child with documented iron deficiency, even in the absence of reduced haemoglobin, because it takes a long time to replenish iron stores by dietary change alone. Behavioural changes and an improved feeling of well being are often noted with iron replacement even in children who were not anaemic.
- For young children, supplemental iron is usually given as ferrous gluconate mixture (daily dose 1 mL/kg of the 300 mg/5 mL preparation) and should be continued for 3 months after the Hb has returned to normal to replenish stores. Alternatives to ferrous gluconate mixture are shown in Table 29.3. The stools may become black/grey. **As iron overdose can be fatal, supplements should be stored in a locked cabinet.**
- Parenteral iron supplementation and blood transfusions are rarely indicated in children. Blood transfusions may be used if a very anaemic child requires urgent surgery or if cardiac failure is present. Transfusion should be slow and only raise the Hb to 60–80 g/L (see Calculating the blood transfusion volume, p. 372).

Vitamin B₁₂ deficiency

B_{12} deficiency in childhood most commonly presents during the first 2 years of life. The most common cause is nutritional, due to undiagnosed maternal B_{12} deficiency in a fully breast-fed child. Transcobalamin II deficiency is uncommon, but is associated with normal serum B_{12} levels, despite severe tissue B_{12} deficiency. Rarer inherited metabolic causes of cellular B_{12} deficiency exist and diagnosis can be masked by therapy. Early involvement of a metabolic physician is imperative for timely diagnosis of these rare conditions.

Table 29.3 Alternatives to ferrous gluconate mixture

Product	Fefol spansules	Ferro-Gradumet slow release tablets	Incremin Iron mixture
Iron contents	Per spansule: Iron sulfate (dried) 270 mg Elemental iron 87.4 mg	Per tablet: Iron sulfate (dried) 325 mg Elemental iron 105 mg	Per 5 mL: Iron pyrophosphate Elemental iron 5 mg
Equivalence to Fergon	1 spansule = 13.2 mL Fergon Half a spansule = 6.6 mL Fergon	1 tablet = 15.9 mL Fergon	5 mL Incremin = 0.76 mL Fergon
Other ingredients	Per spansule: Folic acid 0.3 mg Sucrose		Per 5 mL: Lysine HCl 150 mg Vitamin B_1 5 mg Vitamin B_6 2.5 mg Vit B_{12} 12.5 mcg Alcohol
Administration	Spansules can be pulled apart and the bead content given in a small amount of soft food. Beads should not be crushed or chewed. For a smaller dose, spansule may be opened, beads emptied out and divided to give half the dose. One or half a spansule may be given every second day.	Consider for older children where a whole tablet daily or every second day is an appropriate dose. Tablets should be swallowed whole	Inadequate therapy for established iron deficiency, and should only be used for prophylaxis in selected cases
Note:	Folic acid may mask vitamin B_{12} deficiency		

Any child with failure to thrive or neurodevelopmental abnormalities with an associated haematological abnormality (any cytopenia, macrocytosis or hypersegmented neutrophils) should be suspected of B_{12} deficiency and investigated urgently. The urgency relates to the propensity for rapid neurological deterioration (seizures, apnoea, choreoathetosis) and the lack of reversibility of these symptoms if treatment is delayed.

Investigations
- Bone marrow aspirate can confirm megaloblastosis within an hour to allow therapy to commence immediately.
- Serum homocysteine and urinary methylmalonic acid are also important to establish cellular vitamin B_{12} deficiency.

Haemoglobinopathies
β-Globin thalassemia
β-Thalassemia minor is common and causes hypochromic microcytosis without significant anaemia or clinical symptoms. One clue is an elevated red cell count on the FBE. The diagnosis is confirmed by Hb electrophoresis (or high performance liquid chromatography, HPLC) demonstrating an elevated HbA_2. Iron deficiency obscures the diagnosis by reducing HbA_2 levels, and hence children with thalassemia minor are often unnecessarily treated with iron therapy.

Thalassemia major is now uncommon because of the increased use of antenatal screening and prenatal termination. However, the diagnosis should be considered in the context of hypochromic microcytic anaemia presenting in the second 6 months of life (i.e. after β-globin chain switch has occurred at 6 months). Hepatosplenomegaly, marked erythroblastosis and bizarre red cell forms on the blood film are usually diagnostic.

α-Globin thalassemia
α-Thalassemia traits are relatively common in Asian populations. Hb Barts (four-gene deletion) classically presents with hydrops fetalis at birth. HbH disease (three-gene deletion) usually presents with mild to moderate microcytic anaemia but children are asymptomatic when well. When physiologically stressed, they can become significantly anaemic. Children with α-thalassemia traits (one- or two-gene deletions) may be microcytic (from birth) but not anaemic and are asymptomatic throughout life.

Sickle cell anaemia
Homozygous SS or double heterozygous (HbS/β-thalassemia trait) usually presents after 6 months of age (after β-globin chain switch).

Clinical presentations include:
- Anaemia (haemolysis or aplasia).
- Joint pains (especially small hand and foot joints).
- Acute chest syndrome (pneumonia-like with prominent hypoxia).
- Arterial ischaemic stroke.
- Acute splenic sequestration (rapidly progressive anaemia and splenic enlargement).
- Painful crisis (usually bone or abdominal pain).
- Asymptomatic diagnosis when parents are known carriers.
- Sepsis, especially encapsulated organisms in young infants.

Diagnosis
Diagnosis is made by blood film examination, sickle solubility tests and Hb electrophoresis.

Management
Long-term management includes folate supplementation, penicillin prophylaxis, appropriate vaccinations, and hydroxyurea or transfusion support as required. Acute management of crisis includes hydration, analgesia, transfusion and often antibiotics. Chest syndrome and stroke usually require exchange transfusion. Specialist consultation is required for each presentation.

Haemoglobin C/E
HbC and E are common in Asian populations, and both the heterozygous and homozygous forms are asymptomatic. Blood films may show many target cells. Thalassemia minor and HbC or E double heterozygotes present clinically as thalassemia major.

Haemolysis
Acute haemolysis in childhood is a life-threatening disorder that usually requires admission, thorough investigation and potentially transfusion support. Severe anaemia can develop quickly and frequent clinical review of vital signs and monitoring of Hb is required.

Diagnostic features of haemolysis include anaemia, polychromasia on the blood film, reticulocytosis and hyperbilirubinaemia. Haptoglobin is unhelpful in infants.

Investigations
First line investigations include:
- Blood film examination:
  - Spherocytes: hereditary spherocytosis, Coombs positive, ABO, glucose-6-phosphate dehydrogenase (G6PD).
  - Fragments: microangiopathic haemolysis.
  - Blister/bite cells: oxidative haemolysis (drug or G6PD).
  - Sickle cells.
- Direct Coombs test.
- Heinz body preparation.
- Hb electrophoresis/isopropanol test for unstable Hb.
- G6PD assay.
- Eosin 5 maleimid (E 5M) screening test for hereditary spherocytosis.

Further investigation is often required once the acute episode has resolved, and usually requires input from a specialist.

Potential causes of acute haemolysis are shown in Fig. 29.2.

Transient erythroblastopenia of childhood
This is a form of acquired red cell aplasia predominantly affecting children <7 years old.

Anaemia is normochromic, normocytic and there is no reticulocyte response until the recovery phase commences. Bone marrow aspirate may show red cell aplasia with preservation of other cell lines. The prognosis for previously normal children is excellent, with recovery for most within 2 months. No specific therapy is warranted and blood transfusion is best

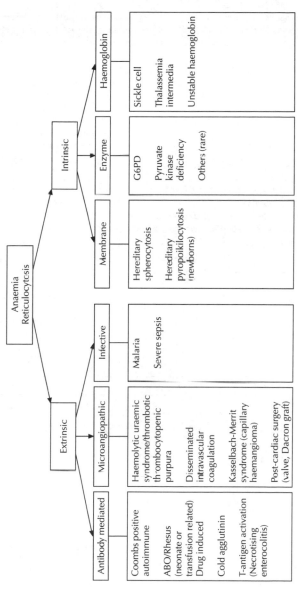

Fig 29.2 Acute haemolysis

avoided if possible (consider if Hb <50 g/L and no reticulocyte response). The differential diagnosis is Blackfan–Diamond syndrome, which usually occurs at a younger age, but may be indistinguishable on peripheral blood and bone marrow aspirate findings.

Coagulation abnormalities

Severe bleeding disorders in childhood can present at any time, although it is usually in the newborn period. Spontaneous bleeding or bruising of multiple ages in unusual sites should raise suspicions of a bleeding tendency. Often coagulopathy screening is required to differentiate a bleeding diathesis from non-accidental injury. Family history, drug history and history of previous surgical challenges (including tooth extraction) are important. Routine coagulation screening preoperatively in well children is rarely indicated and coagulation testing should be guided by the clinical history.

Investigation

First line investigations of a suspected bleeding disorder include:

- Platelet count and blood film.
- Activated partial thromboplastin time (APTT).
- Prothrombin time (PT) or international normalised ratio (INR).
- Fibrinogen.

Interpretation of these investigations is shown in Table 29.4. Further investigations should usually be done in discussion with a haematologist.

Fibrinogen is an acute-phase reactant. In severe sepsis, when fibrinogen should be elevated, a normal level is still consistent with disseminated intravascular coagulation (DIC).

If the investigations above are normal in the setting of clinically abnormal bleeding, consider factor XIII deficiency, Von Willebrand disease, platelet function defects or a capillary fragility syndrome. Specific investigations will be required.

Table 29.4 Investigation of coagulation abnormalities

Screening test result	Causes
Low platelet count	Idiopathic (or immune) thrombocytopenic purpura (ITP) Neonatal alloimmune thrombocytopenia (NAITP) Congenital thrombocytopenia syndromes Chemotherapy/marrow replacement
Isolated prolonged APTT	Factor XI, IX, VIII deficiency Von Willebrand disease Heparin Factor XII (no clinical bleeding)
Isolated prolonged PT/INR	Factor VII deficiency Warfarin
Prolonged APTT, PT Low fibrinogen	Liver disease Disseminated intravascular coagulation (DIC) ± also low platelets Vitamin K deficiency, factor II, V, X deficiency (normal fibrinogen)

In the setting of acute bleeding, if the diagnosis of a specific bleeding disorder is unclear, give 10–20 mL/kg of fresh frozen plasma (FFP) ± platelets.

Generally, children presenting acutely with bleeding disorders should be discussed with a haematologist. Haemophilia A or B, von Willebrand disease and other bleeding disorders are complex disorders requiring specialist management.

General measures

These are applicable to all congenital bleeding disorders.

- Analgesia:
  - Do not give aspirin or other NSAIDs.
  - Narcotic analgesics should only be given as part of a comprehensive pain management plan to avoid overuse.
- Do not give intramuscular injections. Do not do arterial puncture.
- Lumbar punctures should only be done after haematological consultation and appropriate factor replacement.
- Splinting limbs reduces pain.
- Consult with a haematologist about the need for joint aspiration. Beware of the risk of:
  - Volkmann's ischaemic contracture in forearm bleeds.
  - Femoral nerve palsies with retroperitoneal bleeds tracking underneath the inguinal ligament.

Haemophilia A (factor VIII deficiency)
Management of bleeding

- Dosage of factor VIII is usually 30–50 units/kg, which increases factor VIII levels by 60–100%. Note that 1 unit/kg of factor VIII raises levels by 2%. Repeat doses are usually required 8–12 hourly.
- Most bleeding can be controlled with a single dose calculated to increase the factor VIII level to 50%.

Note: A minor head injury can become serious: the factor VIII level should be raised to 100% and the child admitted for observation.

- Recombinant human factor VIII is readily available for haemophilia treatment centres and used for all patients.
- Patients with factor VIII inhibitors may be treated with recombinant factor VIIa (Novoseven). The usual dose of factor VIIa is 90–100 mcg repeated in 2 h.

Mouth bleeding

Use tranexamic acid tablets (see Pharmacopoeia).

Haemophilia B (Christmas disease, factor IX deficiency)

Bleeding is treated with factor IX concentrate (Monofix).
- Requirements: as in haemophilia A.
- Dose: in general 1 unit factor IX/kg increases levels by 1.6%.
- Frequency: injections at 24 h intervals (the half-life for factor IX is 24 h).

Von Willebrand disease

Responds to cryoprecipitate, or to human-derived factor VIII (Biostate). Maintaining adequate supply of Biostate in Australia is difficult and therefore its use usually requires specialist haematologist intervention. Many patients respond to desmopressin (see pharmacopoeia). The half-life of von Willebrand factor is approximately 4 h, but factor VIII levels continue to be increased for 48–72 h after the infusion of cryoprecipitate. Further doses are given if bleeding recurs.

Idiopathic thrombocytopenic purpura

Idiopathic thrombocytopenic purpura (ITP), also known as immune thrombocytopenic purpura, is an acquired thrombocytopenia due to shortened platelet survival (immune mediated) in the absence of other disturbances of haemostasis or coagulation.

In young children, ITP usually presents with bruising and petechiae, often with a history of recent viral infection. In some instances there is oral bleeding, epistaxis, rectal bleeding or haematuria.

Bone marrow biopsy is not necessary where the clinical presentation, FBE and blood film suggests ITP (i.e. no hepatosplenomegaly or lymphadenopathy; no anaemia, leucopenia or blasts).

Although bruising and petechiae can present dramatically, morbidity in ITP is usually minimal. Intracranial haemorrhage is the most serious risk but the probable incidence is <1%.

Management

Controversy surrounds the indications and best form of treatment for children with acute ITP. Without active treatment, most patients' platelet counts return to a satisfactory level within a month.

Careful observation without specific treatment may be appropriate in milder cases. Patients with active bleeding (e.g. mucosal and gastrointestinal) should receive treatment to increase their platelet count more rapidly. Some authorities also recommend treating patients with a platelet count <10–20 × 10^9/L and a florid petechial rash (especially mucosal petechiae).

When treatment is indicated, corticosteroids are usually first line therapy. High dose i.v. immunoglobulin (IVIG) is reserved for the most severe or refractory cases. Various steroid regimens have been used. The following has been demonstrated to raise the count almost as quickly as IVIG: prednisolone 4 mg/kg for 1 week (maximum 75 mg/day), then 2 mg/kg for 1 week followed by 1 mg/kg for 1 week.

While the platelet count is very low, the child should rest quietly at home. As the count rises, more activity is allowed, but contact sports, cycling and rough physical activity should be avoided until the count is normal. Strictly avoid aspirin, NSAIDs and intramuscular/subcutaneous injections (including immunisations) until thrombocytopenia remits.

It is common for thrombocytopenia to recur with further viral infections in the year after diagnosis. Chronic ITP (lasting >6 months) occurs in <10% and requires specialist management. Treatment options include splenectomy and the use of rituximab (monoclonal anti-CD20 antibody). The risk–benefit ratio should be carefully considered and discussed with a haematologist.

Anticoagulation therapy in children

Thromboembolic disease is increasingly frequent in neonates and children, presumably because of increased survival of children with previously fatal primary disorders and the increased use of invasive arterial and central venous catheters, as well as extracorporeal circuits. Consequently the frequency of anticoagulant use in children is increasing, for both treatment and primary prophylaxis.

The coagulation systems of children and adults are physiologically different, which impacts on the use of investigations and the action of anticoagulant medications. Current literature suggests children receiving anticoagulant therapy appear to have higher treatment failure rates and more bleeding complications than adults. Thus anticoagulation in children should be managed only by specialist paediatric haematologists.

The most commonly used anticoagulant agents in children are unfractionated heparin (UFH), low-molecular-weight heparin (LMWH) and warfarin.

- *UFH* is given i.v. and is advantageous because of its rapid onset of action, short half-life and reversibility. However, there is controversy over appropriate therapeutic ranges in children and the interpretation of currently available monitoring tests. Heparin-induced thrombocytopenia appears to be significantly less in children than in adults.
- *LMWH* is frequently used because of its more predictable bioavailability and weight-adjusted dosing schedules, and reduced need for therapeutic monitoring. A number of LMWH preparations are available, but most experience in children is with enoxaparin (Clexane). Twice daily subcutaneous dosing is recommended, but the inability to completely reverse LMWH once given, limits its use in very sick children. Extreme care must be taken when children are having procedures (e.g. lumbar puncture), and at least two doses should be omitted before any procedure. APTT does not reflect the anticoagulant activity of LMWH and may be normal in a fully anticoagulated child. The generally accepted therapeutic range is 0.5–1.0 anti-factor Xa units. Like UFH, LMWH is excreted via the kidneys and half-life may be prolonged in renal disease.
- *Warfarin* is the agent of choice for long-term therapy, but there is a multitude of paediatric-specific issues. There is no paediatric preparation, resulting in complicated dosing schedules. Avoidance of half or quarter tablets can be achieved by variable daily doses (e.g. alternating daily doses, 1 mg one day and 2 mg the next). Monitoring is now significantly easier with 'point of care' capillary blood monitors, although the accuracy is operator dependent and technical limitations remain (especially at higher therapeutic ranges). Life style restrictions are necessary for children on long-term warfarin (mostly avoidance of contact sports), which may impact on adherence.
- *Thrombolytic therapy* in children is reported to cause major bleeding (intracranial or requiring transfusion) in >10%, with variable treatment success rates reported. Discuss this with a paediatric haematologist.

Transfusion therapy

Blood transfusion is common in the tertiary paediatric setting. The most common blood product transfused is packed red cells or packed cell concentrate (PCC). PCC is indicated when acute restoration of oxygen-carrying capacity is required (i.e. to relieve symptomatic or predictably progressive anaemia) or to achieve marrow suppression in chronic ineffective erythropoiesis (e.g. thalassemia major, sickle cell anaemia). Nutritional anaemia rarely, if ever requires transfusion.

> To calculate the desired transfusion volume, the following formula can be used:
> Packed red cells (mL) = weight (kg) × Hb rise required (g/L) × 0.4

Adverse reactions

- *Acute haemolysis:* the most likely life-threatening adverse event, due to an incompatible transfusion. This occurs due to mistaken identification of either the cross-match sample or the unit being transfused to the patient. It is most likely to occur when children of similar names are on the same wards, or in multiple emergencies. It can be prevented by fastidious adherence to identification procedures. Directed donations from parents are reportedly no safer than anonymous homologous transfusions. However, the family may prefer them. Directed donations can only be arranged electively as they require 5 days to process.
- *Non-haemolytic febrile transfusion reaction:* the most common adverse event, due to release of cytokines from white cells within the PCC. Slowing the transfusion rate and premedicating with promethazine (Phenergan) and paracetamol may be helpful. Leucodepletion (via filters) reduces the risk and can also be used to prevent CMV transmission. Leucodepletion is recommended to all children who may require multiple transfusions (although it is arguably beneficial to all patients).
- *Transfusion-related graft versus host disease:* the risk is reduced by **irradiation of blood products before transfusion in all immunocompromised children** (including neonates, oncology patients and some cardiac surgical patients). Irradiation reduces the shelf life of PCC so is usually carried out immediately before release from the blood bank.
- *Bacterial infection:* can present as an acute haemolytic reaction with catastrophic hypotension and fever. Bacterial infection from blood transfusion is much more likely if the PCC has been unrefrigerated for >4 h. Hence, a unit of PCC should not be infused over a longer period than this.
- *Viral infections:* generally rare. In Victoria, since the introduction of nucleic acid testing:
  - The risk of HIV from a blood transfusion is approximately 1 in 9 million.
  - The risk of hepatitis C is 1 in 1 million.
  - Transmission of Creutzfeldt–Jakob disease ('mad cow disease') by transfusion has not been documented in Australia, although there are case reports of this elsewhere in the world.

The most important preventive measure to keep blood safe from viral infection is not laboratory testing, but the use of unpaid volunteer donors and the accurate completion of the donor declaration form.

Oncology

Malignancy in childhood is relatively rare. Approximately 1 in 600 children will develop a malignancy before the age of 15 years. The expeditious investigation and management of the child with a suspected malignancy is a specialised field and should be undertaken under the supervision of a paediatric oncologist.

Table 29.5 Age distribution of common tumour types

	0–4 years	5–9 years	10–14 years
% Total tumours	46	29	25
CNS and eye	44	30	26
Leukaemias	49	30	21
Neuroblastoma	84	11	5
Wilm's tumour	81	18	1
Soft tissue sarcomas	40	34	26

Many paediatric malignancies occur over a relatively restricted age range. A broad understanding of the peak age of occurrence of different tumour types is therefore useful when considering the possibility of malignancy in a child (Table 29.5).

Presentation of childhood malignancies

Malignancy should be considered in children presenting with any of the following:
- Combinations of fever, pallor, bruising or petechiae, and bone pain.
- Lymphadenopathy – marked, progressive or persistent, localised or generalised.
- Hepatosplenomegaly.
- Recurring morning headache, particularly if associated with vomiting or visual disturbance.
- Ataxia, cranial nerve palsies, or other neurological signs, particularly when associated with headache or back pain.
- New onset of dry cough, or stridor, without other symptoms of respiratory infection, particularly if associated with orthopnoea.
- Any unusual mass or swelling.
- Persistent severe unexplained pain, especially bone or joint pain.
- Unexplained weight loss.

When a suspicion of a malignancy arises, discussion with a paediatric oncologist before diagnostic procedures is appropriate.

Emergency presentations

Most children with suspected malignancy can have diagnostic procedures scheduled electively during normal working hours without compromising outcome. However, some presentations require urgent intervention because of potential site-specific and biological behaviours:

Tumour lysis syndrome
Aetiology
- Lysis of tumour cells before or during early stages of chemotherapy, leading to release of intracellular contents into extracellular compartment.

- Common in Burkitt's lymphoma (a rapidly enlarging abdominal mass with ascites and/or pleural effusion), T-cell acute lymphoblastic leukaemia (ALL) and infant ALL, especially when WCC >100 × 10^9/L.

Diagnosis
- Hyperuricaemia and urate nephropathy, may lead to acute renal failre.
- Electrolyte disturbances (acidosis, hyperkalaemia, hypocalcaemia, hyperphosphataemia) may lead to cardiac arrest.

Management/prevention
- Hyperhydration and alkalinisation:
  - Use 5% dextrose with 1/5 normal saline + 60 mmol/L $NaHCO_3$ without K+ at 125 mL/m^2 per hour.
  - Keep urine output >1–2 mL/kg per hour and pH 7.0–7.5.
- Allopurinol 10 mg/kg per day (or urate oxidase); rarely leucophoresis.
- Check electrolytes frequently (6–8 hourly) in first 24–48 h.

Cerebrovascular accident
(see Stroke section in chapter 33, Neurology, p. 464)

Aetiology
- Increased tendency to thrombosis and/or bleeding.
- Usually in patients with leukaemia with one or more of hyperleukocytosis (see above for management), coagulopathy, and thrombocytopaenia.

Symptoms/signs
- Altered conscious state, motor weakness, seizures.

Management/prevention
- CT scan with contrast, MRI, MR angiography (MRA) if venous thrombosis suspected.
- At-risk patients should have coagulation studies carried out promptly.
- Evidence of active disseminated intravascular coagulation (DIC) requires urgent therapy with heparin, fresh frozen plasma (FFP) and platelets.
- Active bleeding secondary to thrombocytopenia alone is relatively rare (unless the platelet count is <10 × 10^9/L).

Respiratory distress/superior vena cava syndrome
Aetiology
- Obstruction of upper airways and venous return due to an anterior mediastinal mass.
- Most commonly T-cell non-Hodgkin's lymphoma (NHL) or ALL, Hodgkin's disease, Germ cell tumour.

Symptoms/signs
- Cough, stridor, orthopnoea (tracheal/bronchial compression).
- Headache, dizziness, facial/neck swelling, suffusion (superior vena caval obstruction).

Note: Minor increase in size of mass, sedation or anaesthesia may result in airway obstruction or right ventricular (RV) outflow tract obstruction.

Management
- Control airway at all times, chest radiograph/CT, echocardiogram to assess venous obstruction, and RV outflow.
- Attempt diagnosis in least invasive way (e.g. bone marrow, lymph node biopsy, pleurocentesis) if possible, empiric therapy if not.

Raised intracranial pressure
Aetiology
- Infratentorial space occupying lesion (tumour) and/or CSF outflow obstruction.
- Most commonly astrocytoma, medulloblastoma, ependymoma.

Symptoms/signs
- Headache, vomiting, cranial nerve palsy or papilloedema.

Management
- Urgent CT/MRI evaluation is required.
- If tumour identified, consider dexamethasone to reduce vasogenic oedema.
- Prompt neurosurgical consultation.
- Emergency shunting may be required before tumour biopsy/removal.

Spinal cord compression
Aetiology
- Extension of extradural tumour into spinal canal or an intramedullary tumour causing cord compression.
- Commonly neuroblastoma, soft tissue sarcomas, lymphomas, astrocytoma, ependymoma.

Symptoms/signs
- Back pain (localised/radicular), motor weakness, sensory loss, change in bowel/bladder function.

Management
- Consider use of dexamethasone to reduce oedema; be aware that steroids may prevent diagnosis of lymphoma, so plan diagnostic procedure accordingly.
- Many extradural tumours respond rapidly to chemotherapy. Prompt radiologic and haematological investigation and biopsy before frank cord compression occurs may enable conservative management without the need for a decompression laminectomy.

Emergencies during therapy
Fever in a patient receiving chemotherapy
Aetiology
Risk factors for infection in immunocompromised patients are:
- *Neutropenia*: A neutrophil count of $<0.5 \times 10^6$/L is associated with a significantly increased risk of bacteraemia and focal infection. This risk is markedly increased with a

neutrophil count $<0.2 \times 10^9$/L. The longer the duration of neutropenia, the higher the risk of infection.

- *Lymphopenia* is associated with increased risk of opportunistic infection such as *Pneumocystis carinii* and reactivation of herpes simplex and herpes zoster viruses.
- *Steroid therapy* is a risk factor for invasive fungal infection.
- *Central venous catheters:* Most children receiving chemotherapy have either a Hickman catheter (externalised central venous catheter, CVC) or an infusaport (completely subcutaneous catheter). Infection may occur at the exit site of a Hickman catheter, along the subcutaneous tunnel or within the lumen of the catheter. The reservoir of the port and associated catheter lumen may become colonised.
- *Breaches of the normal skin and mucosal barriers,* particularly in heavily colonised sites around the perineum, in the mouth, nose and lower gastrointestinal tract, allow organisms access to the bloodstream.

Most children with solid tumours receive intensive myelosuppressive chemotherapy regimens resulting in recurrent neutropenia 1–2 weeks after chemotherapy. Children with acute myeloid leukaemia (AML) have prolonged periods of neutropenia throughout their therapy. Children with ALL are likely to have several phases of treatment in the first 6–8 months that are myelosuppressive, but often have reasonably stable blood counts during maintenance therapy.

Symptoms/signs
Any child receiving an intensive therapy regimen who develops a fever ($>$38.5 °C on one occasion or 38.0 °C on two occasions at least an hour apart) should be presumed to be neutropenic and assessed promptly, with respect to:
- Cardiovascular stability.
- Respiratory status.
- Signs associated with anaemia and thrombocytopenia.
- Possible sites of infection:
  – Upper respiratory tract infection.
  – Dental sepsis.
  – Mouth ulcers including herpetic.
  – Cuts, abrasions, skin sores.
  – Inflamed Hickman/CVC site.
  – Anal fissures.
  – Embolic phenomena of septicaemia/bacterial endocarditis (especially if central line is *in situ*).
  – Lower respiratory tract infections especially *Pneumocystis carinii* pneumonia (fever, cough, tachypnoea, desaturation; clear chest to auscultation; interstitial infiltrate on chest radiograph).
  – Gastrointestinal tract infection including typhlitis (colonic wall inflammation especially caecum).

Investigations
- FBE and differential.
- Blood cultures (from both barrels of a dual-lumen CVC).

- Swabs of local lesions.
- Urine culture.
- Sputum culture in older children.
- Chest radiograph (may be no changes when neutropenic).
- Cross-match.
- Stool for microscopy, culture and viral studies.

Note: Lumbar puncture is contra-indicated, as there is often a coexistent thrombocytopenia.

Management
An initial dose of antibiotics should be given without delay. Delay in administering antibiotics until neutropenia is confirmed may result in progression from bacteraemia to septic shock.

Antibiotic choices must be determined by the infection profile of the unit as well as recent previous infections experienced by the patient, particularly if a CVC is *in situ*.

In the absence of focal signs, one example of an empiric antibiotic regimen is:
- Timentin 50 mg/kg (max. 3 g) i.v. 6 hourly (dose divided between the barrels of a dual-lumen CVC device), **and**
- Gentamicin 7.5 mg/kg (max. 360 mg) i.v. daily (dose divided between the barrels of a dual-lumen CVC device).

Most febrile neutropenic patients will be admitted to hospital and continue i.v. antibiotics until blood cultures have been reported as negative after 48 h.

Some children on maintenance therapy for ALL with previously stable blood counts may present with a mild fever, are assessed as being well and have signs of a respiratory infection or other focal infection. Such children may await the results of a blood count before making a decision regarding oral, i.v. or no antibiotics.

Other issues during treatment
Pain
See also chapter 4, Pain management.
- Pain in patients with cancer is complex and multifactorial; refer promptly for appropriate specialist advice.
- Assessment of the cause will usually allow appropriate therapy to provide relief of symptoms.
- Pain caused by the underlying malignancy at presentation usually responds rapidly to the commencement of chemotherapy, though analgesia may be required while investigations are being carried out, the diagnosis established and treatment commenced.

Nausea and vomiting
- Nausea and vomiting are common side effects of chemotherapy.
- Can now be successfully prevented or ameliorated in most children with the use of a 5HT-receptor antagonist such as ondansetron (0.15 mg/kg) pre-chemotherapy and 8–12 hourly during a course of treatment.
- Highly emetogenic chemotherapy combinations, such as high-dose doxorubicin combined with high-dose cyclophosphamide or cisplatin may require the addition of dexamethasone (0.1 mg/kg i.v. 6 hourly).

- If this combination fails, consider **chlorpromazine** (0.3 mg/kg) i.v., given over 30 min to minimise the risk of hypotension and dysphoria.
  - Other agents used include lorazepam, metoclopramide and domperidone.

Constipation
- Known side effect of vincristine therapy and can be particularly troublesome when the drug is used weekly (as in induction for ALL, Wilm's tumour, rhabdomyosarcoma, and Ewing's sarcoma).
- Instigate prophylaxis with laxatives or stool softener at the beginning of therapy.
- If severe constipation persists despite prophylaxis ± addition of other agents, nasogastric colonic lavage solutions (e.g. Golytely) are usually successful.
- **Suppositories and enemas must not be used** because of the risk of causing small abrasions, which can predispose to secondary local infection and/or septicaemia.

Transfusion of blood products (irradiated and filtered)
- *Packed cells:* generally if Hb < 80g/L; amount (mL) = Hb rise required (g/L) × weight (kg) × 0.4.
- *Platelets:* generally <10 000 (<30 000 for brain tumours); 1 paedi-pack/10 kg.

Extravasation of chemotherapy
- Produces local tissue necrosis (vesicants), burns and minor inflammation (irritants).
- Vesicants include actinomycin-D, anthracyclines, vincristine and vinblastine.
- Cease infusion immediately. Topical dimethylsulfoxide (DMSO), plastic surgeon review if extensive or centrally located.

Haemorrhagic cystitis
- Complication of cyclophosphamide or ifosfamide.
- Manage with vigorous hydration, correction of thrombocytopenia and coagulopathy.

Pneumocystis carinii pneumonia
- All children with acute leukaemia and those on intensive chemotherapy regimens should be started on prophylactic co-trimoxazole (2.5 mg trimethoprim/kg/dose orally b.d. on three consecutive days of the week).
- Consider PCP in an at-risk patient who presents with tachypnoea, lowered oxygen saturations and/or diffuse opacities on chest radiograph.

Infectious disease contacts in immunosuppressed patients
- Varicella and measles may lead to very severe illness in immunocompromised children.
- No effective antiviral agent is available for measles, and it may cause fatal pneumonitis. Although immunity may wane during chemotherapy, prior vaccination or infection is usually protective.
- If the patient's immune status is not known or negative, give herpes zoster immunoglobulin (ZIG) for varicella contact or human immunoglobulin for measles contact within 72 h. Contact must have been directly between the patient and the affected individual during

the period extending from 48 h before the appearance of the rash to 7 days after the appearance of the rash.

Zoster immunoglobulin dose for varicella contact
- Weight <20 kg or <5 years of age: 250 mg i.m. (1 × 2 mL/125 IU vial).
- Weight 20–40 kg or 5–10 years of age: 500 mg i.m. (2 × 2 mL/125 IU vial).
- Weight >40 kg or age >10 years: 750 mg i.m. (3 × 2 mL/125 IU vials).

Immunoglobulin for measles contact
- 0.25 mL/kg i.m. daily for 2 days.

Immunisation during and after therapy
- Response to routine immunisations will not be optimal during therapy. Hence, routine immunisation programmes should be interrupted while the child is on therapy.
- If required for treatment of a tetanus prone wound, tetanus toxoid can be safely given but concurrent use of tetanus immunoglobulin should also be considered.
- **Live virus vaccines must not be given to immunocompromised children.**
- **Siblings of patients should not receive oral polio vaccine (Sabin); give injectable polio vaccine inactivated instead.**
- It is strongly advised that unimmunised, non-immune siblings receive MMR and varicella vaccine.
- All family members including the immunocompromised child should be encouraged to have annual influenza vaccination.
- Approximately 6 months after completion of chemotherapy, interrupted immunisation programmes should be completed. A booster dose of ADT or CDT, Sabin and MMR should be given to those who have previously been fully immunised. Hepatitis B immunisation should be commenced if not previously given.
- Consult with a specialist regarding immunisation after an allogeneic bone marrow transplant.

USEFUL RESOURCES
- *www.cancer.gov/cancertopics/types/childhoodcancers* – US National Cancer Institute.
- *www.childrensoncologygroup.org* – CureSearch Children's Oncology Group.
- *www.aspho.org* – American Society of Pediatric Hematology/Oncology.

CHAPTER 30
Infectious diseases

Nigel Curtis
Mike Starr
Joshua Wolf

Rational antimicrobial prescribing

- Unnecessary antibiotic use for viral illnesses contributes to the increasing problem of antibiotic resistance. Most respiratory tract infections in children, including tonsillitis and otitis media, are self-limiting and do not require antibiotic therapy. If the diagnosis is unclear, it is preferable to repeat the clinical evaluation and simple laboratory tests, rather than use empiric antibiotic therapy 'just in case'.
- Antibiotics do not prevent secondary bacterial infection in viral illnesses.
- The use of antibiotics may make definitive diagnosis and subsequent decisions about management more difficult.
- Empiric antibiotic therapy (i.e. not based on specific aetiological diagnosis) should only be prescribed when a *serious* bacterial infection is suspected (e.g. meningitis) *and* it is not safe or possible to obtain definitive culture specimens or culture results are pending.
- Empiric therapy should be based on the likely cause, local antibiotic resistance patterns and individual host factors (e.g. immunocompromise) in accordance with local guidelines.
- For mild infections, the safest and best-tolerated antibiotic with the narrowest spectrum against the most likely pathogens should be chosen (e.g. trimethoprim for urinary tract infection).
- For serious infections, broad-spectrum agents are chosen until the pathogen and its susceptibility is identified (e.g. cefotaxime for meningitis).
- Theoretical benefits of new antibiotics based on *in vitro* data do not necessarily translate into greater efficacy. Newer antibiotics often offer no advantages, might be expensive with more side effects and have a greater likelihood of leading to resistance or superinfection.

Antibiotic resistance

Although many bacteria are still susceptible to long-established treatments, antibiotic resistance is an increasing problem worldwide. Examples of particular clinical concern include:

- Penicillin (and cephalosporin)-resistant *Streptococcus pneumoniae* (PRP).
- Methicillin (multidrug)-resistant *Staphylococcus aureus* (MRSA).

Paediatric Handbook, 8th edition. By Kate Thomson, Dean Tey and Michael Marks. Published 2009 by Blackwell Publishing, ISBN: 978-1-4051-7400-8.

- Community-acquired non-multiresistant MRSA (CA-MRSA).
- Glycopeptide (vancomycin and teicoplanin) intermediate-resistant *Staphylococcus aureus* (GISA).
- Vancomycin-resistant *Enterococcus* (VRE).
- Multidrug-resistant *Mycobacterium tuberculosis* (MDRTB) and extensively drug-resistant tuberculosis (XDRTB).
- Bacteria that produce inducible *b*-lactamases (IBL) which are always present in bacteria of the 'ESCHAPPM' group comprising *Enterobacter* spp., *Serratia marscesens*, *Citrobacter freundii*, *Hafnia* spp., *Aeromonas* spp., *Providencia* spp., *Proteus vulgaris* and *Morganella morganii*.
- Bacteria that produce extended-spectrum β-lactamases (ESBL), e.g. some *E. coli* and *Klebsiella* spp. which are associated with cephalosporin (and often gentamicin resistance).
- Multidrug-resistant *Salmonella* spp.
- Macrolide-resistant *Streptococcus pyogenes*.

Infections with resistant organisms should be considered in patients who have had prolonged hospitalisation, known exposure to resistant organisms or failed response to initial empiric therapy. Strategies to deal with infections caused by these organisms include using new or broader-spectrum antibiotics, or alternatively using two or more antibiotics concurrently. The choice of empiric therapy becomes increasingly difficult. Specialist consultation is strongly advised.

Approach to the febrile child

Fever is the most common presenting symptom in children in the primary care setting. Although there is no universally accepted definition, fever is generally considered to be present if core temperature (rectal or tympanic) is >38 °C. Axillary and oral temperatures may underestimate body temperature by at least 0.5 °C.

Although tympanic thermometers provide certain advantages over other thermometers (ease of use, rapid results and convenience), several studies have found that they are not as accurate nor sensitive for the detection of fever, particularly in infants <3 months of age. Rectal (neonates), oral and axillary (neutropenic patients) temperatures are preferable for accurate fever detection.

Self-limiting viral infections are the most common cause of fever in children. However, the challenge to the clinician is to identify those children with a more serious cause. Fever in children may be classified into three groups:

- Fever with localising signs.
- Fever without focus.
- Fever (or pyrexia) of unknown origin.

Fever with localising signs

A careful history and examination will identify the source of infection in most patients. These children should be managed according to the individual condition and its severity.

Fever without focus

In a small number of children presenting with fever, no focus is found. Most will have a viral infection, but a more serious illness such as a urinary tract infection (5–8%), occult bacteraemia (<1%) or meningitis may be present. Infants (<12 months old) with rectal temperature >38.0 °C have a higher risk of occult bacteraemia (up to 15%).

Most children who present with fever and no identifiable focus appear otherwise well. History should include details about immunisation status, infectious contacts, travel, diet and contact with animals. A thorough physical examination should be carried out, paying particular attention to:

- *General appearance*: the level of activity and social interaction; peripheral perfusion and colour.
- *Vital signs*: pulse; respiration; blood pressure.
- *Possible clues to source*: full fontanelle, neck stiffness, photophobia; respiratory distress (tachypnoea; grunt; nasal flare; retractions), abnormal chest signs; rhinitis, pharyngitis, otitis or mastoiditis; lymphadenopathy; abdominal distension, tenderness or masses; hepatosplenomegaly; bone and joint tenderness or swelling; skin rashes, petechiae or purpura, or skin infection.
- **Always consider Kawasaki disease in any child with a persistent fever.** It is the only rare cause of persistent fever that requires urgent treatment.

Patients with unexplained fever with a higher likelihood for serious infection include the following patient groups or conditions:

- Neonates and infants <3 months of age.
- Immunocompromised (e.g. congenital immunodeficiency, HIV, neutropenic and other oncology patients, cytotoxic drugs and steroids).
- Asplenic children (congenital, post splenectomy or functional, e.g. sickle cell disease).
- Patients who have received prior oral antibiotics. Many of these patients have a viral infection, but meningitis or other serious bacterial infection must be considered.
- Children with central venous or arterial catheters, or other foreign bodies, including shunts.
- Multiple congenital abnormalities.
- Other specific illnesses (e.g. sickle cell disease, cystic fibrosis or structural cardiac defects (endocarditis)).
- Toxic-appearing children (e.g. those with an altered conscious state, decreased peripheral perfusion (check capillary refill centrally) or purpuric rash).
- Children <6 months of age (higher chance of UTI).
- Children <12 months of age with febrile convulsion, or any children with febrile convulsion lasting longer than 10 min (consider lumbar puncture to exclude meningitis).

These children require admission to hospital, with culture of blood, urine and CSF ('full septic screen') and a chest radiograph if indicated. Antimicrobial therapy should be based on the patient's clinical illness and the local epidemiology of potential pathogens and their antibiotic susceptibility (see Antimicrobial guidelines).

Table 30.1 Management of fever without focus

Age	Investigations	Management
<1 month	FBE; blood, urine and CSF cultures; CXR	• Admit • Empiric i.v. benzylpenicillin and gentamicin, *plus* cefotaxime if meningitis is suspected (see Antimicrobial guidelines)
1 to 3 months	As above (CXR may be omitted if no respiratory symptoms or signs present)	• If WCC 5–15 × 10⁹/L with other investigations normal: discharge and review within 12 h, or sooner if deterioration occurs • If child is unwell, or any results are abnormal: admit and consider empiric antibiotics (see Antimicrobial guidelines)
3 months to 3 years *and well*	Consider urine culture (mandatory if <6 months)	• If <6 months and UTI is suspected from dipstick urine testing: admit for i.v. benzylpenicillin and gentamicin (see Antimicrobial guidelines) • Otherwise: discharge and review within 24 h, or sooner if deterioration occurs

3 months to 3 years and unwell	FBE; blood, urine and CSF cultures; CXR if respiratory symptoms or signs present	• Admit and start empiric antibiotics:
		  – if CSF normal: i.v. flucloxacillin and gentamicin
		  – if CSF abnormal or unavailable: i.v. cefotaxime (see Antimicrobial guidelines)

Notes:
- Fever = rectal temperature >38 °C (>38.9 °C over 3 months of age).
- FBE = full blood examination, including film; CSF = cerebrospinal fluid; WCC = white cell count; CXR = chest X-ray.
- Urine specimens should be obtained by suprapubic aspiration or catheter drainage. Bag specimens are useless in this context.
- Lumbar puncture should not be performed in a child with impaired conscious state or focal neurological signs (see chapter 1, Medical emergencies, chapter 3 Procedures).
- Ceftriaxone can be substituted for cefotaxime (see Antimicrobial guidelines).

In the absence of the above risk factors, a febrile child >6 months of age who appears well but without a focus of infection does not require laboratory testing or treatment, though a urine microscopy and culture may be appropriate.

There is no evidence that oral or parenteral antibiotics prevent the rare occurrence of focal infections from occult bacteraemia; instead, they result in delayed diagnosis, drug side effects, additional costs and the development of resistant organisms. What is required is a careful clinical assessment, review within 24 h and parental education. See Table 30.1 and Box 30.1 on p. 384.

Occult bacteraemia

Infants with bacteraemia may clear the bacteria spontaneously. This is particularly true for pneumococcal bacteraemia. Patients who grow *Streptococcus pneumoniae* in their original blood culture do not require further investigation or treatment if they are now well, remain afebrile and have not received antibiotics, as they have cleared the organism independently. Parents should, however, be asked to bring children back for immediate review if they develop further fever within the following 7 days. Refer for specialist advice if uncertain.

Other pathogens causing occult bacteraemia should be treated with appropriate antibiotics.

Box 30.1 Advice for parents about fever

When caring for your child:

- Make the child comfortable, e.g. dress in light clothing.
- Give small, frequent drinks of clear fluid, e.g. water or diluted juice.
- Fever does not necessarily require treatment with medication. Finding the cause and treating it is often more important.
- Paracetamol may be given if the child is irritable, miserable or appears to be in pain (15 mg/kg p.o. 4 hourly when required, to a maximum of 90 mg/kg per day).
- Giving paracetamol has not been shown to prevent febrile convulsions.
- Do not continue giving regular paracetamol for more than 48 hours without having the child assessed by a doctor.
- Avoid aspirin and other NSAIDs:
  - Aspirin because of risk of Reye's syndrome.
  - NSAIDs because of potential association with invasive staphylococcal and streptococcal disease (including necrotising fasciitis).

Seek immediate medical attention if there is no improvement in 48 hours or at any time if your child:

- Looks 'sick': pale, lethargic and weak.
- Suffers severe headache, neck stiffness or complains of light hurting their eyes.
- Has breathing difficulties.
- Refuses to drink anything.
- Persistently vomits.
- Shows signs of drowsiness.
- Suffers pain.

Partially treated bacterial infection

Patients presenting with fever who have received prior antibiotics should be assessed with a high index of suspicion. Although the child may have a viral illness, partial treatment with antibiotics may mask the typical clinical presentation of a serious bacterial infection, such as meningitis. A full septic screen should be considered even if the child looks well. For this reason, neonates should almost never be treated with oral antibiotics in the community.

Pyrexia (fever) of unknown origin

Pyrexia of unknown origin (PUO) is defined as prolonged fever (usually accepted as 2 weeks or longer) for which history, examination and initial investigations have failed to reveal a cause. In general, PUO in children is more likely to be due to chronic, non-infectious conditions, such as juvenile chronic arthritis and other collagen vascular diseases, inflammatory bowel disease or malignancy. Infectious causes include systemic viral syndromes (such as infectious mononucleosis), upper or lower respiratory infections (e.g. sinusitis), urinary tract infection, CNS infection, bone infection, tuberculosis, abscess (e.g. parameningeal, intra-abdominal), endocarditis and enteric infections (e.g. typhoid fever). The term PUO is often *incorrectly* applied to patients who are suffering a series of simple viral infections.

Febrile neutropenia
See chapter 29, Haematologic conditions and oncology.

Common bacterial infections
Group A streptococcus
Group A β-haemolytic streptococci (GABHS or *Streptococcus pyogenes*) cause a variety of diseases including pharyngotonsillitis (see chapter 24, Ear, nose and throat conditions), impetigo, cellulitis, scarlet fever, otitis media, streptococcal toxic shock syndrome, necrotising fasciitis, glomerulonephritis and rheumatic fever. Group A streptococcal pharyngitis is extremely uncommon in children <5 years of age. *S. pyogenes* is currently always sensitive to penicillin.

Scarlet fever
- *Transmission*: droplet, direct contact.
- *Incubation period*: 2–5 days.
- *Infectious period*: 10–21 days (24–48 h, if adequate treatment).

Clinical features
- *Prodrome*: sudden-onset high fever, vomiting, malaise, headache and abdominal pain.
- *Rash*: appears within 2 h of prodrome, diffuse red flush involving torso and skin folds, blanches, circumoral pallor, strawberry tongue (initially white, then red day 4–5), pharyngotonsillitis, tender cervical/submaxillary nodes.

Complications: otitis media, retropharyngeal abscess, quinsy, rheumatic fever, glomerulonephritis.

Diagnosis: culture of throat swab may confirm clinical impression

Treatment:
- phenoxymethylpenicillin (penicillin V) 250 mg p.o. (<10 years), 500 mg p.o. (>10 years) 12 hourly for 10 days.
- *Control of case*: exclude from school until treated for 24 h.

Differential diagnosis: Kawasaki disease, streptococcal or staphylococcal toxic shock syndrome, viral infection

Acute rheumatic fever
- *Incubation period*: 7–28 days after group A streptococcal infection.

Clinical features
Jones criteria (1992) for initial diagnosis: two major, or one major plus two minor manifestations, plus evidence of antecedent group A streptococcal infection by culture or serology.

- Major manifestations:
  - Carditis (usually mitral regurgitation murmur).
  - Polyarthritis.
  - Erythema marginatum.
  - Subcutaneous nodules.
  - Chorea (does not require evidence of recent GAS infection).
- Minor manifestations:
  - Fever.
  - Polyarthralgia or aseptic mono-arthritis.
  - Raised inflammatory markers (ESR ≥30 mm/h or CRP ≥30 mg/L).
  - Prolonged PR interval on ECG.

Recurrences may be diagnosed with three minor manifestations plus evidence of antecedent group A streptococcal infection without major manifestations, if there are no other more likely diagnoses.

Complications
Increased risk of recurrent disease, particularly for first 5 years after an attack. Heart valve damage may be permanent, especially after severe or recurrent disease, leading to rheumatic heart disease.

Diagnosis
Clinical features (Jones criteria) + culture/serology. Echocardiography may be useful in detecting subclinical lesions or typical rheumatic valvular involvement.

Treatment
- Admission to hospital.
- Phenoxymethylpenicillin (penicillin V): 250 mg p.o. (<10 years), 500 mg p.o. (>10 years) 12 hourly for 10 days or a single i.m. injection of benzathine penicillin G (900 mg, or 450 mg if <30 kg).
- Aspirin:
  - Weeks 1 and 2: 25 mg/kg p.o. 6 hourly (4–8 g/day total in adults) initially.
  - Weeks 3 and 4: Reduce to 15 mg/kg p.o. 6 hourly.
  - May be used to relieve arthritis or fever and leads to resolution of symptoms within 1–2 days (sometimes this response is diagnostic of rheumatic fever).
  - There is no evidence that aspirin affects the long-term outcome.
- Corticosteroids (usually prednisolone 2 mg/kg per day, tapering after 2 weeks) are often used when carditis with cardiac failure is present, although there is no definitive evidence that they improve long-term outcome.
- For severe chorea, haloperidol, sodium valproate or other major tranquillisers have been used with mixed success.

Follow-up
Secondary prophylaxis is essential to prevent subsequent group A streptococcal infections, which may cause recurrences. Phenoxymethylpenicillin (penicillin V) 250 mg p.o. twice daily, or benzathine penicillin G 900 mg i.m. every 3 or 4 weeks. Duration is until 21 years of age

or 5 years after last attack (whichever is later) or to age 35 years if moderate or severe carditis present. Prophylaxis may be lifelong if severe carditis or if patient has required cardiac surgery. Long-term clinical and echocardiographic follow-up is essential.

Post-infectious glomerulonephritis
See chapter 35, Renal conditions.

Streptococcus pneumoniae
Streptococcus pneumoniae (pneumococcus) is a Gram-positive coccus (usually appearing as diplococci) that causes a wide variety of infections including severe, invasive disease (e.g. meningitis, septicaemia, septic arthritis, peritonitis), or mild, often self-limited, invasive disease (occult bacteraemia), pneumonia, otitis media and sinusitis.

Transmission
Droplet.

Epidemiology
The epidemiology of pneumococcal disease in children is changing as a result of the routine use of conjugate pneumococcal vaccine. In trials, the vaccine provided ~70% protection against invasive disease (meningitis, septicaemia), ~50% protection against radiographically proven pneumonia, and <5% protection against otitis media caused by *Pneumococcus*. Routine use of this vaccine in the USA has led to a large decrease in invasive pneumococcal disease in children, particularly in disease caused by penicillin-resistant strains. The incidence of pneumococcal disease is likely to fall in Australia but there remains concern about the possibility of a rise in disease caused by non-vaccine serotypes ('serotype replacement'). Despite the decreasing incidence of pneumococcal disease, this bacterium remains the most common cause of pneumonia, otitis media and meningitis in children.

Most human disease caused by 23 serotypes (of the 90 serotypes that have been described). 7 serotypes (those in the conjugate vaccine) cause about 85% of invasive disease in non-Aboriginal Australian children. Incidence of invasive disease is about 50–100 cases per 100 000 children aged <5 years. Incidence in central Australian Aboriginal children is the highest in the world (~1000–2000 per 100,000 aged <5 years, before the introduction of pneumococcal vaccine). Antibiotic resistance is becoming a problem worldwide – organisms are classified as penicillin susceptible, penicillin-non-susceptible (PNSP), and cefotaxime/ceftriaxone susceptible or resistant. Resistance may be intermediate or high-level.

Clinical features
Pneumonia and otitis media are the most common presentations, followed by septicaemia and meningitis. Soft tissue, bone and joint infections are less common manifestations.

Diagnosis
Meningitis, septicaemia or other sterile site infection is confirmed by culture/Gram stain of appropriate specimen (blood, CSF, joint fluid, peritoneal fluid, etc.). Pneumococcal pneumonia is blood culture positive in only about 10–20% of cases. PCR-based testing of blood and

CSF is available and useful when antibiotics have been initiated before collection of specimens. Pneumococcal urinary antigen has poor specificity in children due to frequent pharyngeal carriage of pneumococcus.

Treatment

Penicillin or amoxicillin is the drug of choice, except in CNS infection with PNSP.

- If non-CNS infection with PNSP, treat with high-dose penicillin (benzylpenicillin 60 mg/kg (max. 2 g) i.v. 4 hourly for invasive disease including pneumonia, or amoxicillin 90–120 mg/kg per day p.o. divided into three or four doses for otitis media or sinusitis).
- If CNS infection with cefotaxime/ceftriaxone-non-susceptible pneumococci, use vancomycin plus rifampicin or, for PNSP with cefotaxime MIC ≤ 2.0 mcg/mL, use high-dose cefotaxime (300 mg/kg per day) as an alternative (see Bacterial meningitis, p. 407). Duration of treatment is 10 days for meningitis and usually 5–7 days for other infections.

Vaccines

The 7-valent conjugate pneumococcal vaccine (7PCV, Prevenar®) has been part of the routine immunisation schedule in Australia since 2005 (2001 for indigenous children). 7PCV is given at 2, 4 and 6 months of age. A fourth dose in the second year of life is recommended for children at high risk of invasive pneumococcal disease, including those with hyposplenism. 9- and 13-valent conjugate vaccines are likely to be available in the near future.

The 23-valent polysaccharide vaccine provides protection against a broader range of serotypes but is not immunogenic in children <18–24 months of age, and protection is not long-lasting (2–3 years). The vaccine is routinely recommended in risk groups such as indigenous Australians, those with respiratory or cardiac co-morbidities, and patients with hyposplenia or certain immunodeficiencies.

Neisseria meningitidis

Neisseria meningitidis (meningococcus) is a Gram-negative diplococcus that mainly causes meningitis or septicaemia, or both. Less commonly, it may cause other infections including conjunctivitis, septic arthritis, pharyngitis, pneumonia, occult bacteraemia. For recommendations specific to meningitis see Bacterial meningitis, p. 407.

- *Transmission*: droplet.
- *Incubation period*: usually hours to 3 days.
- *Infectious period*: as long as carried – may be months. Most virulent within days of acquisition.

Epidemiology

- Peak age groups <2 years and 15–24 years.
- Serogroups B and C are most common in Australia (A, Y and W135 usually confined to travellers).
- Traditionally, group B is most common in young children and group C more common in adolescents.
- Incidence of group C meningococcal infection, which had been steadily rising in Victoria until 2003, has fallen rapidly since the introduction of routine conjugate group C vaccine.
- The case fatality rate has been reported as 5% for group B and 14% for group C infection.

Clinical features
- Meningitis – see below, p. 407.
- Septicaemia: often non-specific prodrome suggestive of viral illness.
- Rapid progression with any or all of the following: fever, rash (classically purpuric or pete-chial, but can be less specific), malaise, myalgia, arthralgia, vomiting, headache, reduced conscious state.
- Chronic meningococcaemia occurs rarely (consider terminal complement deficiency), and may be associated with progressive purpuric rash.

Diagnosis
Initially based on clinical features. Confirmation by culture of blood and/or CSF, preferably collected before first dose of antibiotics, although treatment should not be delayed. Additional tests may include shave biopsy of skin lesions (for Gram stain and culture), PCR on blood, CSF or skin sample.

Treatment
- Shock must be managed appropriately (see chapter 1, Medical emergencies).
- Discuss with Intensive Care for all cases of meningococcaemia and those with meningitis <2 years or very unwell.
- Immediate i.v. antibiotics (cefotaxime 50 mg/kg per dose (max. 2 g) 6 hourly, or if unavail-able, benzylpenicillin 60 mg/kg per dose (max. 2 g) 4 hourly).
- Duration of antibiotics usually 7 days. Can change to i.v. benzylpenicillin when isolate identified as meningococcus. All cases should be notified immediately to statutory health authorities.
- Steroids
  - Meningococcaemia: Consider corticosteroids (hydrocortisone 1 mg/kg i.v. 6 hourly) in severe cases.
  - Meningitis: (Children > 4 weeks old) give dexamethasone 0.15 mg/kg i.v. 6 hourly.
- Immunoglobulin 0.5 g/kg i.v. over 4 hours, is considered in those requiring ICU.

Clearance antibiotics for contacts
Contacts >1 month old should receive prophylaxis (see Table 30.3, p. 412). Patients with invasive disease who have received only penicillin should also receive treatment to eradicate carriage.

Other aspects
Vaccines: Tetravalent polysaccharide vaccine (A, C, Y, W135) protects for a short time (3–5 years) and only in those aged >2 years. Further repeated vaccination is associated with development of tolerance to the vaccine. This vaccine is used for travellers (e.g. to African 'meningitis belt' or attending the Haj) and for controlling outbreaks. It is also used in patients with asplenia in conjunction with conjugate vaccine to provide broader protection. Menin-gococcal group C conjugate vaccine is effective in all age groups and given as part of the routine immunisation schedule to all Australian children at 12 months of age. Children at higher risk should be offered two doses of conjugate vaccine from 2 months of age with a third dose in the second year of life (see chapter 9, Immunisation).

Staphylococcus aureus

Staphylococcus aureus is a Gram-positive coccus that causes a wide variety of invasive and non-invasive disease.

Epidemiology

S. aureus is a common commensal, being present in the nose of about 1/3 of individuals. Both hospital- and community-acquired multi-resistant *S. aureus* (MRSA) are increasing problems.

Clinical features

Causes a variety of diseases including impetigo, boils and abscesses, cellulitis (including periorbital cellulitis), osteomyelitis, septic arthritis, endocarditis, pneumonia, food poisoning, bacteraemia, septicaemia and toxic shock syndrome. *S.aureus* is responsible for scalded skin syndrome in younger children. Staphylococcal infection may be accompanied by significant constitutional symptoms (e.g. myalgia) in addition to localising features.

Diagnosis

- Sterile site infection is confirmed by appropriate culture/Gram stain.
- Patients with *S. aureus* bacteraemia should undergo careful examination to exclude focal infection.

Treatment

- Surgical drainage is often necessary for abscesses and other foci of infection. Anti-staphylococcal antibiotics include flucloxacillin, cefalexin, cefazolin and clindamycin. MRSA is resistant to all penicillin and cephalosporin antibiotics.
- Community-acquired MRSA is often sensitive to a wide range of antibiotics including clindamycin, co-trimoxazole, ciprofloxacin, vancomycin, teicoplanin, rifampicin and fusidic acid. (*Note*: ciprofloxacin, rifampicin or fusidic acid should never be used as monotherapy for *S. aureus* as resistance develops rapidly.)
- Hospital-acquired MRSA is often only sensitive to vancomycin and teicoplanin. Although vancomycin may be necessary to treat some MRSA infections, it is not as effective as flu-cloxacillin for the treatment of susceptible patients.
- *S. aureus* (MSSA). Prolonged duration of treatment may be required to prevent recurrence.

Mycoplasma pneumoniae

- *Transmission*: droplet.
- *Incubation period*: 1–4 weeks.
- *Infectious period*: unknown, likely to be many months; typically infects all members of a family over a period of weeks/months although most are asymptomatic.
- *Epidemiology*: all ages (*not* just >5 years).

Clinical features

- *Pneumonia*: malaise, fever, headache, non-productive cough for 3–4 weeks (may become productive); 10% have rash (usually maculopapular); chest radiograph may demonstrate unilateral lobar or bilateral diffuse changes; bronchitis, pharyngitis, otitis media.

- *CNS manifestations* (uncommon; likely post-infectious): aseptic meningitis, meningo-encephalitis, encephalitis, polyradiculitis/Guillain–Barré syndrome, acute cerebellar ataxia, cranial nerve neuropathy, transverse myelitis, acute disseminated encephalomyelitis and choreoathetosis.

Complications
Idiopathic thrombocytopenic purpura.

Diagnosis
- *Serology*: Not useful in acute setting. Infection can be diagnosed by fourfold rise in IgG over 2–4 weeks; IgM alone has very poor specificity in children as positive results occur in ~30% of healthy preschoolers.
- Polymerase chain reaction (PCR) of respiratory specimens or CSF is now the gold standard but suffers from relatively poor sensitivity (sputum ~70%, NPA ~50%, throat swab ~38%).

Treatment
- Roxithromycin 2.5–4 mg/kg (max. 150 mg) p.o. 12 hourly for 10 days is recommended, although its role is uncertain.
- Macrolides (e.g. azithromycin) are recommended in CNS disease although their role in this situation is also unclear.

Viral infections
Cytomegalovirus
Cytomegalovirus (CMV) is a ubiquitous herpes virus. It persists in latent form after primary infection and reactivation can occur years later, particularly with immunosuppression.

Transmission
- *Horizontal*: salivary contamination or sexual transmission; blood transfusion/organ transplantation.
- *Vertical*: transplacental, intrapartum via passage through infected genital tract and post-natal via ingestion of CMV-positive breast milk.

Incubation period
Unknown; infection usually manifests 3 weeks to 3 months after blood transfusion and 4 weeks to 4 months after tissue transplantation.

Clinical features
Vary with age and immunocompetence of child; asymptomatic infection is most common. Cytomegalovirus mononucleosis: cervical lymphadenopathy; hepatosplenomegaly in children, fever in adults. Note, clinical signs of CMV infection are similar to graft rejection in transplant patients. Both events peak 30–90 days after transplantation.

Diagnosis

Identification of the virus by culture or PCR of urine or saliva in the first 3 weeks of life is diagnostic of congenital disease; after this period, positive results may represent postnatally acquired infection. PCR of stored dried blood spots taken for the neonatal screening test may aid the diagnosis.

Distinguishing past from active infection can be difficult. Viral culture (rapid enhanced tissue culture immunofluorescence) or PCR of urine, saliva and even blood may be misleading as CMV can be excreted intermittently for life after primary infection, especially in immunocompromised patients. Leucocyte antigenaemia assay (degree of antigenaemia) correlates with the severity of CMV disease and is therefore a good means of predicting disease and monitoring progression in immunocompromised patients.

Complications

- Encephalitis, myocarditis, pneumonia, haemolytic anaemia, thrombocytopenia are rare manifestations.
- Primary CMV infection has been described in conjunction with Guillain–Barré syndrome and other peripheral neuropathies.
- Pneumonia, retinitis, hepatitis and colitis in immunocompromised.
- Congenital infection: >90% appear normal at birth: CNS sequelae in 10–20% of these (mainly sensorineural hearing loss); 5% present early with petechiae, hepatosplenomegaly, microcephaly and thrombocytopenia and have high rates of neurological sequelae.

Treatment

- Ganciclovir or valacyclovir for active CMV disease in the immunocompromised. Cytomegalovirus hyperimmune globulin is also sometimes used in these patients.
- Ganciclovir therapy should be considered in any neonate with symptomatic congenital CMV to reduce the risk of hearing loss and other neurological sequelae.

Enterovirus (non-polio)

Coxsackie A, B and echoviruses are important causes of childhood infections, especially in the summer months. These include a wide range of clinical presentations, including non-specific febrile illness; pharyngitis; herpangina; hand, foot and mouth disease; gastroenteritis; aseptic meningitis; encephalitis; myocarditis; pericarditis and several forms of viral exanthem (maculopapular, vesicular, petechial). Infection in agammaglobulinaemic patients can cause particularly severe or persistent meningoencephalitis. In neonates, enteroviral infection may be difficult to distinguish clinically from bacterial sepsis.

Hand, foot and mouth disease

- *Cause*: coxsackie A virus (usually A16).
- *Transmission*: direct contact/droplet.
- *Incubation period*: 3–6 days.
- *Infectious period*: until blisters have gone.

Clinical features
Vesicles on cheeks, gums, sides of the tongue; papulovesicular lesions of palms, fingers, toes, soles, buttocks, genitals, limbs (may look haemorrhagic); sore throat; fever and anorexia.

Diagnosis
Tests are usually unnecessary as the clinical picture is sufficient for diagnosis.

Control of case
Exclusion is unnecessary (as virus is excreted in faeces for weeks).

Treatment
Symptomatic.

Epstein–Barr virus (infectious mononucleosis)
- *Incubation period*: 30–50 days.
- *Infectious period*: unknown, viral excretion from oropharynx for months.

Clinical features
Glandular fever: Fever, malaise, exudative tonsillopharyngitis, generalised lymphadenopathy and hepatosplenomegaly. Highly variable clinical course: acute phase lasts 2–4 weeks and convalescence may take weeks to months. May be associated with hepatitis or CNS involvement. In immunocompromised (particularly transplant patients), can cause severe lymphoproliferative disease.

Diagnosis
Atypical lymphocytes in the peripheral blood. Monospot test in blood for heterophile antibody identifies 90% of cases in older children and adults, but lacks sensitivity in children under 4–5 years of age. Serology is the gold standard. PCR of blood or tissue may be helpful in transplant patients.

Complications
Upper airway obstruction; dehydration from poor oral intake (uncommon). An unknown minority may develop symptoms of chronic fatigue syndrome. See also chapter 15, Adolescent health.

Treatment
Symptomatic: prednisolone 1 mg/kg (max. 50 mg) oral, daily may be considered in patients hospitalised for airway obstruction. Amoxicillin and ampicillin cause florid rash in up to 90% of children with EBV infection.

In patients with splenomegaly, avoidance of contact sports is recommended for 3–4 weeks after the onset of the illness to prevent splenic rupture.

Herpes simplex virus (HSV)
Manifestations of HSV infection include skin and mucous membrane involvement, gingivostomatitis (mainly HSV-1), genital herpes (mainly HSV-2), eczema herpeticum (see chapter 23, Dermatologic conditions), herpetic whitlow and eye involvement. HSV encephalitis is an

important treatable condition that must not be missed (see p. 413 and chapter 33, Neurologic conditions, p. 461). Pneumonia and disseminated infection occur in the immunocompromised. Congenital infection also occurs. Infection can be primary (e.g. gingivostomatitis) or from a reactivation of the latent virus (e.g.cold sores).

Primary herpes gingivostomatitis

- *Transmission*: droplet, direct contact.
- *Incubation period*: 2–14 days
- *Infectious period*: indeterminate; virus can be excreted for at least 1 week, occasionally months. Shed intermittently with or without symptoms (including cold sores) for years afterwards.

Clinical features
Fever, irritability, cervical lymphadenopathy, halitosis, diffuse erythema and ulceration within the oral cavity (buccal mucosa, palate, gingiva and tongue) and mucocutaneous junction. Duration 7–14 days.

Diagnosis
Immunofluorescence or culture of vesicular scrapings.

Complications
Poor oral intake; autoinoculation resulting in herpetic whitlow, keratitis or genital herpes; eczema herpeticum; dissemination (particularly in immunocompromised).

Treatment
Symptomatic: topical anaesthesia (e.g. 1–2% lignocaine [lidocaine] gel, xylocaine viscous), analgesia (paracetamol), fluids and a soft diet. Aciclovir, valaciclovir or famciclovir should be considered if immunocompromised.

HSV in pregnancy
Primary infection during the first 20 weeks of gestation is associated with an increased risk of spontaneous abortion, stillbirth and congenital disease. Beyond 20 weeks, premature labour and growth retardation are more common. Primary infection after 34 weeks is associated with high rates of neonatal disease.

Neonatal HSV
Transmission

- *Intrapartum* (70–85%): perinatal acquisition from maternal genital tract; usually presents day 5–19.
- *Postnatal* (10%): usually presents day 5–19.
- *Intrauterine* (5%): transplacental; usually presents within 48 h of birth.

Transmission is 10 times more likely to occur with primary than with recurrent infection, both of which may be asymptomatic in women. More than 70% of women who give birth to infants with neonatal HSV infection give no history of genital HSV in themselves or their partners. The risk of infection to a baby of an asymptomatic woman with a history of recurrent genital herpes is <3%.

Clinical features
Neonatal infection presents in three ways:
- *Localised skin, eye and/or mouth ('SEM') disease* (45%). Onset 7–14 days. Death is rare; 30% or more of patients eventually develop evidence of neurological impairment.
- *CNS disease* (50%). Onset 14–21 days, in the form of encephalitis or a more disseminated disease. Mortality is 15%; 50–60% of survivors have psychomotor retardation, with or without microcephaly, spasticity, blindness, etc.
- *Disseminated disease* (20%). Onset 5–10 days. Involves any organ but primarily liver and adrenals; encephalitis occurs in 70% or more of patients. Presentation includes irritability, seizures, respiratory distress, jaundice, coagulopathy, shock and characteristic vesicular rash. *Note*: About 20% of babies never have skin lesions. Mortality is 50–60% (in spite of treatment) and neurological sequelae in 40%.

Diagnosis
Viral isolation from neonatal vesicular fluid, mouth or conjunctival swabs, stool, urine, leucocytes and maternal genital tract swabs. HSV antigens are detected by immunofluorescence. Serology is not always helpful, as maternally acquired IgG confounds interpretation in the neonate and IgM may not be produced until 2 weeks after the onset of illness. Detection of viral DNA by PCR (especially in CSF to detect subclinical CNS disease) is helpful. Changes on EEG, CT and MRI may all provide supporting evidence of HSV infection.

Complications
Overall mortality (following treatment) is 15–20% and 40–50% of infants have some neurological impairment.

Treatment
Aciclovir 20 mg/kg i.v. 8 hourly (see Antimicrobial guidelines, Appendix 3) for at least 14 days (SEM disease) or 21 days (CNS or disseminated disease). Suppressive treatment with aciclovir, for 6–12 months, should be considered for CNS or disseminated disease.

Prevention
20% of newborns born to women with primary HSV will be infected, even if delivered by Caesarean section.

HSV encephalitis
See Encephalitis, p. 413 and chapter 33, Neurologic conditions, p. 461.

Human herpes virus 6 (roseola infantum)

95% of children are infected with human herpes virus 6 (HHV-6) by the age of 2 years. Up to 30% will present with the clinical features of roseola. HHV-7 has also been shown to be the cause in a small number of children. HHV-6 infection may also present as an acute febrile illness without a rash.

- *Transmission*: direct contact/droplet (asymptomatically shed).
- *Incubation period*: 9–10 days.
- *Infectious period*: unknown (greatest during period of the rash).

Clinical features

Roseola: fever with occipital lymphadenopathy; then rapid defervescence corresponding with appearance of a red, maculopapular rash over trunk and arms lasting 1–2 days.
Note: Many children are started on antibiotics for the fever and then misdiagnosed as having a drug reaction when the rash appears.

Diagnosis

Investigations do not usually alter management, but serology and PCR are available.

Complications

Febrile convulsions (HHV-6 is thought to be the cause of up to 1/3 of febrile convulsions in children <2 years of age), aseptic meningitis, encephalitis (rare), hepatitis.

Treatment

Symptomatic.

Influenza virus

- *Cause*: influenza A or B virus.
- *Transmission*: direct contact/droplet.
- *Incubation period*: 1–4 days
- *Infectious period*: 3–7 days after onset of symptoms. Longer in immunocompromised.

Epidemiology

Continuous genetic re-assortment of influenza A viruses can lead to epidemics; the degree of cross-immunity from previously circulating strains and vaccines determines whether this occurs. Large-scale epidemics (pandemics) occur when there is no protection from previous exposure. Although the virus may cause disease at any time, seasonal epidemics occur during the winter months.

Clinical features

Variable. Severity of illness is dependent on partial immunity from previous exposure to related influenza viruses and vaccines. Asymptomatic infection occurs. Commonly presents with fever and rigors; respiratory symptoms including coryza, pharyngitis, cough, pneumonia, wheeze or croup; headache, myalgias, fatigue. Vomiting and diarrhoea are less common.

Complications

Important complications include bacterial superinfection with pneumonia (especially *S. aureus*), otitis media or sinusitis; neurological: encephalitis, meningitis, encephalopathy; myositis and cardiomyopathy. Death occurs in ~1% of hospitalised children.

Diagnosis

- Rapid diagnosis by immunofluorescence or PCR on respiratory specimens (nasal swab or NPA) may lead to early treatment.
- Viral culture is also important for epidemiology.

Control of case

Exclude from school until resolution of symptoms.

Treatment

- Neuraminidase inhibitors (zanamavir, oseltamivir) reduce the severity and length of illness by up to 36 h if started within 48 h, but earlier initiation is associated with the best outcome. **Routine treatment of influenza in immunocompetent patients is not recommended.**
- Neuraminidase inhibitors (oseltamivir ≥1 year of age, zanamavir ≥7 years of age) should be considered in children with laboratory-confirmed influenza, who are immunocompromised or who have chronic medical conditions.

Prevention

Vaccines can be used to prevent influenza in children.

- Trivalent inactivated intramuscular vaccine is ~65% protective against influenza and prevents ~30% of influenza-like illnesses, but efficacy varies from year to year. Annual vaccination with vaccine containing the most recent strains is necessary to provide continued protection. Two doses at least one month apart are recommended for children <9 years who are receiving influenza vaccine for the first time.
- Live attenuated vaccine is more effective (~79% protective) but is not yet available in Australia.

Neuraminidase inhibitors may be used to prevent influenza in children at risk of complications.

Measles virus (rubeola)

As a result of widespread measles immunisation, this disease is now seen infrequently. However, outbreaks continue to occur in most parts of the world.

- *Transmission*: droplet, direct contact.
- *Incubation period*: 7–18 days (usually 14 days) to the appearance of a rash.
- *Infectious period*: 1–2 days before the onset of symptoms to 4 days after the onset of the rash.

Clinical features

- *Prodrome*: fever, conjunctivitis, coryza, cough and Koplik spots (white spots on a bright red buccal mucosa).

- *Rash*: appears 3–4 days later; erythematous and blotchy; starts at hairline and moves down the body, then becomes confluent; lasts 4–7 days; may desquamate in the second week.

Diagnosis
Serology (IgM is usually detectable 1–2 days after onset of rash, and almost always 4 days after), immunofluorescence and culture or PCR on nasopharyngeal aspirate.

Complications
Otitis media (1/4), pneumonia (1/25), encephalitis (1/2000), subacute sclerosing panencephalitis (SSPE) (1/25 000).

Treatment
Symptomatic: vitamin A should be considered for young infants with severe measles, the immunocompromised and those with vitamin A deficiency.

Control of case
Exclude from school for at least 5 days from the appearance of the rash.

Contacts
- Measles, mumps, rubella (MMR) vaccine should be given within 72 h of exposure, to unimmunised children >9 months of age (another dose should be given at 12 months of age or 4 weeks after the first dose, whichever is the later).
- If MMR is contraindicated, or if >72 h since exposure, normal human immunoglobulin should be given i.m. within 7 days (see chapter 29, Haematologic conditions and oncology).
- Exclude from school for 2 weeks if unimmunised.

Parvovirus B19 (erythema infectiosum, slapped cheek disease, fifth disease)
- *Transmission*: droplet, direct contact.
- *Incubation period*: 4–21 days.
- *Infectious period*: highly infectious until rash appears (50% of adults are immune).

Clinical features
Fever in 15–30%; non-specific prodrome. The rash has three stages:
- *Slapped cheek appearance* (1–3 days).
- *Maculopapular rash*: on proximal extensor surfaces, flexor surfaces and trunk; fades over next few days, then central clearing, forming a reticular pattern (after 7 days).
- *Reticular rash*: reappears with heat, cold and friction (weeks/months).

Diagnosis
Mainly clinical. PCR on blood and serology.

Complications

Arthritis; aplastic crisis in children with chronic haemolytic anaemia; bone marrow suppression; fetal hydrops.

Treatment

Symptomatic.

Control of case

School exclusion is inappropriate as the patient is no longer infectious once the rash appears.

Contacts

Pregnant contacts should seek advice regarding the unlikely possibility of intrauterine infection as treatment of fetal infection may prevent sequelae.

Rubella virus

- *Transmission*: droplet, direct contact.
- *Incubation period*: 14–21 days.
- *Infectious period*: 5 days before to 7 days after rash.

Clinical features

- 25–50% have no symptoms.
- *Rash*: small, fine, discrete pink maculopapules; starts on face and spreads to chest and upper arms, abdomen and thighs, all within 24 h.
- *Prodrome*: (1–5 days) low-grade fever, malaise, headache, coryza, conjunctivitis (more common in adults), postauricular/occipital/posterior triangle lymphadenopathy precedes rash by 5–10 days.

Diagnosis

Serology.

Complications

Congenital rubella syndrome: >25% affected if mother infected during 1st trimester; 10–20% have single congenital defect if infection occurs at 16–40 days.

Control of case

Exclude from school for at least 5 days from the onset of the rash.

Contacts

Check serology if pregnant. Immunoglobulin given after exposure in early pregnancy may not prevent infection or viraemia, but may modify risk of abnormalities in the baby.

Varicella zoster virus (chickenpox, shingles)

- *Incubation period*: 10–21 days. Shorter incubation in the immunocompromised. Zoster immune globulin (ZIG) may prolong incubation to 28 days.

- *Infectious period*: 1–2 days before appearance of the rash until the rash is fully crusted.

Clinical features
Fever, irritability, anorexia and lymphadenopathy. A pruritic rash develops over the next 3–5 days, which progresses from maculopapular to vesicular, followed by crusting by 5–10 days. Lesions appear in crops with a central distribution. Affects scalp, face, trunk, mouth, conjunctivae and extremities.

Diagnosis
Clinical diagnosis is usually sufficient. Immunofluorescence and culture or PCR of vesicular scrapings, or serology.

Complications
Secondary bacterial infection of skin lesions (most commonly group A streptococcus or *S. aureus*) or bacterial pneumonia; neurological (cerebellitis, transverse myelitis, Guillain–Barré syndrome); dissemination (pneumonitis, hepatitis, encephalitis) in patients with abnormal T-cell immunity. Herpes zoster ('shingles'), resulting from a reactivation of the latent virus, is more common in children who have had chickenpox in infancy or who have been exposed *in utero*.

Treatment
- Aciclovir, famciclovir or valaciclovir in patients with impaired T-cell immunity. Antiviral treatment is **not** indicated in the immunocompetent child.
- Antibiotics for secondary bacterial skin infection (e.g. flucloxacillin).
- **Aspirin is contraindicated because of the association with Reye's syndrome.**
- Other NSAIDs (including ibuprofen) should be avoided because of possible increased risk of invasive group A streptococcal disease.
- Paracetamol can be used.

Prevention
ZIG within 96 h of exposure (6 mL for adults, 4 mL for children 6–12 years of age, 2 mL for children up to 5 years of age). Indicated in the following patients in contact with varicella (or direct contact with shingles):
- Immunocompromised children (e.g. HIV, immunosuppressive therapy (including high-dose steroids; prednisolone 2 mg/kg or more per day) and patients with transplants, lymphoma, leukaemia or severe combined immune deficiency).
- Newborn infants whose mothers have varicella onset from within 7 days before delivery to 2 days after delivery.
- Infants under 28 days of age with non-immune mothers exposed to varicella.
- Hospitalised premature infants with no maternal history of varicella.
- Hospitalised premature infants <28 weeks gestation or <1000 g, regardless of maternal history.

Varicella vaccine
See chapter 9, Immunisation.

Infectious diarrhoea

See also chapter 27, Gastrointestinal conditions.

Infectious diarrhoea continues to cause significant morbidity in children from developed and developing countries. In Australia, approximately 20 000 children (15/1000) <5 years of age are admitted to hospital each year with acute gastroenteritis. Rotavirus is the causal agent in up to 2/3 of hospitalised children where a pathogen is identified. Other important pathogens in hospitalised children include caliciviruses, enteric adenoviruses, astroviruses, *Salmonella* spp., *Campylobacter jejuni*, *Giardia intestinalis (lamblia)*, *Cryptosporidium parvum*, enteropathogenic (and other) *Escherichia coli*, *Shigella* spp. and *Yersinia enterocolitica*.

- Children <5 years of age with rotavirus-positive gastroenteritis are unlikely to have another pathogen isolated from their faeces.
- It is unusual to find a protozoal parasite in the setting of acute diarrhoea.
- Repeat stool investigations are not helpful except in patients with chronic diarrhoea, suspected *Salmonella* carriage or parasitic infection.
- The cause of infectious diarrhoea can often be identified by simple laboratory studies but rarely alters management.
- Most bacterial causes of diarrhoea are self-limiting and do not usually require antibiotic therapy, even if blood or mucus is present. As with viral gastroenteritis, the primary aim of treatment is to achieve and maintain adequate hydration. Antibiotics should be considered for the immunocompromised and neonates.
- Nosocomial infection is common. Hence, adequate infection control measures established by the hospital are essential in preventing spread.

Rotavirus

- *Incubation period*: illness usually begins 12 h–4 days after exposure.
- *Infectious period*: most children shed the virus in the stools for up to 10 days; however, about 1/3 with severe primary rotavirus infection continue shedding for >21 days.

Clinical features

Major cause of severe diarrhoea in children causing over 50% of hospitalisations for acute gastroenteritis in children <5 years. Also a common cause of nosocomial infection. Annual peak period of infection occurs in the winter–spring period. Presents with diarrhoea, vomiting (may precede diarrhoea) and fever lasting for up to 1 week. Respiratory symptoms are common. May be complicated by dehydration, electrolyte imbalance and acidosis.

- *Diagnosis*: enzyme immunoassay and latex agglutination assay.
- *Treatment*: supportive, with particular attention to hydration.
- *Vaccine*: two safe and efficacious rotavirus vaccines are available. There is reasonable evidence that intussusception is not associated with these new vaccines (a concern with previous vaccines).

Adenovirus

Similar presentation to rotavirus, but there is no seasonality. It is more common under 12 months of age. Diarrhoea and vomiting may last longer and high fever is less common.

Salmonella (non typhi)

Clinical features

Broad spectrum of clinical syndromes including asymptomatic carriage, gastroenteritis, bacteraemia and focal infections (e.g. bone and joint). Age-specific attack rates are highest in children <5 years of age (peak at <1 year of age) and the elderly. Invasive infections and mortality are more common in infants, the elderly and those with underlying diseases.

Diagnosis

Does not usually alter management, but serology and PCR are available.

Treatment

Antibiotic treatment is not usually indicated for uncomplicated gastroenteritis as it may prolong excretion. Antibiotic treatment is indicated for bacteraemia, systemic involvement or infection in infants <3 months of age, those with underlying disease (e.g. immunocompromised) and elderly people. The choice and duration of treatment depends on the clinical manifestation and antibiotic susceptibility.

Campylobacter jejuni

More common >5 years of age. Causes diarrhoea with visible or occult blood, abdominal pain, malaise and fever. Antibiotic treatment is not usually necessary, except in special circumstances where the elimination of the carrier state is important, such as infection in food handlers.

Giardia intestinalis (lamblia)

Transmission

The most common parasite identified in stool specimens from children. More common in children (and staff) in childcare centres and returned travellers. The major reservoir and means of spread is contaminated water and, to a lesser extent, food. Person-to-person spread also occurs.

Clinical features

There is a broad spectrum of clinical manifestations, but the most common are: diarrhoea (usually persistent), abdominal distension, flatulence, abdominal cramps and weight loss/failure to thrive.

Diagnosis

Confirmed by microscopy of stool specimens. These do not usually contain blood, mucus or leucocytes. Repeat specimens may be necessary.

Treatment

Metronidazole 30 mg/kg (max. 2 g) p.o. daily for 3 days **or** tinidazole 50 mg/kg (max. 2 g) p.o. as a single dose are effective treatments for symptomatic giardiasis.

Dientamoeba fragilis
Transmission

This parasite is thought to be transmitted with the eggs of *Enterobius vermicularis* (pinworm).

Clinical features

Symptoms include acute or chronic diarrhoea and abdominal pain, although many infected children are asymptomatic. May be associated with eosinophilia.

Treatment

May be treated with metronidazole (dose as above) although treatment is unnecessary in asymptomatic patients where the organism is found incidentally.

Escherichia coli

There are at least five categories of diarrhoea-producing *E. coli*:

- Enterohaemorrhagic *E. coli* (EHEC): haemolytic uraemic syndrome (HUS), haemorrhagic colitis.
- Enteropathogenic *E. coli* (EPEC): watery diarrhoea in children <2 years of age in developing countries.
- Enterotoxigenic *E. coli* (ETEC): the major cause of traveller's diarrhoea (usually self-limiting).
- Enteroinvasive *E. coli* (EIEC): usually watery diarrhoea, but may cause dysentery.
- Enteroaggregative *E. coli* (EAEC): chronic diarrhoea in infants and young children.

Antibiotic treatment is not usually indicated for diarrhoea caused by *E. coli* and may be associated with increased rates of HUS in EHEC infection.

Clostridium difficile
Transmission

Acquired from the environment or by faecal–oral transmission from a colonised host. Up to 50% of healthy neonates and infants <2 years of age are colonised, in contrast to 5% of those >2 years of age.

Clinical features

Rare cause of diarrhoea in those <12 months of age. Only clinically significant diarrhoea or colitis should be considered to be caused by *Clostridium difficile*. Pseudomembranous colitis usually occurs in patients on antibiotics (particularly penicillins, clindamycin and cephalosporins).

Treatment
- Cessation of antibiotics, **and**
- Oral metronidazole 7.5 mg/kg (max. 400 mg) p.o. 8 hourly for 10 days, **and**
- Consider probiotics – *Saccharomyces* spp. (baker's or brewer's yeast) or *Lactobacillus* spp.

Failure of treatment or recurrence may be due to reinfection, non-compliance, continued antibiotic use, or, rarely, a metronidazole-resistant organism. Options in this context include repeat metronidazole, oral vancomycin (not i.v.) or probiotics.

Enterobius vermicularis (threadworm, pinworm)

The most common worm infection in Australia. The highest rates of infection occurs in school-age children, followed by preschoolers. In some groups, nearly 50% of children are infected.

Transmission
Eggs survive up to 2 weeks on clothing, bedding or other objects. Eggs often remain under the fingernails. Reinfection by autoinfection is common. Infection often occurs in more than one family member.

Incubation period
At least 1–2 months from the ingestion of eggs until the adult female migrates to the perianal region to deposit eggs.

Infectious period
Eggs are infective within a few hours of being deposited on the perianal skin.

Clinical features
Causes pruritus ani and vulvae.

Diagnosis
Visualisation of worms in the perianal region (at night) or microscopy of eggs collected on sticky tape briefly applied to perianal skin in the morning.

Treatment
Mebendazole 50 mg (<10 kg), 100 mg (>10 kg) p.o. (not in pregnancy or in those <6 months of age) or pyrantel 10 mg/kg (max. 750 mg) p.o. as a single dose, followed by a second dose 2 weeks later. All family members should be treated.

Hepatitis

See also chapter 27, Gastrointestinal conditions.

Hepatitis A
Hepatitis A virus (HAV) is the most common viral hepatitis; it is particularly prevalent in developing countries.
- *Transmission*: faecal–oral route.
- *Incubation period*: usually about 4 weeks (2–7 weeks).

- *Infectious period*: viral shedding lasts 1–3 weeks; the highest titres in stool occur 1–2 weeks before the onset of illness, corresponding to the highest risk of transmission; lowest risk after onset of jaundice.

Clinical features
Usually an acute self-limited illness; mild, non-specific symptoms without jaundice in infants and preschoolers; fever, malaise, jaundice, anorexia and nausea in older children and adults.

Complications
Relapse (unusual), fulminant hepatitis (rare).

Diagnosis
Serology for HAV-specific IgM and IgG.

Treatment
Supportive.

Control of case
Children should be excluded from childcare or school for 7 days from the onset of illness, although the virus is excreted for many weeks.

Prevention
Inactivated HAV vaccine is recommended for travellers to endemic areas and patients with chronic liver disease (e.g. hepatitis B or C infection) or transfusion dependent illness.

Hepatitis B
Hepatitis B virus (HBV) infection is endemic worldwide. The prevalence of HBV and carriage rates vary in different parts of the world. The carriage rate is about 0.2% in Australians of European origin, and >10% in some indigenous populations. Rates are highest in those born in Asian or Mediterranean countries.

Transmission
Blood or body fluids that are HBsAg positive; vertical transmission occurs in infants born to HBsAg-positive mothers; there is a high risk of horizontal transmission in the first 5 years of life.
- *Incubation period*: 7 weeks–6 months.
- *Infectious period*: from several weeks before the onset until documented clearance of virus.

Clinical features
Symptomatic acute hepatitis (jaundice, anorexia, malaise and nausea) in adults; usually asymptomatic in young children, particularly in those <1 year of age.

Complications

The carrier state is associated with 25% mortality from hepatocellular carcinoma or chronic liver disease; lifelong follow-up is indicated. Those infected as infants or young children are more likely to become carriers and develop fatal complications as adults: 70–90% of infants infected at birth become chronic HBV carriers (particularly if the mother is HBeAg positive), in contrast to only 5% of adults. The remainder eliminate the virus and have no long-term effects.

Diagnosis

Test for:

- HBsAg (active disease).
- HBsAb (protection by vaccine or natural infection).
- HBeAg or HBV PCR (increased infectivity and risk of sequelae).
- HBcAb (past or present HBV infection).

Treatment

No specific therapy for HBV is available; α-interferon and nucleoside analogues may resolve chronic infection but are less effective if infection is acquired during childhood. Hepatitis A vaccination is recommended.

Prevention

- In Australia, recombinant HBV vaccine is currently recommended for all infants from birth, pre-adolescents, as well as those at high risk. Infants born to HBsAg-positive mothers should be given HBV-specific immunoglobulin plus a full course of HBV vaccination. They should be tested at 12–18 months with HBsAg and HBsAb.
- See needle-stick injuries (p. 419) for management of exposure to infected blood or body fluid.

Hepatitis C

Hepatitis C virus (HCV) causes acute and chronic hepatitis. The carriage rate is about 0.3% in apparently healthy new blood donors in Australia, but this probably underestimates the prevalence in the population, which may be around 1%.

Transmission

Parenteral exposure to HCV-infected blood and blood products; vertical transmission occurs from about 6% of HCV-positive mothers (higher if the mother is co-infected with HIV). Avoid use of fetal scalp electrodes; breast-feeding is not contraindicated but temporary avoidance is recommended if bleeding or cracked nipples; sexual transmission is rare.

- *Incubation period*: 6–7 weeks (range 2 weeks–6 months).
- *Clinical features*: mild, insidious hepatitis; usually asymptomatic in children.
- *Complications*: persistent infection in >85% (most children with chronic infection are asymptomatic); 65–70% develop chronic hepatitis, 20% develop cirrhosis. Uncommonly, hepatocellular carcinoma can develop in the absence of chronic hepatitis.
- *Diagnosis*: current or past infection is detected by serology (anti-HCV antibodies); current infection is confirmed by PCR for HCV RNA.

- Treatment:
  - Patients must be screened for chronic hepatitis, cirrhosis and hepatocellular carcinoma.
  - Optimal treatment regimens are under investigation. Hepatitis A and B vaccination is recommended.

Hepatitis E

Hepatitis E virus (HEV) is an uncommon cause of hepatitis, which occurs predominantly in tropical countries, especially in parts of India. Cases have been reported in travellers returning from these regions.

- *Transmission*: faecal–oral route, by contamination of water.
- *Incubation period*: 2–10 weeks.
- *Infectious period*: excreted in stool for 2 weeks after the onset of symptoms.
- *Clinical features*:
  - Similar to HAV infection. Most infected children have asymptomatic infection or mild gastrointestinal symptoms.
  - Mortality is rare, except in pregnant women.
- *Diagnosis*:
  - HEV-specific IgM.
  - PCR of stool and serum.
- *Prevention*: food and water safety in endemic countries.

Bacterial meningitis
Bacterial meningitis is a medical emergency.

Clinical features

- In infants, non-specific e.g. fever, lethargy, irritability or vomiting.
- In older children, headache, vomiting, drowsiness, photophobia and neck stiffness may be present. Kernig sign (inability to extend the knee when the leg is flexed at the hip) and Brudzinski sign (bending the head forward produces flexion of the legs) may be positive.

Diagnosis

Diagnosis is confirmed by examination of the cerebrospinal fluid (CSF), unless lumbar puncture (LP) is contraindicated (see chapter 3, Procedures). If LP is deferred or reveals no organism, identification of the pathogen may still be possible through:

- Blood cultures – often positive.
- PCR on blood or CSF for enterovirus, HSV and other viruses, TB, *N. meningitidis and S. pneumoniae*.
- Blood smear for Gram stain.
- Skin scraping or aspirate of purpuric lesions for *N. meningitidis* on Gram stain, PCR or (less likely) culture.
- Throat swab.

Antibiotics must be given immediately after the collection of appropriate cultures, but should not be delayed if the LP is to be deferred. Antibiotics should be rationalised to more specific treatment based only on *final* CSF or blood culture results.

Interpretation of cerebrospinal fluid findings

CSF findings should always be interpreted in the light of the clinical setting (see Table 30.2).

Cell count

- **Perform microscopy without delay**. Cell lysis begins shortly after collection: neutrophils may decrease by up to 1/3 after 1 h and by 1/2 after 3 h (lymphocytes may decrease by ~10% after 2 h).
- Macroscopic appearance of CSF may be misleading: $200–500 \times 10^6$/L cells are required before CSF appears cloudy to the naked eye.
- In early bacterial meningitis there may be no increase in the CSF cell count.
- CSF contaminated by blood can be difficult to interpret. There is no reliable rule to correct for red blood cells (RBC) in CSF, although a ratio of one white blood cell to 500–700 red blood cells is sometimes used. Similarly, 0.01 g/L protein for every 1000 RBCs may be allowable. It is safer to be cautious and interpret the CSF as if it has *not* been contaminated with blood.
- Even in bacterial meningitis, the CSF cell count may remain normal in up to 4% of young infants and up to 17% of neonates.
- Presence of neutrophils in the CSF should always raise concern (except in neonates, see Table 30.2).
- In early viral (typically enteroviral) meningitis, the CSF findings can mimic bacterial meningitis with a neutrophil predominance. This shifts to a lymphocytic picture after 6–8 h.
- In bacterial meningitis there can be a shift to a lymphocyte predominance after 48 h of therapy.
- *Listeria* infection is associated with a lower neutrophil rise than other causes of bacterial meningitis.
- Gram stain may be negative in up to 60% of cases of bacterial meningitis even without prior antibiotics.
- Antibiotics usually prevent the culture of bacteria from the CSF, but they do not significantly alter the CSF cell count nor biochemistry in samples taken early. In 'partially treated meningitis' the CSF should be interpreted like any other CSF.
- Seizures do *not* cause an increased CSF cell count.
- In neonates, interpretation of CSF may be difficult. Normal values for CSF cell counts and biochemistry differ from those of older infants (typically they have higher cell count and protein and lower glucose, particularly in premature neonates) (see Table 30.2).

Biochemistry

- CSF protein is normal in about 40% of school-age children with bacterial meningitis.
- CSF glucose is normal in about 1/2 of school-age children with bacterial meningitis.

Table 30.2 Classical cerebrospinal fluid (CSF) findings

	Neutrophils (× 10⁶/L)	Lymphocytes (× 10⁶/L)	Protein (g/L)	Glucose (CSF:blood ratio)
Normal (>1 month of age)	0	≤5	<0.4	≥0.6 (or ≥2.5 mmol/L)
Normal term neonate	Higher than for older infant/child	<20–30	Higher than for older infant/child usually <1	Lower than for older infant/child
Bacterial meningitis	100–10 000 (but counts may be normal)	Usually <100	>1.0 (but protein may be normal)	<0.4 (but glucose may be normal)
Viral meningitis	Usually <100	10–1000 (but counts may be normal)	0.4–1 (but protein may be normal)	Usually normal
TB meningitis	Usually <100	50–1000 (but counts may be normal)	1–5 (but protein may be normal)	<0.3 (but glucose may be normal)
Encephalitis	Usually <100		0.4–1 (but protein may be normal)	Usually normal
Brain abscess	Usually 5–100		>1 (but protein may be normal)	Usually normal

- CSF glucose may be decreased in mumps meningitis and lymphocytic choriomeningitis, as well as in bacterial and TB meningitis.

Adjunctive steroid treatment of meningitis
- There is now sufficient evidence to recommend the routine use of adjunctive steroid therapy for bacterial meningitis in children >4 weeks old, as this can reduce the risk of hearing loss.
- Steroids are recommended at the time of LP where there is a strong clinical suspicion of meningitis.
- Antibiotics should not be delayed for >30 min to enable administration of steroids.
  - *Initial dose*: dexamethasone 0.15 mg/kg i.v. ideally given 15 min before, but up to 1 h after, the first dose of antibiotics.
  - *Ongoing dose*: dexamethasone 0.15 mg/kg i.v. 6 hourly should be continued for 4 days (unless bacterial meningitis has been excluded).

Antibiotic treatment of meningitis
Age >2 months
The incidence of bacterial meningitis has fallen dramatically since the introduction of conjugated *Haemophilus influenzae* type b (Hib) vaccine. The major pathogens are now *Streptococcus pneumoniae* and *Neisseria meningitidis*.

Penicillin (and cephalosporin)-resistant pneumococci (PRP) are an increasing problem worldwide. Local patterns of resistance dictate treatment.

- *Initial therapy*: cefotaxime 50 mg/kg (max. 2 g) i.v. 6 hourly.
- In areas with a significantly high incidence of PRP, or when PRP are suspected, vancomycin 15 mg/kg (max. 500 mg) i.v. 6 hourly should be added to a third generation cephalosporin as empiric therapy.
- *Continued therapy*: antibiotic treatment is adjusted according to culture and sensitivity results to complete (i.v. therapy):
  - 7 days for *N. meningitidis*.
  - 10 days for *S. pneumoniae*.
  - 7–10 days for Hib.
- If there is prolonged or secondary fever, or where sensitivity testing indicates the pneumococcal isolate has reduced susceptibility to third-generation cephalosporins, LP should be repeated to detect treatment failure, and CT brain should be considered, looking for abscess or empyema formation.
- For sensitive *S. pneumoniae* or *N. meningitidis*: benzylpenicillin 60 mg/kg (max. 2 g) i.v. 4 hourly, or amoxicillin 50 mg/kg (max. 2 g) i.v. 4 hourly, or continue with cefotaxime.

Age <2 months
The organisms responsible for meningitis in this age group can be either neonatal pathogens (e.g. group B streptococcus (GBS), *Escherichia coli* and other enteric Gram negatives, and *Listeria monocytogenes*), or those more commonly detected in older children (e.g. *Streptococcus pneumoniae*, *Neisseria meningitidis*, Hib).

- *Initial therapy*: i.v. benzylpenicillin, cefotaxime and gentamicin (see Antimicrobial guidelines, Appendix 3).
- *Continued therapy*: treatment is adjusted according to culture and sensitivity results. Gentamicin is used for its synergistic action with penicillin for the treatment of GBS and *Listeria* meningitis. Therapy should be continued for:
  - 2–3 weeks in GBS and *Listeria* meningitis
  - At least 3 weeks in Gram-negative coliform meningitis.

Meningitis associated with shunts, neurosurgery, head trauma and CSF leak
In addition to the organisms discussed above, meningitis in these circumstances can be caused by *Staphylococcus aureus*, coagulase negative staphylococci and (with a ventriculo-peritoneal shunt *in situ*) Gram-negative bacilli including *Pseudomonas aeruginosa*.

- *Initial therapy*: vancomycin 15 mg/kg (max. 500 mg) i.v. 6 hourly **plus**:
  - (with ventriculo-peritoneal shunt) ceftazidime 50 mg/kg (max. 2 g) i.v. 8 hourly
  - (without ventriculo-peritoneal shunt) cefotaxime, 50 mg/kg (max. 2 g) i.v. 6 hourly

Antibiotic prophylaxis for contacts of meningitis cases
See Table 30.3.

General measures
Requirement for intensive care
Admission to ICU should be discussed with a specialist in the following circumstances:
- Age <2 years.
- Coma.
- Cardiovascular compromise.
- Intractable seizures.
- Hyponatraemia.

Fluid management
Careful fluid management is important in the treatment of meningitis as many children develop the syndrome of 'inappropriately' increased antidiuretic hormone secretion (SIADH). The degree of fluid restriction varies with each patient according to their clinical state. Hypovolaemia should be corrected with 10 mL/kg of normal saline repeated as required. A patient who is not in shock and has a normal serum sodium should usually be given 50% maintenance fluid requirements as initial management. If the serum sodium is <135 mmol/L give 25–50% of maintenance requirements. Serum sodium should be measured every 6–12 h for the first 48 h and the total fluid intake adjusted accordingly.

Observations
Neurological observations and blood pressure should be done every 15 min for the first 2 h and then at intervals determined by the child's conscious state. Head circumference should be monitored daily. Weight is measured daily or more frequently if required.

Seizures
Hypoglycaemia, electrolyte imbalance (especially hyponatraemia) and raised intracranial pressure should be excluded before attributing seizures to the underlying infection or febrile convulsion. Control of seizures is vital and specialist consultation is advised.

Analgesia
Ensure adequate analgesia; children in the recovery phase may have significant headache.

Fever persisting for >7 days
May be due to nosocomial infection, subdural effusion or other foci of suppuration. Uncommon causes include inadequately treated meningitis, a parameningeal focus or drugs.

Outcome/follow-up
All patients require a hearing assessment 6–8 weeks after discharge, or sooner if hearing loss is suspected.

More than 1/4 survivors have mild disabilities that adversely affect school performance and behaviour. Consequently, all children surviving bacterial meningitis should be regularly

Table 30.3 Prophylaxis regimens for contacts of meningitis cases

Organism	Antibiotic	Those requiring prophylaxis
Haemophilus influenzae type b	Rifampicin 20 mg/kg (max 600 mg) p.o. daily for 4 days *Infants <1 month of age*: Rifampicin 10 mg/kg p.o. daily for 4 days *Pregnancy/contraindication to rifampicin*: Ceftriaxone 250 mg i.m. daily for 2 days	• Index case and all household contacts if household includes other children <4 years of age who are not fully immunised. • Index case and all household contacts in households with any infants <12 months of age, regardless of immunisation status. • Index case and all household contacts in households with a child 1–5 years of age who is inadequately immunised. • Index case and all room contacts, including staff, in a childcare group if index case attends >18 h/week and any contacts <2 years of age who are inadequately immunised. • **AND** children who are not up to date with Hib should be immunised.
Neisseria meningitidis	Rifampicin 10 mg/kg (max 600 mg) p.o. 12-hourly for 2 days *Infants <1 month of age*: Rifampicin 5 mg/kg p.o. 12-hourly for 2 days *Pregnancy/contraindication to rifampicin*: Ceftriaxone 250 mg (>12 y) or 125 mg (<12 y) i.m. as a single dose *or* Ciprofloxacin 500 mg (>12 y) or 250 mg (6–11 y) p.o. as a single dose	• Index case (if treated only with penicillin) and all intimate household or day care contacts who have been exposed to index case within 10 days of onset. • Any person who gave mouth-to-mouth resuscitation to the index case.
Streptococcus pneumoniae	Nil	• No increased risk to contacts.

Notes:
• It is important that rifampicin is given early to both the index case and contacts, especially for *N. meningitidis* disease, because of the rapidity with which secondary cases may develop.
• As prophylaxis is not infallible, any febrile household contact should seek urgent medical attention.
• Nasopharyngeal carriage of Hib is not eradicated by a single injection of ceftriaxone.
• Rifampicin interferes with the metabolism of several medications, including the oral contraceptive pill (alternative contraception should be instituted), anticonvulsants, warfarin and chloramphenicol.
• Rifampicin colours body fluids red, e.g. urine, saliva, tears (soft contact lenses may be damaged), sweat, etc.

reviewed during their early school years. Less common sequelae include epilepsy, visual impairment and cerebral palsy.

Prevention
Many cases of meningitis are now preventable. All parents should be encouraged to have their children fully immunised (see chapter 9, Immunisation).

Other CNS infections
Viral meningitis
The most common causes of viral meningitis or meningoencephalitis are enteroviruses (Coxsackie and echoviruses) and HHV-6 (see p. 396). Most cases are self-limiting; however, their clinical presentation can mimic bacterial meningitis. Enterovirus may be isolated from throat swabs and stools, and PCR of the CSF may be positive. Treatment is symptomatic except in the rare instance of infection in the immunocompromised where i.v. immunoglobulin (IVIG) may be used. Positive enteroviral PCR on CSF in a child with a consistent clinical presentation can allow for early cessation of antibiotics and discharge from hospital.

Tuberculous meningitis
Tuberculous meningitis is uncommon in Australia. It often presents in an insidious manner and can be difficult to recognise. Large volumes of CSF are required (at least 10 mL) for diagnosis by microscopy and culture of mycobacteria, or mycobacterial PCR (which is not necessarily more sensitive). Treatment with combination antitubercular antibiotics plus corticosteroids should be started early and requires specialist advice.

Encephalitis
Encephalitis is most commonly caused by HSV-1 or 2, EBV, VZV, enterovirus, adenovirus, influenza virus or *Mycoplasma pneumoniae*. Encephalitis usually presents with one or more of the following: fever, headache, vomiting, change of behaviour, drowsiness, convulsions (particularly focal), focal neurological deficits and signs of raised intracranial pressure. CSF findings are non-specific (see Table 30.2). CT or MRI of the brain and EEG may be more helpful.

The recognition of herpes encephalitis is critical because treatment with aciclovir is indicated. Focal seizures and neurological signs are more typical of herpes encephalitis but clinical presentation, especially early in the disease, is not specific to a particular pathogen. Therefore, any child with encephalitis of an uncertain cause should be started on i.v. aciclovir (see Antimicrobial guidelines, Appendix 3). If the patient does not regain consciousness over a short period of time, i.v. aciclovir should be continued until:
- An alternative diagnosis is reached; **or**
- Herpes encephalitis is excluded by:
  - Absence of typical clinical features.
  - Normal serial MRI scans.
  - Normal serial EEG.

- Negative PCR for HSV on CSF obtained >72 h into the illness (this may necessitate a repeat LP).

Macrolides (e.g. azithromycin) are sometimes used in encephalitis due to *M. pneumoniae* but their benefit is uncertain.

Brain abscess

Brain abscess classically presents with fever, headache and focal neurological deficit. Although it is rare, early recognition is important because most cases are readily treated and delayed diagnosis can be disastrous. Diagnosis is by brain CT or MRI. Empiric treatment to cover the major aetiological pathogens is flucloxacillin 50 mg/kg (max. 2 g) i.v. 4 hourly, cefotaxime 50 mg/kg (max. 2 g) i.v. 6 hourly **and** metronidazole 15 mg/kg (max. 1 g) i.v. stat, then 7.5 mg/kg (max. 500 mg) i.v. 8 hourly (see Antimicrobial guidelines). Aspiration for diagnosis or neurosurgical intervention is usually necessary.

Kawasaki disease

Kawasaki disease (KD) is a systemic vasculitis that predominantly affects children under 5 years of age. Although the specific causal agent remains unknown, it is believed that KD is initiated by an infectious agent, although it is not transmitted from person to person. Early recognition and treatment are essential to reduce the risk of life-threatening complications.

Diagnosis

Diagnosis is often delayed because the features are similar to those of many viral exanthems. The diagnostic criteria for KD are:

- Fever for 5 days or more; **plus**
- Four of the following five features:
  - Polymorphous rash.
  - Bilateral (non-purulent) conjunctivitis.
  - Mucous membrane changes; e.g. reddened or dry cracked lips, strawberry tongue, or a diffuse redness of oral or pharyngeal mucosa.
  - Peripheral changes; e.g. erythema of the palms or soles, oedema of the hands or feet and desquamation *in convalescence*, particularly involving skin of hands, feet or perineal region.
  - Cervical lymphadenopathy (>15 mm in diameter, usually unilateral, single, non-purulent and painful).
- Exclusion of diseases with a similar presentation: staphylococcal infection (e.g. scalded skin syndrome and toxic shock syndrome), streptococcal infection (e.g. scarlet fever and toxic shock-like syndrome, but not just isolation from throat), measles, adenovirus and other viral exanthems, leptospirosis, rickettsial disease, Stevens–Johnson syndrome, drug reaction and juvenile chronic arthritis.

The diagnostic features of KD can occur sequentially and may not all be present at the same time. *Note*: that these children are **frequently inconsolably irritable**.

Particular clinical vigilance is needed to recognise patients with 'incomplete' or 'atypical' KD. Such patients do not fulfil the formal diagnostic criteria, but are still at risk of developing coronary artery aneurysms. Other relatively common features include arthritis, diarrhoea and vomiting, coryza and cough, and hydropic gallbladder.

Investigations
Laboratory features may include neutrophilia, raised erythrocyte sedimentation rate (ESR) and C-reactive protein (CRP), mild normochromic, normocytic anaemia, raised transaminases, hypoalbuminaemia and marked thrombocytosis in the second week.

Complications
Up to 30% of untreated children develop coronary artery dilation or aneurysm formation. This can occur up to 6–8 weeks after the onset of the illness. Echocardiography should therefore be done at least twice: at presentation and, if negative, again at 6–8 weeks to exclude coronary artery involvement. Coronary artery aneurysms can be associated with severe early ischaemic heart disease.

Management
Management includes early (preferably within the first 10 days of the illness) administration of IVIG (single dose of 2 g/kg i.v. over 10 h) and aspirin (3–5 mg/kg p.o. once a day (anti-platelet dose) for at least 6–8 weeks; maximum dose 150 mg). There is no evidence that using high (anti-inflammatory) dose aspirin decreases the risk of aneurysm development over and above that prevented by IVIG. However, some guidelines suggest using high dose aspirin (10 mg/kg p.o. 8 hourly) until defervescence. Paracetamol can be used for symptomatic relief.

A repeat dose of IVIG (2 g/kg) should be given to patients who fail to defervesce within 24 h after the completion of the first dose. Refractory cases with continuing fever and other signs of inflammation subsequent to this need specialist advice for further treatment that may include high-dose steroids (e.g. methylprednisolone 30 mg/kg i.v.).

Treatment with IVIG is highly effective in preventing the potentially devastating complication of coronary artery involvement. Treatment should still be undertaken in patients presenting after 10 days of illness if they have evidence of ongoing inflammation (fever, raised acute phase markers).

Cervical lymphadenitis
This is usually caused by an infection or inflammation of the lymph nodes. Malignancy is much less common.

Infectious causes
Acute bilateral lymphadenitis
- Viral upper respiratory tract infections.
- Systemic viral infections (e.g. EBV and CMV: may have generalised lymphadenopathy and hepatosplenomegaly).

- Kawasaki disease: may present initially as cervical lymphadenitis alone (see p. 414 above).

Acute unilateral lymphadenitis
- Group A streptococcus or *Staphylococcus aureus*: 40–80% of acute unilateral lymphadenitis; occurs at 1–4 years of age; fever, tenderness, overlying erythema; may be associated with cellulitis.
- Anaerobic bacteria: older children with dental caries or periodontal disease.
- Group B streptococcus may have overlying cellulitis (neonates).

Subacute/chronic unilateral lymphadenitis
- *Bartonella henselae* (cat-scratch disease): occurs about 2 weeks after a scratch or lick from a kitten or dog, usually involves axillary nodes, tender nodes; there may be a papule at infection site.
- *Mycobacterium avium complex* (MAC – formerly known as MAIS): patient usually 1–4 years of age, afebrile, systemically well and not immunocompromised; node usually unilateral, slightly fluctuant, non-tender, sometimes tethered to underlying structures and with violaceous hue to overlying skin.
- *Toxoplasma gondii*: systemic features (fatigue, myalgia), there may be generalised lymphadenopathy.
- *Mycobacterium tuberculosis*: usually a contact history; affects older children; systemic symptoms (e.g. fever, malaise, weight loss), non-tender nodes.
- HIV.

Management
Acute bilateral lymphadenitis without other signs (e.g. pallor, bruising or hepatosplenomegaly) is usually of viral cause and needs no specific treatment or investigation. Acute unilateral lymphadenitis with a fluctuant node needs incision and drainage (contra-indicated in suspected TB as may result in sinus formation). Otherwise, acute unilateral lymphadenitis is treated with oral flucloxacillin 25 mg/kg (max. 500 mg) p.o. 6 hourly for 10 days (see Antimicrobial guidelines, Appendix 3), with review in 48 h.

Cellulitis
Clinical features
- An infection of cutaneous and subcutaneous tissue characterised by erythema, warmth, oedema and tenderness.
- Predisposing factors include a break in the skin (e.g. insect bite, trauma) or a pre-existing skin lesion.
- May be associated with regional lymphadenopathy, fever, chills and malaise.
- It may be associated with deeper involvement including necrotising fasciitis, osteomyelitis and septic arthritis.
- Usually caused by *Streptococcus pyogenes* or *Staphylococcus aureus*.

- *Haemophilus influenzae* type b (Hib) is uncommon but should be considered in non-immunised children <5 years. It is often accompanied by bacteraemia or meningitis, or both.

Diagnosis

Cultures of blood, skin aspirate or skin biopsy are positive in about 25% of cases.

Management

- Flucloxacillin 25 mg/kg (max. 500 mg) p.o. 6 hourly.
- Parenteral therapy is needed if there is fever, rapid progression, lymphangitis or lymphadenitis. Non-immunised children <5 years with facial cellulitis should be treated with cefotaxime 50 mg/kg (max. 2 g) i.v. 6 hourly, **and** flucloxacillin.

Toxin-mediated disease

Gram-positive bacteria (group A β-haemolytic streptococci and *Staphylococcus aureus*) can cause disease as a result of production of protein (superantigen) toxins.

Clinical features

Fever, erythematous rash, conjunctivitis, reddened mucous membranes, strawberry tongue and prolonged capillary refill time. A range of clinical presentations may be seen. At the most severe end of the spectrum, capillary leak leads to hypotension, shock and multi-organ failure (toxic shock syndrome).

This condition may also be associated with the use of tampons and specific information should be sought.

Diagnosis

Early diagnosis depends on recognition of clinical features. Culture results may help to confirm the diagnosis later.

Management

A critical part of early management is to remove any possible focus of infection (including retained tampon if appropriate).

Early recognition of shock with appropriate fluid management and intensive care is important. Antibiotics should include an anti-staphylococcal agent (e.g. flucloxacillin 50 mg/kg (max. 2 g) i.v. 4 h, see Antimicrobial guidelines). Treatment should also include clindamycin (to inhibit bacterial toxin and host cytokine production) and i.v. immunoglobulin (as an immunomodulatory agent).

HIV infection and AIDS
Cause

Acquired immunodeficiency syndrome (AIDS) is caused by human immunodeficiency virus (HIV).

Transmission

Perinatal (vertical) transmission is the most common mechanism of paediatric HIV infection.

Incubation period

It is important to distinguish between infection with HIV, which may be asymptomatic during a variable latent period, and the progressive immunological derangement that leads to AIDS. Perinatally infected infants may be asymptomatic for several months or years.

Risk groups

- Infants of mothers who are known to be HIV positive or who are members of a high-risk group (e.g. sex workers, i.v. drug users and those with bisexual partners).
- I.v. drug users.
- Men who have sex with men.
- Sexual contacts (including sexually abused children) of individuals with HIV.
- Transfusion recipients, particularly patients with congenital bleeding disorders who received blood products before 1985.
- Individuals from countries with a high prevalence of HIV infection.

Clinical features

Clinical presentations of HIV infection include prolonged fever, failure to thrive or weight loss, generalised lymphadenopathy, hepatosplenomegaly, parotitis, chronic or recurrent diarrhoea, recurrent otitis, chronic candidiasis and chronic eczematous rash.

The indicator diseases for the diagnosis of AIDS in children include candidiasis, lymphoid interstitial pneumonitis, recurrent episodes of serious bacterial infection, opportunistic infection (e.g. *Pneumocystis carinii* pneumonia and disseminated *Mycobacterium avium complex* disease), CMV retinitis, cerebral toxoplasmosis, progressive neurological disease and malignancy (e.g. primary brain lymphoma).

Diagnosis

Patients (± their families) require counselling and informed consent before testing for HIV, which should be done on a confidential basis. Specific antibody detection is a sensitive indicator of HIV infection in adults and children, but passively transferred maternal antibodies may persist for up to 18 months in infants. Prior to 18 months, ultrasensitive HIV PCR is the best available test to confirm the diagnosis of HIV infection. The disease is monitored using a combination of CD4+ T-cell count and quantification of HIV RNA (viral load). Patients may also have lymphopaenia, abnormal T-cell subsets and hypergammaglobulinaemia.

Management

A multidisciplinary approach by a specialised team is vital for the unique needs of these patients and their families. Medical management of HIV-positive patients includes:
- Antiretroviral drugs (highly active antiretroviral treatment, HAART).

- Prevention of opportunistic and other infections (immunisation and prophylactic antimicrobials).
- The early diagnosis and aggressive management of opportunistic infections.

Control

Antiretroviral therapy given to the HIV-infected woman during pregnancy and delivery, and to the newborn, complete avoidance of breast-feeding (where formula Is available and safe) and with other measures can decrease the rate of transmission to the child from 25–35% to <2%. Recognition of HIV-infected pregnant women is therefore critical.

Antiretroviral therapy and other interventions (e.g. immunisation, *Pneumocystis* prophylaxis) can have a significant impact on disease progression.

Needle-stick injuries
Community acquired needle-stick injurles

The risk of seroconversion to HIV, HBV or HCV from a community-acquired needle-stick injury is very low. Exposed individuals should be reassured. Immunity to hepatitis B should be confirmed, and if incomplete, hepatitis B vaccine should be given. Unless the injury is considered to be particularly high risk, no further management is required at the time. Follow-up should be arranged for counselling and serology if required. Tetanus toxoid ± immunoglobulin should be considered.

Occupational needle-stick injuries
Standard precautions

- All sharp objects and body fluids should be considered as potentially contaminated.
- Avoid contact with blood and other body fluids by:
  - Using protective barriers (e.g. gloves) if contact is likely.
  - Immediately cleaning up accidental spills.

Managing needle-stick injury or exposure to blood/blood-stained body fluid

- Squeeze the puncture wound.
- Wash blood off the skin with soap and water.
- Rinse blood from the eyes and mouth with running water.
- Document the date and time of exposure, details of incident, names of the source and exposed individuals.
- Inform source individual of exposure.
- Assess the risk of HIV, HBV and HCV in the source individual (see below).
- If indicated, test known source for HBV surface antigen (HBsAg), HCV antibody (anti-HCV Ab) and antibodies to HIV-1 and HIV-2 (HIV Abs). Obtain consent from the source individual.
- Even if the source individual is not infected with a blood-borne pathogen, storage of a serum specimen from the exposed person is recommended.
- Follow-up should be arranged for counselling (of the exposed person).

Medicine and Surgery

Table 30.4 Evaluation of needle-stick injury sources

High risk of HIV and HBV	High risk of HCV
• Unsafe sex, particularly with multiple (or homosexual) partners • Intravenous drug users (IVDU) (particularly if they share equipment) and their sexual partners • Family members of an infected person • Individuals from communities with high HIV prevalence	• Recipients of blood products prior to 1985 • IVDU past or current (particularly if they share equipment)

Table 30.5 Management of needle-stick injury

Exposure	Virus	Bloods to take from the exposed individual	Bloods to take from the source individual	What to give the exposed individual
High-risk	Hepatitis B	Anti-HBsAb (urgent)	HBsAg (urgent)	*HBV immune*: Nil *HBV non-immune*: • Source HBsAg positive/unknown ⇒ HBV immunoglobulin (*within 48 h*)* + HBV vaccine • Source HBsAg negative ⇒ HBV vaccine
	Hepatitis C	ALT + hold serum	Anti-HCV Ab (urgent)	Nil
	HIV	Hold serum	HIV Ab (urgent)	HIV prophylaxis† if source is HIV positive and/or risk of transmission is significant
Low-risk	All viruses	Anti-HBsAb (if unsure of HBsAg immunity) Hold serum		*HBV immune*: Nil *HBV non-immune*: HBV vaccine

* HBV immunoglobulin should be given as soon as possible, but can be deferred for 48 h, while awaiting results of serology to confirm affected individual's immunity (when checking whether a vaccinated individual has maintained immunity or whether the individual is immune from previous infection).
† Urgent expert advice should be sought.

- Give HBV-specific immunoglobulin ± HBV vaccine if appropriate (see Tables 30.4, 30.5).
- HIV post-exposure prophylaxis is only required if source is HIV Ab positive, or if the source is unknown and HIV is considered likely.

Assessing risk

A significant exposure is considered to have occurred if there has been:

- An injection of blood/body fluid (particularly if >1 mL).
- A skin-penetrating injury with a sharp that is contaminated with blood/body fluid.
- A laceration from a contaminated instrument.
- A direct inoculation in the laboratory with contaminated material.
- A contaminated wound or skin lesion.
- Mucous membrane/conjunctival contact with blood/body fluid.

The incidence of HBV, HCV and HIV in Victorian i.v. drug users is 1.8, 10.7 and 0.2 per 100 person–years, respectively. The estimated risk of virus transmission from an occupational needle-stick injury from a *known positive donor* (e.g. in Victoria) is:

- HBV: 6–30%
- HCV: 0–7%
- HIV: ~0.4%.

Note: These figures are for needle-stick injury from a positive source. When the source is unknown, the actual risk of infection for the affected individual depends on the probability of infection in the source population.

USEFUL RESOURCES
- *http://www.health.vic.gov.au/ideas/bluebook/* – Australian national information on infectious diseases and their control, from the Department of Human Services. Has detailed information on most infections.
- *http://www.cdc.gov* – The US Centers for Disease Control and Prevention has an enormous array of information on infectious diseases and travel medicine.

CHAPTER 31

Metabolic conditions

Avihu Boneh
George Werther

Metabolic diseases, although rare individually, in aggregate are an important cause of illness in Western society. Some newborns admitted with a clinical presentation of 'neonatal septicaemia' will eventually be found to have an inborn error of metabolism.

Assessment

A high index of suspicion is the primary rule in the diagnostic approach to metabolic disorders.

The presenting symptoms of metabolic diseases are non-specific (see Table 31.1). Children presenting *in extremis* must be resuscitated quickly, but with attention to procuring blood samples before administration of drugs/fluids. Discuss with a senior. See chapter 1, Medical emergencies.

History must be thorough and include:
- The pregnancy, delivery, neonatal period, dietary history (food refusal or craving), medications, and motor and cognitive development.
- The family history, with particular note of consanguinity, relatives with seemingly unrelated disorders (e.g. 'retardation'), maternal morbidity during pregnancy (e.g. severe chronic vomiting, liver disease and intercurrent infections), miscarriages, unexplained deaths of newborns and sudden infant death syndrome (SIDS), as well as other children having similar clinical signs in the family.
- Physical examination: some findings may be suggestive of a metabolic disease. These are summarised in Table 31.2.

Laboratory investigations

Blood, urine and CSF samples collected at the time of presentation may be diagnostic and are invaluable. Always attempt to collect these samples *before* commencing treatment, but do not delay treatment in crisis situations.

Paediatric Handbook, 8th edition. By Kate Thomson, Dean Tey and Michael Marks. Published 2009 by Blackwell Publishing, ISBN: 978-1-4051-7400-8.

Table 31.1 Clinical features suggestive of a metabolic disease

Age	Clinical signs	Possible diagnosis
Day 1 of life	Seizures	Persistent hyperinsulinaemia Mitochondrial cytopathy Disorders of purines and pyrimidines
Neonatal period*	Vomiting, feed refusal, changes in respiration, prolonged jaundice, lethargy or irritability, movement disorder, seizures, hypo/hypertonia, changes in the level of consciousness	Organic acidaemias, Non-ketotic-hyperglycinaemia Urea cycle defects Fatty acid oxidation defects Galactosaemia Mitochondrial cytopathy Disorders of purines and pyrimidines
1st year of life	Same as above, plus: Failure to thrive, motor/cognitive developmental delay or regression	Organic acidaemias Urea cycle defects Fatty acid oxidation defects Lysosomal storage diseases
Early childhood	Mental retardation, seizures, behavioural abnormalities, learning difficulties, autistic features	Organic acidaemias Urea cycle defects Fatty acid oxidation defects Amino-acidopathies Lysosomal storage diseases Adrenoleucodystrophy
Any age group**	Acute decompensation: change in consciousness, seizures, movement disorder, change in respiration	Organic acidaemias Urea cycle defects Fatty acid oxidation defects Adrenal insufficiency

* Symptoms should be considered in relation to the child's age (in days), fasting, food intake (i.e. specific sugars, protein and fat) and changes in diet.
** May follow an intercurrent infection, prolonged fasting, a large meal with high protein content, and so on.

There are four initial questions to be answered:
- Is there acidosis, and is it of metabolic origin?
- Is there hypoglycaemia?
- Is there hyper- or hypoketonaemia?
- Is there hyperammonaemia?

The tests listed in Table 31.3 should be done to answer these questions. See Table 31.4 for interpretation of laboratory results.

In addition to these tests, brain CT or MRI (looking for brain oedema) and abdominal Doppler ultrasonographic examination (looking for porto-caval shunting as a cause of hyper-ammonaemia) may be helpful in the diagnostic process.

Table 31.2 Physical examination: potential signs of metabolic disease

General appearance	Growth parameters: height and weight Dysmorphism
Skin	Rash Odour Hyperkeratosis Pigmentation Signs of chronic scratching
Head and neck	Craniomegaly Dysmorphism Bulging fontanelle Clefts (mid-line defects) Signs of rickets Abnormal eye movement
Chest	Signs of lung disease
Heart	Cardiomegaly Signs of cardiac failure
Abdomen	Hepato ± splenomegaly Signs of liver disease
Genitalia	Ambiguous genitalia
Skeleton	Signs of rickets Bone or joint pain, contractures Abnormal spine posturing/vertebral disease
Muscles	Muscle mass, wasting
Neurological	Muscle strength, tone Sensation Reflexes (tendon and primitive) Movement disorders Ataxia

Table 31.3 Investigation of suspected metabolic disease

	First-line tests	**Second-line tests***
Blood	Acid–base (arterial or capillary) Electrolytes Glucose Ammonia Lactate (check specification with the Biochemistry Laboratory of your service, place on ice) Acylcarnitines (blood spots on a Guthrie (PKU) card) Insulin Cortisol Growth hormone	Complete blood count Plasma amino acids (place on ice) Pyruvate (place on ice) FA/ketones (specify: beta-hydroxy butyrate and acetoacetate, place on ice) Liver transaminases Urea, creatinine, calcium, phosphate Uric acid Cholesterol Freeze additional plasma for further testing
Urine	pH, glucose, ketones, protein (ward test) Reducing substances (ward test) Organic acids (keep frozen if not analysed immediately)	Freeze additional urine for further testing
CSF	Glucose, protein, lactate	Freeze additional CSF for further testing (amino acids, neurotransmitters, etc.)

* Check with the laboratory for the preferred sample.
Do not discard any blood, urine or CSF taken at time of metabolic decompensation and hypoglycaemia. Send any excess to the laboratory marked 'excess – store'.

Table 31.4 Interpretation of laboratory results

Metabolic condition	**pH**	**Glucose**	**Ketones**	**Ammonia**
Urea cycle defects	N or ↑	N	N	↑↑
Organic acidaemias	↓	↑, N or ↓	N or ↑	↑
Ketolysis defects, MSUD	N or ↑	N or ↑	↑↑	N
FA oxidation defects	N or ↓	N or ↓	N or ↓	N or ↑
Hyperinsulinaemia	N	↓↓	N	N or ↑

FA, fatty acid; MSUD, maple syrup urine disease; N, normal.

Hypoglycaemia
Definition
A blood sugar level of <2.5 mmol/L. If suspected clinically and on a glucometer, it must be confirmed with a true blood glucose measurement in the laboratory.

Causes
See Table 31.5. The two most common causes of hypoglycaemia beyond the neonatal period are:

- Hyperinsulinism in the first 2 years. This usually results in persistent, severe hypoglycaemia and may lead to permanent brain damage, as the brain depends on glucose in the first 2–3 years of life. Urinalysis for ketones is negative. Treat with glucose at >10 mg/kg per min.
- 'Ketotic hypoglycaemia' (or 'accelerated starvation'): the cause is unclear, and this entity may simply be one end of the normal spectrum or reaction to fasting
  - Usually >2 years old.
  - Often small for age, ± past history of small for gestational age.
  - Poor oral intake in 24 hours prior to hypoglycaemia.
  - Documented hypoglycaemia.
  - Early morning seizure.
  - Spontaneous remission by 8 years.
  - Exclude hypopituitarism or adrenal insufficiency.

Specific signs and symptoms
Infantile/neonatal
- Apnoea/tachypnoea/cyanotic spell.
- Hypotonia, poor crying and feeding.
- Irritability, tremor and seizures.

Childhood
- Catecholamine mediated: hunger, pallor, sweating, tremor and tachycardia.
- Neuroglycopenic effects: altered conscious state, abnormal behaviour, seizure.

Relevant history
- Gestation and birthweight.
- Previous episodes.
- Relationship to meals/feeds and duration of fasting.
- Age at onset of hypoglycaemia.
- Family history of neonatal deaths and affected relatives.
- Drugs – alcohol and insulin.
- Intercurrent illness.

Specific examination features
- Growth parameters (height, weight and head circumference). Overgrowth may suggest hyperinsulinism; underweight ketotic hypoglycaemia.

Table 31.5 Causes of neonatal/childhood hypoglycaemia

Transient neonatal:	
↓ Substrate/enzyme function	Premature/SGA RDS
↑ Glucose utilisation	Sepsis, hyperinsulinism (Beckwith–Wiedeman, IDM, Rh disease)

Persistent neonatal, recurrent childhood:	
↑ *Glucose utilisation* Ketone −ve	Hyperinsulinism Salicylate poisoning Sepsis
↓ *Hepatic glucose production* Ketone +ve ± ↑ lactate	Glycogen storage disease Gluconeogenic defect Galactosaemia Fructose intolerance Inborn errors of amino acid metabolism (maple syrup urine disease) Severe liver disease (Reye's syndrome)
↓ *Production of alternative fuels* Ketone −ve	Fatty acid oxidation defects (medium chain acyl coA dehydrogenase def.) Ketogenesis defects
Hormonal deficiency Ketone +ve	Cortisol (1°/2° to ACTH deficiency) Growth hormone
Drugs Ketone +ve/−ve	Alcohol Salicylates Propranolol Valproate Oral hypoglycaemics

IDM, infant of a diabetic mother; RDS, respiratory distress syndrome; SGA, small for gestational age.

- Midline defects (e.g. cleft lip, central incisor and micropenis) may suggest hypopituitarism.
- Muscle bulk, power and tone (glycogen storage disease).
- Hepatomegaly (e.g. glycogen storage disease and galactosaemia).
- Jaundice (e.g. galactosaemia, citrullinaemia type 2).

- Cataracts (e.g. galactosaemia).
- Unusual odours (e.g. ketones and maple syrup) suggesting metabolic disease.
- Ambiguous genitalia (congenital adrenal hyperplasia with adrenal crisis).

Investigation

Before i.v. glucose is given (and usually before the true blood glucose is available), blood and urinary samples *at the time of hypoglycaemia must* be obtained as these are essential for diagnosis. See Table 31.3 for first-line tests to be done.

Some hospitals have sets of the required tubes, labelled 'Hypoglycaemia Kit', but if not have a staff member look up the tubes required, while you are cannulating, collecting samples and treating the hypoglycaemia. Specimens *should be taken and returned on wet ice as soon as possible* to the laboratory.

Do not discard any blood or urine taken at time of hypoglycaemia – send any excess to the laboratory marked 'excess – store'.

Management

- *Neonate:* i.v. 200–300 mg (2–3 mL/kg of 10% dextrose) over 5 min, then 5–10 mg/kg per min.
  Note: **10%** dextrose solution at **0.1 mL/kg per min** will supply **10 mg/kg per min**.
- *Older children:* i.v. 200 mg (1 mL/kg of 20% dextrose) over 5 min, then 3–5 mg/kg per min until stable.

General treatment guidelines

Always discuss with metabolic physician.

There are three basic guidelines in the treatment of metabolic conditions:

- Enhance the disposal of the accumulating toxic metabolites. Adequate fluid intake is important, particularly as many of the toxic metabolites are excreted by the kidney. Correct dehydration and replace ongoing losses (diarrhoea, fever, etc.). Haemofiltration should be considered in severe cases or when there are indications of rapid accumulation of toxic metabolites (rapid deterioration in the level of consciousness, increasing intracranial pressure, etc.).
- Avoid catabolism, which can lead to an ongoing accumulation of these metabolites. It is of the utmost importance to provide the patient with an adequate amount of calories for age and weight. I.v. glucose infusion (10–20% solution) is usually a safe mode of treatment. I.v. fat solutions (Intralipid, 10 or 20% solutions) may serve as a good source of calories in a small fluid volume. Do not use i.v. fat solutions if you suspect a fatty acid oxidation disorder. I.v. amino acids can usually be given at a low dose (e.g. 0.5 g/kg per day for a newborn) to enhance anabolism, unless there is hyperammonaemia.
- Enhance enzymatic activity, whenever possible. Treatment with some vitamins and co-factors may be indicated to enhance the disposal of toxic metabolites or to enhance residual enzymatic activity. These are listed in Table 31.6. Treatment with carnitine and biotin is considered 'rescue treatment'. These should be used even if the diagnosis is unknown, following proper blood, urine and, if indicated, CSF sampling. Consult with the metabolic physician.

Table 31.6 Treatment with vitamins and other supplements (rescue treatment in bold)

Compound	Dose	Indication
Carnitine	100–300 mg/kg per day (oral) 15–60 mg/kg per day (i.v.)	Organic acidaemias Fatty acid oxidation disorders
Thiamine (B₁)	100–300 mg per day (i.v. or oral)	MSUD, PDH deficiency MRC disorders
Riboflavin (B₂)	100–300 mg/day	Glutaric acidurias MRC disorders
Pyridoxine (B₆)	100–300 mg/day (i.v. or oral)	Homocystinuria Seizures
Cobalamin (B₁₂)	1 mg/day as hydroxycobalamin (i.m.)	Homocystinuria and MMA, combined or separately
Biotin	10–20 mg/day (i.v. or oral)	Hyper-lactataemia Biotinidase deficiency Holocarboxylase synthetase deficiency
Vitamin C	250 or 500 mg/day or 100 mg/kg per day (oral)	MRC disorders Organic acidaemias
Vitamin K (menadione)	10 mg/day (oral) or 1 mg/day i.m.	MRC disorders
Coenzyme Q	50–300 mg/day	MRC disorders
Folic acid	5 mg/day	MRC disorders with anaemia Some amino-acidopathies
Folinic acid	5–7.5 mg/day	Bioamine-neurotransmitter defects
Glycine	200 mg/kg per day	May be given in some cases instead of carnitine

MMA, methylmalonic aciduria; MRC, mitochondrial respiratory chain; MSUD, maple syrup urine disease; PDH, pyruvate dehydrogenase.

Urgent autopsy for suspected metabolic disease
- Collect samples as soon as possible after death, preferably within 2 h.
- Note the time between death and freezing or the attainment of the samples.
- Obtain blood, urine, CSF and bile samples, if possible (see Table 31.3), for further metabolic analysis. A vitreous humour specimen should be obtained if urine is unavailable.

- Obtain a skin biopsy for fibroblast culture. One piece of full-thickness skin (2–3 mm surface diameter) in a tissue culture medium bottle, or a viral medium bottle or sterile normal saline without preservatives. Store in a refrigerator at 4 °C. *Do not freeze this sample.*
- Organ biopsies for light microscopy should be placed in aluminium foil or Parafilm®, frozen immediately (on dry ice) and put in screw-cap tubes. Store in a freezer at −70 °C. Note the time of sampling.
- Organ biopsies for electron microscopy should be placed in a glutaraldehyde bottle. Store in a refrigerator at 4 °C. *Do not freeze this sample.*
- Muscle samples are preferably from the quadriceps. If the parents object to the two incisions (the muscle and liver), suggest a right upper quadrant incision to take samples from the liver, rectus muscle and skin biopsy.
- Blood for DNA tests: 10 mL of heparinised blood (no mixing beads or separating gel) can be sent at room temperature if they are expected in the laboratory within 24 h, or frozen.

Note: To avoid mistakes in obtaining and handling of samples please consult with the metabolic physician to your service.

USEFUL RESOURCES
- *www.rch.org.au/nets/handbook* – Follow the link to Metabolic Diseases.
- *http://emedicine.com/emerg/topic768.htm* – Summary article of inborn errors of metabolism.

CHAPTER 32
Neonatal conditions

Peter McDougall
Rod Hunt

Routine care

The vast majority of deliveries are uncomplicated and do not require medical intervention. The baby will start breathing spontaneously and will be kept adequately warm by being swaddled and cuddled by the mother. Early contact helps with establishing bonding and breast-feeding.

The first minutes
Establishing breathing

The major stimuli to start breathing include cooling of the face and physical stimuli as well as hypoxia and acidosis. Babies usually start breathing within seconds of birth. If the baby is not breathing, drying with a towel is a very effective stimulus.

Heat loss after birth

Evaporative cooling occurs very quickly after birth. It is minimised by drying and wrapping the baby in warm towels. A well, term infant will be kept warm by being swaddled and cuddled by the mother. The baby's rectal temperature should stabilise around 37 °C (±0.3 °C) by 1 h of age. A baby who becomes cold may need controlled warming under a radiant heater or in an incubator and should always be assessed for illness. Both hypothermia and hyperthermia are bad for babies.

The umbilical cord

This is clamped and cut cleanly close to the skin just after birth. The cut end and the base of the cord must be kept clean and dry. Antiseptic solution, such as chlorhexidine in alcohol, may be applied daily until the cord stump drops off. Omphalitis may occur if this is not done. The plastic clamp can be removed after 2 days.

The first hours

After the infant's temperature is stable, s/he can be washed with soap and water. There is no hurry to do this. Record the heart rate, colour, respiratory rate and effort, at frequent intervals, depending on the infant's condition.

Often the baby will be very alert and breast-feeds should be started at these times.

Paediatric Handbook, 8th edition. By Kate Thomson, Dean Tey and Michael Marks. Published 2009 by Blackwell Publishing, ISBN: 978-1-4051-7400-8.

Vitamin K

All infants, regardless of size, maturity, or ill health, should receive vitamin K mixed micelles (Konakion) 0.1 mL i.m. This eradicates haemorrhagic disease of the newborn. Claims associating i.m. vitamin K and childhood cancer have not been substantiated. An increased incidence of both early and late haemorrhagic disease of the newborn occurs in breast-fed infants who received either an oral or inadequate i.m. dose, or no prophylactic vitamin K. Parents who insist on their infant having oral vitamin K must be given instructions that it must be given for three doses at 2-weekly intervals from birth.

The first day

After an initial period of alertness the infant will sleep for long periods and may not be too demanding with feeds. However, the infant must:

- *Suck and swallow easily*: if s/he does not, consider unrecognised prematurity, a congenital abnormality, hypoglycaemia or infection.
- *Pass urine*: many babies pass urine at birth and it is missed. If a boy does not pass urine in the first 24 h, consider posterior urethral valves. This requires careful urological investigation. A reasonable screening test is to ultrasound the bladder and see if it empties completely with micturition.
- *Pass meconium within the first 48 h*: if not, consider bowel obstruction or Hirschsprung disease.

The first examination

The purpose of this examination is to detect congenital abnormalities, reassure the parents and to discuss their concerns. Many major abnormalities will have been seen on antenatal ultrasound, but not all.

- *Observation*: before disturbing the baby observe the posture, behaviour, general appearance, colour and well-being.
- *Chest*: while the baby is quiet examine the heart sounds, rate, presence of femoral pulses and the pulse characteristics. Many babies have a very soft murmur in the first few days. If it sounds pathological, is associated with other signs or persists, then refer to a cardiologist. Normal babies breathe so shallowly when they are sleeping that it can be difficult to see. Recession and laboured breathing are the most important signs of respiratory distress. In babies the rate and depth of each breath can be very variable.
- *Head and neck*: look for scalp defects; fractures; haematomas; lacerations; eye size, anatomy and red reflex; neck cysts, lumps or fistulae; cleft palate; tongue size and shape; ear position, shape, size and tags or fistulae and facial symmetry when crying. A cephalohaematoma is a soft boggy swelling over one bone (usually the parietal) due to blood under the periosteum. It needs no treatment. **Beware of a generalised boggy swelling all over the scalp in a shocked baby**. It may be a subgaleal haemorrhage. Babies can bleed profusely into these and they are a neonatal emergency.
- *Abdomen*: feel for masses (liver, spleen, kidneys, bladder and ovaries), distension and tenderness. Examine the genitalia, anus and inguinal and umbilical region for herniae. The umbilicus should be clean and dry. The liver is often just palpable or percussible in normal babies.

- *Limbs*: examine for abnormal fingers, hands, toes and feet; posture of the hands and feet; and the flexibility of the joints.
- *Hips*: carefully examine for congenital dislocation by observation and specific palpation (see chapter 34, Orthopaedic conditions).
- *Measurement*: naked weight, length and head circumference should be recorded and plotted on the growth chart in the baby's record book.

The first week

- *Feeding*: will be established during this time. After an initial phase of waking frequently until lactation is established, the breast-fed baby should establish a regular cycle of waking for feeds, followed mostly by sleeping. However, even in the first week of life, some babies will stay awake after some feeds. Some babies will sleep for 4 h; others will wake frequently for small feeds. After an initial weight loss of up to 10% over the first few days, the baby's weight should stabilise and then increase towards the end of the first week.
- *Stools*: change over the first 4–5 days from black, sticky meconium, to dark-green, yellow-green and finally to loose yellow once full breast-feeding is established. The frequency of bowel actions varies, but is usually once per feed after feeding is established.
- *Urine*: production is usually low in the first few days, but increases after feeding has been established, with a urinary frequency of usually at least once per feed.
- *Jaundice*: occurs in >50% of babies after the first 24 h of age; see p. 438.
- *Screening*: is done on the third day for cystic fibrosis, hypothyroidism, phenylketonuria, and other metabolic conditions from a heel prick. Results are available approximately 1 week after sampling. Negative (normal) results are not notified, but the laboratory will contact the baby's doctor regarding the management of children with positive (abnormal) results and advise on appropriate management. This usually involves an immediate referral to a tertiary paediatric hospital for further testing and treatment.

Behaviour and sleep

In the first days, babies mostly sleep and eat. They spend little time awake when not feeding, unless inadequate milk supply leads to hunger. Their sleep cycles through quiet and active phases and may switch from one type of sleep to the other every 5–10 min. In quiet sleep babies appear to sleep deeply, breathe quietly and regularly and do not move much. They often appear quite pale in this phase of sleep and their limbs are cool to touch. Parents occasionally mistake this appearance for apnoea. In active sleep (rapid eye movement [REM] sleep), they breathe erratically, make various noises (including crying, vocalising and yawning), have many body movements and may seem to be waking up. It is in this phase of sleep that babies frequently have short periods (up to 10 s) of apnoea. This behaviour is normal but can be confusing and frightening to parents.

The first month

The baby should be weighed and measured weekly to ensure adequate nutrition. The results must be recorded and plotted on growth charts. Weight gain for term babies varies from 150–250 g per week.

Maternal concerns about the baby usually relate to crying, not sleeping enough, not gaining weight, rashes or poor feeding. (See chapter 6, Nutrition; chapter 11, Common behavioural and developmental problems; and chapter 12, Sleep problems.)

Neonatal resuscitation

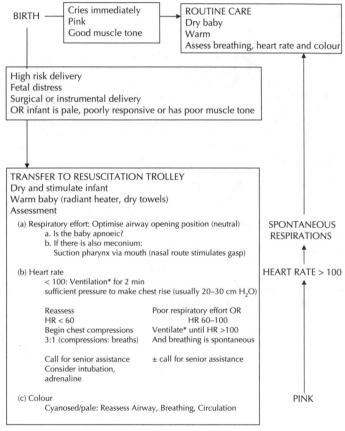

Fig. 32.1 Neonatal resuscitation. (Adapted from the Australian Resuscitation Council Neonatal Guidelines, Section 13, February 2006.) See also Neonatal Handbook website http://www.rch.org.au/nets/handbook

* Ventilation is provided by positive pressure ventilation delivered with bag and mask, or Neopuff.

- Increasingly it has been recognised that the traditional practice of resuscitation with 100% oxygen may **not** be beneficial and a systematic review demonstrates that resuscitation with air, rather than oxygen, reduces perinatal mortality. It should be noted that 'normal' oxygen saturations in the preterm infant are as low as 40% for the first 4 min of life, with those in the term infant ranging from 60% at 1 minute to 90% at 5 min, without intervention with supplemental oxygen. Currently, resuscitation with 100% oxygen, or medical air, is acceptable.
- The most common cause for failure of resuscitation is inadequate ventilation. This can be due to a poor seal at the facemask or inadequate pressure. Sometimes pressures up to 50 cm H_2O are required for the first few breaths.
- A baby who does not respond and has a slow heart rate (<60 bpm) needs cardiac massage and may need infusions of bicarbonate, blood or adrenaline to improve cardiac output depending on the underlying problem. Chest compressions should be provided with positive pressure ventilation in a ratio of 3:1.
- In general, admission to a neonatal intensive care unit is required if spontaneous ventilation is not established by 5 min of age.
- The Apgar score is used to assess the condition of the baby at 1, 5 and occasionally 10 min of age (see Table 32.2). The total score ranges from 0 to 10. A score between 7 and 10 indicates the infant is well. A score between 4 and 7 indicates the baby needs assistance. A score between 0 and 3 indicates severe cardiorespiratory depression. In practice it is best to describe exactly what was happening to the infant.
- Naloxone is rarely required. It should only be given if a mother has received narcotics within 2 h of delivery. When using naloxone, be aware that the effect can wear off quickly and the baby may then develop apnoea, the most serious sign of narcotic overdose. Do not use naloxone if there is a possibility of maternal narcotic abuse (risk of fulminant withdrawal in the baby).

Variations from normal

When the baby is fully examined, normal variants or minor problems are often noted. If they are obvious to the doctor, most will be obvious to the parents who often need explanation and reassurance.

Table 32.1 Endotracheal tubes

Weight	ETT size	Tie at lips
<1000 g	2.5 mm	6.5–7.0 cm
1000–2000 g	3.0 mm	7–8 cm
2000–3000 g	3.0/3.5 mm	8–9 cm
>3000 g	3.5/4.0 mm	>9 cm

Table 32.2 The Apgar score

Sign	0 (absent)	1 (present but depressed)	2 (normal)
Heart rate	Absent	<100	>100
Respiratory effort	Absent	Slow, irregular	Good, crying
Muscle tone	Limp	Some flexion	Active
Response to stimulation	No response	Grimace	Cry
Colour	Pale, blue	Centrally pink, blue periphery	Pink

Reproduced with permission from *Pediatrics,* Oct, 1994, **94**: 558–565.

Skin

- *Naevus flammeus* ('*stork-bite*'): dilated capillaries, on the nape of the neck and on the bridge of the nose, eyelids and adjacent forehead. They fade over 6–12 months.
- *Milia*: small white blocked sebaceous glands on the nose. They disappear over the first month.
- *Miliaria*: there are two types – 'crystallina' and 'rubra'. Miliaria crystallina are beads of sweat trapped under the epidermis and are most prominent on the forehead in babies who are overheated. Miliaria rubra, also called 'heat rash', usually appear after a few weeks of age, fluctuate over 2–3 weeks and then disappear. They are related to an increasing activity of the sweat glands. They are prominent on the face, in babies who are overheated.
- *Erythema toxicum* ('*toxic erythema*' or '*urticaria of the newborn*'): these are red 'urticarial' spots over the baby's trunk that peak at 2–3 days of age and generally resolve by the first week of life, but occasionally runs a fluctuating course over a few weeks. They are harmless and of unknown cause. New lesions have a broad erythematous base up to 2–3 cm diameter with a 1–2 mm papule or pustule. The diagnosis can be made with confidence on clinical appearance alone. The differential diagnosis is staphylococcal skin infection, which is persistent and purulent. An examination of the fluid reveals neutrophils and Gram-positive cocci in infection, or eosinophils and no organisms in erythema toxicum.
- '*Mongolian*' *blue spot*: this condition results in areas of increased melanin deposition over the lower back and sacrum. It can be more extensive and is sometimes mistaken for bruising. It is present in most babies born to dark-skinned parents. It gradually lightens over a few years, as the rest of the skin becomes more pigmented.
- *Dry skin*: babies who are post-term have a thicker epidermis and hence drier-looking skin after birth. This dry skin may occasionally crack and bleed around the hands and feet during the first few days. Emollients will help. Otherwise the dry skin should be allowed to peel off naturally, which may take up to 1–2 months.

Deformities

- *Moulding*: the skull moulds to enable the head to be delivered. This changes to a normal shape over the first few days. In addition there may be postural deformities of the face, skull and limbs that are related to the baby's position in the uterus. These gradually improve after birth, but sometimes they do not disappear completely – very few people are symmetrical, especially in their face.
- *Positional talipes*: is quite common. The foot is deformed from being compressed in the uterus. To determine whether this is pathological, test the range of movements of the foot. A normal foot can be flexed and extended so that the angle with the shin is less or more than 90°. The forefoot should be mobile. A fixed deformity should be referred to a paediatric orthopaedic surgeon for management (see chapter 34, Orthopaedic conditions).

Other

- *Puffy eyelids/scalp oedema*: the newborn infant has excess body fluid at birth. Fluid accumulates easily in the eyelids and, after lying on one side, the lower eye may be more swollen. Scalp oedema is common in the first few hours after a normal birth, but can persist for several days. This needs further investigation if it persists, or is generalised.
- *Bruising/petechiae/subconjunctival haemorrhages*: the part of the baby that was presenting during delivery is commonly bruised. If the cord was wrapped tightly around the neck, the baby may have petechial haemorrhages on the face and head (traumatic cyanosis). Subconjunctival haemorrhages occur in up to 25% of babies delivered normally and do not adversely affect vision. They may persist for up to 2 weeks and must not be confused with postnatal trauma. Bruising is common after forceps deliveries, particularly over bony prominences, but disappears over the first week of life. Less commonly after forceps deliveries, firm nodules may be noted in the subcutaneous tissue over similar sites. This is subcutaneous fat necrosis and resolves spontaneously over the first month of life.
- *Sucking blisters*: these are common on the lips, particularly the upper lip and need no treatment.
- *Epstein's pearls*: these are small white cysts on the hard palate in the midline. They are benign and disappear in the first weeks after birth.
- *Breast hyperplasia*: a breast bud is palpable in most term babies, regardless of gender. The breasts may become enlarged during the first week and milk may be observed. They should be left alone and the swelling will subside over several months. However, a breast that is swollen, hot, red and tender may be infected.

Common minor problems

- *Hiccups*: these occur frequently after a feed. They are not caused by inadequate burping and are harmless.
- *Snuffles*: these occur in about 1/3 of normal babies in the few weeks after birth. Despite the noise, the baby is otherwise quite well and is able to feed normally. The problem diminishes with time as the baby's feeding becomes more efficient and the nasal passages enlarge. It is only important if it interferes with the baby's ability to suck.

- *Vomiting*: small vomits are harmless. The serious signs are vomit that is bile-stained (grass green), blood-stained, projectile, persistent or associated with frequent choking or failure to thrive. Bile-stained vomiting must be referred to a tertiary paediatric centre for an upper barium study.
- *Bleeding umbilical cord*: small amounts of bleeding occur rarely as the cord is separating and require no treatment. More profuse bleeding may indicate a bleeding disorder.
- *Umbilical hernia*: this is present in approximately 25% of babies and resolves in almost all. Consider surgical referral if present beyond 2 years.
- *Vaginal skin tag*: a small tag of vaginal skin commonly protrudes between the labia in newborn girls. It is benign and disappears as the labia enlarge.
- *Vaginal discharge*: a small amount of vaginal mucus is universal. In some it can be bloodstained during the first week as the endometrium involutes.
- *Red urine*: a red-orange discoloration of the napkin when the urine is concentrated (common in the first few days of life) may be mistaken for blood, but is usually due to urates.
- *Clicky hips*: some ligamentous clicking is common in all large joints, including the hips. It can be considered normal in the absence of any abnormal movement of the femoral head, restriction of hip movement, strong family history, or breech presentation. However, if there is any doubt, hip ultrasound is indicated.

Jaundice

Jaundice is common in the newborn period and is almost always caused by unconjugated hyperbilirubinaemia. The clinical importance of jaundice depends on the time at which it is observed and the gestational age of the baby. Jaundice needs to be taken seriously; if the bilirubin level is too high (>340 µmol/L) brain damage (kernicterus) may occur.

The first 24 hours

- Jaundice in the first 24 h is abnormal. The infant must be admitted to a special care nursery and investigated urgently.
- It is mostly caused by haemolysis, usually ABO or rhesus incompatibility between mother and fetus. Severe haemolysis leads to a rapid rise in serum bilirubin over a few hours.
- The following investigations are required urgently: the mother's and baby's blood group, the baby's serum bilirubin (total and unconjugated), direct Coombs' test, haemoglobin, white cell count, and platelets. The mother's red cell antibodies may need to be tested.
- Further investigations are needed if there is no haemolysis, or conjugated hyperbilirubin-aemia is present.
- Phototherapy should be commenced if the bilirubin level is >150 µmol/L in the first 24 h in a term infant.
- An immediate exchange transfusion may be required if the jaundice is due to rhesus incompatibility and the infant is anaemic (Hb < 110 g/L). This primarily corrects the anaemia and removes antibodies. Further exchange transfusions may be required to control the jaundice.

- Frequent monitoring of bilirubin levels is essential as rapid changes may occur. The results should be plotted on a chart and an 'action level' for exchange transfusion established so that mistakes are not made.

Days 2–7
Jaundice is considered to be 'physiological' if the following criteria are satisfied:
- The jaundice appeared on day 2–4.
- The baby is not premature.
- The baby is well (afebrile, feeding well and alert).
- The baby is passing normal-coloured stools and urine.
- There are no other abnormalities.
- Bilirubin levels are not above treatment threshold.

About 1/3 of term babies become visibly jaundiced by 2–4 days of age. Jaundice is visible once serum bilirubin is >85–120 µmol/L. In physiological jaundice, serum bilirubin rarely exceeds 220 µmol/L. If the unconjugated bilirubin is >220 µmol/L, other causes, including infection, should be considered.

Well, term infants with no haemolysis are at minimal risk of kernicterus. Infants who are at higher risk of kernicterus are:
- Unwell infants (particularly those exposed to hypoxic insults).
- Infants with haemolysis.
- Preterm infants.

These infants should have treatment started at lower bilirubin levels. For guidelines in management of jaundice, see Tables 32.3, 32.4 and 32.5.

In most places, a centralised tertiary neonatology service is available to give phone advice and coordinate retrievals. Paediatricians seeking advice about issues such as exchange transfusions are encouraged to contact their local service.

Prolonged jaundice (>14 days)
In a well infant, prolonged neonatal jaundice is usually secondary to breast-feeding and is benign. A serum bilirubin should be checked to determine whether hyperbilirubinaemia is conjugated or unconjugated.
- *Unconjugated bilirubinaemia*: hypothyroidism, infection or red cell enzyme abnormalities should be considered.
  - A sudden onset of jaundice at this age is suggestive of haemolysis caused by a red blood cell enzyme abnormality, most frequently glucose-6-phosphate dehydrogenase (G6PD) deficiency. Urgent admission to hospital is indicated.
- *Conjugated bilirubinaemia (>25% total or >25 µmol/L)*: is uncommon and always pathological. Consider biliary atresia (the stools are acholic – grey), neonatal hepatitis, a choledochal cyst obstructing the bile duct, galactosaemia or parenteral nutrition.

See also chapter 27, Gastrointestinal conditions, p. 348.

If the above are excluded and the baby is well and breast-feeding, the likely diagnosis is breast-milk jaundice. This occurs in approximately 10% of breast-fed infants, is not associated

Table 32.3 Management of non-pathologic jaundice in healthy term infants

Age (h)	Serum bilirubin (µmol)			
	Consider phototherapy	Phototherapy	Exchange transfusion if intensive phototherapy fails	Exchange transfusion and intensive phototherapy
<24*	–	–	–	–
25–48	>170	>260	>340	>430
49–72	>260	>310	>430	>510
>72	>290	>340	>430	>510

From American Academy of Pediatrics Guidelines (reproduced with permission from *Pediatrics,* Oct, 1994, **94**: 558–565).

In cases of pathologic jaundice, these guidelines are modified and treatment is typically more aggressive.

* Pathologic jaundice is clinical jaundice at less than 24 h of age, and/or bilirubin rising at greater than 8.5 µmol/L/hr, and/or true haemolysis.

Table 32.4 Management of jaundice in preterm infants: guidelines for phototherapy

Age (h)	Serum bilirubin (µmol)		
	<1500	Weight (g)1500–2000	>2000
<24	>70	>70	>85
24–48	>85	>120	>140
49–72	>120	>155	>200
>72	>140	>170	>240

Reproduced with permission from *Pediatrics,* Oct, 1994, **94**: 558–565.

Table 32.5 Management of jaundice in preterm infants: guidelines for exchange transfusion

Age (h)	Serum bilirubin (µmol)		
	<1500	Weight (g)1500–2000	>2000
<24	>170–255	>255	>270–310
24–48	>170–255	>270	>290–320
49–72	>255	>290	>310–340

For high-risk premature infants: use lower end of range and weight, next lower weight category, and next lower age category in that order.

Premature LGA infants: use average birthweight for gestational age.

These 3 tables and guidlines can be found at www.rch.org.au/nets/handbook

with kernicterus and does not need any treatment. Reassurance that breast-feeding should continue is very important.

Prolonged jaundice (after the first few days of life) can usually be managed as an out-patient, but may require readmission for investigation or treatment

Respiratory distress

Most major causes of respiratory distress will present within the first hours of life. The signs are:

- Increased work of breathing (recession of the lower chest wall and upper abdomen).
- Rapid breathing (>60 breaths/min).
- Expiratory grunt.
- Central cyanosis.

Babies need to be considered for level 3 neonatal intensive care if they require >40% oxygen to maintain saturations >88% (usually measured by pulse oximetry).

Common pulmonary diseases

Respiratory distress syndrome (RDS) or hyaline membrane disease

- RDS is primarily caused by immaturity. The incidence increases with decreasing gestation. It usually affects babies <30 weeks' gestation, but it can occur in term babies, especially those delivered by elective Caesarean section. Due to immaturity of surfactant lung structure and fluid clearance, the lungs do not expand easily nor evenly. This causes damage to the epithelium and protein exudes on to the surface, forming hyaline membranes.
- Respiratory distress (oxygen requirement, work of breathing) typically increases over 12–24 h before improvement is seen. Rapid deterioration may occur leading to respiratory failure (rising arterial CO_2 level).
- The diagnosis is made by clinical features and chest radiograph, which has a generalised fine reticulogranular ('ground glass') appearance with air bronchograms.
- Respiratory support with oxygen, assisted ventilation (CPAP, IPPV) and surfactant therapy may be required.

Transient tachypnoea of the newborn or 'wet lung syndrome'

- This is caused by delayed clearance of fetal lung fluid and commonly occurs in babies born near term by elective Caesarean section. It presents as mild respiratory distress and lasts for up to 1–2 days.
- It is diagnosed by chest radiograph, which demonstrates coarse streaking of lung fields with fluid in the fissures. The baby is usually not very ill, needing <30% oxygen.

Bacterial infections

- Group B β-haemolytic streptococcus (GBS) is the most common and serious cause of pneumonia and septicaemia in the newborn. It is acquired around the time of birth from a colonised mother. Other organisms, including *E. coli*, can also cause pneumonia.
- Pneumonia presents early with severe and progressive respiratory failure. If not treated immediately there is rapid progression to collapse and death.
- Later infections can present with lethargy, temperature instability, poor feeding, respiratory difficulty, apnoea or poor perfusion.
- The chest radiograph of GBS infection is similar to severe RDS and is not diagnostic.
- Because of the rapid and severe nature of GBS septicaemia, all babies with early-onset respiratory failure must be treated with penicillin and gentamicin until the cause is confirmed.

Meconium aspiration syndrome

- Hypoxia before delivery may cause the baby to gasp *in utero* and inhale meconium. This causes respiratory difficulty. It is associated with pulmonary hypertension and right-to-left shunting.
- The chest radiograph shows hyperinflation and patchy consolidation (pneumothorax and pneumomediastinum may follow) or a diffuse hazy appearance.
- Oxygen is the mainstay of therapy, but other respiratory support (CPAP or ventilation) may be required. Antibiotics are given to counter infection.

Pneumothorax

- May occur spontaneously at birth, or secondary to other lung disease. It is a serious cause of respiratory distress and vital to be recognised and treated early.
- The diagnosis is by chest radiograph. Transillumination using a cold light source can be useful.
- The main treatment is an intercostal catheter with an underwater drain at low negative pressure.
- Asymptomatic pneumothorax usually needs no treatment.

Tension pneumothorax

- This is a medical emergency.
- If a baby is deteriorating rapidly despite full resuscitation this diagnosis should be considered, particularly if there is poor air entry on auscultation to one or both sides of the chest. There may be no time for a chest radiograph.
- In the event of severe deterioration, aspirate the chest using a 25-gauge scalp vein needle attached via a three-way tap to a 10 mL syringe. The needle is inserted into the second or third intercostal space in the midclavicular line. Aspirate the chest with the 10 mL syringe.
- This manoeuvre may be life saving and is followed by insertion of an intercostal catheter.

Upper airway obstruction
- *Nasal*: may be due to an upper respiratory tract infection, choanal atresia (obstruction to the back of the nose) or traumatic deviated nasal septum. It presents with difficulty in breathing or feeding. Suspect choanal atresia/stenosis when the baby's condition improves with opening the mouth. Choanal atresia is diagnosed when a 10-French suction tube cannot be passed from the nose to the nasopharynx.
- *Oral*: macroglossia may be associated with Beckwith–Wiedemann syndrome or hypothyroidism. Micrognathia may result in a tongue that obstructs the pharynx. Pierre Robin sequence is an association of mandibular hypoplasia (micrognathia), cleft palate and upper airways obstruction caused by the tongue falling back into the cleft palate. The severity of the upper airways obstruction can vary from mild to severe. There is usually a soft inspiratory stridor associated with subcostal and intercostal indrawing of variable severity. Babies with mild upper airways obstruction feed reasonably well, gain weight and usually need no intervention other than prone posturing. However, babies who feed poorly, vomit and fail to thrive usually have significant airways obstruction. These babies often adopt an extensor posture in an attempt to relieve their obstruction. Presentation at 2–4 weeks of age with these features is not uncommon. Insertion of a nasopharyngeal tube is necessary to relieve airway obstruction. Babies needing prolonged treatment with a nasopharyngeal tube respond well to mandibular distraction surgery. Tracheostomy is rarely needed.
- *Larynx*: laryngomalacia, subglottic stenosis, laryngeal inflammation or occasionally vocal cord palsy, present with inspiratory stridor and suprasternal and lower chest indrawing.
- *Trachea*: tracheal obstruction presents with an inspiratory and expiratory wheeze and lower chest indrawing. It may be due to tracheomalacia or a vascular ring.

Non-pulmonary causes of respiratory difficulty
Cardiac
- Left-to-right shunts or left-sided obstructions cause pulmonary oedema.

Pulmonary hypertension
- Presents with an increased oxygen requirement and little respiratory difficulty. Chest radiograph often reveals clear lung fields.

Management of respiratory diseases
Before birth
- If possible, anticipate high-risk babies and transfer to a hospital with a level 3 nursery for delivery and neonatal care.
- Betamethasone given to mothers with threatened preterm labour reduces the severity of hyaline membrane disease, halves the mortality and incidence of brain haemorrhages and improves long-term outcome.

General care
- Observation, usually in an incubator.
- Temperature control is essential – aim for a rectal temperature of 37 °C (±0.3 °C) or axillary temperature range 36.8 °C (±0.3 °C).

- Measure blood glucose, electrolytes, full blood count and CRP.
- Take a blood culture (but not an LP in the acute stage).
- Avoid enteral feeds initially as they worsen respiratory distress via splinting the diaphragm.
- Give i.v. fluids.
- Treat with benzylpenicillin and gentamicin until blood cultures are negative.

Respiratory care
- A chest radiograph provides the diagnosis in most cases of respiratory difficulty in neonates.
- Monitor cardiorespiratory and blood gas measurements.
- *Arterial pH* should be maintained at 7.35–7.45. A level of 7.25 (or just under) may be acceptable, depending on the circumstances.
- *Arterial Pco_2* should be 40–60 mmHg.
- *Arterial Po_2.* A low Po_2. means the baby is hypoxic. If the pH is also low, the baby may have a metabolic acidosis and a higher level of inspired oxygen is required. If this does not improve oxygenation, suspect cyanotic heart disease as a cause (see chapter 21, Cardiac conditions).
- *Arterial bicarbonate* should be 22–26 mmol/L. A low level is due to a metabolic acidosis. The pH will also be low unless the baby has compensated by blowing off CO_2.
- *Base excess* should be between +3 and −3. If low it indicates a metabolic acidosis. A level of −5 is usually tolerated in small babies without a significant change in pH.

Note: If arterial blood gases cannot be obtained, sample the capillary blood. This is simple and rapid to do, providing some information about acid–base status and CO_2 levels to guide further therapy, while tertiary assistance is sought.

- In ventilated babies with RDS, especially those <30 weeks' gestation, surfactant should be given via the endotracheal tube as early as possible.
- The inspired oxygen requirement is initially determined using a pulse oximeter. Aim for an oxygen saturation of 88–95%.
- Arterial blood gases should be measured in babies needing >30% oxygen. Aim for a PaO_2 level of 50–80 mmHg.
- Nasal continuous positive airway pressure (CPAP) is effective for treating RDS or apnoea. It should be used early for any baby who is grunting or showing increased respiratory effort (starting at 7 cm H_2O).
- The decision to ventilate a baby is made on the following criteria:
  - Apnoea not responding to simple treatment.
  - Unsatisfactory arterial blood gases: pH <7.25 with a Pco_2 >60 mmHg, or inspired oxygen >60% despite treatment with CPAP (up to 10 cm H_2O).

Hypoglycaemia
This is defined as a true blood glucose of <2.5 mmol/L. Dextrostix or BM stix are only useful for screening purposes. If these suggest hypoglycaemia, a true blood glucose must be measured.

Blood glucose should be measured before 1 h of age for infants with the following conditions: infants of diabetic mothers, infants weighing <10th centile, prematurity, large for gestational age, shock, seizures and infants receiving i.v. infusions.

Clinical features

There are no specific clinical features of hypoglycaemia. The infant may be asymptomatic, or may have apathy, hypotonia, poor feeding, temperature instability, apnoea, jitteriness or convulsions.

Management

- Asymptomatic infants with a true blood glucose of 1.5–2.5 mmol/L: give early, frequent small milk feeds at 90 mL/kg per day. If no response occurs within 2 h, give i.v. 10% dextrose.
- If the blood glucose is <1.5 mmol/L i.v. dextrose should be given. A bolus of 10% dextrose, 2 mL/kg, should be followed by an infusion providing 5–10 mg/kg per min of glucose. The response to therapy should be monitored by frequent blood glucose measurements.
- To calculate an infusion of 10 mg/kg per min:
  - Remember a fluid bag of 10% dextrose = 10 g/100 mL = 0.1 g/mL = 100 mg/mL of dextrose.
  - Hence, 10 mg/kg per min = 0.1 mL/kg per min of 10% dextrose infusion.
- If the blood glucose is <1 mmol/L and it is difficult to insert an i.v. line, give 0.3 units/kg of glucagon i.m. pending successful insertion of the line, or transfer to a higher level of care.
- Further investigation and treatment is necessary if the glucose requirement is 10 mg/kg per min or greater (see chapter 31, Metabolic conditions).

Neonatal infection

Infection is one of the most common preventable causes of neonatal mortality and morbidity. Infection may be acquired from the mother before or at birth (early onset) or postnatally from the environment by droplet spread or handling (late onset). The most frequently encountered bacteria are:

- *Early onset:* Group B β-haemolytic streptococcus (GBS), *Escherichia coli* and *Listeria monocytogenes.*
- *Late onset:* Coagulase-negative staphylococci, *Staphylococcus aureus*, GBS, *Klebsiella* spp. and *Pseudomonas* spp.

The most serious viral infection is herpes simplex virus (HSV), but other viruses, especially respiratory syncytial virus (RSV), can cause problems in neonatal nurseries, or soon after discharge home in ex-premature infants. There are also occasional outbreaks of enteroviral infections in the community causing significant illness in babies.

Clinical features

The early symptoms and signs may be subtle, but if ignored, rapid progression to overwhelming sepsis may occur.

The following are important warning signs of infection: respiratory difficulty, poor feeding, vomiting, abdominal distension and tenderness, drowsiness, floppiness, pallor, apnoea, seizures, temperature instability, tender limb. In particular poor feeding is a frequent early sign of infection.

Investigations

If one or more of the warning signs are present it is important to investigate infection. This includes:

- *Blood culture*: arterial or venous, at least 2–4 mL.
- *Urine*: suprapubic aspiration (SPA) under ultrasound imaging if possible. If unsuccessful pass a catheter using a 5-French gauge tube after adequate preparation of the genitalia. A bag collection of urine is rarely helpful.
- Throat and rectal swabs and swabs of any obviously infected lesion.
- Cultures or specific PCR for viral infections.
- Lumbar puncture if meningitis is suspected. This should **always** be done in the presence of fever in a newborn.

Management

Any ill neonate should be admitted to hospital for investigation and treatment.

- Start with i.v. benzylpenicillin and gentamicin.
- Add i.v. cefotaxime if meningitis is suspected (see Antimicrobial guidelines) and i.v. metronidazole if abdominal sepsis is suspected.
- If there is any possibility that the baby may have HSV (i.e. the mother has active genital herpes), give aciclovir.
- Antibiotics may be subsequently tailored according to culture results (see Antimicrobial guidelines).
- Careful attention to temperature stability, respiratory status, fluid and electrolytes, blood pressure, blood glucose and haematology is essential.

Neonatal seizures
Clinical features

- *Subtle*: deviation of the eyes, staring, abnormal sucking, lip smacking or cycling movements of the limbs.
- *Tonic*: stiffening of limbs, frequently associated with apnoea and eye deviation.
- *Clonic*: movement of one or all limbs that persists despite holding the limb.

These can be distinguished from 'jitteriness' or tremulousness, which have no ocular phenomena, are stimulus-sensitive and can be stopped by gentle passive flexion of the limbs.

- *Benign sleep myoclonus*: occurs in neurologically normal infants only during sleep. The electroencephalogram (EEG) is normal and no treatment is necessary. It can be exacerbated by benzodiazepines and usually resolves by 2 months of age.

Aetiology

The aetiology can usually be determined for neonatal seizures. Causes include:

- Hypoxic ischaemic encephalopathy: seizures occur within 24 h of the hypoxic episode, often within the first 4–6 h.
- Intracranial haemorrhage (subdural, subarachnoid, intraventricular or parenchymal).
- Infection: bacterial or viral meningitis.
- Stroke.
- Metabolic:
  - Hypoglycaemia.
  - Hypocalcaemia/hypomagnesaemia.
  - Hypo- or hypernatremia.
  - Kernicterus.
  - Inborn errors of metabolism (characterised by intractable seizures, with progressive loss of consciousness, or metabolic acidosis), including:
    Pyridoxine dependency.
    Urea cycle disorders.
    Non-ketotic hyperglycinaemia.
    Fatty acid oxidation defects.
    Amino acid/organic acid/hyperammonaemia.
- Drug withdrawal.
- Developmental brain abnormalities.
- Autosomal dominant neonatal seizures.

Investigations

- Bloods:
  - Immediately check blood glucose.
  - Electrolytes including calcium and magnesium.
  - Blood gases.
  - Blood cultures.
- Metabolic screen: blood ammonia, lactate, amino acids, carnitine and urinary organic acids. See also chapter 31, Metabolic conditions, p. 425.
- Urine analysis including ketones and reducing substances.
- Lumbar puncture and viral investigations.
- Cranial ultrasound.
- Cranial CT scan to exclude intracranial haemorrhage that may warrant neurosurgical intervention.
- MRI brain scan to determine extent of injury in hypoxic–ischaemic encephalopathy (HIE) (usually done around day 5); to exclude stroke where focal seizures are occurring, or for suspected developmental brain abnormality.
- EEG to detect seizure activity and to aid prognosis. Where conventional EEG is not immediately available, bedside amplitude integrated EEG (aEEG) may be useful in the detection of some seizures.

Management
Admission to a neonatal intensive care unit is mandatory for all neonates with seizures. Attention to normoglycaemia, optimal ventilation, blood pressure control, and fluid and electrolyte balance is essential.

Anticonvulsants
- *Phenobarbitone:* 20 mg/kg i.v. over 30 min (beware – this dose may cause apnoea in a non-ventilated baby). A further 10 mg/kg may be given for refractory seizures followed by 5 mg/kg per day.
- *Phenytoin:* 20 mg/kg, i.v. over 1 h.
- *Clonazepam:* up to 0.25 mg. This may cause apnoea. Careful monitoring and the availability of mechanical ventilation are essential.
- *Pyridoxine:* 50–100 mg i.v. or p.o. should be considered for intractable seizures. Where possible, conventional EEG should be obtained both before and after administration of the first dose of pyridoxine.

Most infants can be weaned from anticonvulsant therapy within a few days of their last seizure. Some infants who have residual seizures or abnormal neurological signs with an abnormal EEG will require ongoing treatment and specialist referral.

Neonatal abstinence syndrome
This occurs in babies born to women who are chemically dependent and who may use multiple substances. These babies exhibit signs of withdrawal and may require treatment. The features of withdrawal are assessed using a standardised scoring system (commonly adapted from the system devised by Finnegan).
- **Do not use naloxone at delivery in these babies; it may precipitate acute withdrawal associated with seizures.**
- The onset of withdrawal is variable:
  - *Heroin:* 48–72 h.
  - *Methadone:* may be delayed for up to 1–2 weeks.
- Withdrawal may be less evident in premature infants.

Clinical features
Neurological signs
- Hypertonia, tremors, hyperreflexia.
- Myoclonic jerks, seizures (1–2% heroin, 7% methadone).
- Irritability, restlessness, high-pitched cry.
- Sleep disturbance.

Autonomic system dysfunction
- Nasal stuffiness, sneezing, yawning.
- Low grade fever, sweating.

- Skin mottling.
- Gastrointestinal abnormalities:
  - Regurgitation, vomiting, diarrhoea.
- Poor feeding, dysmature swallowing.
- Failure to thrive.
- Respiratory symptoms:
  - Tachypnoea.
  - Increased apnoea.
- Skin excoriations (especially around the anus).

Management of opiate withdrawal may involve the administration of morphine to assist gradual withdrawal.

Note: The selective serotonin reuptake inhibitors (SSRIs) commonly used to treat depression were once thought to be entirely safe from the perspective of the fetus. However, a minority of exposed newborns will develop seizures in the first few days of life as a consequence of withdrawal from SSRIs. These seizures are usually short lived (days) and the long-term neurodevelopmental outcome is thought to be normal.

Postnatal depression

Mild to moderate postnatal depression (PND) occurs in about 1 in 6 women. A smaller number experience severe PND, which may be a risk to the life of both mother and baby. PND can have profound effects on a family and on the child's development. The diagnosis may not always be obvious, so a high level of awareness is required when assessing any baby in the first months of life. Infants of mothers with PND may present with feeding problems, failure to thrive or excessive crying.

Clinical features

Clinical features in the mother may include:
- Lowered mood/fearfulness.
- Anxiety.
- Disorganisation.
- Inattentiveness to the baby.
- Recurrent presentations to healthcare professionals.

Management

- Recognise and acknowledge the problem. The Edinburgh Postnatal Depression Scale is a useful 10-item screening instrument that is easy to administer, score and interpret.
- Arrange or refer to appropriate counselling.
- Medication is often necessary.
- Referral to a mother and baby unit or psychiatric hospital facility is often beneficial.

Maternal mastitis

Mastitis is common in breast-feeding women.

- It presents with aches, pains and fever; women often think they have flu.
- An examination reveals a tender engorged segment in one or both breasts.
- The organism is usually *Staphylococcus aureus*.

Management

- Prompt treatment is important to prevent abscess formation.
- Oral antibiotics – flucloxacillin 500 mg p.o., 6 hourly.
- Paracetamol and increased fluids.
- Breast-feeding should continue.
- Thorough emptying of the affected breast (the baby is more efficient at this than expression).

Problems of the ex-very low birthweight infant

Although it is not the intention of this chapter to discuss the problems of managing very-low-birthweight (VLBW) infants (birthweight <1500 g), it is important to be aware of some of the problems that occur after discharge from the neonatal unit.

Bronchopulmonary dysplasia

This is a common chronic lung disease occurring for a few months in very premature infants after RDS. It is characterised by an abnormal chest radiograph and oxygen dependency after 36 weeks' gestation. Most infants with bronchopulmonary dysplasia (BPD) can be weaned from oxygen treatment within 4 weeks of the expected date of delivery. A small number require oxygen therapy for months and some are managed at home in oxygen. Consideration should be given to the timely immunisation of these infants against influenza. The first dose is given after 6 months chronological age, at the appropriate season, with a booster 1 month later. Pavilizumab (monoclonal antibody to RSV) is also considered in some infants, but is currently not cost-effective.

These babies are particularly susceptible to respiratory infections in the first 18 months of life and may deteriorate rapidly and need re-admission to hospital. If a baby is feeding poorly because of dyspnoea, is in respiratory distress, has apnoeic episodes or is drowsy, urgent admission to hospital is indicated. In the absence of these signs the infant may be managed at home, but the parents need to be informed of the warning signs and the child should be reviewed frequently.

Necrotising enterocolitis

This is due to inflammation of the intestine in the early neonatal period. While many babies recover with conservative management (nil orally, i.v. alimentation and antibiotics), some develop necrosis that necessitates bowel resection. The risks to these babies after discharge from hospital are:

- *Stricture formation*: this can present weeks or months after the initial episode. The presenting features of obstruction include bile-stained vomiting, distension, constipation and failure to thrive.
- *Gastroenteritis*: this can produce severe dehydration very rapidly in a baby who has had a bowel resection. Admission to hospital for i.v. fluids is mandatory.

Hearing and visual deficits

These are common problems and must be carefully screened and assessed soon after discharge from hospital. Currently, infants discharged home from a NICU usually have hearing screening, but those who are transferred to a level 2 nursery at another hospital may not undergo testing. Eventually hearing screening will be universal in Australia.

Further common problems

- *Inguinal hernias*: require prompt surgical referral as they frequently strangulate. See chapter 38, Surgical conditions.
- *Immunisation*: hepatitis B vaccination is recommended just after birth or at 32 weeks if born prematurely. All other immunisations are given at the appropriate postnatal age according to the immunisation schedule. The doses should not be delayed or reduced because of either size or prematurity. A booster for hepatitis B may be required at 12 months of age. Refer to chapter 9, Immunisation.
- *Apnoea*: this is a common problem until about 34 weeks' gestation. However, ex-VLBW infants are at increased risk of apnoea until 3 months past their due date, after general anaesthesia, or with respiratory infections. Close monitoring is advised at these times.
- *Haemangiomas (strawberry naevi)*: these appear after birth as small, raised, red, lobulated and compressible lesions that increase in size over a few months. They are more common in premature infants, but also occur in term babies. Most involute during the first 2 years. Failure to involute or difficult locations (e.g. near the eye) require urgent referral to a dermatologist for laser or intralesional steroid therapy (see chapter 23, Dermatologic conditions).

USEFUL RESOURCES
- *www.rch.org.au/nets/handbook/* – Victorian Newborn Emergency Transport Services handbook.
- American Academy of Pediatrics Guidelines. From *Pediatrics* 1994; 94: 558–565, Oct. (tables reproduced with permission).
- *http://www.neonatology.org/* – Excellent collection of resources including clinical teaching, links, important papers.
- *http://depts.washington.edu/nicuweb/* – From the Department of Neonatal Pediatrics, University of Washington; protocols, references and links.

CHAPTER 33

Neurologic conditions

Andrew Kornberg
Simon Harvey
Mark Mackay
Wirginia Maixner

Febrile convulsions

- Febrile convulsions (FC) are usually brief, generalised seizures associated with a febrile illness, in the absence of any CNS infection or past history of afebrile seizures.
- Most FC occur in the context of a genetically determined, age-dependent seizure disorder in which the child has a tendency to have seizures with fever.
- *Simple FC* are brief, generalised and single.
- *Complex FC* are either focal, >15 min, or multiple in a 24 h period.
- FC occur in 3–4% of children aged 6 months to 5 years and are recurrent in 1/3.
- In otherwise healthy children, FC are not accompanied by an increased risk of intellectual disability, cerebral palsy, other neurological disorders or death. However, there is a modest increase in the risk of epilepsy.

Management

- Stop a continuing convulsion (>10 min duration) with i.v. or rectal diazepam 0.2–0.4 mg/ kg (max. 10 mg).
- General temperature-lowering measures such as removing clothing and administering paracetamol 15 mg/kg may help reduce symptoms of fever.
- A careful search for the cause of fever is required. Most will be due to viral respiratory infections.
- A lumbar puncture need not be done routinely following a simple FC, but meningitis should be considered in any unwell child, especially when there is a persistently depressed conscious state and in children with multiple or prolonged convulsions. The younger the child, the higher the index of suspicion of meningitis.

Recurrence of FC is more likely if seizures occur in early infancy and if there is a family history of FC. As FC are usually benign and as anticonvulsants may have significant side effects and do not alter long-term prognosis, they are not routinely recommended for children with

Paediatric Handbook, 8th edition. By Kate Thomson, Dean Tey and Michael Marks. Published 2009 by Blackwell Publishing, ISBN: 978-1-4051-7400-8.

recurrent FC. In some circumstances (e.g. children with a history of prolonged FC) parents may be taught to administer rectal diazepam or buccal midazolam.

About 3% of children with FC subsequently develop afebrile seizures (epilepsy). This is in comparison to the prevalence of epilepsy of 0.5% of all children. The risk is greater with:

- Previous abnormal neurological development.
- A history of epilepsy in first-degree relatives.
- Prolonged (>10 min) FC.
- Focal features present during, or after, the FC.
- Multiple convulsions during a single febrile episode.

When counselling parents, remember that many will have felt that their child nearly died. The very low risk of neurological complications, the excellent prognosis for eventual remission of FC, but the 1 : 3 risk of FC recurrence, need to be emphasised. Advice on the management of future febrile illnesses and FC is required. A follow-up visit is recommended to review FC and minimise the development of 'fever phobia' in the parents. An electroencephalogram (EEG) is of little value in single or recurrent, simple or complex FC.

Epilepsy

Epilepsy (defined as two or more unprovoked seizures) occurs in approximately 0.5% of children. Seizures may be focal (partial) and/or generalised and the aetiology may be idiopathic (genetic) or symptomatic (malformation, tumour, scar, degenerative).

Benign focal (idiopathic partial) epilepsies of childhood

- Onset is typically in mid-childhood (peak 7 years).
- Seizures are commonly nocturnal or early morning. In the centro-temporal (Rolandic) variety, they are usually focal motor or sensory phenomena related to the face, mouth or jaw. The occipital variety may have visual manifestations. Secondarily generalised tonic–clonic seizures may also occur.
- On EEG, spike discharges typically occur in the centrotemporal or occipital region.
- Imaging is only necessary if clinical or EEG features are atypical or if seizure control is difficult.
- The prognosis is excellent as the seizures are usually infrequent and remit before the teenage years.
- Treatment is only indicated in children with frequent or prolonged seizures. Low-dose carbamazepine or sodium valproate is used for 1–2 years given the spontaneous remission of seizures.

Idiopathic generalised epilepsies

- This term describes a group of recognisable childhood epilepsies characterised by recurrent generalised tonic–clonic, absence or myoclonic seizures of presumed genetic cause.
- The first seizure usually occurs at 4–16 years of age, in an otherwise normal child who may have a history of prior FC.
- The EEG invariably shows intermittent generalised spike wave patterns.
- The prognosis is generally good for seizure control and remission in later childhood or adulthood.

- Idiopathic generalised epilepsy syndromes include childhood and juvenile absence epilepsies, juvenile myoclonic epilepsy, and epilepsy with isolated tonic–clonic seizures.

Symptomatic focal epilepsies

- This term describes a heterogeneous group of seizure disorders in which children have focal (partial) seizures from particular brain regions, due usually to an underlying developmental (congenital) or acquired lesion.
- Complex partial seizures and focal motor seizures are the main seizure type. The former is usually manifest by arrest of activity, staring, autonomic disturbances, semi-purposeful automatic movements (automatisms) and altered conscious state, sometimes preceded by an aura. Specific seizure manifestations depend on the brain region involved. Seizures may secondarily generalise.
- Seizures typically occur in clusters and may be difficult to treat.
- Children may have associated learning and behavioural problems, due to dysfunction in the affected brain region or the pervasive effect of uncontrolled seizures and medications.
- An EEG may show localised epileptic activity. Structural pathology is sought using MRI.

Symptomatic generalised epilepsies

- These are usually severe seizure disorders affecting infants and young children in which uncontrolled generalised seizures are associated with generalised epileptic disturbances on EEG and global developmental delay or regression.
- Examples include West and Lennox–Gastaut syndromes. The characteristic seizures in these syndromes are epileptic spasms (clusters of brief tonic seizures that are usually generalised and in flexion), drop attacks and tonic–clonic seizures, generally difficult to control with medication.

Status epilepticus

See chapter 1, Medical emergencies.

Anticonvulsant therapy
Indications for commencing anticonvulsants

- After the first afebrile seizure, only 1/3 of children experience further episodes. Therefore treatment is not normally commenced unless there are features to suggest an increased risk of recurrence.
- Children with absence, myoclonic, complex partial seizures and epileptic spasms have usually had multiple seizures at presentation and require treatment.
- It is important to characterise the epileptic syndrome from history, EEG and sometimes imaging. This guides prognosis and the need for treatment.

- About 50% of childhood epilepsies have a favourable course from the outset, 25% gradually improve with time, and 25% are refractory to treatment.

The decision to investigate and treat a child following a seizure depends on many factors.
- Children with FC do not generally need EEG or imaging investigation.
- An EEG should generally be done in any child with a definite, non-febrile, seizure, whether generalised or partial. EEG aids in the characterisation of seizures and epilepsies, but should not be used to distinguish seizures from nonepileptic events.
- Brain imaging is reserved for children with epilepsy in whom there is suspicion from history, examination or EEG that there may be an underlying cerebral lesion. Children with typical forms of uncomplicated and well-controlled idiopathic focal or generalised epilepsy do not require imaging. MRI is more sensitive than CT scan in identifying cerebral lesions, particularly subtle abnormalities of the cerebral cortex.

Antiepileptic medication is only indicated in children at risk of recurrent epileptic seizures (see Table 33.1).

Principles of anticonvulsant therapy
- *Monotherapy:* most patients are well controlled with one anticonvulsant.
- *Titrate slowly:* most antiepileptic medications are commenced at a low dose and titrated up to the maintenance dose, to avoid side effects during their introduction ('start low and go slow').
- *Changing medications:* introduce or change one anticonvulsant at a time, except in emergency situations.
- *Dosage variation:* individuals vary greatly in dosage requirements and tolerance. Young children and infants typically require relatively large doses.
- *Monitoring:* if seizure control is inadequate, or non-adherence or clinical toxicity is suspected, anticonvulsant blood levels may be measured for phenytoin, phenobarbitone, carbamazepine and valproate. Routine monitoring of phenytoin and phenobarbitone levels are indicated, especially in young infants and intellectually disabled older children in whom side effects may not be identified as easily. Other drugs are generally monitored with attention to usual prescribed doses and clinical markers.
- *Poor response to medication:* if seizure control is poor, the diagnosis and the choice of medication should be reviewed.

Depending on the type of epilepsy, one to several years free of seizures are generally required before anticonvulsants are withdrawn. This is done gradually over several months.

Parents also need to be instructed in the first aid management of seizures, and be given a plan for what to do when seizures recur. Safety precautions such as supervision in water

Table 33.1 Guidelines for the use of common anticonvulsants

	Generalised tonic–clonic seizures	Partial: simple, complex or 2° generalised	Absence (typical and atypical) myoclonic, tonic	Spasms and tonic seizures	Side effects (common or severe)
Carbazepine (Tegretol, Tegretol CR)	++	+++	Avoid	Avoid	Drowsiness, irritability, GIT, rash
Clobazam (Frisium)	+	+	+	+	Drowsiness, irritability
Clonazepam (Rivotril)	+	+	+	+	Irritability and behaviour disorder, increased secretions
Diazepam (Valium)	–	–	–	–	Drowsiness, respiratory depression
Ethosuximide (Zarontin)	–	–	+	–	GIT, thrombocytopenia
Gabapentin (Neurontin)	–	++	Avoid	Avoid	Drowsiness, dizziness, ataxia, fatigue
Lamotrigine (Lamictal)	++	++	++	+	Skin rash (3%) – may be severe. Increased risk if rapid introduction or on concurrent sodium valproate
Levetiracetam (Keppra)	+	++	–	–	Behaviour disturbance
Nitrazepam (Mogadon)	–	–	–	+	Drowsiness, increased bronchial secretions
Oxcarbazepine (Trileptal)	+	++	Avoid	Avoid	Drowsiness, hyponatraemia

(Continued)

Table 33.1 *Continued*

	Generalised tonic–clonic seizures	Partial: simple, complex or 2° generalised	Absence (typical and atypical) myoclonic, tonic	Spasms and tonic seizures	Side effects (common or severe)
Phenobarbitone	++	+	–	–	Cognitive, irritability, overactivity or drowsiness
Phenytoin sodium (Dilantin)	++	++	–	–	Gum hyperplasia, ataxia, nystagmus, serum sickness-like illness, cognitive, rash
Pregabalin (Lyrica)	–	+	–	–	Weight gain
Sodium valproate (Epilim)	+++	++	++	+	Nausea, anorexia, vomiting, weight gain, severe hepatotoxicity (rare)
Tiagabine (Gabitril)	–	+	Avoid	Avoid	Headache, dizziness
Topiramate (Topamax)	+	++	–	+	Weight loss, sedation, cognitive nephrolithiasis, paraesthesia
Vigabatrin (Sabril)	–	+	Avoid	++	Excitation, agitation, drowsiness, dizziness, headache, weight gain, visual field constriction

Notes:
- Table shows relative effectiveness of each drug against each of the major seizure types. It does not represent a comparison of one drug against another.
- Table represents suggestions only. Final decision of most appropriate anticonvulsant should take into consideration the patient's age, neurological status, co-morbidities, epilepsy syndromes, EEG, patient and parent attitudes and potential side effects.
- Anticonvulsants listed as to 'avoid' can potentially exacerbate seizures.
- Sodium valproate should be used with caution in children <3 years old, particularly if multiple anticonvulsants are used and underlying cerebral pathology is present.
- Cognitive side effects are seen with all anticonvulsants (particularly benzodiazepines and barbiturates).
- For status epilepticus, refer to chapter 1, Medical emergencies.

and avoidance of heights need to be discussed. Driving and other lifestyle and vocational restrictions apply to older teenagers and adults with epilepsy.

Non-epileptic paroxysmal events

- Many children referred for assessment of epilepsy do not have epilepsy, but rather a non-epileptic paroxysmal disorder such as syncope, breath-holding spells, parasomnias or non-epileptic staring.
- In differentiating epileptic from non-epileptic events, the description of the event is important, including the circumstances in which the event occurred and the details of what the child was doing immediately before the event.
- Most non-epileptic paroxysmal disorders can be diagnosed on history alone, or with the aid of a home video recording of a typical event. In some circumstances video-EEG monitoring may be required.
- The long Q–T syndrome should be considered in any episode of fainting or seizure that is not clearly due to typical breath-holding, vasovagal syncope or a definable epilepsy syndrome.

Table 33.2 lists some of these events and their salient features.

Weakness of acute onset

The acute onset of symmetrical limb weakness usually has a peripheral neuromuscular or spinal cord origin. Toxins (e.g. snake or tick bite), metabolic disturbance, systemic illness and psychogenic causes need to be considered under appropriate circumstances. Oral polio vaccine is a rare cause of acute flaccid paralysis.

Two key questions require urgent consideration:

- Is there a treatable cause?
- Is there respiratory or bulbar dysfunction of sufficient degree to warrant management in an intensive care unit?

Myasthenia gravis

- This diagnosis should be considered in any child with relatively acute-onset limb weakness, particularly if accompanied by ptosis, eye movement disorder, pharyngeal or respiratory insufficiency.
- A diagnostic/therapeutic trial of parenteral anticholinesterase is warranted if myasthenia is a possibility.

Guillain–Barré syndrome

- Presents with weakness (ascending progression may be less clear in young children), pain and sensory loss. Weakness may be misinterpreted as ataxia.
- The child should be transferred to a tertiary referral centre at the time of diagnosis, as respiratory weakness may occur rapidly
- Gamma-globulin or plasma exchange need to be commenced early if they are to be effective.

Table 33.2 Non-epileptic paroxysmal events

	Syncope	Breath-holding attacks	Shuddering	Benign paroxysmal vertigo	Self-stimulation	'Daydreams'	Confusional arousals*	Nightmares
Age	All ages	Infancy	Infancy	Preschool	Preschool	School	Preschool/school age	All ages
Circumstances	Always triggering factor or situational	Always upset or a trigger is needed	Any time, anywhere	Any time, anywhere	Any time, anywhere	Commonly school, watching TV, times of inactivity	First 1/3 of sleep (non-REM)	Second 1/2 of sleep (REM)
Frequency	Occasional	Varies greatly	Sometimes many per day	1/month or less	Daily or less	Varies, but not large numbers per day	Nightly or less. Rarely >1/night	Nightly or less
Onset	Gradual or sudden	Sudden, with or without crying	Sudden	Sudden	Sudden	Vague	Sudden	Sudden
Recovery	Gradual	Slow if hypoxic seizure occurs	Rapid	Rapid	Rapid	Vague. May be 'snapped out'	Returns to sleep	Remains asleep
Duration	Seconds to minutes	Seconds to minutes	Seconds	1–5 min	Minutes to hours	Seconds to minutes	Minutes	Minutes

(Continued)

Table 33.2 *Continued*

	Syncope	Breath-holding attacks	Shuddering	Benign paroxysmal vertigo	Self-stimulation	'Daydreams'	Confusional arousals*	Nightmares
Impairment of consciousness	Yes	Usually	No	No	No	Apparent but not real	Apparently awake but does not respond	Asleep
Observations	May describe light-headedness, dizziness or loss of vision. Tonic or tonic-clonic seizure may occur at end	Cyanotic or pale, limp, may develop opisthotonos /seizure	Rapid shivering movement maximal in head, trunk and arms	Frightened, pale, holds on to objects to maintain balance or falls	Posturing with stiffening and while lying on side or supine, leaning against firm edge. Irregular breathing, flushing, sweating	Blank staring but no motor automations or blinking despite long episodes. Not precipitated by hyperventilation	Screaming, crying inconsolably, may get out of bed. Appears terrified	Nil
Post-event impairment	Minimal	Mild unless hypoxic seizure occurs	No	No	No	No	No recollection of event	Good recall of event

* Including sleep-walking and night terrors.

Infant botulism

- Suspect in children 2–9 months of age with constipation and rapid onset of weakness, particularly with ophthalmoplegia and bulbar/respiratory weakness.
- A child with suspected infant botulism should be transferred urgently to a centre capable of undertaking long-term ventilation.

Spinal cord compression

- Persistent or severe back pain and stiffness are ominous symptoms requiring prompt attention.
- Myelopathy should always be considered when there is paraparesis or quadriparesis without neurological dysfunction at higher levels.
- Brisk deep tendon reflexes or extensor plantar responses may not be prominent early and a sensory level is often the most important clue to a myelopathy.
- The confirmation or exclusion of trauma, tumour, abscess, haematoma or skeletal pathology is an urgent priority.
- Spinal imaging with MRI is required even when acute 'transverse' myelopathy is suspected.
- Steroid therapy is important in spinal cord compression, before decompression.

Encephalopathies

- Encephalopathies are characterised predominantly (but not exclusively) by cerebral hemispheric dysfunction producing at least two of the following:
  - Altered conscious state.
  - Altered cognitive state/personality.
  - Seizures.
- The onset can be acute, subacute or chronic.
- Causes can be grouped into infective (or post-infective), hypoxic, traumatic, epileptic, metabolic, migrainous, raised intracranial pressure and drug or toxin exposure. The primary cause may be systemic or originate in the CNS (see also chapter 30, Infectious diseases, Encephalitis, p. 413).

Examination

Impaired conscious state or cognitive function is the cardinal sign. There may be widespread upper motor neurone signs. Meningism may or may not be present.

Investigations

Investigations are guided by history and examination. Consider the following:
- Electrolytes.
- Toxin and metabolic screen.
- Cerebrospinal fluid (microscopy and culture; viral and mycoplasma PCR).
  Note: For contra-indications to lumbar puncture see chapter 3, Procedures.
- EEG.

- Neuroimaging: CT can exclude a mass lesion or acute bleed, but MRI is preferable in most circumstances. MRI of the brain and spinal cord may show multifocal demyelination in acute disseminated encephalomyelitis (ADEM).

Management

- Early specialist referral – early neurosurgical referral if raised intracranial pressure is suspected.
- Seizure control.
- Identify and treat the primary cause.
- Consider empiric antimicrobials e.g. cefotaxime and aciclovir (see chapter 30, Infectious diseases).
- If ADEM is suspected, consider high-dose i.v. corticosteroids.

Acute disseminated encephalomyelitis

Acute disseminated encephalomyelitis (ADEM) is a monophasic inflammatory condition of the CNS that most commonly affects children and young adults. The usual presentation is with altered conscious state and multifocal neurological disturbance. It typically occurs following a viral prodrome and has been described following a variety of infections including measles, varicella, EBV, *Mycoplasma pneumoniae* and non-specific febrile illnesses.

Clinical

- A prodrome of ataxia before onset is typical.
- Encephalopathy: may vary in severity from irritability to coma.
- Multifocal neurological abnormalities such as ataxia, hemiparesis, optic neuritis, cranial nerve palsies and bladder dysfunction.
- A characteristic feature of ADEM is the evolution of symptoms and signs over time: new neurological symptoms and signs appear over the first few days (compared to other types of encephalitis where the onset is usually explosive without new manifestations after 24–48 h).

Investigation

MRI is the investigation of choice and usually demonstrates white matter changes (although grey matter involvement is not uncommon).

Management

General principles as above. Steroids are used in the treatment of ADEM despite the lack of controlled studies to prove their efficacy. Anecdotal evidence of their benefit is now strong. Steroid therapy may improve the patient's condition but withdrawal of treatment while the disease is still active may result in the return of original symptoms, or the development of new symptoms.

Early studies found a mortality rate of up to 20% with a high incidence of neurological sequelae in those who survived. Recent case reports and small series suggest a more favourable prognosis, with most individuals recovering fully. Residual deficits in higher cognitive function may occur.

Chronic and recurrent headache

- Migraine is the most common identifiable cause of recurrent or chronic headache in childhood.
- In adolescence, muscle contraction (tension-type) headache is also common.
- Although rare, raised intracranial pressure and systemic illness must also be considered.

History

- Determine the location of the headache and its quality, duration, frequency and time of onset.
- Identify trigger factors (food, sleep deprivation), associated symptoms (e.g. nausea or vomiting, visual disturbance and localising or focal symptoms) and the disruption to normal activities.
- Inquire whether the symptoms are progressive and if there is a history of recent head injury; development of visual, gait or coordination difficulties; or changes in personality or intellectual functioning; or a family history of migraine or cerebral tumours.
- Take a detailed social history.
- Consider recording symptoms in a 'headache diary'.

Distinguishing features

- *Tension headache:* tends to be persistent but usually does not interfere with sleep.
- *Migraine:* tends to have a fluctuating temporal pattern.
- *Migraine without aura:* usually frontotemporal or bilateral in older children. It is frequently accompanied by nausea and vomiting, followed by lethargy or sleep. Marked pallor is common and there is commonly a positive family history.
- *Migraine with aura or prolonged neurological symptoms:* uncommon in young children.
  - Aura is not often reported by young children.
- *Intracranial pathology:* suggested by recurrent morning headaches; headaches that are intense, prolonged and incapacitating or that show a progressive change in character over time. Other features include abnormal examination findings, unusual migraine description and failure to respond to simple treatment measures. Such patients require urgent specialist referral.

Examination

- Do a thorough neurological examination, including examination of visual acuity and fields, eye movements, optic fundi, coordination and gait. Measure head circumference and blood pressure.
- Auscultate the skull for intracranial bruits; palpate over the sinuses, cervical spine and teeth.
- Assess the child's growth and pubertal status; inspect the skin for neurocutaneous stigmata.

Management of migraine

- Reassure the child and parents that migraine is not usually a serious condition.
- In an acute attack, all that is usually required is trigger avoidance, stress management and the early use of paracetamol 15 mg/kg per dose orally, 4 hourly (max. 90 mg/kg per 24 h). NSAIDs (e.g. ibuprofen 2.5–10 mg/kg per dose (max. 600 mg) oral 6–8 hourly) can also be useful. The role of sumatriptan in childhood is not yet clear. In children with severe vomiting and oral agents are not tolerated, metoclopramide and chlorpromazine can be used.
- Prophylactic therapy for those with severe or frequent attacks is best used in consultation with a specialist. Propranolol or pizotifen are commonly used. Sodium valproate, cyproheptadine, verapamil, clonidine and amitriptyline can also be effective in some children.
- 2/3 of children cease having attacks but 50% of these have recurrences in adult life.

Abnormal head shape

Craniosynostosis is an uncommon disorder of childhood affecting 4/10 000 children. It is a condition of premature fusion of the cranial sutures resulting in an abnormal head shape.

- The resulting head shape depends on which suture fuses. The common shapes are:
  - Scaphocephaly (sagittal suture).
  - Brachycephaly (coronal suture).
  - Plagiocephaly (lambdoid suture). Most children with plagiocephaly have a postural deformation rather than craniosynostosis.
- The main problem is cosmetic. Only a small proportion have raised intracranial pressure.

Management

- Frank sutural synostosis requires surgical correction.
- Postural lambdoid plagiocephaly is not associated with sutural fusion and does not require surgery. It may partially correct spontaneously with changes in sleeping position. The asymmetric head shape becomes less obvious with hair growth.

Childhood stroke
Background

- Although considered rare by adult standards, childhood stroke is more common than brain tumours and amongst the top ten causes of death in childhood.
- Subtypes include arterial ischaemic stroke (AIS), cerebral sinovenous thrombosis (CSVT) and haemorrhagic stroke (HS).
- Mode of presentation, risk factors, aetiology, recurrence rates and outcome are dependent on stroke subtype and age.
- Neuroimaging is required to confirm the diagnosis and to differentiate from other paroxysmal neurological disorders.

Aetiology
- Arteriopathies – transient (e.g. post varicella, dissection) or progressive (e.g. Moya Moya disease) in AIS.
- Congenital heart disease in AIS and CSVT.
- Thrombophilias in AIS and CSVT.
- Head and neck/ENT infections in CSVT.
- Metabolic.

Clinical features
- *Neonates:* commonly present non-specifically with seizures, lethargy and apnoea. Focal neurological signs are rarely evident.
- *Older infants:* typically present with congenital hemiplegia, early hand preference and lateralised neurological deficits.
- *Patients with CSVT:* commonly present non-specifically with seizures and signs of raised intracranial pressure.

Diagnosis
- Urgent imaging:
  - CT head – sufficient to exclude haemorrhage (but may potentially miss AIS or CSVT).
  - MRI or MRA head – if not done immediately should be done <48 h.
- ECG and transthoracic echocardiogram:
  - To look for structural heart defects and patent PFO with paradoxical embolisation.
- Prothrombotic work-up:
  - Preferably taken before anticoagulation.
  - Includes antithrombin, protein C, protein S, plasminogen, activated protein C resistance (APCR), prothrombin gene *20210A*, anticardiolipin antibody (ACLA), lupus anticoagulant, serum homocysteine.

Management
General management
- Measures that improve outcome in adults include correction of fever, maintaining normal glycaemia, normal blood pressure.
- Oxygen – to keep Sao_2 >95% through first 24 h.
- Close observations – initially hourly neurological observations.
- Keep nil by mouth until assessment by speech pathologist.
- If seizures, load with i.v. phenytoin (or phenobarbitone in neonates).
- Rehabilitation: early referral should be made once the child is stable.

Acute antiplatelet/anticoagulant treatment should be discussed with the neurologist and haematologist on call.

For neonates with AIS
- Aspirin or anticoagulation for 6–12 weeks is recommended for neonates **with cardioembolic AIS**.

- Do **not** use anticoagulation or aspirin for **non-cardioembolic AIS** unless there are recurrent events.

For children with AIS
- Initial treatment with aspirin, 1–5 mg/kg per day, unfractionated heparin (UFH) or low-molecular-weight heparin (LMWH) for 5–7 days while being investigated for cardioembolic sources and vascular dissection.
- Treatment should be continued with LMWH or warfarin for another 3–6 months if dissection or cardioembolic source is confirmed.
- Conversion to aspirin, 1–5 mg/kg per day is recommended for all other children for a minimum of 2 years.

For children with CSVT
Anticoagulation is usually recommended, except if associated with a significant haemorrhage, patient is hypertensive or other risks for bleeding are present.
- For CSVT **without** significant intracranial haemorrhage:
  - Initially with UFH or LMWH.
  - Subsequently with LMWH or warfarin for a minimum of 3 months (neonates 6 weeks to 3 months).
- For CSVT **with** significant intracranial haemorrhage:
  - Radiological monitoring at 5–7 days and anticoagulation if thrombus propagation occurs.

Head injuries
Assessment
- Determine the nature of the injury, its severity, the time of occurrence and the clinical course before the consultation.
- Always consider inflicted injury (child abuse) in infants and young children with head injury (see chapter 17, Child abuse).
- Assessment using the Glasgow coma chart is essential (see Table 33.3).
- General and neurological examination findings will provide a baseline for further assessment and must be carefully recorded. In the unconscious patient the presence of brain stem signs must be assessed.
- In all but minor cases of head injury, cervical spine injury must be assumed until excluded.

Radiological examination
- A skull radiograph is not done routinely in patients presenting with a non-localised head injury and is not used to determine whether a child requires admission. If a child is assessed as being clinically unwell after a head injury, they should be transferred immediately to a centre with paediatric neurosurgical expertise; the transfer should not be delayed by the taking of a skull radiograph.
- If the child is unwell enough to warrant a skull radiograph, they should be in hospital under observation. There is no place for a skull radiograph 'just in case'. The only exception

Table 33.3 Level of consciousness – Glasgow coma scale

Eye opening		Verbal response (modifications for small children in italics)		Motor response	
Spontaneous	4	Orientated *Appropriate words or social smile, fixes, follows*	5	Obeys commands	6
To speech	3			Localises to stimuli	5
		Confused *Cries but consolable*	4	Withdraws to stimuli	4
To pain	2			Abnormal flexion	3
		Inappropriate words *Persistently irritable*	3		
Nil	1			Extensor responses	2
		Incomprehensible words *Restless & agitated*	2		
		Nil	1	Nil	1

is the child with a large scalp haematoma who is otherwise perfectly well, where a depressed skull fracture cannot be excluded clinically.
- A cervical spine radiograph is necessary when there is a suggestion that the spine may have been injured and in all patients with moderate to severe head injuries.
- A CT scan is indicated in all patients with significant head injury, particularly if there is the possibility of an intracranial haematoma, as suggested by severe headache and vomiting, a depressed conscious state or focal neurological signs.
- An MRI is indicated in those children in whom there is suspicion of a spinal cord injury or a vascular injury or anomaly.

Blunt head injury
This form of injury is due to an impact on a flat surface that produces an acceleration–deceleration type of injury.

Effects
- *Scalp haematomas*: are common in the infant or young child. They may be responsible for a significant reduction in the circulating blood volume.
- *Skull fracture*: significant injuries may not necessarily have a skull fracture, but the majority do. Conversely, a skull fracture may not be associated with significant brain injury. The fracture is usually linear and it may extend to the skull base. The involvement of the nasal, paranasal or middle ear spaces implies that the injury is compound, with a risk of infection. Check for CSF rhinorrhoea or otorrhoea.
- *Concussion*: the most common and least serious type of traumatic brain injury. Involves transient loss of brain function, such as loss of awareness or memory of the event. The duration of unconsciousness is an indicator of the severity of the concussion.

- *Localised brain damage*: this is due to either local deformity at impact (which is not generally an important factor except for some injuries in infancy) or surface laceration of the brain due to brain movement within the skull.
- *Intracranial haemorrhage*: subarachnoid and subdural haemorrhages are usually due to a surface laceration of the brain. In extradural haemorrhage, a dural vessel is torn by distortion at or near the point of impact, especially if on the lateral aspect of the head.
- Intracerebral haemorrhage may result from local damage or a shearing injury within the brain.

Clinical course
Most patients rapidly recover from the effects of concussion in 12–24 h. A delay or reversal of recovery suggests haemorrhage, brain swelling, infection or an extracranial complication – most commonly an impairment of ventilation (hypercarbia → brain swelling).

Management
Mild
- A brief loss of consciousness (<5 min) without other neurological symptoms or signs suggests a mild injury and these patients can be sent home after an initial 4 h observation in emergency.
- Explanation and written information must be given to the parents regarding signs suggesting deterioration and indications for re-presentation (see below).
- The patient should be reviewed the following day, either by the local medical officer or in emergency.

Blows to the side of the head are potentially serious and these patients should be admitted.

Serious
A more serious head injury is indicated by:
- A longer period of unconsciousness.
- Increasingly severe headache with or without vomiting.
- A deterioration in the conscious state, behaviour or vital signs.
- Neurological defects.
- Bleeding or CSF leak from the nose or ear.
- Severe bleeding from a scalp wound.
- A superficial haematoma on the side of the head. This may be associated with an extradural haematoma, even if no fracture is seen on the radiograph.

Children with these signs will require admission and must be observed carefully for at least 48 h.

Delayed presentation
This can be grouped into four categories:

- Clinical features of potentially serious head injuries – admit.
- Patients with a wide linear fracture and a large scalp haematoma – admit.
- Patients with a skull radiograph showing a narrow linear fracture, but who do not require admission on clinical grounds – discuss with a neurosurgeon and consider early involvement of a paediatrician.
- Apparently well patients – send home after appropriate advice, with instructions to return immediately if there is any deterioration.

Localised head injury
In these injuries the damage is predominantly confined to a focal area of the head. Injuries of this type are relatively more common in children than in adults.

Effects
- Simple or compound depressed fractures are common.
- Infection may occur with compound injuries.
- Focal contusion or laceration of the brain may be present to a varying size or depth, and may produce neurological signs or seizures.
- Concussion may be absent.

Management
- Radiographs are always required and should be done as part of the admission including, where indicated, tangential views. CT is indicated in focal injuries.
- Admission for neurosurgical assessment and monitoring is required in most cases.
- To prevent wound infection all patients with external compound head injuries should receive antibiotics (flucloxacillin i.v., with contamination add gentamicin i.v. and metronidazole i.v.) and the wound covered by a head dressing. Prophylactic antibiotics are not indicated, however, for patients with internal compound fractures (base of skull) with CSF leaks. These patients should be observed closely and, if they develop a fever with no obvious focus, given empirical antibiotics (e.g. flucloxacillin 50 mg/kg (max. 2 g) i.v. 4–6 hourly and cefotaxime 50 mg/kg (max. 2 g) i.v. 6 hourly).

Box 33.1 Minor head injuries: discharge instructions for parents

For the next 24 hours keep a careful watch over the patient, who should be roused at least every 2 hours. The child must be reassessed immediately if you notice any of the following:

- The child becomes unconscious or more difficult to rouse.
- The child becomes confused, irrational or delirious.
- There are convulsions or spasms of the face and limbs.
- The child complains of persistent headache or has neck stiffness.
- Repeated vomiting.
- Bleeding from the ear or recurrent watery discharge from the ear or nose.

Care of the unconscious patient
- Maintain the airway.
- Observe for vital and basal neurological signs.
- Protect the cervical spine.
- Ensure temperature regulation.
- Fluid and electrolyte balance.
- Nasogastric aspiration to avoid the inhalation of gastric contents (orogastric if the base of the skull is definitely or possibly fractured).

Anticipate complications
Early evaluation is essential to assess the development of complications, such as compression and infection. Observing for complications associated with extracranial injury is also important. The patient who is not improving should be referred to a neurosurgeon.

Cerebrospinal fluid shunt problems
Subacute shunt obstruction
Cause
- *Upper end block*. The tube is too long or blocked by the choroid plexus.
- *Lower end block*. The tube is too short or blocked by abdominal tissues.
- *Fracture/disconnection*.

Symptoms
- Headache.
- Drowsiness.
- Vomiting.
- Seizures.
- The same as a previous episode.

Signs
General
- Increased fontanelle tension.
- Abnormal cranial percussion note.
- Focal neurological signs.
- Change in vital signs.
- Deterioration in the conscious state.
- Recent increase in head circumference in infants.

Specific
- *Upper end block*. The pump depresses but it does not refill.
- *Lower end block*. The pump is difficult to depress. A radiograph of the chest or abdomen will give an indication of the length of the tube.
- *Fracture/disconnection*. The signs depend on the site of the disconnection. Ventricular tube disconnection is unusual and has the same signs as upper end block. Pump discon-

nection produces local swelling. Fracture along the course of the tubing may produce local swelling. Radiographs may demonstrate a disconnection.

Assessment

The neurosurgeon will want to know:

- Type of shunt: atrial or peritoneal.
- Symptoms and signs, including the state of the pump and shunt tubing.
- Findings on plain radiograph, CT head or ultrasound.

Shunt infection

These infections are often indolent and should be suspected in any child with a shunt who is constitutionally unwell with fevers. There may be associated obstruction, with symptoms and signs as above.

USEFUL RESOURCES

- *http://www.rch.org.au/cep/* – Children's epilepsy program includes information about epilepsy, tests, treatments; proformas for seizure diary and management plan and links to other resources.
- *http://www.pedisurg.com/PtEduc/Craniosynostosis.htm* – Texas Pediatric Surgical Associates – Includes diagrams and discussion about surgical management.
- *http://www.headaches.org/education/Educational_Modules* – A series of education modules provided by the US National Headache Foundation.

CHAPTER 34
Orthopaedic conditions

Kerr Graham
Peter Barnett

Neonatal orthopaedic conditions
Developmental dysplasia of the hip

This condition was previously known as congenital dislocation of the hip; however, not all cases are present at birth and the hips are not necessarily dislocated. Risk factors are breech delivery, oligohydramnios, Caesarean section, family history, congenital anomalies (especially foot abnormalities), being first-born and female.

Diagnosis
General screening

All neonates should have a clinical examination for hip joint instability – the Ortolani and Barlow tests. The baby should be relaxed. With the knee flexed, the thumb is placed over the lesser trochanter and the middle finger over the greater trochanter. The pelvis is steadied with the other hand and the flexed thigh is abducted and adducted. Any clunk or jerk where a dislocation reduces allowing the hip to abduct fully, is a positive Ortolani's sign. The demonstration of acetabular dislocation by levering the femoral head in and out of the acetabulum is a positive Barlow's sign (see Fig. 34.1).

Selective screening

Infants in high-risk groups and those with an abnormal routine clinical screening examination should have an ultrasound examination of their hips.

- As clinical diagnosis can be difficult and ultrasound has diagnostic limitations, the repeated examination of children with risk factors during the first year of life is important.
- When the ossification nucleus of the femoral head develops, between 3 and 9 months, the preferred mode of imaging changes from ultrasound to plain radiograph. Generally use ultrasound up to 6 months of age and radiography thereafter.

Management
The earlier the diagnosis, the easier the management.
- Most neonates can be successfully treated by abduction bracing with a Pavlik harness.
- Operative treatments, including open reduction, may be required with later diagnosis.

Paediatric Handbook, 8th edition. By Kate Thomson, Dean Tey and Michael Marks. Published 2009 by Blackwell Publishing, ISBN: 978-1-4051-7400-8.

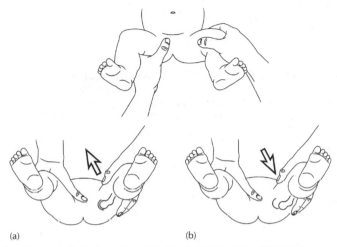

(a)　　　　　　　　　　　　　(b)

Fig. 34.1 Screening for developmental dysplasia of the hip. (a) Ortolani's sign, (b) Barlow's sign

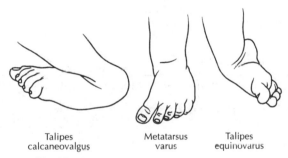

| Talipes calcaneovalgus | Metatarsus varus | Talipes equinovarus |

Fig. 34.2 Congenital foot deformities

Club foot (congenital talipes equinovarus)

Most infants with abnormal-looking feet are said to have 'talipes'. However, the majority have postural problems such as talipes calcaneovalgus (excessive dorsiflexion and eversion), metatarsus varus (adduction of the forefoot) or postural talipes equinovarus (see Fig. 34.2). These deformities are usually mild and mobile; that is, they correct easily and fully with the pressure of one finger. They resolve spontaneously with no treatment.

The true club foot deformity is more severe and is often stiff. The foot is in equinus, with the hind foot in varus and the forefoot supinated.

Management
- All require manipulation and casting.
- Soft tissue surgery is required for many.
- Bone surgery is required for a few.

Torsional and angular deformities in children

Many children are seen with normal angular or torsional variants of the lower limbs. It can be difficult to distinguish physiological variation from pathological conditions. The range of 'normality' is wide, but physiological variations can result in as much parental anxiety as pathological disorders.

Intoeing

Intoeing in childhood can be due to metatarsus varus, internal tibial torsion or medial femoral torsion. See Table 34.1, Figs 34.3 and 34.4.

Out-toeing

Infants and toddlers have restricted internal rotation at the hip because of an external rotation soft tissue contracture, not retroversion of the femur.

Infants

- Present with a 'Charlie Chaplin' posture between 3–12 months.
- The child weight-bears and walks normally.
- Resolution occurs with no treatment.

Table 34.1 Intoeing in childhood

	Metatarsus varus	**Internal tibial torsion**	**Medial femoral torsion**
Synonyms	Metatarsus adductus		Inset hips
Age at presentation	Birth	Toddler	Child
Site of problem	Foot	Tibia	Femur
Examination	Sole of foot bean shaped	Thigh–foot angle is inwards	Arc of hip rotation favours internal rotation
Management	Observe or cast	Observe and reassure	Observe, rarely surgery
When to refer if not resolved	3 months after presentation	6 months after presentation	8 years after presentation

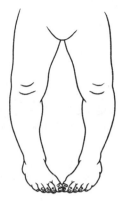

Fig. 34.3 Internal tibial torsion

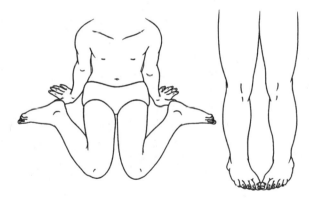

Fig. 34.4 Medial femoral torsion

Children
- May be due to neurologic disorder.
- Surgery may be necessary.

Bow-legs (genu varum)
The vast majority are physiological. Rare causes include skeletal dysplasias, rickets and Blount's disease (tibia vara).

Presentation
- Toddlers are usually bowed until 3 years of age.
- Physiological bowing is symmetrical, not excessive and improves with time.

Management
Monitor intercondylar separation (ICS; see Fig. 34.5). Refer when ICS is >6 cm, is not improving or is asymmetric.

Knock-knees (genu valgum)
Again, the vast majority are physiological. Rare causes are rickets and trauma.

Presentation
- Children are usually knock-kneed from 3 to 8 years.
- Physiological knock-knee is symmetrical, not excessive and improves with time.

Management
- Monitor the intermalleolar separation (IMS; see Fig. 34.5).
- Refer if IMS >8 cm.

Note: Most children with bow-legs or knock-knees are normal, with <1% having an underlying problem.

Flat feet (pes plano valgus)
This condition is painless and asymptomatic.
Note: If painful or stiff, referral is needed.

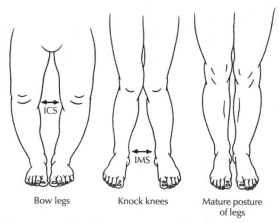

Bow legs   Knock knees   Mature posture of legs

Fig. 34.5 Postural variants in the lower limbs

Causes
- Physiological (in the vast majority): all newborns have flat feet due to fat that fills the medial longitudinal arch; 80% of children develop a medial arch by their sixth birthday.
- Tarsal coalition (in older children and adolescents only).

Management
- No treatment is required unless the condition is painful or stiff.
- The condition is unaffected by orthotics or exercises.
- Most cases resolve spontaneously.

Trauma

The management of fractures and dislocations is an integral part of the overall management of the trauma patient. Common fractures in children involve the wrist, elbow, clavicle, distal tibia, fibula and femur. Each has distinct management strategies but there are common themes.

Assessment

Patients presenting with a suspected fracture or dislocation require a full evaluation of the fracture and exclusion of damage to other structures.

An accurate history of the mechanism of injury will determine which structures may potentially be damaged.

Box 34.1 Consider child abuse in infants with fractures (see chapter 17, Child abuse)

The following details must be sought for every child presenting with an injury: age, developmental stage (including motor capabilities), where injury occurred, whether witnessed (by whom), what actually happened, what is suspected if not witnessed, any delay in presentation, history of previous injuries. Inconsistency of the history between carers or on repeated telling should raise concern.

Examination
- Closed or open fracture (the latter will require operative intervention).
- Deformity or swelling. *Note*: Acute swelling in children usually indicates a fracture.
- Neurological status distal to the injury.
- Peripheral pulses – if the blood flow to the limb is compromised, emergency orthopaedic consultation is necessary.
- Associated injuries.

Management
- The affected limb should be splinted by a board or plaster slab before radiography.
- Analgesia (usually parenteral) is required (e.g. morphine 0.05–0.1 mg/kg dose i.v.). See chapter 4, Pain management.
- A radiograph should be obtained of the suspected fracture site, with additional views to include the joints above and below the suspected fracture site. Anteroposterior and lateral views should be obtained.

- If the arm appears bent on examination or if the angle between the shaft of the bone and the fractured fragment is >15–20°, manipulation of the fracture needs to occur before the placement of a plaster. Forearm fractures in children 5 years or older can usually be manipulated using a local anaesthetic block (e.g. Bier's block, see chapter 3, Procedures).
- If the fracture involves both cortices of the bone, plaster the joints above and below (e.g. above the elbow for a forearm fracture).
- A simple undisplaced greenstick or buckle fracture can be treated in a short cast/backslab.

Home treatment after a full plaster
- Elevate the limb above the heart level for the next 24–48 h.
- *Forearm:* a sling should only be worn after this period and the hand should not be below the elbow while in the sling.
- *Lower limb:* crutches should only be used by children over 6–7 years of age, who are co-ordinated enough to use them.
- Written plaster instructions should be explained and given to parents.

Follow-up
For patients who have had a manipulation of fracture or a fracture involving both cortices of the bone, a repeat radiograph should be obtained in 1 week to ensure the correct position is maintained. Plaster should remain in place for 3–6 weeks, depending on the degree of injury and bone involved. Following the removal of the cast, the bone is still at risk of re-fracture for the next 8–12 weeks; therefore, contact sports are not recommended during this period.

Box 34.2 Description of fractures

It is helpful to use a specific, technical vocabulary to describe fractures for the purposes of documentation, and discussion with colleagues. Important features include:

- *The anatomical site of the fracture:* Which bone? Which side? For example, right humerus or left tibia. In most long bones it is helpful to specify whether the fracture is in the upper, middle or distal third of the bone.
- *The fracture type:* i.e. open or closed. An open fracture has a wound which communicates with the exterior, a closed fracture has an intact soft tissue envelope.
- *The appearance of the fracture line:* e.g. transverse, oblique, spiral or comminuted (more than one fragment).
- Whether there is a *specific type of fracture*. Children's bones are more elastic and less brittle than adult bones. Consequently they are more likely to bend and buckle, rather than crack or break. This results in two common patterns of fracture that are seen in children and not in adults:
  - Greenstick fractures.
  - Buckle fractures.

(Continued)

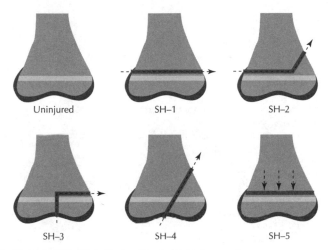

Fig. 34.6 Salter–Harris (SH) classification of growth plate injuries

---

Box 34.2 (*Continued*)

- *The displacement of the fracture*, e.g. undisplaced, angulated or displaced. Angulation is described by drawing a line along both major fragments and measuring the angle of intersection. Displacement is best described by comparing the position of the bone ends with the width of the bone at that point e.g. half a diameter displaced or completely displaced.
- Fractures of the expanded ends of long bones are usually described as *metaphyseal*, and injuries to the growth plate are described according to the Salter–Harris classification (see Fig. 34.6).

From these terms, a complete description of any fracture can be given that should be meaningful to a colleague who has not seen the radiographs. For example, a femoral shaft fracture might be described as a closed, displaced, midshaft fracture of the left femur with 30° of angulation and one complete diameter of displacement.

Specific management of some common fractures
Clavicle

- Sling for 2–3 weeks.
- Inform the parents that a lump will develop at the fracture site which may be visible for up to 1 year.
- No contact sports for 6 weeks.
- No follow-up radiograph is necessary in children, but it is required in adolescents.

Humerus
Surgical neck
- *Undisplaced*: sling for 3 weeks.
- *Displaced*: frequently treated with a collar and cuff and refer for follow-up.

Shaft
- Check the integrity of the radial nerve.
- *Undisplaced*: collar and cuff. A U-shaped plaster slab may be applied to the humerus to reduce movement and minimise knocks.
- *Transverse, displaced or comminuted*: refer for an immediate orthopaedic consultation.

Supracondylar
- Check the integrity of the radial artery, radial nerve, median nerve and ulnar nerve. **If there is vascular compromise, extend the elbow until perfusion returns.**
- *Undisplaced*: collar and cuff (under clothing) or backslab with the elbow flexed to at least 90° for 3–4 weeks.
- *Angulated, displaced or comminuted*: refer for an immediate orthopaedic consultation.
- Immobilisation with a backslab provides excellent analgesia. Most children with minimal or no displacement may only need paracetamol to supplement the immobilisation to achieve adequate comfort. Children with more displacement, however, are likely to require a dose of opiate analgesia while awaiting theatre.
- Consider intranasal fentanyl (1.5 mcg/kg, half in each nostril). See chapter 4, Pain management, p. 63.

Epiphyseal and intra-articular
Refer for an immediate orthopaedic consultation.

Radius and ulna
Shaft
- *Undisplaced*: above-elbow plaster, follow up with an orthopaedic opinion.
- *Displaced*: refer for an immediate orthopaedic consultation.

Distal end
- *Undisplaced and non-deformed clinically*:
  - If a single cortex only is involved, use a short arm cast/backslab for 3–4 weeks.
  - If both cortices are involved, plaster above the elbow – refer for an orthopaedic opinion within a week with repeat radiograph.
- *Displaced and clinically deformed*: use local anaesthesia manipulation and plaster (LAMP) in the emergency department.
- *Totally displaced* with fracture ends not touching: use general anaesthesia manipulation and plaster (GAMP) in theatre.

Metacarpals

- Check carefully for rotation at the fracture site. This is assessed clinically by asking the patient to keep the fingers of the hand side-by-side and flexing them together. Rotation is seen where the affected finger crosses over the adjacent finger.
- *Undisplaced*: volar slab; follow up with an orthopaedic opinion.
- *Displaced*: refer for an immediate orthopaedic consultation.

Phalanges (hand)

- Check carefully for rotation at the fracture site.
- Intra-articular fractures require anatomical reduction.
- *Undisplaced*: strap to the adjacent finger for 3–4 weeks.
- *Displaced*: refer for an immediate plastic surgical consultation; some may be reduced under regional nerve block (see chapter 3, Procedures).

Femur

- Isolated femur fractures in young children rarely cause hypotension; however, in adolescents and patients with multiple trauma an i.v. line should be inserted.
- Ensure adequate analgesia with nitrous oxide, opioids and a femoral nerve block (see chapter 3, Procedures).
- Apply simple skin traction, refer for an immediate orthopaedic consultation.

Tibia

- *Undisplaced proximal or midshaft*: above-knee plaster, follow up with an orthopaedic opinion within 1 week (there is a risk of valgus deformity).
- *Undisplaced distal*: below-knee plaster, follow up with an orthopaedic opinion.
- *Displaced*: will need manipulation, refer for an immediate orthopaedic consultation.

Toddlers' fracture

- This is a clinical diagnosis in a young child where a fractured tibia is suspected on clinical grounds (i.e. non-weight-bearing after a fall or tender tibia/fibula on palpation), but no abnormality is detected on radiograph. Exclude septic arthritis/osteomyelitis.
- Apply an above-knee plaster for pain relief, or allow weight-bearing as the child desires if the pain is minimal.
- Limping may continue for 6 weeks.

Ankle

- *Undisplaced*: below-knee plaster, follow up with an orthopaedic opinion.
- *Displaced*: will need manipulation, refer for an immediate orthopaedic consultation.

Metatarsals

Undisplaced: lower leg plaster slab, followed by elevation, follow up with an orthopaedic opinion within 1 week.

Ankle injury

True sprains or soft tissue injuries are more common in adolescents. Pre-adolescent children who have open growth plates commonly sustain a growth plate injury and should be treated in a plaster cast for 2–3 weeks.

Clinical assessment

- Mechanism of injury – it is usually caused by an inversion injury to the ankle.
- Was the patient able to bear weight immediately after the injury?
- Where is the swelling most prominent?
- What is the point of maximal tenderness?

Investigation

Radiographs are required if:

- Deformity is present.
- Maximal tenderness occurs over the distal tibia or fibula.
- The patient is unable to weight-bear.

Note: If the patient is tender over the growth plate of the tibia or fibula and the radiographs are normal, the patient has a Salter–Harris type 1 epiphyseal (growth plate) injury and it should be treated in a below-knee plaster. However, if there is a large amount of swelling use a plaster slab.

If none of the above conditions apply, the treatment will depend on the severity of symptoms.

Management

Mild–moderate sprain

Remember the RICE acronym:

- *Rest*: weight-bearing should occur when comfortable to do so.
- *Ice*: should be applied for 15 min every 2–3 h during the first 48 h, then heat can be applied.
- *Compression*: should be accomplished with either a firm bandage or a plaster slab.
- *Elevation*: the limb should be elevated on a few pillows whenever possible to allow the swelling to subside.

Severe sprain

Treat like a fracture:

- Use below-knee plaster (or if the swelling is severe, a plaster slab followed by a full plaster) for 2–4 weeks.
- No weight-bearing for the first week.
- Gradual rehabilitation should occur after several days of rest. This includes gentle weight-bearing and ankle exercises to strengthen the damaged ankle ligaments (initially plantar- and dorsiflexion exercises as soon as possible; later toe raises, inversion/eversion and proprioception exercises when the pain has subsided).

Pulled elbow
Pathology
Dislocation of the radial head.

Clinical features
- This injury usually occurs at the age of 1–3 years.
- The cause of injury is usually another person pulling the child's arm forcefully. There may be a crack or popping sound at the time. Occasionally, it may occur after a fall.
- The arm is held pronated and slightly flexed (i.e. limp by their side as if they are ignoring it).
- The child is not distressed and is not using the apparently lifeless limb.
- Palpation from the clavicle to the wrist does not demonstrate any swelling or tenderness.
- Supination of the arm causes pain.

Investigations
If the symptoms are typical of a pulled elbow, no investigations are necessary.

Management
- Hold the child's hand as if to shake it and with your other hand encircle the elbow with the thumb over the annular ligament of the radius.
- Gently apply traction and supinate the hand. Flex the forearm at the elbow all the way to the shoulder. You should feel a pop as the radial head is relocated.
- The child should be moving the arm normally within 10–15 min. If there has been a delay in relocation it may take longer for the child to resume using the arm.

Note: If the history is not typical, there is swelling or your attempts at reduction fail, a radiograph of the elbow should be obtained to exclude a radial head fracture.

Limp in childhood
Limp is a common presenting complaint in childhood (see Table 34.2).

Clinical assessment
- Is the limp acute, subacute or chronic?
- Is there associated pain or fever?
- Are there other constitutional symptoms?
- Have there been previous episodes of pain or limp?
- What position is the leg held in (e.g. flexed and externally rotated)?
- Does joint movement or bony pressure cause pain?
- Is there limitation of movement?

Table 34.2 Differential diagnosis of limp in childhood

Acute	Subacute	Chronic
Fracture	Juvenile rheumatoid arthritis	Cerebral palsy
Irritable hip	2Tumour/leukaemia	Developmental dysplasia of the hips
Septic arthritis	Acute or chronic SCFE	Perthes' disease
Osteomyelitis		Chronic SCFE

SCFE, slipped capital femoral epiphysis.

Investigations

- Full blood examination (FBE), differential, erythrocyte sedimentation rate (ESR) and C-reactive protein (CRP).
- Plain radiograph of the joint or affected limb.
- Ultrasound of hip if it is painful (looking for fluid in the joint).
- Bone scan.

Management

This will depend on the underlying problem:

- Slipped capital femoral epiphysis (SCFE), tumours, Perthes' disease or developmental dysplasia of the hip should be referred immediately to an orthopaedic surgeon.
- Toddlers' fractures may be occult and not seen on a radiograph. If the child is afebrile then observation is appropriate.
- A bone scan should be arranged if the limp persists or symptoms worsen.

Irritable hip (transient synovitis)

The usual presentation is a child who is constitutionally well with a partial limp and difficulty walking ± a painful hip. This is a common condition which needs to be distinguished from the others listed in Table 34.2. Although it is the most common reason for limp in the pre-schooler, irritable hip is a diagnosis of exclusion.

Usual clinical features

- Occurs in 3–8 year olds.
- History of a recent viral illness.
- Absence of trauma.
- Child is able to walk, but with pain.
- Severity of the symptoms may vary with time.
- Child is afebrile and appears well.
- There is a mild to moderate decrease in the range of motion due to pain, particularly internal rotation.

Note: The less movement in the joint, the more likely the cause is infective.

Investigations

- These are the same as for limp (see previous; ultrasound usually demonstrates an effusion).
- Results are normal for radiographs, FBE, ESR (<20) and CRP (<8).

Note: The history, symptoms and signs of an irritable hip overlap with septic arthritis, which is a serious condition requiring urgent treatment. If there is any suspicion of bone or joint sepsis, paediatric orthopaedic consultation is required and admission to hospital should be arranged.

Management

Rest and simple analgesics. The more the child can rest, the quicker the recovery. Patients may have a relapse if they increase their activity too quickly. Occasionally, these patients need to be admitted to hospital for bed rest and observation.

Acute bone and joint sepsis: septic arthritis and osteomyelitis

Septic arthritis (SA) and osteomyelitis (OM) can affect any joint or bone, but most commonly involve the lower limbs. **Septic arthritis is an orthopaedic emergency. Drainage and antibiotics are essential to prevent long-term morbidity**.

Clinical features

- Acute onset of limp/non-weight-bearing/non-movement of the limb (may be delayed in OM).
- Pain is localised to the joint or the metaphysis of the bone. Hip pain may be referred to knee.
- Irritability and poor feeding in infants.
- Temperature is usually >38.5 °C.
- Joint is held in a mid-range position.
- Pain on all movements with a decreased range of movement (severe in SA).

Investigations

As for limp – see p. 484.

- Usually ESR is >20–30 and CRP is >20.
- White cell count (WCC) is raised in SA and is usually raised in OM.
- A bone scan may be indicated if the diagnosis is not clear.

Management

- **Urgent paediatric orthopaedic consultation and possibly surgery is required.**
- Admit to hospital; keep nil orally.
- Collect all possible specimens for culture **before** starting antibiotics, including blood culture (all patients) and fluid from the involved joint (consult with the orthopaedic team before starting antibiotics).
- I.v. antibiotics to cover *Staphylococcus aureus*. Cover should be broadened in neonates and children who have not had Hib vaccine to include *Haemophilus influenzae* and other Gram-negative organisms. See Antimicrobial guidelines.

- Duration of antibiotics: For uncomplicated, acute haematogenous septic arthritis and osteomyelitis, i.v. antibiotics are required until defervescence, improvement in symptoms and signs and evidence of reduced inflammatory markers (CRP falls before ESR). This is often 3–5 days. Oral antibiotics are then administered to complete a minimum 3-week course. For disease with any evidence of complication (duration of symptoms ≥14 days, changes of chronicity on plain radiograph, any underlying disease, penetrating injury or delayed response to treatment) i.v. treatment should be prolonged for at least 7–14 days and the total duration of treatment should be at least 4–6 weeks.

Perthes' disease

This is a specific hip disease of childhood. Affected children have a generalised disorder of growth with a tendency to low birthweight and delayed bone age. The pathology is avascular necrosis of the capital femoral epiphysis followed by a sequence of changes including resorption of necrotic bone, reossification and remodelling. This sequence of events is seen radiologically as density of the capital epiphysis, patchy osteolysis, new bone formation and remodelling with a variable degree of femoral head deformity.

Clinical features

- Age range: 2–12 years, but the majority present between 4 and 8 years.
- Sex ratio: 5 males to 1 female, 20% bilateral.
- Symptoms: pain and limp, usually for at least 1 week.
- Signs: restriction of hip motion.

Investigations

- Radiograph.
- A bone scan is useful in the early stages before the signs are clear on radiograph.

Management principles

- Resting the hip in the early irritable phase.
- Regaining motion if the hip is stiff.
- Containing the hip by bracing or surgery in selected patients.

Slipped capital femoral epiphysis

Can occur acutely or chronically. Early detection will prevent later morbidity.

Clinical features

- Age: this occurs in late childhood to early adolescence. Maximum incidence in girls aged 10–12 years and boys 12–14 years.
- Weight is usually >90th percentile.
- Pain in the hip or knee (often pain only in the knee).
- Limp.
- The hip appears externally rotated and shortened.
- Decreased hip movement, particularly internal rotation.
- Can be bilateral.

Investigation
Take a radiograph of the pelvis and a frog-leg lateral of the affected hip.

Management
- The patient should not weight-bear if this diagnosis is considered.
- Urgent orthopaedic referral and surgery to prevent further slipping is required. Most children can be managed with pinning *in situ*.

Scoliosis
Definitions
- Scoliosis is a curvature in the spine when viewed from the frontal (coronal) plane.
- A *structural scoliosis* occurs when the curvature has an element of rotation and may progress with growth.
- A *non-structural scoliosis* may be secondary to a problem outside the spine, such as unequal leg lengths.

Detection
The most common type of scoliosis is adolescent scoliosis, affecting girls in 90% of cases. Because abnormal spinal curvatures start small and may progress with time and growth, efforts have been made to detect the condition at an early stage by school screening programmes. This is usually done by the forward bend test, in which the examiner observes the spine from behind as the subject bends forwards. Flexion of the spine usually demonstrates the deformity much more clearly because of the asymmetry of the ribs and chest wall. Very small curves are relatively common and it can be difficult to decide when a radiograph is required, which curves are likely to progress and which require brace treatment or surgery. The risk of curve progression is related to the age at presentation and the size and cause of the curve.
- 10% of normal adolescents have a curve of 5° or more, but only 2% have curves of >10°.
- Scoliosis is also common in some developmental disorders such as Rett syndrome and complicates many conditions that affect mobility, e.g. spina bifida, cerebral palsy and Duchenne's muscular dystrophy.

Management
All children with scoliosis should be referred to a paediatric orthopaedic surgeon.
- If the curvature <20°: observe.
- If the curvature is 20–40°: a brace is recommended.
- If the curvature is >40°: surgery is required.

USEFUL RESOURCES
- *http://www.rch.org.au/gait* – The Hugh Williamson Gait Analysis Laboratory includes case studies and summaries of research undertaken.

CHAPTER 35

Renal conditions

Colin Jones

Significant renal disease in childhood usually presents in one of the following ways:
- Antenatal ultrasound abnormality of the urinary tract.
- Urinary tract infection (UTI).
- Functional voiding disorder – see chapter 13, Constipation and continence.
- Proteinuria (including nephrotic syndrome).
- Haematuria.
- Hypertension.
- Acute renal failure.
- Chronic renal failure.

Antenatal abnormalities
See Fig. 35.1.

Urinary tract infections
Clinical features
Infants and younger children
- Fever can be the sole symptom.
- Non-specific symptoms such as lethargy, irritability, vomiting and poor feeding are common.
- Offensive urine is neither sensitive nor specific for UTIs in children.

Older children
- Fever, dysuria, urgency, frequency, incontinence, macroscopic haematuria, abdominal pain.

Remember that finding a UTI in a sick child does not exclude another site of serious infection (e.g. meningitis).

Risk factors
- Previous UTI.
- Structural abnormality of renal tract, e.g. duplex systems, posterior urethral valves.

Paediatric Handbook, 8th edition. By Kate Thomson, Dean Tey and Michael Marks. Published 2009 by Blackwell Publishing, ISBN: 978-1-4051-7400-8.

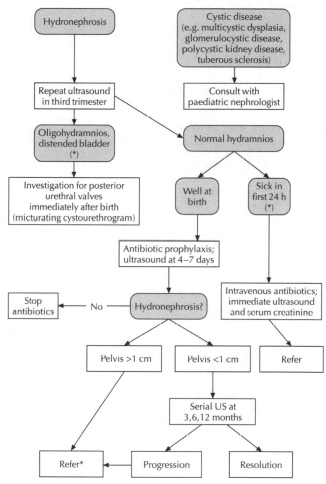

* Consult a paediatric nephrologist or urologist early in all cases

Fig. 35.1 Antenatal abnormalities

- Vesico-ureteric reflux (VUR).
- Strong family history.

Pathogens
- *Escherichia coli* (80%).
- *Enterococcus faecalis* (10%).
- Other Gram-negatives – *Klebsiella, Proteus, Enterobacter, Citrobacter.*
- Other Gram-positives – *Staphylococcus saprophyticus.*

Associated renal tract abnormalities
40% of children with UTI have underlying renal tract abnormalities:
- VUR 40%
- Reflux-associated nephropathy (renal scarring) 12%.
- Pelvic-ureteric junction (PUJ) or vesico-ureteric junction (VUJ) obstruction 4–6%.
- Other congenital abnormalities.

Diagnosis
Urine infections are diagnosed by bacterial growth on midstream urine (MSU), catheter (CSU) or suprapubic aspirate (SPA) specimens of urine. A clean catch specimen is prone to contamination.

Urine 'ward test' strips
These are useful as a screening test in a child with low suspicion of a UTI (>6 months, without known renal tract abnormality and with an alternative focus for fever). Ward test should not be used in a child with a high chance of a UTI. The ward test strips for leucocytes or nitrites are negative in up to 50% of UTIs in children. This is because the production of nitrites by bacteria is time-dependent and infant bladder capacity necessitates frequent voiding.

Bag urine specimen collection
- Do not send for culture.
- Use for chemical strip screening only.
- In sick infants or those where the suspicion of UTI is high (e.g. renal tract anomaly or previous UTI), a bag specimen **should not** be taken, as it only delays the diagnosis. A SPA (preferred) or CSU sample should be obtained as part of the septic workup (see chapter 30, Infectious diseases).

Midstream urine specimen collection
This can be obtained from children who are able to void on request (usually by 3–4 years of age). The child's genitalia are first washed with warm water. In girls the labia should be separated. The child is asked to void. After passing the first few millilitres, a specimen is collected.
- A pure growth of 10^8 c.f.u./L in a MSU is proof of a UTI.
- A pure growth of $>10^5$–10^8 c.f.u./L in a MSU is suggestive of a UTI (correlate with clinical setting).

Catheter specimen collection

See chapter 3, Procedures.

- These are useful in infants after a failed SPA or in older children who are unable to void on request. A pure growth of >105 c.f.u./L indicates infection.

Suprapubic aspirate collection

See chapter 3, Procedures.

- This is the preferred method of urine collection in infants. Aspirated urine should be sterile; hence any pure growth of bacteria indicates infection.

Other investigations

- Blood culture and electrolytes.
- Do not omit a lumbar puncture in a sick child just because UTI has been diagnosed. **All infants <3 months with UTI should have a lumbar puncture.** Consider a lumbar puncture in all infants aged 3 months–2 years with UTI.

Management

- Most infants <12 months of age with a UTI require benzylpenicillin 60 mg/kg i.v. (max. 2 g) 6 hourly and gentamicin 7.5 mg/kg i.v. (<10 years) or 6.0 mg/kg i.v. max. 240 mg (>10 years) daily.
- In children who are well and not vomiting (even those with clinical pyelonephritis), a course of oral antibiotics has been shown to be as effective as i.v. antibiotics (see Antimicrobial guidelines). Antibiotic sensitivity should be checked when available (usually at 48 h).
- In children at high risk of recurrent UTI (see Risk factors, p. 488) prophylactic antibiotics should be commenced immediately after the treatment antibiotic course has finished. Their role in children <12 months with first episode is debated.
- If used, prophylactic antibiotics should be continued until the minimal initial imaging investigations have been done (see below). A decision regarding continuing prophylaxis is then made on the basis of the anatomy of the urinary tract and other clinical indicators (see Fig. 35.2). The guidelines recently released by the UK National Institute for Health and Clinical Excellence (NICE) recommend fewer investigations than in many previous guidelines and remain somewhat controversial. See also Antimicrobial guidelines. The use of prophylactic antibiotics is an area of controversy with ongoing research.
- For neonates <1 month old or preterm infants, discuss with a specialist.

Subsequent investigations (see Fig. 35.2)

- The extent to which a child should be investigated following a UTI is of international debate, and should be tailored for the individual patient.
- Ultrasound:
  - All children <6 months old presenting with a first UTI should have an ultrasound (refer to National Institute for Health and Clinical Excellence (NICE) UK guidelines).
  - Consider an ultrasound in children >6 months old presenting with a first UTI.

Imaging strategies

Children with cystitis/lower urinary tract infection should undergo ultrasound (within 6 weeks) only if they are younger than 6 months or have had recurrent infection. No other investigations are required for any child with cystitis/lower urinary tract infection unless they have recurrent UTI and/or abnormality on ultrasound. In which case late DMSA should be considered

Children younger than 6 months	Responds well to treatment within 48 hours without any features for atypical and/or recurrent UTI	Atypical UTI	Recurrent UTI
Ultrasound during the acute infection	No	Yes[b]	Yes
Ultrasound within 6 weeks	Yes[a]	No	No
DMSA 4–6 months following the acute infection	No	Yes	Yes
MCUG	No	Yes	Yes

[a] If abnormal consider MCUG.
[b] In a child with a non-E. coli UTI, responding well to antibiotics and with no other features of atypical infection, the ultrasound can be requested on a non-urgent basis to take place within 6 weeks.

Children 6 months or older but younger than 3 years	Responds well to treatment within 48 hours without any features for atypical and/or recurrent UTI	Atypical UTI	Recurrent UTI
Ultrasound during the acute infection	No	Yes[b]	No
Ultrasound within 6 weeks	No	No	Yes
DMSA 4–6 months following the acute infection	No	Yes	Yes
MCUG	No	No[a]	No[a]

[a] While MCUG should not be performed routinely it should be considered if the following features are present: dilatation on ultrasound; poor urine flow; non-E. coli infection; family history of VUR.
[b] In a child with a non-E. coli UTI, responding well to antibiotics and with no other features of atypical infection, the ultrasound can be requested on a non-urgent basis to take place within 6 weeks.

Children 3 months or older	Responds well to treatment within 48 hours without any features for atypical and/or recurrent UTI	Atypical UTI	Recurrent UTI
Ultrasound during the acute infection	No	Yes[ab]	No
Ultrasound within 6 weeks	No	No	Yes[a]
DMSA 4–6 months following the acute infection	No	No	Yes
MCUG	No	No	No

[a] Ultrasound in toilet-trained children should be performed with a full bladder with an estimate of bladder volume before and after micturition.
[b] In a child with a non-E. coli UTI, responding well to antibiotics and with no other features of atypical infection, the ultrasound can be requested on a non-urgent basis to take place within 6 weeks.

Definitions

Atypical UTI* includes:
- seriously ill
- poor urine flow
- abdominal or bladder mass
- raised creatinine
- septicaemia
- failure to respond to treatment with suitable antibiotics within 48 hours
- infection with non-E. coli organisms.

Recurrent UTI
- two or more episodes of UTI with acute pyelonephritis/upper urinary tract infection, or
- one episode of UTI with acute pyelonephritis/upper urinary tract infection plus one or more episode of UTI with cystitis/lower urinary tract infection, or
- three or more episodes of UTI with cystitis/lower urinary tract infection.

*Presence of any of these features should be documented

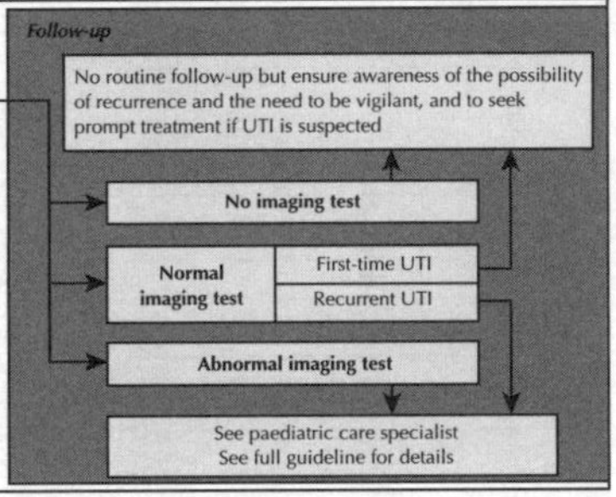

Follow-up

No routine follow-up but ensure awareness of the possibility of recurrence and the need to be vigilant, and to seek prompt treatment if UTI is suspected

No imaging test	First-time UTI
	Recurrent UTI

Normal imaging test
Abnormal imaging test

See paediatric care specialist
See full guideline for details

Fig. 35.2 Imaging strategies for children presenting with UTI

Reproduced with permission from the UTIC guideline, commissioned by NICE to the National Collaborating Centre for Women and Children's Health (NCC–WCH), UK

- Dimercaptosuccinic acid (DMSA) scan:
  - This nuclear medicine scan is done at least 6 months after the UTI to look for renal parenchymal defects (primarily renal scarring).
- Micturating cystourethrogram (MCU):
  - Performed to detect VUR.
  - It also provides good anatomic detail of the bladder and urethra.
  - Radiographic contrast is instilled in the bladder via a urethral catheter and subsequent radiographs taken to image the bladder and urethra.
- Siblings of children with VUR:
  - In children with VUR, their siblings will also have (or have had) VUR in 50%.
  - Consider an ultrasound scan in such cases.

Proteinuria
Isolated proteinuria
See Fig 35.3.

Nephrotic syndrome
Diagnosis
The diagnosis of nephrotic syndrome is made on the basis of proteinuria (>40 mg/m^2 per hour on a recumbent urine, usually >3 g/1.73 m^2 per day; urine protein/Cr ratio >0.4 g/mmol; usually 3+ to 4+ on dipstick testing), generalised oedema, hypo-albuminaemia (<25 g/L) and hypercholesterolaemia (>4.5 mmol/L).

Investigations
- Electrolytes, urea, creatinine.
- Albumin.
- C3, C4, CH50.
- Cholesterol.
- ANA, Igs.

Management
Exclude life-threatening complications
- Sepsis (e.g. peritonitis) – secondary to urinary loss of immunoglobulins.
- Symptomatic hypovolaemia (e.g. cool extremities and postural hypotension) – secondary to loss of albumin and subsequent contraction of intravascular space.
- Symptomatic oedema (e.g. marked ascites, respiratory distress with pleural effusions and skin breakdown).
- Symptomatic thromboembolism (e.g. venous sinus thrombosis: convulsions and a reduced conscious state; deep venous thrombosis and pulmonary embolism) – secondary to increased hepatic synthesis of plasma fibrinogens, urinary loss of antithrombin III and haemoconcentration.

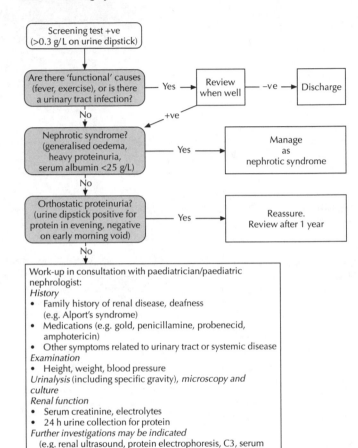

Fig. 35.3 Isolated proteinuria

Admit to hospital
• For initial observation and patient and family education

Medication
Note: Minor variations in protocol may exist between centres.
• Prednisolone:
  – 60 mg/m² per day as a single dose up to max. 80 mg/day for 4 weeks.
  Then:

- 40 mg/m^2 per alternate day for 4 weeks.
- 20 mg/m^2 per alternate day for 4 weeks.
- 15 mg/m^2 per alternate day for 4 weeks.
- 10 mg/m^2 per alternate day for 4 weeks.
- 5 mg/m^2 per alternate day for 4 weeks.

- Phenoxymethylpenicillin: 12.5 mg/kg (max. 1 g) oral twice daily until oedema clears (to prevent pneumococcal sepsis).
- Aspirin: 10 mg/kg per alternate day until oedema clears (to reduce the incidence of arterial thromboses).

Note: The long-term prognosis of nephrotic syndrome is dependent on the response to prednisolone.

For m^2 formulae, see Appendix 4, p. 614.

Treatment of complications

- *Symptomatic oedema*: concentrated albumin (i.e. 20%) 1 g/kg (5 mL/kg), i.v. over 4 h with frusemide 1 mg/kg at 2 and 4 h after the start of the infusion.
- *Circulatory insufficiency*: concentrated albumin (i.e. 20%) 1 g/kg (5 mL/kg), i.v. over 4 h. (Administer frusemide only if the circulation is markedly improved at the end of the infusion – it is dangerous in hypovolaemic patients.)
- *Thromboembolism*: systemic anticoagulation with heparin, followed by warfarin for 3–6 months.
- *Sepsis*: high-dose antibiotic therapy to cover *Streptococcus pneumoniae*, *Haemophilus influenzae* and *Escherichia coli* (e.g. cefotaxime 50 mg/kg (max. 2 g) i.v. 6 hourly).
- *Suspected primary peritonitis*:
  - Peritoneal tap to establish diagnosis.
  - If early diagnosis and minimal symptoms, antibiotic therapy alone may be sufficient.
  - Usually requires laparotomy for a peritoneal lavage.

Additional treatments

If the patient does not respond to steroids, refer to a specialist for consideration of cyclophosphamide or cyclosporin A treatment.

Indications for renal biopsy

- Age: <1 year of age.
- Failure to respond to prednisolone within 3–4 weeks of treatment using 60 mg/m^2 per day, either at diagnosis or with relapse.
- Nephritic/nephrotic syndrome (increased blood pressure, moderate haematuria and renal impairment without evidence of peripheral circulatory insufficiency).
- Low complement (C3).

Relapse

Most (75%) patients relapse.

- This is usually precipitated by a febrile illness or an allergic reaction.
- Four days of heavy proteinuria (>100 mg/dL; i.e. 3+ to 4+ on urine dipstick) distinguishes relapse from transient proteinuria associated with a febrile illness.

- Treat with: prednisolone 60 mg/m² per day till proteinuria dip test result in 0, trace or +. Then:
  - 40 mg/m² alternate day for 2 weeks.
  - 20 mg/m² alternate day for 2 weeks.
  - 15 mg/m² alternate day for 2 weeks.
  - 10 mg/m² alternate day for 2 weeks.
  - 5 mg/m² alternate day for 2 weeks.

Also use penicillin and aspirin if the patient becomes oedematous (see p. 495).

Indications for referral
Refer to a specialist in cases of:
- Nephritic/nephrotic syndrome.
- Complications.
- Failure to respond to steroids in 2–3 weeks.
- Frequent relapsing nephrotic syndrome or steroid dependence.

Haematuria
Causes of macroscopic haematuria
- Infection.
- Glomerulonephritis (GN):
  - Post infectious GN (common)
  - IgA GN (common)
  - Rapidly progressive crescenteric GN (rare but important), e.g. SLE, antineutrophil cytoplasmic antibody (ANCA) GN.
- Trauma.
- Calculi.
- Tumour.

Causes of microscopic haematuria
- Febrile illness.
- Thin membrane nephropathy.
- Causes of macroscopic haematuria (as above).

See Fig. 35.4.

Hypertension
Measurement of blood pressure
- Use a cuff with a bladder that covers at least 75% of the length of the upper arm.
- Take in the right arm, with the patient sitting; if initially increased, retake after resting quietly.

Definition
The 95th percentiles for blood pressure (BP) at different ages in childhood are shown in Table 35.1.

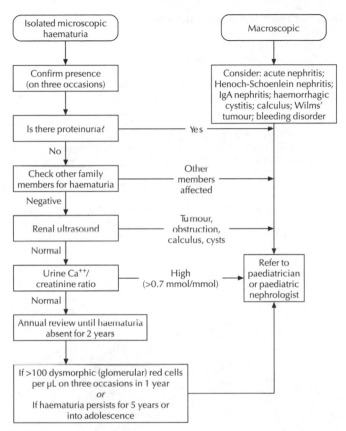

Fig. 35.4 Haematuria assessment

Table 35.1 95th centiles (systolic/diastolic) in childhood

Newborn	95/70
0–6 years	115/75
6–13 years	120/80
13–16 years	135/85
16–18 years	140/90

Causes of hypertension in adolescents

- Obesity – common.
- Essential hypertension – common.
- Continuation of causes for younger children – uncommon.
- Blood pressure 'tracks' poorly (i.e. only 20–40% of children with BP higher than the 80th percentile still remain in that group 10 years later). Children placed on medication for essential hypertension should undergo a trial of no treatment after their BP has been controlled for 9 months.
- In asymptomatic hypertension, the BP should be lowered slowly. (Although there is no research evidence currently proving a long-term benefit.)
- Blood pressure reduction slows the progression of renal impairment in people with renal disease. Children with renal impairment should have their BP target range set at less than the mean BP for their age.
- Hypertensive children should be referred to a specialist for investigation for causes outlined in Tables 35.2 and 35.3.
- An angiotensin-converting enzyme (ACE) inhibitor is the usual drug of choice and should be started in low doses then increased, with monitoring of potassium and creatinine.

Table 35.2 Causes of secondary hypertension in pre-adolescent children

Renal (75%)	Post-infectious glomerulonephritis
	Chronic glomerulonephritis
	Obstructive uropathy
	Polycystic kidney disease
	Autosomal recessive
	Autosomal dominant
	Reflux nephropathy
	Renovascular
	Haemolytic uraemic syndrome
Cardiovascular (15%)	Coarctation of the aorta
Endocrine (5%)	Phaeochromocytoma
	Hyperthyroidism
	Congenital adrenal hyperplasia
	Primary hyperaldosteronism
	Cushing's syndrome
Other (5%)	Neuroblastoma
	Neurofibromatosis
	Glucocorticoids
	Increased intracranial pressure

Table 35.3 Initial investigation of established hypertension

Urine	MSU, careful urinalysis (dipstick) Microscopy Urinary catecholamines
Blood	Creatinine Potassium Bicarbonate
Imaging	Renal ultrasound DMSA scan

Management
Asymptomatic hypertension
Refer to a specialist.

Symptomatic hypertension
This requires immediate treatment:
- In a conscious child, who is not vomiting, give a crushed nifedipine tablet by nasogastric tube or swallowed with water. The dose is nifedipine 5 mg oral (<2 years of age); nifedipine 10 mg oral (>2 years of age). Repeat 20 minutely, titrating to BP control.
- In a child with impaired consciousness or vomiting either:
  - Labetalol 0.2 mg/kg i.v. push over 2 min. If no response in 5–10 min, increase to 0.4 mg/kg (max. 60 mg), **or**
  - Nitroprusside 0.3–8.0 mcg/kg per min constant infusion (need ICU monitoring), **or**
  - Diazoxide 1 mg/kg i.v. push repeated 5–10 minutely to 5 mg/kg.
- Hypertension due to catecholamine production: phentolamine 0.1 mg/kg i.v. bolus (to 5 mg), followed by labetalol.
- Head trauma/increased intracranial pressure: labetalol or nitroprusside. *Note*: Nifedipine/diazoxide contra-indicated.

Glomerulonephritis
Glomerulonephritis presents as either proteinuria, haematuria, hypertension, acute renal failure or chronic renal failure (see appropriate sections). See Table 35.4.

Acute renal failure
Definition
Acute renal failure is the change in glomerular filtration such that the renal solute load (electrolytes, other ions and nitrogenous wastes) cannot be excreted. There are two main forms:
- *Oliguric*: acute reduction in urine output to <0.5 mL/kg per hour. This form is more complex to manage (see Fig. 35.5).
- *Polyuric*: often subacute and clinically unapparent, until the fluid intake is reduced and the patient becomes dehydrated due to an inappropriately high urine output.

Table 35.4 Types of glomerulonephritis

Type of glomerulonephritis (GN)	Clinical features
Thin membrane nephropathy	Microscopic haematuria (often other family members affected, normal BP, normal renal function and no proteinuria)
Minimal lesion GN	Nephrotic syndrome (oedema, proteinuria, hypoalbuminaemia)
Post-infectious GN	Nephritic syndrome – microscopic haematuria (often macroscopic), hypertension, oliguria, renal impairment 2–3 weeks following infection
IgA nephropathy	Microscopic haematuria and episodes of haematuria coincident with mucosal infection and loin pain
HSP nephritis	Haematuria, +/– nephrotic/nephritic features (as above), following rash and sometimes abdominal pain or arthralgia/arthritis.
Chronic GN (focal segmental glomerulosclerosis membrano-proliferative GN, membranous GN)	Chronic nephritic – nephrotic syndrome usually with nephrotic features dominating
Acute severe nephritis (SLE nephritis, crescentic GN, ANCA +ve GN, some HSP GN)	Acute nephritic/nephrotic syndrome usually with nephritic features dominating

ANCA, Anti-neutrophil cytoplasmic antibody;
GN, Glomerulonephritis;
HSP, Henoch Schoenlein purpura.

Causes
Pre-renal
- Dehydration (e.g. gastroenteritis).
- Shock.
- Sepsis.
- Nephrotic syndrome.

Renal
- Crescentic glomerulonephritis: acute post-infectious glomerulonephritis, membranoproliferative glomerulonephritis, Henoch-Schonlein purpura, and anti-neutrophil cytoplasmic antibody-associated haemolytic uraemic syndrome.
- Acute tubular necrosis.
- Crush injury (myoglobinuria).

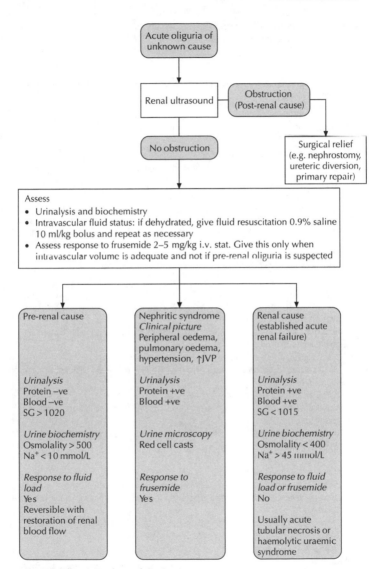

Fig. 35.5 Differentiation of types of oliguria

- Urinary tract infection with septicaemia.
- Nephrotoxin (e.g. gentamicin).

Post-renal
Obstruction, especially to a single kidney. The cause is usually apparent from the clinical context of the illness.

Management
Water
Limit to insensible losses (300 mL/m^2) plus urine output.

Sodium
- *Oliguric*: minimal Na$^+$ intake.
- *Polyuric*: measure the urine [Na$^+$] and volume of urine. Generally, about 75 mmol/L is required.

Potassium
There should be no i.v. or oral intake until losses of K$^+$ are established.

Hyperkalaemia
- Repeat venous or arterial serum K$^+$ urgently. Arrange haemofiltration or dialysis in the patient who has renal failure.
- ECG: peaked T waves, wide QRS, increased PR interval, decreased P and R waves, ST segment depression and a prolonged QT interval.
- If K$^+$ > 7 mmol/L with ECG changes:
  - *10% calcium gluconate* 0.5 mL/kg i.v. over 3–5 min (do not mix with bicarbonate). Works in seconds.
  - *Salbutamol:* spacer and inhalation: <6 years 6 puffs, >6 years 12 puffs; ICU i.v. 5 µg/kg per min for 60 min then 1 µg/kg per min. Works within 30 min and lasts some hours.
  - *Insulin plus concurrent glucose infusion:* 0.1 U/kg rapid-acting insulin and 2 mL/kg 50% dextrose. Works in minutes.
  - Arrange dialysis urgently if renal failure.
- If K$^+$ > 7 mmol/L, no ECG changes:
  - *NaHCO$_3$ 1–3 mmol/kg* (shifts K$^+$ intracellularly); however, there is the risk of hypocalcaemic tetany with decreased pH. This works rapidly (within the hour) if the child is acidotic.
  - *Dextrose* 0.5 g/kg per hour (10% dextrose at 5 mL/kg/h) until blood glucose reaches 14 mmol/L (shifts K$^+$ intracellularly). Works within the hour.
  - Arrange dialysis urgently in setting of renal failure.
- If K$^+$ >6 mmol/L:
  - *NaHCO$_3$* to correct coexistent acidosis.

– *Na+–K+ exchange resin*, e.g. Resonium A, 1 g/kg p.o. (action within 6–12 h) or p.r. (action within 30 min; may repeat in 1–2 h).
– Arrange dialysis in setting of renal failure.

Acidosis

Correct with bicarbonate **(mmol = base deficit × weight × 0.3)** over 4 h as long as:

- The patient is not severely hypocalcaemic (HCO_3 may lower calcium and cause convulsions).
- The accompanying Na^+ load does not cause fluid overload (e.g. hypertension and pulmonary oedema).

Hypocalcaemia

This is usually due to increased serum phosphate. There is a danger of metastatic calcification if the $Ca^{2+} \times PO_4^{3-}$ product is >5–6.

Management

- Low-phosphate diet.
- Calcium carbonate (phosphate binder).
- Symptomatic hypocalcaemia may require i.v. calcium gluconate.
- Consider dialysis.

Uraemia

- An acute rise in serum urea to >30 mmol/L may cause CNS symptoms.
- Protein restriction and high-quality protein food are required.
- High-carbohydrate diet.

Indications for dialysis/haemofiltration

- Fluid overload (hypertension or pulmonary oedema) not responding to frusemide.
- Hyperkalaemia.
- Severe metabolic acidosis.
- Progressive uraemia.
- Dialysable nephrotoxin.
- Hyperammonaemia.
- The reduction of intravascular volume to facilitate total parenteral nutrition or blood transfusion.

Chronic renal failure
Presentation

- Growth failure.
- Rickets.
- Anaemia: normochromic, normocytic.
- Radiological studies: small kidney, with other renal disease; e.g. obstruction uropathy.

- Proteinuria.
- Urinary tract infection.

Diagnosis

Increased serum creatinine, urea, and phosphate; metabolic acidosis.

Management

Investigation of the cause and treatment of chronic renal failure should be done in conjunction with a specialist.

USEFUL RESOURCES
- *http://www.nice.org.uk* – Use the search tool to reach Urinary Tract Infection (UTI) in Children Guideline.
- *http://kidneyatlas.org* – Free online atlas of kidney disease: 5 volumes can be downloaded as pdf files.
- *http://www.paediatriconcall.com/fordoctor/pedcalc/bp.asp* – A blood pressure calculator. See also RCH Clinical Practice Guidelines [Hypertension] for blood pressure centile charts as pdf files.

CHAPTER 36
Respiratory conditions

John Massie
Sarath Ranganathan

Respiratory illness accounts for at least 50% of all acute paediatric presentations. Infants and young children tire quickly and can rapidly present in acute respiratory failure. The assessment and management of acute respiratory distress is also considered in chapter 1, Medical emergencies, p. 1.

Respiratory conditions result in:
- Airway compromise (e.g. asthma, bronchiectasis, croup). This results in noisy breathing (stirtor above the larynx, stridor if extrathoracic or wheeze if intrathoracic).
- Parenchymal compromise (e.g. pneumonia). This may directly affect the blood–gas barrier and result in hypoxaemia.
- Mixed picture of airway and parenchymal compromise (e.g. bronchiolitis).

Asthma
Establishing the diagnosis and pattern of asthma
The two main components of asthma pathology include:
- Airway inflammation.
- Reactive airways (bronchoconstriction).

The important clinical features are:
- Wheeze.
- Shortness of breath.
- Chest tightness.
- Cough.
- Response of symptoms to short acting bronchodilators.
- Ask also for interval symptoms, e.g. symptoms at night (waking the patient), early in the morning, at rest during the day, during physical activity/sport.

Note: Cough alone, in the absence of wheeze, is rarely asthma.

Common triggers of asthma are:
- Upper respiratory tract infections (URTs).
- Exercise.
- Exposure to cold air.
- Allergen exposure.

Paediatric Handbook, 8th edition. By Kate Thomson, Dean Tey and Michael Marks. Published 2009 by Blackwell Publishing, ISBN: 978-1-4051-7400-8.

Important clinical settings where asthma is more common:
- Individuals with allergic disease (perennial rhinitis, hay fever, eczema).
- First-degree relatives with asthma and/or atopic disease.

There may be few physical findings between acute attacks. Undertreated or chronic asthma may be associated with:
- Hyperinflation.
- Chest wall abnormalities, e.g. pectus carinatum or flaring of the lower ribs (Harrison's sulci).
- Expiratory wheeze (generalised).
- Slowed growth parameters.
- Side effects of medication (e.g. oral candidiasis in those taking inhaled steroids).

Keep in mind other diagnoses if there are atypical findings, such as digital clubbing (suppurative lung disease), tracheal shift (mediastinal mass) or localised wheeze (inhaled foreign body).

In most cases the diagnosis of asthma in children is a clinical diagnosis.
- Although wheezing is a cardinal feature of asthma, there are a number of other causes for wheeze. In particular, wheeze in young children is common and may be due to small airway calibre rather than asthma. Infant and preschool patterns of wheeze include transient early wheeze and viral-associated wheeze. Most children with these patterns have stopped wheezing by 6 years of age.
- The natural history for most children with episodic (infrequent or frequent) asthma is that it will improve over time.
- The diagnosis of asthma is not always straightforward and a therapeutic trial of bronchodilator is sometimes required. In this case it is important that the treating doctor, referring doctor and family recognise that the trial of treatment does not lead to an inappropriate diagnostic label of asthma. An apparent response to therapy may be the natural course of the underlying disease as improvement occurs. An escalating requirement for treatment should trigger the need for reassessment (e.g. pneumothorax).

Investigations
Usually no investigations are required, but tests that may help with the diagnosis and management of asthma include:

Spirometry
- Children over the age of 6 years can learn to do spirometry accurately. However, it is important to note that peak flow measurements are unreliable in children and have a minimal role in diagnosis or in monitoring progress.
- Airway obstruction is defined as FEV_1 <80% (predicted), FEV_1/FVC <75%, MMEF 25–75 <67% (predicted).
- If there is evidence of airway obstruction then bronchodilator reversibility should be assessed (an improvement of FEV_1 of 12% in absolute values).
- In most cases spirometry is unhelpful during an acute admission unless there is a difference between the perceived symptoms and objective clinical measures.

Exercise challenge
- May be used in children able to do accurate spirometry.
- 70% of children with asthma have exercise-induced bronchoconstriction.
- 15% reduction in FEV_1 following exercise is considered significant.
- Graded dose inhalation of dry powder mannitol is a new alternative to the exercise challenge.
- Other challenges such as histamine and methacholine are not used in clinical practice for children.

Chest radiograph (CXR)
- CXR is not routinely required in either the acute or interval management of asthma.
- CXR may be required if there is evidence of an acute complication (e.g. mucous plugging) or patients with difficult-to-control, persistent asthma (particularly if they have not had a previous CXR).
- CXR is helpful if symptoms and signs are not wholly explained by asthma and may be caused by another disease (e.g. mediastinal mass, suppurative lung disease or foreign body).

Management of acute asthma
Also see chapter 1, Medical emergencies, p. 10, for the management of critical asthma.

Assessment of the severity of an attack
The severity of acute asthma can be classified as mild, moderate, severe or critical. The most reliable indicators are mental state and work of breathing (comprising accessory muscle use and recession). See Table 36.1.

Patients with an acute exacerbation of asthma requiring salbutamol every 3 h at home should be assessed by their Local Medical Officer or in the emergency department. Parents who are familiar with their child's asthma can initiate prednisolone at home at the start of an exacerbation, although there is limited evidence for this practice.
- The initial arterial O_2 saturation (Sao_2) in air, heart rate and ability to talk should be used as additional features in assessing the severity of acute asthma.
- Wheeze intensity, central cyanosis, pulsus paradoxus, peak expiratory flow are not reliable for the assessment of the severity of acute asthma.
- Arterial blood gases, CXR and spirometry should not be routinely used in assessing the severity of acute asthma

Table 36.1 Assessment of the severity of an acute asthma attack

Sign	Mild	Moderate	Severe	Critical
Mental state	Normal	Normal	Agitated	Confused/drowsy
Work of breathing	Normal	Mildly increased	Moderately/markedly increased	Maximally increased or exhausted

Table 36.2 Treatment of an acute asthma attack

	Mild	Moderate	Severe	Critical
Oxygen	No	No	If SaO$_2$ < 92%	Yes
Inhaled β$_2$-agonist (e.g. salbutamol)	6–12 puffs pMDI/spacer[1] once review after 20 min	6–12 puffs pMDI/spacer[1] 3 times in 1st hour (20 minutely) review 10 min after 3rd dose	6–12 puffs pMDI/spacer[1] 3 times in 1st hour (20 minutely) review 10 min after 3rd dose[2]	Nebulised continuous salbutamol[3]
Ipratropium	No	No	2 or 4 puffs pMDI/spacer[4] 3 times in 1st hour only (20 minutely)	Nebulised (25 mcg) –3 times in 1st hour only (20 minutely, add to salbutamol)
Corticosteroids	Usually no	Oral prednisolone 1 mg/kg/dose once daily for up to 3 days	Oral prednisolone 1 mg/kg/dose – once daily for up to 3 days – i.v. if vomiting	I.v. methylprednisolone 1 mg/kg/dose – 6 hourly on day 1
I.v. β$_2$-agonist (e.g. salbutamol)	No	No	No	Consider if poor response to initial therapy[5]
Aminophylline	No	No	No	Consider if poor response to initial therapy[6]
Observation/admission	Usually discharge home after initial observation	Observe for at least 1 h then decide need for hospital admission	Admit to hospital Frequent review	Arrange admission to ICU

[1] Salbutamol (100 mcg/puff) delivered by pMDI and spacer – 6 puffs if <6 yo, 12 puffs if ≥6 yo.

[2] Reduce frequency of β2-agonist if improving. If no change, continue 20 minutely β2-agonist. If deteriorating, treat as critical.

[3] Salbutamol 0.5% solution delivered by nebuliser.

[4] Ipratropium (40 mcg/puff) delivered by pMDI and spacer – 2 puffs if <6 yo, 4 puffs if ≥6 yo.

[5] Salbutamol 5 mcg/kg per min for 1 h i.v. (load), then 1 mcg/kg per min infusion.

[6] Aminophylline loading dose 10 mg/kg (max. 250 mg) over 1 h (if patient previously taking theophylline, measure serum level to decide need for loading dose); then infusion 1.1 mg/kg per hour if age 1–9 years, 0.7 mg/kg per hour if 10+ years. Aminophylline and salbutamol must be given by separate i.v. lines.

Hospital discharge and home treatment

Patients should be discharged from medical care when they are stable and can be cared for at home. This usually corresponds to a requirement for salbutamol 3–4 hourly or less frequently and no oxygen requirement for 24 h. Education of caregivers is an important component of this process.

Writing an individual asthma action plan assists caregivers in treating asthma in the current and subsequent episodes. The key elements in the plan are:
- Daily treatment.
- Treatment of minor symptoms.
- Treatment before exercise if it is a known trigger.
- Treatment of acute exacerbation.
- Emergency plan.

Drug delivery

Ensure that delivery devices are appropriate to the patient's age. Selection of appropriate delivery system is crucial for good asthma management. Allow older children and adolescents to choose the inhaler and tailor the medication to the delivery system.
- All metered-dose inhaler doses are given through a spacer. In young children a mask is firmly applied to the face, and older children put their lips around a mouthpiece.
- Shake the puffer initially and then after every three puffs.
- Load with one puff at a time (and repeat).
- If the child uses tidal breathing, allow 5–6 breaths. If the child is able to take larger breaths (this is best), wait until they take 1–2 breaths.
- Frequency: in hospital, doses may be given frequently as indicated by severity and response. The use of oxygen between treatments does not preclude using a spacer.
- Spacers should be washed in household detergent weekly to reduce static and then air-dried (spacers should not be rinsed, rubbed or towel dried).

Table 36.3 Drug delivery devices

Delivery system	Age
Pressurised metered dose inhaler (pMDI)	>8 (reliever only, mild symptoms)
PMDI + small volume spacer Mask No mask	 0–3 years 3–5 years
PMDI + large volume spacer	>5 years
Turbuhaler	>8 years
Accuhaler	>8 years
Autohaler	>8 years

Table 36.4 Patterns of asthma and interval treatment

Classification of pattern	Common features	Preventer	Symptom controller	Reliever
Infrequent episodic	Episodes 6–8 weeks apart or more Attacks usually not severe Symptoms rare between attacks Normal examination and lung function between episodes	Nil	Nil	Short-acting β₂-agonist as needed*
Frequent episodic	Attacks <6 weeks apart Attacks more troublesome Increasing symptoms between attacks Normal examination and lung function between episodes	Inhaled corticosteroids (most patients will be well controlled on 100–200 mcg/day fluticasone (or equivalent) or montelukast	Nil	β₂-agonist as needed*
Persistent	Daytime symptoms >2 days/week Nocturnal symptoms >1 night/week Attacks <6 weeks apart May have abnormal lung function Multiple Emergency Department visits or hospital admissions	If mild, montelukast Inhaled corticosteroids (most patients will be well controlled on 100–200 mcg/day fluticasone or equivalent)	If on ≥250 mcg/day fluticasone and poorly controlled: add a long-acting β₂-agonist (maximum effective dose of fluticasone is 500 mcg/day) If symptoms poorly controlled on maximum inhaled therapy reconsider the diagnosis, adherence, drug delivery and consider referral to a paediatric respiratory physician	Short-acting β₂-agonist as needed*

> All asthma preventers and symptom controllers prescribed as pressurised metered dose
> inhalers (pMDIs) should be delivered through a spacer regardless of the age of the patient.
> All patients using ICS should rinse their mouths afterwards, regardless of the inhaler.

Principles of interval asthma management

After establishing the diagnosis it is important to determine the pattern of asthma in order
to prescribe the appropriate treatment (see Tables 36.4 and 36.5).

A number of issues should be attended to at subsequent check-ups, including:

- Symptom review, in particular nocturnal and exercise symptoms.
- Review of asthma action plan and medication regimen.
- Adherence with medication.
- Avoiding precipitants (e.g. allergens).
- Avoidance of cigarette smoking (active and environmental).
- Monitoring of growth and development.

Acute viral bronchiolitis
Aetiology

Respiratory viruses are the most common cause of bronchiolitis in young infants. The most
common is respiratory syncytial virus (RSV). Bronchiolitis is a generalised lower respiratory
tract infection, but RSV infection can also cause lobar pneumonia.

Clinical features

- Cough, wheeze, tachypnoea, apnoeas, fever and poor feeding in an infant.
- There may be signs of respiratory distress including tracheal tug, recession, use of accessory
  muscles, grunting.
- Crackles and wheeze on auscultation
- Severe bronchiolitis is associated with respiratory failure
- Young infants (<6 weeks) are at risk of apnoeas.

Management

See Fig. 36.1.

- CXR and nasopharyngeal aspirates are not routine investigations for bronchiolitis.
- Infants <3 months and those with severe bronchiolitis are more likely to become hyponatraemic (due to the syndrome of 'inappropriate' increased ADH secretion (SIADH)) and
  warrant close attention to fluid balance. See also p. 73, Fluid and electrolyte therapy.

Pneumonia
Aetiology

- Respiratory viruses are the most common cause of pneumonia in young infants in developed countries. There is generally only mild to moderate constitutional disturbance. There
  may be scattered inspiratory crackles on auscultation.

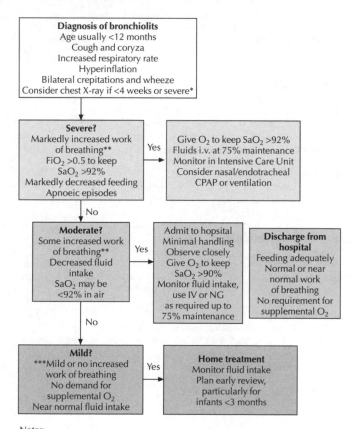

Diagnosis of bronchiolits
Age usually <12 months
Cough and coryza
Increased respiratory rate
Hyperinflation
Bilateral crepitations and wheeze
Consider chest X-ray if <4 weeks or severe*

Severe?
Markedly increased work of breathing**
FiO₂ >0.5 to keep SaO₂ >92%
Markedly decreased feeding
Apnoeic episodes

Yes →

Give O₂ to keep SaO₂ >92%
Fluids i.v. at 75% maintenance
Monitor in Intensive Care Unit
Consider nasal/endotracheal CPAP or ventilation

No ↓

Moderate?
Some increased work of breathing**
Decreased fluid intake
SaO₂ may be <92% in air

Yes →

Admit to hopsital
Minimal handling
Observe closely
Give O₂ to keep SaO₂ >90%
Monitor fluid intake, use IV or NG as required up to 75% maintenance

Discharge from hospital
Feeding adequately
Normal or near normal work of breathing
No requirement for supplemental O₂

No ↓

Mild?
***Mild or no increased work of breathing
No demand for supplemental O₂
Near normal fluid intake

Yes →

Home treatment
Monitor fluid intake
Plan early review, particularly for infants <3 months

Notes:
* Routine CXR is not required for children with typical clinical features.
** Use the respiratory rate, accessory muscle use and recessions to judge the work of breathing.
*** Very young infants and infants with a co-morbidity (e.g. cardiac disease, Down syndrome, chronic lung disease etc.) are at greatest risk of severe disease. These infants may need admission for observation even if they have mild bronchiolitis. Administration of β2 agonists may be distressing for young infants and is of no proven value.

Fig. 36.1 Assessment and management of acute viral bronchiolitis

- *Mycoplasma pneumoniae* is the most common pathogen in children >5 years old and is an under-recognised cause of pneumonia in younger children. Typically symptoms develop over several days before the cough, often with a systemic illness. Cough is prominent and crackles may be focal or widespread. Children are usually unwell, may have headache and focal signs are present in the chest.
- *Streptococcus pneumoniae* is the most common bacterial pathogen in all age groups, followed by non-typeable *Haemophilus influenzae* and *Staphylococcus aureus*. Group A β-haemolytic streptococcus is less common but may cause severe pneumonia. Many older children can be managed at home, but most <24 months should be admitted to hospital.

Clinical features
- Tachypnoea, fever and cough. There may be signs of respiratory distress.
- Focal signs in the chest may be difficult to detect in young infants.
- A diagnosis of pneumonia, especially in younger children, can often only be made with radiological confirmation.
- CXR changes do not distinguish viral from bacterial pneumonia, although lobar changes are more likely to be caused by *Streptococcus pneumoniae*.
- Young infants and those with severe disease are at risk of the syndrome of 'inappropriate' ADH secretion (SIADH). Monitor sodium and consider limiting parenteral fluids. See also p. 73, Fluid and electrolyte therapy.

Management
See Fig. 36.2.

Pharyngitis/tonsillitis, acute otitis media and URTI
See chapter 24, Ear, nose and throat conditions.

Laryngotracheobronchitis (croup)
See Fig. 36.3.

Epiglottitis
See also chapter 1, Medical emergencies.

Aetiology
Usually due to *Haemophilus influenzae* type b (Hib). The incidence of acute epiglottitis has fallen markedly in countries where Hib immunisation is widespread. However, it continues to occur (child not immunised, immunisation failure, other bacteria) and if the diagnosis is not made promptly, the child is likely to die.

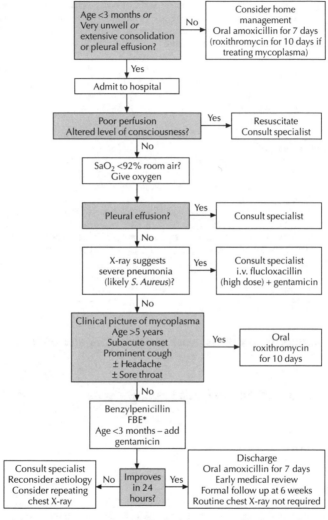

* Other investigations as indicated. Blood culture positive in less than 5% of cases; Nasopharyngeal aspirate for viral identification not usually helpful; mycoplasma serology may be helpful if diagnosis in doubt.

Fig. 36.2 Management of pneumonia (previously well patient >1 month old)

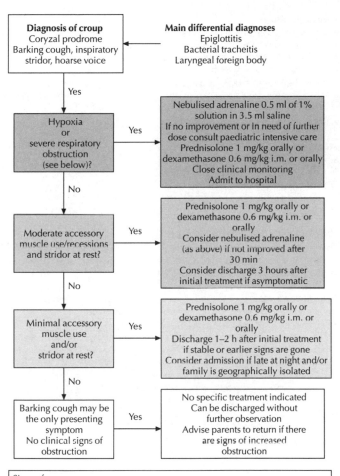

Diagnosis of croup
Coryzal prodrome
Barking cough, inspiratory
stridor, hoarse voice

Main differential diagnoses
Epiglottitis
Bacterial tracheitis
Laryngeal foreign body

Yes

Hypoxia
or
severe respiratory
obstruction
(see below)?

Yes

Nebulised adrenaline 0.5 ml of 1%
solution in 3.5 ml saline
If no improvement or in need of further
dose consult paediatric intensive care
Prednisolone 1 mg/kg orally or
dexamethasone 0.6 mg/kg i.m. or orally
Close clinical monitoring
Admit to hospital

No

Moderate accessory
muscle use/recessions
and stridor at rest?

Yes

Prednisolone 1 mg/kg orally or
dexamethasone 0.6 mg/kg i.m. or
orally
Consider nebulised adrenaline
(as above) if not improved after
30 min
Consider discharge 3 hours after
initial treatment if asymptomatic

No

Minimal accessory
muscle use
and/or
stridor at rest?

Yes

Prednisolone 1 mg/kg orally or
dexamethasone 0.6 mg/kg i.m. or
orally
Discharge 1–2 h after initial treatment
if stable or earlier signs are gone
Consider admission if late at night and/or
family is geographically isolated

No

Barking cough may be
the only presenting
symptom
No clinical signs of
obstruction

Yes

No specific treatment indicated
Can be discharged without
further observation
Advise parents to return if there
are signs of increased
obstruction

Signs of
Hypoxia: agitated, distressed, cyanosis, Sa_{O_2} <92% in air
Severe obstruction: marked accessory muscle use/recessions
Note: **Risk factors for severe disease**: subglottic stenosis (either congenital or
prolonged intubation), age <6 months, Down syndrome (or other neurological
abnormalities). Consider admission for such children even with mild symptoms

Fig. 36.3 Management of croup

Clinical features

Epiglottitis differs from laryngotracheobronchitis in the following ways:

- Cough is not a prominent feature.
- Most children appear toxic because of associated sepsis.
- The onset is with fever and lethargy. Symptoms of respiratory obstruction develop after 2–6 h. There may be a history of a preceding upper respiratory tract infection.
- The stridor is soft, and the expiratory element is often dominant with a snoring or gurgling quality.
- Difficulty in swallowing with drooling of saliva is common.

Management

See chapter 1, Medical emergencies.

Treatment of contacts

Rifampicin prophylaxis 20 mg/kg (max. 600 mg) p.o. daily for 4 days.

Whooping cough (pertussis)

Whooping cough continues to be widespread in many communities because of suboptimal uptake of childhood immunisation and waning immunity in adolescents and adults immunised as children (the current vaccines give protection for only 5–10 years).

Clinical features

- Starts with a coryzal illness that resembles an URTI (infectious period).
- The cough continues for many weeks to months, is paroxysmal and may be associated with facial suffusion and vomiting. In some children the paroxysm is terminated by an inspiratory whoop. The cough is often only recognised as pertussis at this stage (paroxysmal phase).
- The child appears well between coughing paroxysms.
- In small infants, pertussis can present with apnoea alone.

Diagnosis

- Diagnosis can be made on clinical grounds.
- Lymphocyte count may be markedly elevated ($>20 \times 10^9$/L).
- In the acute phase the diagnosis can be confirmed by identifying *Bordetella pertussis* from a nasopharyngeal aspirate (culture, immunofluorescence, PCR).
- Pertussis serum IgA is specific (but not sensitive) for past infection. It may be elevated after 3 weeks and persist for 2 years. It is rarely positive from infants <2 years of age.

Management

- No pharmacological agents improve the clinical course of whooping cough.
- Clearance of nasal carriage of *B. pertussis* has been best studied with erythromycin estolate for 14 days, but the estolate preparation is no longer available in Australia. Com-

parative studies suggest that a shorter course of clarithromycin is as effective as, and possibly more effective than, erythromycin. The current recommendation is clarithromycin 7.5 mg/kg (max. 500 mg) twice daily for 7 days.

- Treatment of household and other close contacts has not been proved to be effective, but contact prophylaxis is recommended if a contact is in the late phase of pregnancy or there is an incompletely immunised child in the family. Use clarithromycin (same dosage) for 7 days.
- Admission: infants <6 months, apnoea, cyanosis, not coping with the cough, poor feeding, systemically unwell.
- In hospital, careful observation, including the use of an apnoea monitor. If paroxysms occur frequently and are associated with marked cyanosis, nursing in oxygen may be of some help.
- Infants with proven pertussis should continue with routine vaccinations (which will include DTPa).

Cough

Cough is a common symptom in children. The degree to which a family becomes concerned about the frequency and severity of a child's cough seems to be extremely variable. There is often a poor correlation between a parental report of cough and objective measures.

Acute cough

The cause of an acute onset cough is generally easy to recognise, most commonly with a respiratory infection, asthma or inhaled foreign body.

Persistent or recurrent cough

The history and characteristics of the cough are usually the keys to diagnosis. Whilst asthma, gastro-oesophageal reflux and postnasal drip are the three favoured diagnoses in adults, these occur less commonly in children. In children think of:

- Onset in infancy (and barking): tracheomalacia.
- Dry (worse at night): post-viral cough, chronic non-specific cough of childhood, asthma.
- Dry (paroxysmal): pertussis.
- Wet (productive): suppurative lung disease (chronic suppurative bronchitis, cystic fibrosis, immunodeficiency, primary ciliary dyskinesia, inhaled foreign body).
- Onset in older childhood (honking): psychogenic.

Asthma

Although cough can be a troublesome symptom of asthma, it rarely occurs without some evidence of airways obstruction (e.g. wheeze). There is considerable doubt as to whether the entity of 'cough variant asthma', in which cough is the only symptom of asthma, exists in children. Be very reluctant to diagnose asthma in the absence of evidence of airways obstruction. The management of asthma is based on the severity and duration of the airways obstruction, not on the cough.

Physical examination

This is usually normal, but key findings include:
- Poor growth and nutrition.
- Digital clubbing (suppurative lung disease).
- Chest wall deformity (pectus carinatum suggesting chronic airway obstruction).
- Localised wheeze (inhaled foreign body).

Investigations

Specific investigations for persistent cough depend on the clinical suspicion after history and examination. In some circumstances it can be reassuring to the family to have a normal CXR and lung function.

Cough management

- The most important aspect of management is to make a diagnosis and explain its nature to the parents. The effects of passive smoking should be discussed.
- Most cough suppressants provide only partial relief.
- A foreign body must be removed bronchoscopically.
- It is often much more difficult to control the cough of asthma than the wheeze.

Foreign body in the bronchial tree
Clinical features
Symptoms

- Coughing or choking episodes while eating solid foods (classically nuts), or while sucking a small plastic toy or similar object. This history should never be dismissed.
- Persistent coughing and wheezing.
- Beware of the sudden onset of a first wheezing episode in a toddler in whom there is no history of allergy, especially if it follows a choking episode.
- Parents may not volunteer the history of possible inhalation (many foreign body aspirations are not witnessed).

Signs

- There may be no physical signs or alternatively reduced breath sounds over the whole or part of one lung.
- Wheeze.

Investigations

A CXR is taken in full inspiration and full expiration to exclude obstructive hyperinflation or an area of collapse. The radiograph should include the nasopharynx to the chest. Normal radiographs do not exclude a foreign body.

Management

Bronchoscopy is indicated for all patients with a suspected inhaled foreign body. There should be a high index of suspicion as aspirated foreign body is frequently missed.

- Bronchoscopy in children is difficult and it requires an expert paediatric endoscopist teamed with an experienced paediatric anaesthetist. It should only be done in a major children's hospital. Rigid bronchoscopy is the procedure of choice.
- In most cases the removal of the foreign body improves symptoms and there is rarely an indication for corticosteroids or antibiotics.

Cystic fibrosis
Background
Cystic fibrosis (CF) is the most common life-shortening inherited disease of childhood. The incidence is 1:2500 and carrier frequency in people of European origin is 1:25.

Screening
- Newborn screening for CF detects 90% of affected babies. All babies have a heel prick on day 2–4 and the blood placed on a filter paper card. Serum trypsinogen is measured by immunoreactive assay (IRT). Babies with an IRT >99th percentile have gene mutation testing for 12 common CF gene mutations. Babies with 2 CF gene mutations have CF and are referred to the CF clinic. Babies with 1 CF gene mutation are referred for a sweat test at an approved laboratory. Those with a positive sweat test are referred to the CF clinic. Those with a negative sweat test are healthy carriers and their families referred for genetic counselling.
- Most babies with an elevated IRT and no CF gene mutations do not have CF.
- This screening test can miss babies who have a falsely low IRT or an uncommon gene mutation. (The 12 most common CF gene mutations are tested; >1200 have been identified.) Internationally many countries do not include CF in the newborn screening programme. Screening began in the late 1980s/early 1990s in most Australian states. For these reasons any child with a suspicious clinical history should be referred for a sweat test.

Diagnosis
- Classic clinical features of CF include:
  - Suppurative lung disease.
  - Pancreatic exocrine insufficiency (85% of patients), which manifests as steatorrhoea and failure to thrive.
  - Multifocal biliary cirrhosis.
  - Meconium ileus.
  - Male infertility (absent vas deferens).
  - Elevated sweat electrolytes (occasionally presenting as hyponatraemic, hypochloraemic metabolic alkalosis).

Family history
- CF gene mutation analysis. The diagnosis and management of CF is complex and best achieved in a specialist CF centre.

- Genetic counselling for the extended family of patients with CF is offered routinely but most babies with CF are born to families with no history of CF. For this reason pre-conceptual and pre-natal carrier testing of all prospective parents is available.

Management
- Nutrition:
  - High-fat, high-calorie diet.
  - Pancreatic enzyme replacement.
  - Vitamin supplementation (A and E, occasionally D).
- Salt supplementation.
- Pulmonary care:
  - Chest physiotherapy, usually at least once daily.
  - Antibiotics and treatment regimes are largely dependent on which organism colonises and infects the lungs (see Table 36.6). Bronchoalveolar lavage is done soon after diagnosis and then annually until the child can expectorate sputum. Cough suction specimens are also taken at each clinic visit.
  - The acquisition of chronic *P. aeruginosa* infection is associated with deterioration in lung function and a poorer prognosis. An aggressive antibiotic approach may prevent chronic infection and limit airway disease. **The aim of treating infection early is to eradicate *Pseudomonas aeruginosa* when first identified.**

Upper respiratory tract infections (URTIs)
- A viral infection may predispose CF patients to secondary bacterial infection, so oral antibiotics are used aggressively (Table 36.6).
- For mild URTI, we recommend 2 weeks of anti-*Staphylococcal* and *Haemophilus* cover (e.g. Augmentin).
- If a child chronically infected with *Pseudomonas* develops a cold or an infective acute exacerbation, 2 weeks of oral ciprofloxacin is indicated. If symptoms persist, admit for i.v. antibiotics. It is accepted practice to give two antibiotics – usually combining an aminoglycoside (gentamicin, tobramycin, amikacin) with a penicillin/β-lactam combination (Timentin = ticarcillin/clavulanic acid) or third-generation cephalosporin (ceftazadime) to minimise the development of antimicrobial resistance (see Fig. 36.4). Nebuliser therapy can be stopped during i.v. therapy.

Successful eradication
- At least three negative cultures one month apart, **or**
- One negative culture from bronchoalveolar lavage **and** one other negative culture 1 month apart.

Non-pulmonary complications of CF
Distal intestinal obstruction syndrome (DIOS)
- The accumulation of tenacious, muco-faeculent masses in the distal ileum or caecum which may become adherent and calcify.

Table 36.5 Management of bacterial infection in CF

	Staphylococcus aureus	Haemophilus influenzae	Pseudomonas aeruginosa
Prophylaxis	Antibiotic prophylaxis against infection with S. aureus is given soon after diagnosis for 1 year or until cultures in early infancy are clear	Antibiotic prophylaxis against infection with H. influenzae non-type B is given soon after diagnosis for 1 year or until cultures in early infancy are clear	Not used
Acute infection	2 weeks oral antibiotics	2 weeks (co-amoxiclav, e.g. Augmentin) if Haemophilus is isolated in sputum. Continue for a further 2 weeks if symptoms persist If symptoms persist after a total of 4 weeks, consider i.v. antibiotics A bronchoalveolar lavage is indicated in patients not responding to treatment	See Fig. 36.4. If child is quite well and treatment adherence is good, the initial 2 weeks of intravenous therapy is omitted First-line i.v. therapy is ticarcillin and tobramycin pending sensitivities
Chronic infection	Patients should remain on prophylactic anti-staphylococcal antibiotics where (1) S. aureus is regularly cultured in sputum, (2) annual bronchoalveolar lavage is positive on two consecutive occasions, or (3) symptoms return when anti-staphylococcal antibiotics are stopped If patients develop an intercurrent respiratory tract infection, change to another anti-staphylococcal agent for 2 weeks If this is unsuccessful, i.v. ticarcillin and gentamicin (pending sensitivities) for 2 weeks may be necessary. Consider a bronchoscopic lavage in patients not responding to rule out Pseudomonas infection After treatment, oral antibiotics are recommended	In those patients who repeatedly have H. influenzae cultured in their sputum consider long-term prophylaxis (e.g. Augmentin) Augmentin is also the antibiotic of choice for acute exacerbations in those with chronic H. influenzae infection	Three consecutively positive cultures obtained at least 1 month apart Long-term nebulised tobramycin is then commenced If patients continue to deteriorate then switch to either nebulised colistin, nebulised preservative-free tobramycin (TOBI), or oral ciprofloxacin alternating with nebulised tobramycin on a monthly basis An exacerbation is characterised by an increase in cough, sputum production, change in sputum colour, loss of weight, decreased activity and deterioration in lung function. Fever may occur but is not typical

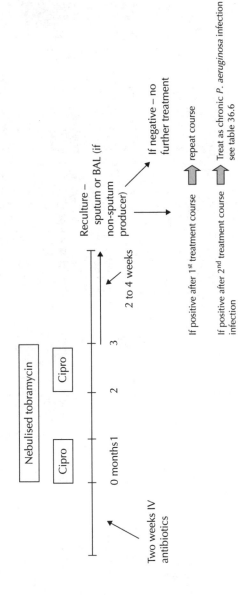

Fig. 36.4 Treatment of an acute infection with *Pseudomonas*

- The cause is unclear but appears to be associated with dehydration, fever, reduction of enzyme supplementation, liver disease and the use of anticholinergic and opiate drugs.
- Although it occurs most frequently in those >15 years, it can occur at any age.
- DIOS presents acutely with signs of abdominal obstruction or more commonly, sub-acutely with cramping abdominal pain and relative constipation. A mass is often palpable in the right iliac fossa. The management varies according to severity (see Table 36.7).
- Other conditions which should be considered in the differential diagnosis include:
  - Constipation.
  - Intussusception.
  - Acute appendicitis.
  - Acute pancreatitis.
  - Volvulus.
  - Strictures of the colon or ileocaecal junction.
  - Obstruction due to adhesions or strictures.

Table 36.6 Management of DIOS

Acute presentations	Investigation	Treatment
Mild episodes		
Mild abdominal pain No obstruction May be recurrent (out- patient management)	Nil	Rehydration Lactulose 10–20 mL b.d. Acetylcysteine 100 mg 3 times daily Consider adding oral gastrografin
Severe episodes		
Abdominal pain with distension and constipation No obstruction No peritonism (consider admission)	Full blood count Urea & electrolytes Abdominal radiograph (classically, speckled faecal gas pattern in right lower quadrant with dilated small-bowel loops)	Rehydration Lactulose 20 mL 3 times a daily Klean-Prep or ColonLytely via NG tube until clear fluid passed PR* Consider gastrografin enema (under radiological guidance)
Obstruction present		
Admit to ward	Full blood count Urea & electrolytes Abdominal radiograph	Rehydration 'Drip and suck' Inform surgeons Consider gastrografin enema (under radiological guidance)

* Monitor for hypoglycaemia in those with diabetes or liver disease.

Other considerations in DIOS
- Check dose of pancreatic enzymes.
- Check timing of enzymes and consider possible mismatch in gastric emptying between food bolus and pancreatic enzymes.
- Check adherence to medications.
- Ensure adequate dietary fibre and fluid intake.
- Ensure patient has a well-established toilet routine.
- Consider adding ranitidine or omeprazole if evidence of ongoing malabsorption.

Congenital lung disease
- Congenital lung malformations are associated with failure of normal lung development.
- Airways develop early in gestation (by 17 weeks). Abnormal development may lead to a number of congenital cystic lung diseases:
  - Pulmonary sequestration.
  - Congenital cystic adenomatoid malformation.
  - Bronchogenic duplication cyst.
  - Congenital lobar emphysema.
- Alveolar development is predominantly postnatal but is influenced *in utero* by space-occupying lesions (congenital diaphragmatic hernia) and oligohydramnios (e.g. Potter's syndrome).

CHAPTER 37

Rheumatologic conditions

Roger Allen
Jane Munro

Musculoskeletal symptoms and signs are common in children and adolescents and may be the presenting feature of a broad spectrum of conditions. Clinical features and laboratory findings may be relatively non-specific in rheumatological conditions and it is important to look for disease patterns when evaluating the presenting complaint and conducting a systems review.

Evaluation of arthritis/arthralgia
History
- Check the nature of onset – is it acute or insidious?
- **Acute onset monoarticular arthritis associated with fever is septic until proved otherwise.**
- Check the timing of symptoms during the day – as a general guide:
  - Early morning stiffness = inflammatory.
  - Post-activity pain = mechanical.
- Check duration of illness – if >6 weeks it is less likely to be reactive/postviral arthritis.
- Are there any intercurrent infections (respiratory, enteric or skin)? Postviral infections are probably the commonest cause of transient arthritis.
- Has the child been taking any medications (e.g. cefaclor)?
- What does the child, or parent, consider to be the most symptomatic site – is it in the joint, muscle, adjacent bone or a more diffuse area?
- Check for extra-articular symptoms – ensure a thorough systems review and keep the three following diagnoses in mind:
  - Systemic lupus erythematosus (SLE).
  - Acute lymphoblastic leukaemia (ALL).
  - Inflammatory bowel disease (IBD).
- Assess whether the normal physical activities or interests have been interrupted.
- Assess the functional milieu of the patient (e.g. school progress, family and peer relationships, stress experiences).
- Check the family history for other types of inflammatory arthritis, particularly the spondyloarthropathies, autoimmune disorders and pain syndromes (e.g. fibromyalgia or other models for pain behaviour).

Paediatric Handbook, 8th edition. By Kate Thomson, Dean Tey and Michael Marks. Published 2009 by Blackwell Publishing, ISBN: 978-1-4051-7400-8.

Examination

Observe the patient as they move about the room, looking for limitations or alterations in function, and be opportunistic when examining them.

- Examine all joints, not only the site of the presenting complaint. There may be inflammation without symptoms in juvenile idiopathic arthritis (JIA).
- Aim to localise the site of maximal discomfort (e.g. is it the joint capsule, adjacent bone or muscle belly, tendon or ligament attachments?).
- Examine for signs of systemic diseases with an articular component and extra-articular features of JIA. In particular, examine the skin, eyes, abdomen, nails and lymph nodes.

A musculoskeletal assessment should include:

- *Joints:* signs of inflammation such as swelling or tenderness, the range of movement and deformity.
- *Entheses:* bone attachment sites of ligaments/tendons (e.g. Achilles tendon).
- *Tendon sheaths* of fingers and toes (e.g. dactylitis in psoriasis).
- *Gait:* antalgic (pain) or limp, Trendelenburg's sign.
- *Muscles:* tenderness, wasting or weakness, e.g. inability to toe or crouch walk (walking in a full-squat position).
- *Patellar tracking pattern* – does the patella move vertically on walking?
- *Shoe sole* and heel-wearing pattern.
- *Leg length* measurement.
- *Spinal flexion*, including Schober's test (the measurement of the lumbosacral range should increase by at least 6 cm on maximal flexion; the starting range is between the lumbosacral junction and a point 10 cm above).
- *Growth parameters*.

The PGALS is an excellent screening tool for joint exammation. See Table 37.1.

Investigations

There is no single diagnostic test for JIA.

Often useful

- Full blood examination (FBE), erythrocyte sedimentation rate (ESR) and C-reactive protein (CRP). Normal inflammatory markers do not exclude the diagnosis.
- Synovial fluid culture – if sepsis is considered.
- Antinuclear antibody (ANA) – beware of over-interpretation as up to 20% of normal children may have a low positive ANA.

Occasionally useful

- Rheumatoid factor – in polyarticular patients, older children or if the pattern of disease appears unusual.
- HLA-B27 – if spondyloarthropathy is suspected. Remember almost 9% of the White population are positive.
- Imaging – consider plain radiograph, bone scan and ultrasound. In early arthritis, plain films usually give no more information than a careful examination. They may be useful for

Table 37.1 The Components of paediatric Gait, Arms, Legs, Spine screen (pGALS)

SCREENING QUESTIONS
- ☐ Do you have any pain or stiffness in your joints, muscles or your back?
- ☐ Do you have any difficulty getting yourself dressed without any help?
- ☐ Do you have any difficulty going up and down staris?

GAIT
- ☐ Observe the child walking
- ☐ 'Walk on your tip-tones/walk on your heels'

ARMS
- ☐ 'Put you hands out in front of you'
- ☐ 'Turn your hands over and make a fist'
- ☐ 'Pinch you index finger and thumb together'
- ☐ 'Touch the tips of your fingers with your thumb'
- ☐ Squeeze the metacarpophalangeal joints
- ☐ 'Put your hands together/put your hands back to back'
- ☐ 'Reach up and touch the sky'
- ☐ 'Look at the ceiling'
- ☐ 'Put your hands behind your neck'

LEGS
- ☐ Feel for effusion at the knee
- ☐ 'Bend and then straighten your knee' (active movement of knees and examiner feels for crepitus)
- ☐ Passive flexion (90 degrees) with internal rotation of hip

SPINE
- ☐ 'Open your mouth and put 3 of your (*child's own*) fingers in your mouth'
- ☐ Lateral flexion of cervical spine – 'Try and touch your shoulder with your ear'
- ☐ Observe the spine from behind
- ☐ 'Can you bend and touch your toes?' Observe curve of the spine from side and behind

Reproduced with permission from Foster, H.E., Kay, L.J., Friswell, M., Coady, D., Myers, A. Musculoskeletal screening examination (pGALS) for school-age children based on the adult GALS screen. *Arthritis Care Research* (2006) **55(5)**; 709–716.

difficult sites such as the hip, or if there is a long history of arthritis. MRI can be occasionally useful but is not usually an appropriate initial investigation.
- Diagnostic aspirate – worthwhile if sepsis or haemarthrosis is considered, but will not necessarily differentiate between other inflammatory arthritides.
- Specific bacterial/viral studies – if the clinical picture is suggestive (e.g. ASOT, antiDNase B, *Yersinia* and parvovirus serology), see Postinfectious arthritis, p. 529.

Not useful
- Serum uric acid.

Causes of arthritis/arthralgia in childhood
Juvenile idiopathic arthritis (previously juvenile rheumatoid arthritis and juvenile chronic arthritis)
Assessment
- Age of onset <16 years of age.
- Minimum duration of arthritis – 6 weeks.
- **Most acute non-septic arthritis is not JIA.**

Disease subtypes
- *Oligoarticular*: affects 4 joints or fewer:
  - Young, often ANA-positive females (can get asymptomatic uveitis that does not correlate with activity of arthritis – screen 3 monthly).
  - Older, typically HLA-B27-positive males (who may have an evolving spondyloarthropathy).
- *Polyarticular*: affects 5 joints or more; rheumatoid factor positive or negative.
- *Systemic*: joint involvement plus fever, rash and lymphadenopathy.

It is useful to look for:
- Features suggestive of a spondyloarthropathy: enthesitis, sacroiliitis or acute uveitis.
- Nail pits/scalp rash (indicative of psoriasis).
- Rash of Still's disease (faint urticarial-like erythema) – mostly when febrile.
- Uveitis (especially oligo-JIA patient) by slit-lamp.
- Inflammatory features, including subtle behavioural features such as withdrawal from activity, excessive irritability or sleep disruption.

Management
Depends on the clinical picture of disease severity and subtype.

Principles
- Preserve joint function.
- Control pain.
- Manage complications.

Multidisciplinary approach, including physiotherapy, occupational therapy, and psychosocial support. Physical therapy is essential to maintain joint range and function. Splinting should be considered where appropriate.

Medication
- Initially NSAIDs, e.g. naproxen, indomethacin, diclofenac, piroxicam or ibuprofen.
- Then usually low-dose methotrexate to minimise joint destruction.
- Other options include corticosteroids in systemic JIA and intra-articular corticosteroid injections (used early in mono- or pauciarticular arthritis). These are usually performed under GA or procedural sedation and analgesia (e.g. nitrous oxide)

Enthesitis-related arthropathies (spondyloarthropathies)

- Uncommon (more frequent in males) with onset >10 years of age.
- HLA-B27 positive (80%), often raised inflammatory markers.
- Intermittent episodes of enthesitis (tender at tendon insertions) and low back pain/sacroiliitis.
- Acute uveitis (usually clinically evident).
- Management: NSAIDs such as naproxen; sulfasalazine in refractory cases.

Henoch–Schönlein purpura (HSP)

A small-vessel vasculitis.

Clinical features

- Most common age of onset 2–8 years.
- Evolving crops of palpable purpura – predominantly buttocks and legs.
- Abdominal pain (occasionally melaena) may precede rash.
- Large joint migratory arthritis of variable duration and severity.
- Nephritis.
- Other (e.g. oedema dorsum of the feet and hands, acute scrotal swelling and 'bruising', fever and fatigue).
- Exclude other causes of purpura (see chapter 23, Dermatologic conditions).

Investigations

- Full blood examination (to exclude thrombocytopenia).
- Urinalysis – haematuria/proteinuria.
- Renal function – urea/creatinine and urinary protein estimation.

Management

- Supportive – bed rest and analgesia.
- Corticosteroids – may reduce the duration of abdominal pain, but it is uncertain if they significantly affect other features.
- Refer to a specialist if renal dysfunction, hypertension or surgical complications develop.

Irritable hip (transient synovitis)

See chapter 34, Orthopaedic conditions.

Septic arthritis

See chapter 34, Orthopaedic conditions.

Kawasaki disease

See chapter 30, Infectious diseases.

Postinfectious arthritis
Acute rheumatic fever

See chapter 30, Infectious diseases.

Reactive arthritis
Poststreptococcal reactive arthritis
- Afebrile symmetrical non-migratory poly- or pauciarticular arthritis.
- Arthritis responds slowly to NSAIDs.
- Carditis may occur and form part of a spectrum with acute rheumatic fever.
- Consider penicillin prophylaxis if carditis is present.

Postenteric reactive arthritis
- Mainly *Salmonella, Shigella* and *Yersinia* (also reported with *Campylobacter* and *Giardia*).
- It is clinically similar to the spondyloarthropathies; i.e. predominantly lower limb (including sacroiliitis), enthesitis is common and positive family history (especially if HLA-B27 positive). However, it may not present with all the classic clinical features.
- Consider Crohn's disease or ulcerative colitis.
- Associated features – acute anterior uveitis and sterile pyuria.
- Treatment – NSAIDs: indomethacin 0.5–1.0 mg/kg (max. 75 mg) p.o. 8 hourly is often the most effective.

Postviral arthritis
- Many viral illnesses are associated with arthritis.
- It is uncertain in most situations whether it is the primary (infective) or secondary (reactive) event; e.g. Epstein–Barr virus, rubella, adenovirus, varicella (beware septic arthritis secondary to infected skin lesion), parvovirus B19 and hepatitis B.
- A transient arthritis often follows a non-specific 'viral' illness, the confirmation of which may be difficult and unnecessary.
- Treatment: NSAIDs probably shorten the duration.

Non-inflammatory causes of joint pain
Benign nocturnal limb pains ('growing pains')
- Onset at 3–7 years, often occurs in the evenings and at night.
- Well between attacks.
- Recurrent pain mainly involving the knee, calf and shin.
- No symptoms or signs of inflammation either on history or examination.
- Investigations (if carried out) are normal.
- Management involves analgesia (usually paracetamol), ibuprofen and reassurance; heat and massage/rubbing often help.

Benign hypermobility
Common, particularly in the older child/adolescent (<7 years of age all the features are normal variants).

Typical sites
- Hyperextension of the fingers parallel to the forearm.
- Apposition of the thumb to the anterior forearm.
- Hyperextension of the elbows, knees, or both >10°.
- Excessive dorsiflexion of the ankles.
- Hip flexion allowing the palms to be placed flat on ground.

Clinical features
- Pain occurs typically in the afternoon or after exercise and occurs mostly in the lower limbs.
- The child may have features of patello-femoral dysfunction.
- The child may have transient joint effusions.
- Management: symptomatic treatment and reassurance.

Complex regional pain syndrome
See chapter 4, Pain management.

Other rheumatological disorders

Maintain an index of suspicion regarding other rheumatological disorders (e.g. SLE, derma-
tomyositis and other connective tissue disorders).

Enquire about the following symptoms:
- Lethargy, weight loss, mouth ulcers, alopecia or frontal hair breaking.
- Recurrent fevers.
- Raynaud's phenomenon, rashes or photosensitivity.
- Ophthalmological symptoms: red sore eyes, change in vision or dry eyes.
- Weakness.
- Consider investigating with: C3, C4, ANA, dsDNA, ENA, CK, LDH or LFT.

USEFUL RESOURCES
- *www.arc.org.uk/arthinfo/emedia.asp* – Arthritis research campaign with link to DVD on administration of pGALS

CHAPTER 38

Surgical conditions

John Hutson
Tom Clarnette

Inguinoscrotal conditions

The underlying pathological basis of an inguinal hernia, an encysted hydrocele of the cord or a scrotal hydrocele is the persistence of a patent processus vaginalis after the completion of testicular descent.

The causes of groin lumps in neonates are:
- Inguinal hernia – if irreducible, irritable baby, tender lump in the groin, unable to get above it.
- Encysted hydrocele of the cord, unable to be reduced – e.g. well baby, mobile lump.
- Undescended testes.
- Lymphadenitis with abscess formation – rare condition, often not diagnosed until operation.

Inguinal hernia (see Fig. 38.1a)
- Occurs when the patent processus vaginalis is large enough to allow bowel, omentum or ovary (in females) to protrude through the inguinal canal and sometimes, in males, down to the scrotum.
- The younger the child, the greater the risk of bowel or ovary becoming strangulated.
- Bowel strangulation in boys compresses the testicular vessels and may result in testicular ischaemia.
- Surgery is always required to prevent strangulation and this is done as a day case, except when the baby is <4 weeks of age.

Reducible inguinal hernia
See Table 38.1.

Irreducible inguinal hernia
- Urgent surgical referral is indicated.
- Most irreducible inguinal hernias can be manually reduced by a surgeon and surgery carried out within 48 h.
- Pain relief is appropriate to aid with reduction.
- The use of ice packs or traction is inappropriate.

Paediatric Handbook, 8th edition. By Kate Thomson, Dean Tey and Michael Marks. Published 2009 by Blackwell Publishing, ISBN: 978-1-4051-7400-8.

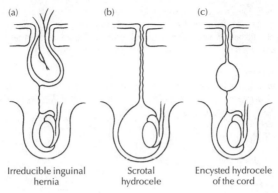

(a)   (b)   (c)

Irreducible inguinal hernia   Scrotal hydrocele   Encysted hydrocele of the cord

Fig 38.1 Inguinoscrotal conditions

Table 38.1 Reducible inguinal hernia

Age at presentation	Timing of surgical consultation	Appropriate operating time
Birth–6 weeks	Day of diagnosis	Next available list
6 weeks–6 months	Within few days	Within 2 weeks
6 months–6 years	Within 2 weeks	Within 2 months

Scrotal hydrocele, encysted hydrocele of the cord (see Fig. 38.1b,c)

In these conditions, the patent processus vaginalis is narrow and enables peritoneal fluid, but not abdominal contents, into the cord structures. A patent processus vaginalis often closes of its own accord in the first 18 months of life.

The important clinical signs of a scrotal hydrocoele are:

- Brilliantly transilluminable swelling.
- Narrow cord above the swelling.
- Swelling does not empty on squeezing and a normal testicle is felt in it.
- Non-tender.

If a hydrocele persists beyond 1 year of age, surgery is recommended and an inguinal herniotomy (i.e. division of patent processus vaginalis) is done as a day case.

Undescended testes

- *Congenital:* When the testis cannot be brought to the bottom of the scrotum, it is 'undescended'. This is caused by incomplete migration of the gubernaculum to the scrotum. An assessment should be made by a paediatric surgeon between 3–6 months of life and an orchidopexy done at 6–12 months of age as a day case.

- *Acquired:* Some boys present with undescended testis later in childhood (4–10 years). This is the result of failure of elongation of the spermatic cord with age, caused by persistence of a fibrous remanent of the processus vaginalis. Surgery is recommended, if the testis does not remain in the bottom of the scrotum, to optimise fertility.

Acute scrotum

A child with a painful, tender or red scrotum should be seen by a surgeon as a matter of urgency. Without surgical exploration, it is usually impossible to differentiate between the two common causes:

- Torsion of the testis.
- Torsion of the testicular appendage.

Torsion of the testis

- Can occur at any age, but is most common in babies and adolescents.
- In older children it is characterised by more severe pain and vomiting.
- A testis lying horizontally in the scrotum indicates an anatomical predisposition to torsion and may cause intermittent testicular pain.
- **Ultrasound is unreliable in distinguishing between torsion of the testis and torsion of the testicular appendage and often delays critical operative treatment.**

Other causes

- Epididymo-orchitis is a rare disease in prepubertal boys who do not have urinary tract infections and should not be considered part of the initial differential diagnosis.
- Mumps orchitis is not seen before puberty. Do not treat with antibiotics.

The penis
The foreskin/prepuce

The foreskin is normally adherent to the glans at birth and remains so for a variable period of time. It is usually fully retractable by 3 years of age, but partial adherence is still normal up to 10 years of age. There is no need to retract the foreskin in preschool children.

Smegma deposits

- Present as firm yellow-white masses beneath the prepuce in non-retractile foreskins (see Fig. 38.2a).
- Often confused with tumours or cysts of the penis, but are a normal variant and require no treatment.

Balanitis

- This is an infection under the foreskin with redness, inflammation, swelling and sometimes a white exudate (see Fig. 38.2b).
- Immediate treatment with local penile toilet, i.e., soaking in an antiseptic solution, local antiseptic ointment (e.g. neomycin eye ointment) beneath the foreskin and topical hydrocortisone 1% are used in mild cases. Oral antibiotics (e.g. co-trimoxazole) may also be added.

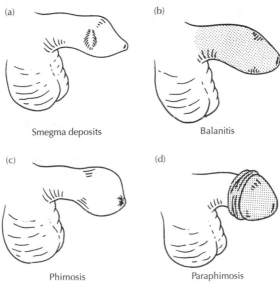

(a) Smegma deposits
(b) Balanitis
(c) Phimosis
(d) Paraphimosis

Fig 38.2 Conditions of the penis

- If the whole penile shaft skin is red and swollen to the pubis, i.v. antibiotics may be required.

Phimosis

- This is scarring of the preputial opening, which causes:
  - Urinary obstruction.
  - Ballooning of the foreskin on micturition.
- It is often the end result of recurrent episodes of balanitis (see Fig. 38.2c).
- It usually requires circumcision if severe, although mild cases respond to topical 0.5% betamethasone valerate cream applied four times daily for 14 days.

Paraphimosis

- Acutely painful condition, which results from a retracted foreskin trapped behind the glans, forming an oedematous ring constricting the exposed and swollen glans penis (see Fig. 38.2d).
- Manual reduction should be attempted in all cases.
- To facilitate the procedure, use topical local anaesthetic cream (e.g. EMLA cream) 5 min before reduction.
- **Ice and adrenaline-containing creams should not be applied**.
- Failure to reduce the paraphimosis requires urgent surgical consultation.

Circumcision
- The indications for circumcision are phimosis and recurrent balanitis.
- There is no indication for neonatal circumcision.
- Hypospadias is an absolute contraindication, as the foreskin may be required for penile reconstruction.
- **Circumcision is not required for cleanliness** and <10% of Australian boys are currently being circumcised.
- It is an unnecessary operation with complications of surgery and anaesthesia.

Umbilical hernia
- Common finding in newborn children; usually resolves in the first 12 months of life.
- If persists, operation as a day case is recommended before starting school.
- The operation is primarily cosmetic, although strangulation can occur during adult life (particularly during pregnancy).

Acute abdominal pain
Abdominal pain is a common symptom in children. Acute appendicitis must be distinguished from common causes of abdominal pain, including gastrointestinal and urinary tract infection and constipation.

Appendicitis
- The symptoms and signs of appendicitis are related to the degree of peritoneal irritation and the position of the appendix.
- Diagnosis is straightforward if there is localised peritonitis with guarding in the right iliac fossa; however, peritonitis may not occur in retrocaecal appendicitis and in pelvic appendicitis there may be only vague suprapubic tenderness.
- Repeated clinical examination and abdominal ultrasound may help identify these difficult cases. Rectal examination should not be done in children.
- Diagnosing appendicitis in the young child (<4 years of age) is difficult. It is important to refer a child who complains of persistent abdominal pain, even if this is associated with vomiting or diarrhoea. In particular, suspect significant peritonitis if the child does not allow abdominal examination.

Differentials
- Urinary tract infection may be excluded by urine testing (see chapter 35, Renal conditions). Blood, protein and white cells may all be present in the urine in acute appendicitis. Nitrites are more specific for urinary tract infections.
- Gastrointestinal infections often produce a local ileus but no peritonitis and are frequently distinguished by 'squelchiness' (secondary to air and fluid) in the right iliac fossa on examination.

Intussusception

- Consider in children aged 3 months to 2 years presenting with vomiting, intermittent abdominal pain and lethargy/pallor.
- These early symptoms should be acted on, rather than awaiting the classic 'red currant jelly stool', which is a feature of advanced disease.
- The abdominal mass is central, beneath the rectus abdominis on the right side, and is often difficult to feel.
- Ultrasound should be done to confirm the diagnosis. Contrast enema should not be used in the presence of peritonitis, significant dehydration or established bowel obstruction.
- **An infant with suspected intussusception requires urgent surgical assessment and radiological investigations for diagnosis and treatment.**
- Although an ultrasound may confirm the diagnosis, a contrast air or barium enema is required to reduce the intussusception.

These procedures should only be undertaken by experienced radiologists with a surgical team immediately available at a tertiary centre.

Vomiting in infancy
Malrotation and volvulus

- Green vomiting without an obvious septic cause is an indication for urgent surgical consultation, to exclude intestinal malrotation and the associated lethal complication of midgut volvulus. In regional settings, consider doing an urgent contrast study first, if surgical review is not immediately available.
- Initially, there may not be any clinical signs of abdominal disease. Abdominal distension is not usually seen in the early stages of presentation.
- Urgent surgical referral is necessary.

Pyloric stenosis

- Usually presents between 2 and 6 weeks of age (chronological age, regardless of prematurity).

Table 38.2 Vomiting in infancy

Green vomit	Curdled milk
Differential diagnosis: • Malrotation • Infection (gastroenteritis/meningitis/UTI) • Small bowel obstruction (rare)	Differential diagnosis: • Pyloric stenosis • Gastro-oesophageal reflux • Infection (UTI/gastroenteritis/meningitis)
Management (*after exclusion of major sepsis*): URGENT SURGICAL REFERRAL	Projectile vomiting ± weight loss/gastric peristalsis: URGENT SURGICAL REFERRAL

- It may be difficult to diagnose and should be suspected when vomiting is projectile and if failure to thrive is present.
- Gastric peristalsis occurs due to pyloric obstruction and is clearly visible on the baby's abdominal wall. When seen, it should prompt surgical referral.
- If the stomach is not grossly distended with fluid and/or air, the pyloric tumour is readily palpable.
- Ultrasound is only required if the diagnosis is unclear and the pyloric tumour cannot be felt.

Metabolic complications

- Vomiting in these infants results in loss of gastric fluid (water and HCl). The kidneys can initially conserve H^+, but once the baby becomes dehydrated, water and Na^+ are conserved in exchange for K^+ and H^+. The resulting condition is hypovolaemia with alkalosis, low chloride and potassium. Even if serum K^+ is normal, there is a total body potassium deficiency.
- A metabolic alkalosis (chloride < 100 mmol/L, pH > 7.45, bicarbonate > 32 mmol/L and sodium < 130 mmol/L) is present only in significant cases. Inappropriate rehydration with low-sodium-containing fluids can result in cerebral oedema.

Management

- **An appropriate fluid for resuscitation is 0.45% (1/2 normal) saline with 5% dextrose. Potassium should be added once the baby is passing urine** (refer to Table 38.3).
- If the baby's weight before the onset of symptoms is known, fluid deficit is easily calculated. Maintenance requirements may be calculated at 100 mL/kg per 24 h.
  - For example: a baby normally weighing 3 kg now weighs 2.7 kg.
  - Deficit 300 gram (10% dehydration): replacement required 300 mL.
  - Maintenance required: 300 mL/24 h.
  - For resuscitation over 12 h, 450 mL is required in this period, i.e. 38 mL/h.
- For a simple guideline to facilitate fluid calculations if the baby's weight is not known see Table 38.3.

Neck lumps

- *Cervical adenopathy:* Enlargement of cervical lymph nodes is common with upper respiratory infections.
- *Abscess:* Consider bacterial infection with abscess formation in infants and children with large (2–4 cm) tender masses. There is often no overlying redness in cervical abscesses because the lymph nodes are beneath the deep fascia. Skin involvement occurs late in the disease. Fluctuance is the indication for surgical referral for incision and drainage.
- *Mycobacterial lymph node infection* (e.g. *Mycobacterium avium complex*): consider with evolution of indolent, non-tender, persistent lymphadenopathy in children 1–3 years of age. Purple discolouration in the overlying skin indicates an abscess, which requires surgical treatment.
- *Other:* large (>3–4 cm) or suspicious lymph nodes need a biopsy to exclude malignancy.

Table 38.3 Fluid calculations in pyloric stenosis

Clinical state	Fluids preoperative period/first 12–16 h	Monitoring
Mildly dehydrated <5%		
Clinically well, reduced urine output	No bolus required	Check O$_2$ saturations
	1/2 normal saline & 5% dextrose with 20 mmol/l KCL in each litre	Monitor pulse, urine output
Electrolytes usually normal	Rate = 1.5 × maintenance for 12 h	Glucose, U&E, creatinine 12-hourly
Moderately dehydrated 5–10%	Bolus normal saline 20 ml/kg in 30 min	Monitor O$_2$ saturations, pulse, BP and urine output
Mildly lethargic, pale, dry mouth	Then 1/2 normal saline & 5% dextrose with 30 mmol/l KCL in each litre	Glucose, U&E, creatinine 6–12-hourly
Poor urine output	Rate = 2 × maintenance for 12 h	
Low chloride +/– sodium		
Severely dehydrated 10%	Bolus normal saline 20 ml/kg in 30 min	Monitor O$_2$ saturations, pulse, BP and urine output
Lethargic, pale, mottled, dry mouth, no urine, tachycardia & may have low BP	Then 1/2 normal saline & 5% dextrose with 30 mmol KCL in each litre	Glucose, U&E, creatinine 4–6-hourly
Low chloride & sodium +/– low potassium	Rate = 2 × maintenance	
	Continue up to 16 h or further if clinically indicated	

Table 38.4 Rectal bleeding

Sick neonate	Necrotising enterocolitis (NEC) Malrotation Severe enteritis
Well neonate	Ingested maternal blood Bleeding disorder Anal fissure
Well child: bright red blood	Anal fissure Polyp (with mucus)
Well child: dark blood	Meckel's diverticulum Peptic ulcer/varices Inflammatory bowel disease

Rectal bleeding

See Table 38.4. See also chapter 27, Gastrointestinal conditions.

Urgent neonatal surgical conditions
Important warning signs

- Excessive drooling of frothy secretions from the mouth may suggest oesophageal atresia.
- Bile-stained or green vomiting is always abnormal (malrotation may be present and requires urgent treatment).
- Delayed passage of meconium (beyond 24 h) is abnormal and may indicate Hirschsprung disease.
- Inguinoscrotal hernias need urgent attention to avoid strangulation.

All the conditions below require urgent paediatric surgical consultation and transfer to a tertiary centre.

Oesophageal atresia

Excessive drooling or frothy, mucousy secretions from the mouth in a newborn suggests an inability to swallow. The test for oesophageal atresia is to pass a 10-French gauge catheter (which will not curl up) gently through the mouth.

- In the baby with oesophageal atresia, the catheter stops at 10 cm from the gums.
- In a normal baby, it passes to 20–25 cm and returns acid on litmus testing.
- First aid includes:

Table 38.5 Urgent neonatal conditions:

Symptom	Diagnosis	Investigation	Management
Excessive drooling Feed intolerance	Oesophageal atresia	Passage of 10 F catheter by mouth, stops at ~10 cm	Oropharyngeal suction
Respiratory distress with scaphoid abdomen	Diaphragmatic hernia	Abdominal and chest X-rays – bowel loops in chest	O_2 No bag and masking Nasogastric tube
Intestinal contents in a sac	Exomphalos (consider Beckwith-Weidemann syndrome, especially if infant is large)	Blood glucose	10% IV dextrose Temperature control Nasogastric tube
Prolapsed intestinal contents	Gastroschisis	–	Cover with kitchen wrap Temperature control Nasogastric tube
Green vomiting	Malrotation Bowel obstruction	Abdominal X-ray U&Es (barium study only after surgical referral)	Nasogastric drainage

    – Nil orally.

    – I.v. fluids.

    – Frequent oropharyngeal suction (every 10–15 min), to prevent aspiration.

- **Urgent transfer is required.**

Diaphragmatic hernia

- Respiratory distress in a newborn with a scaphoid abdomen suggests diaphragmatic hernia.
- Cardiac displacement and a chest radiograph showing bowel loops in the chest (left side more commonly) confirms the diagnosis.
- First aid is described in Table 38.5.
- If mechanical ventilation is required, only provide this via tracheal intubation; bag and mask ventilation may exacerbate respiratory distress by distending the bowel.

Exomphalos/gastroschisis

- These anterior abdominal wall defects place the child at risk of heat and water loss from the exposed surface of the sac (exomphalos) or bowel (gastroschisis).
- First aid is described in Table 38.5.

Sacrococcygeal teratoma

- Any lump over the coccyx of the baby should be assumed to be a teratoma until proven otherwise.
- Needs immediate referral at birth.

Ambiguous genitalia

Genitalia that are frankly ambiguous need urgent consultation with an experienced paediatric endocrinologist or surgeon on the first day of life (see chapter 25, Endocrine conditions).

- An enlarged clitoris in an apparent female is also abnormal and needs immediate referral.
- Hypospadias may overlap with ambiguous genitalia. This needs a careful initial assessment; if the diagnosis of hypospadias has been made, someone has already assumed the gender is male.
- If one or both testes are undescended, or the scrotum is bifid, or both, the baby should be treated as having ambiguous genitalia until proven otherwise, with immediate referral for further investigation.

CHAPTER 39
Prescribing for children

Noel Cranswick
Andrew Rechtmann

Knowledge of drug administration in children and infants is essential to the practice of paediatrics. Most registered medicines do not have indications or dosing for children.

Drug choice and dose
There are many issues that influence drug choice and dose in paediatric practice. Pharmacokinetic parameters change with age and dosage regimens need to take into account factors such as growth, organ development and sexual maturation.

Unlicensed and off-label drug use
These are commonplace in paediatric practice as a result of inadequate paediatric data.
- *Unlicensed drug use* is the use of
  - a drug that has not been approved by the Therapeutic Goods Administration (TGA), **or**
  - an untested formulation of an approved drug, **or**
  - a non-pharmacopoeial substance as a medicine.
- *Off-label prescribing* is the use of a drug in a manner other than that recommended in the manufacturer's product information.

Dosing considerations
- Most medicines in children are dosed by weight. Always attempt to obtain accurate weight and height data before calculating the appropriate initial dose.
  - Consider using ideal body weight in obese children (BMI > 95th% for age and sex).
- A few medications, especially cytotoxic drugs, may only have dosing information by surface area (see Appendix 4).
- Child's weight (in kg) can be estimated by the formula (age + 4) × 2.
  - Remember to confirm an accurate weight at the first available opportunity.
- In emergencies, standardised centile charts for weight and height may be utilised for these calculations.

See general guidelines in Table 39.1.

Paediatric Handbook, 8th edition. By Kate Thomson, Dean Tey and Michael Marks. Published 2009 by Blackwell Publishing, ISBN: 978-1-4051-7400-8.

Table 39.1 Guidelines for best prescribing practice

- DO check the dose:
  - Use a calculator for dosing by weight/BSA
  - Ensure it doesn't exceed the maximum adult dose
- DO check for allergies and contra-indications
- DO write legibly
- DO write UNITS (not IU) after insulin doses
- DO include generic drug name, dose, frequency, route, and date of start, finish or review
- DO write a leading zero before a decimal point, e.g. 0.6 milligrams not .6 milligrams
- DO NOT write a trailing zero after a whole number, e.g. 8 milligrams not 8.0 milligrams
- DO NOT abbreviate drug names, e.g. AZT could be azathioprine or azithromycin

Adverse drug reactions

- Are common but under-recognised in children.
- All suspected and proven adverse drug reactions (ADR) should be reported, even if seemingly trivial.
- Suspected allergic reactions should be assessed and followed up (e.g. by a drug allergy clinic).
- When an avoidable ADR is identified, patients should be given a permanent record (e.g. card or medical alert bracelet) as appropriate.

The important points to document on history are:
- The specific illness the medication was prescribed for (intercurrent viral infections may also cause urticaria).
- The name of the medication and preparation.
- Whether this was the first exposure to the medication.
- How many doses were given before a reaction occurred.
- The time of onset of the reaction from the last dose given.
- The symptoms of the reaction and its total duration.

There are two main types:

Type A adverse drug reaction
- These are predictable from the known pharmacology of the drug and are dose dependent.
- Examples include opiate sedation and tachycardia with β_2-agonists.

Type B adverse drug reaction
- These are less common, unpredictable (idiosyncratic) and dose-independent.
- They are often serious and usually require ceasing the drug, e.g. Stevens–Johnson syndrome (most commonly associated with anticonvulsants).

Therapeutic drug monitoring

- Relatively few drugs need therapeutic drug monitoring.
- It is beneficial in drugs with a narrow therapeutic index, or where serum levels are well-correlated with efficacy or toxicity.
- Therapeutic drug monitoring can be useful for:
  - Antibiotics, e.g. gentamicin, vancomycin.
  - Anticonvulsants, e.g. phenytoin, phenobarbitone.
  - Immunosuppressants, e.g. tacrolimus, cyclosporin, methotrexate.
  - Drug overdose, e.g. paracetamol, iron.
- Routine testing is not beneficial for:
  - Carbamazepine.
  - Valproate.
- Timing of samples for monitoring will vary depending upon the actual drug but accurate recording of the drug dose, administration time and sample time is essential.

Drug errors

- Paediatric patients are at high risk of drug errors.
- Certain drugs are commonly associated with medication errors in children (e.g. opiates, paracetamol, antibiotics, 50% dextrose and electrolytes such as i.v. Ca^{2+} and Mg^{2+}). Extra care should be taken when prescribing or administering these medicines.
- When prescribing for children, the following factors should be taken into consideration:
  - Children's doses vary widely and so there is no standard dose (as there is with adults).
  - Clarify if drug doses are given in mg/kg per day in divided doses (or mg/kg per dose given x times per day).
  - Calculations are required for most childhood dosing and errors may occur during this step.
  - Some paediatric preparations may cause confusion in those unfamiliar with their use, e.g. i.v. versus enteral paracetamol, or Painstop Night-Time which contains three active agents.
  - The small doses used in children may cause measuring and administration errors.
  - Misplacing or misreading of decimal points can lead to error.

Drug interactions

- Drug interactions are always possible when using more than one medicine.
- Only a few drug combinations result in clinically significant sequelae.
- Be aware that drug interactions are more common when:
  - More drugs are prescribed – where possible, aim for monotherapy.
  - Patients are sick, especially with multiple organ pathologies.
- Drugs with a narrow therapeutic window are more likely to result in more significant interactions.

Complementary medicines

Specific history of these should be sought, as:

- Complementary medicines and many herbal products are available 'over the counter' or through alternative medicine practitioners.
- Families often do not offer this information.
- Such products can be involved in adverse drug reactions and interactions.

Examples of potential drug interactions

- *St John's wort:* anticoagulants, antidepressants, digoxin, MAO inhibitors, dextromethorphan, decreases effects of cyclosporin and antiviral drugs, and prolongs effect of general anaesthetics.
- *Ginseng:* anticoagulants, stimulants, antihypertensives, antidepressants, phenelzine, digoxin, potentiates effects of corticosteroids and oestrogens.
- *Ginger:* anticoagulants, antihypertensives, cardiac drugs, hypoglycaemic drugs and enhances effects of barbiturates.

USEFUL RESOURCES

- *http://www.drugdoses.net* – For information regarding and purchase of Frank Shann's drug doses book.
- *http://www.australianprescriber.com/* – An independent journal with articles relevant to both paediatric and adult prescribing.
- *http://www.tga.gov.au/docs/html/mip/medicine.htm* – Prescribing medicines in pregnancy.

Growth charts

Girls in utero 24 - 42 weeks & post natal 0 - 3 years

Intrauterine Growth Curves (Composite Male/Female)

Measuring Technique: As for ages 0-36 months (see over page).

Additional Notes: Gestational ages are recorded in completed weeks from the first day of the mother's last menstrual period.
Foetal growth is influenced by many factors including age, body weight, height, parity, ethnic origin of the mother and sex of the foetus.
Corrections for some of these factors are found in the quoted reference.

Data Source: Kitchen, W. H. *et al.* 1983, 'Revised intrauterine growth curves for an Australian hospital population', *Aust. Paediatr. J.* 19: 157-161.

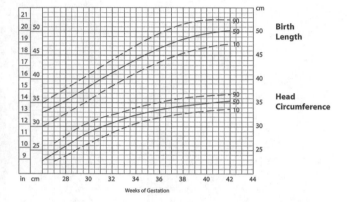

Birth Length

Head Circumference

Weeks of Gestation

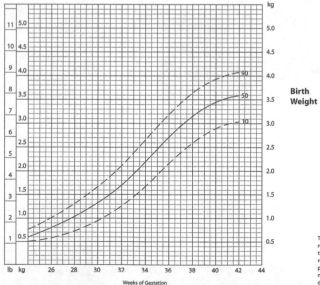

Birth Weight

Weeks of Gestation

Girls in utero 24-42 weeks & post natal 0-3 years

Surname	Identification No.
Given Names	Date of Birth

Weight Percentile for Girls 0-3 years

Weight should be taken in the nude, or as near thereto as possible. If a surgical gown or minimum underclothing (vest and pants) is worn, then its estimated weight (about 0.1 kg) must be subtracted before weight is recorded. Weights are conventionally recorded to the last completed 0.1 kg above the age of six months. The bladder should be empty.

Endorsed By

Australasian Paediatric Endocrine Group

Simplified Calculation of Body Surface Area (BSA)

$$BSA\ (m^2) = \sqrt{\frac{Ht\ (cm) \times Wt\ (kg)}{3600}}$$

Reference: Mosteller, R. D. 1987, 'Simplified calculation of body surface area', *N. Engl. J. Med.*, 317: 1098.

DATE	AGE	LENGTH	WEIGHT	HEAD CIRCUM.

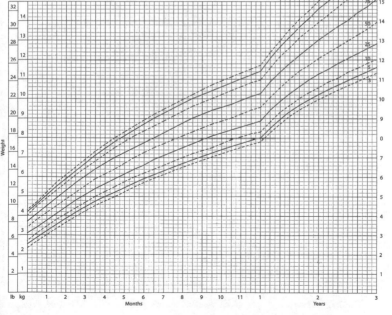

Length Percentile for Girls 0-3 years

Mother's Height

Father's Height

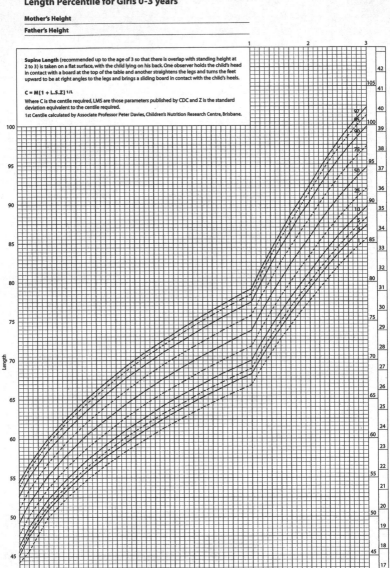

Supine Length (recommended up to the age of 3 so that there is overlap with standing height at 2 to 3) is taken on a flat surface, with the child lying on his back. One observer holds the child's head in contact with a board at the top of the table and another straightens the legs and turns the feet upward to be at right angles to the legs and brings a sliding board in contact with the child's heels.

$$C = M[1 + L.S.Z]^{1/L}$$

Where C is the centile required, LMS are those parameters published by CDC and Z is the standard deviation equivalent to the centile required.

1st Centile calculated by Associate Professor Peter Davies, Children's Nutrition Research Centre, Brisbane.

Length

Months

Years

Head Circumference

Measuring Technique: The tape should be placed over the eyebrows, above the ears and over the most prominent part of the occiput taking a direct route. A paper tape is preferable to plastic, which stretches unacceptably under tension. The maximum measurement should be recorded to the nearest 0.1 cm.

In utero 28 - 40 weeks, 0-12 months

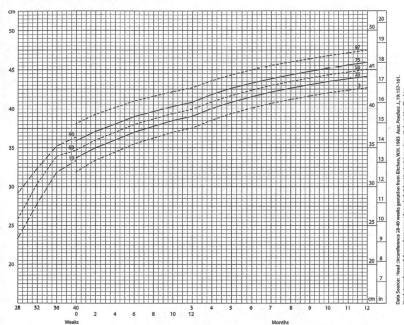

Data Source: Head Circumference 28-40 weeks gestation from Eitchen, W.H. 1983. Aust. Paediatr. J. 19: 157-161.
Head circumference 0-3 years from www.cdc.gov/nchs/about/major/nhanes/growthcharts/datafiles.htm

1 - 3 years

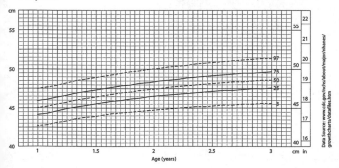

Data Source: www.cdc.gov/nchs/about/major/nhanes/
growthcharts/datafiles.htm

Boys in utero 24-42 weeks & post natal 0-3 years

Intrauterine Growth Curves (Composite Male/Female)

Measuring Technique: As for ages 0-36 months (see over page).

Additional Notes: Gestational ages are recorded in completed weeks from the first day of the mother's last menstrual period.
Foetal growth is influenced by many factors including age, body weight, height, parity, ethnic origin of the mother and sex of the foetus.
Corrections for some of these factors are found in the quoted reference.

Data Source: Kitchen, W.H. *et al.* 1983, 'Revised intrauterine growth curves for an Australian hospital population', *Aust. Paediatr. J.* 19: 157-161.

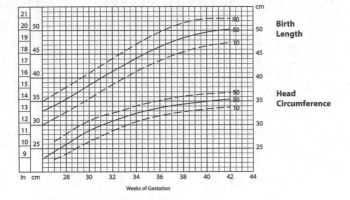

Birth Length

Head Circumference

Weeks of Gestation

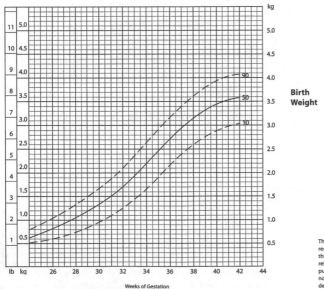

Birth Weight

Weeks of Gestation

Boys in utero 24-42 weeks & post natal 0-3 years

Surname _____

Identification No. _____

Given Names _____

Date of Birth _____

Weight Percentile for Boys 0-3 years

Weight should be taken in the nude, or as near thereto as possible. If a surgical gown or minimum underclothing (vest and pants) is worn, then its estimated weight (about 0.1 kg) must be subtracted before weight is recorded. Weights are conventionally recorded to the last completed 0.1 kg above the age of six months. The bladder should be empty.

Endorsed By

Australasian Paediatric Endocrine Group

Simplified Calculation of Body Surface Area (BSA)

$$BSA\ (m^2) = \sqrt{\frac{\text{lt (cm) x Wt (kg)}}{3600}}$$

Reference: Mosteller, R. D. 1987, 'Simplified calculation of body surface area', *N. Engl. J. Med.*, 317: 1098.

DATE	AGE	LENGTH	WEIGHT	HEAD CIRCUM.

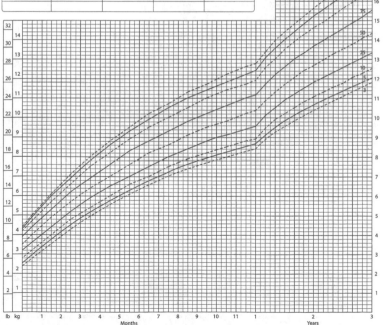

Data Source: www.cdc.gov/nchs/about/major/nhanes/growthcharts/datafiles.htm

Length Percentile for Boys 0-3 years

Mother's Height

Father's Height

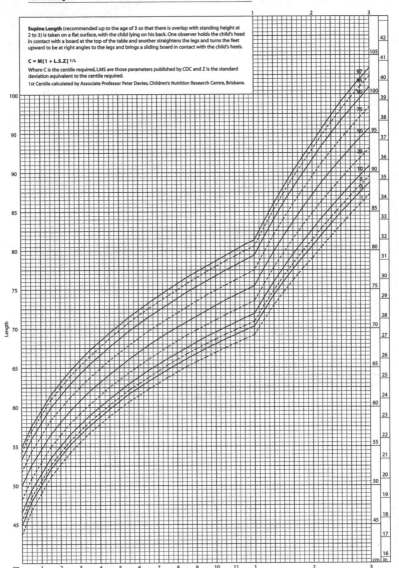

Supine Length (recommended up to the age of 3 so that there is overlap with standing height at 2 to 3) is taken on a flat surface, with the child lying on his back. One observer holds the child's head in contact with a board at the top of the table and another straightens the legs and turns the feet upward to be at right angles to the legs and brings a sliding board in contact with the child's heels.

C = M[1 + L.S.Z] ¹/ᴸ

Where C is the centile required, LMS are those parameters published by CDC and Z is the standard deviation equivalent to the centile required.

1st Centile calculated by Associate Professor Peter Davies, Children's Nutrition Research Centre, Brisbane.

Data Source: www.cdc.gov/nchs/about/major/nhanes/growthcharts/datafiles.htm

Head Circumference

Measuring Technique: The tape should be placed over the eyebrows, above the ears and over the most prominent part of the occiput taking a direct route. A paper tape is preferable to plastic, which stretches unacceptably under tension. The maximum measurement should be recorded to the nearest 0.1 cm.

In utero 28-40 weeks, 0-12 months

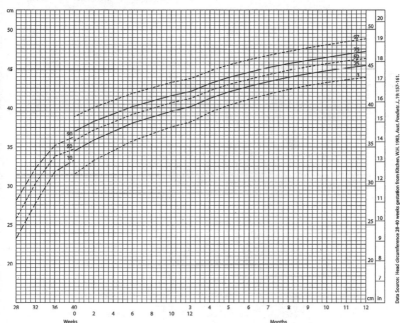

Data Source: Head circumference 28-40 weeks gestation from Kitchen, W.H. 1983, *Aust. Paediatr. J.*, 19:157-161.
Head circumference 0-3 years from www.cdc.gov/nchs/about/major/nhanes/growthcharts/datafiles.htm

1-3 years

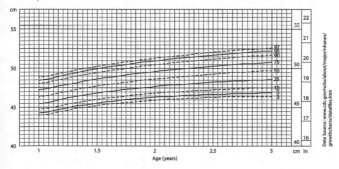

Data Source: www.cdc.gov/nchs/about/major/nhanes/growthcharts/datafiles.htm

Girls 2 -18 years

Stages of Puberty

Ages of attainment of successive stages of pubertal sexual development are given in the Height Percentile chart.
The stage Pubic Hair 2+ represents the state of a child who shows the pubic hair appearance stage 2 but not stage 3 (see below).

The centiles for age at which this state is normally seen are given, the 97th centile being considered as the early limit, the 3rd centile as the late limit. The child's puberty stages may be plotted at successive ages (Tanner. 1962, *Growth at Adolescence*, 2nd edn).

Pubic Hair Development

Stage 1. Pre-adolescent. The vellus over the pubes is not further developed than that over the abdominal wall, i.e. no pubic hair.

Stage 2. Sparse growth of long, slightly pigmented downy hair, straight or slightly curled, chiefly along labia.

Stage 3. Considerably darker, coarser and more curled. The hair spreads sparsely over the junction of the pubes.

Stage 4. Hair now adult in type, but area covered is still considerably smaller than in the adult. No spread to the medial surface of thighs.

Stage 5. Adult in quantity and type with distribution of the horizontal (or classically 'feminine') pattern. Spread to medial surface of thighs but not up linea alba or elsewhere above the base of the inverse triangle (spread up linea alba occurs late and is rated stage 6).

Breast Development Stages

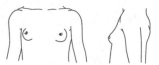

Stage 1. Prepubertal

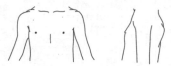

Stage 2. Elevation of breasts and papilla

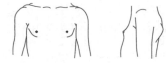

Stage 3. Further elevation and areola but no separation of contours

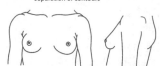

Stage 4. Areola and papilla form a secondary mound above level of the breast

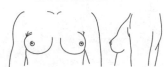

Stage 5. Areola recesses to the general contour of the breast

Pubic Hair Stages

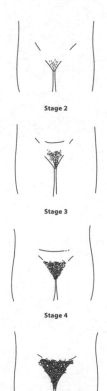

Stage 2

Stage 3

Stage 4

Stage 5

Girls 2-18 years

Reproduced with permission of Pfizer Australia

Endorsed By **A**ustralasian **P**aediatric **E**ndocrine **G**roup

Surname _____

Given Names _____

Identification No. _____

Date of Birth _____

Weight Percentile

Weight should be taken in the nude, or as near thereto as possible. If a surgical gown or minimum underclothing (vest and pants) is worn, then its estimated weight (about 0.1 kg) must be subtracted before weight is recorded. Weights are conventionally recorded to the last completed 0.1 kg above the age of six months. The bladder should be empty.

Body-Mass Index

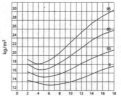

DATE	AGE	HEIGHT	WEIGHT	HEAD CIRCUM.	PUBERTAL STAGES		
					BREAST	PUBIC HAIR	MENARCHE

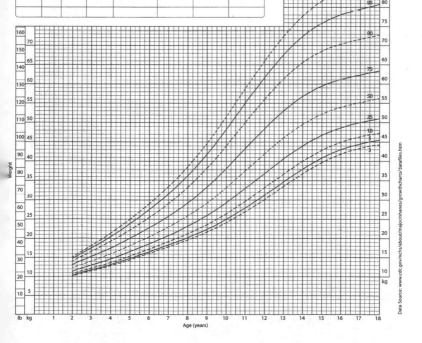

Height Percentile

Mother's Height

Father's Height

Simplified Calculation of Body Surface Area (BSA)

$$BSA (m^2) = \sqrt{\frac{Ht (cm) \times Wt (kg)}{3600}}$$

Reference: Mosteller, R. D. 1987, 'Simplified calculation of body surface area', *N. Engl. J. Med.*, 317: 1098.

Supine Length (recommended up to the age of 3 so that there is overlap with standing height at 2 to 3) is taken on a flat surface, with the child lying on her back. One observer holds the child's head in contact with a board at the top of the table and another straightens the legs and turns the feet upward to be at right angles to the legs and brings a sliding board in contact with the child's heels.

Standing Height (recommended from age 2 onwards) should be taken without shoes, the child standing with her heels and back in contact with an upright wall. Her head is held so that she looks straight forward with the lower borders of the eye sockets in the same horizontal plane as the external auditory meati (i.e. head not with the nose tipped upward). A right-angled block (preferably counterweighted) is then slid down the wall until its bottom surface touches the child's head and a scale fixed to the wall is read. During the measurement the child should be told to stretch her neck to be as tall as possible, though care must be taken to prevent her heels coming off the ground. Gentle but firm pressure upward should be applied by the measurer under the mastoid processes to help the child stretch. In this way the variation in height from morning to evening is minimised. Standing height should be recorded to the last completed 0.1 cm.

$C = M[1 + L.S.Z]^{1/L}$

Where C is the centile required, LMS are those parameters published by CDC and Z is the standard deviation equivalent to the centile required.

1st Centile calculated by Associate Professor Peter Davies, Children's Nutrition Research Centre, Brisbane.

Represents 50th centile height attained for an individual girl entering puberty at the average time based on longitudinal data. All other centiles are based on cross-sectional data.

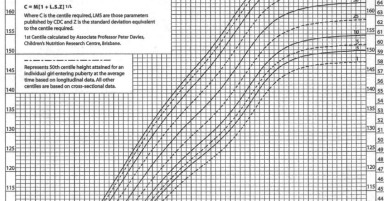

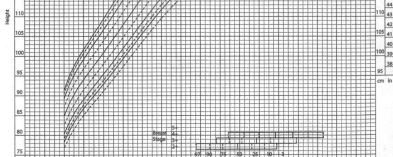

Height

Age (years)

Head Circumference

Measuring Technique: The tape should be placed over the eyebrows, above the ears and over the most prominent part of the occiput taking a direct route. A paper tape is preferable to plastic, which stretches unacceptably under tension. The maximum measurement should be recorded to the nearest 0.1 cm.

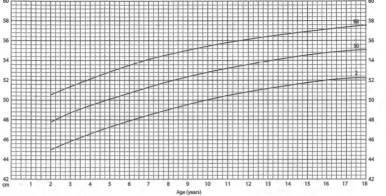

Data Source: 2–5 yr: Jones, D.L. 1973. *NSW Health Communication Publication.* 5–18 yr: Nellhaus, G. 1968. *Pediatrics,* 41:106–114.

Height Velocity

The standards are appropriate for velocity calculated over a whole year period, not less, since a smaller period requires wider limits (the 3rd and 97th centiles for whole year being roughly appropriate for the 10th and 90th centiles over six months). The yearly velocity should be plotted at the mid-point of a year. The centiles given in black are appropriate to children of average maturational tempo, who have their peak velocity at the average age for this event. The red line is the 50th centile line for the child who is two years early in maturity and age at peak height velocity, and the blue line refers to a child who is 50th centile in velocity but two years late. The arrows mark the 3rd and 97th centiles at peak velocity for early and late maturers.

Centiles for
girls maturing
at average time

97 and 3 centiles at peak
height velocity for
Early (+ 2SD) maturers
Late (– 2SD) maturers

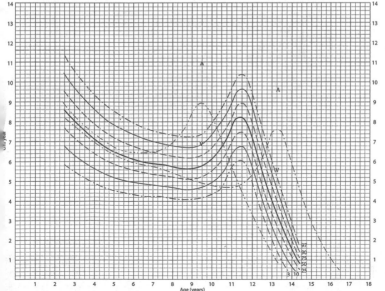

Data Source: Tanner, J. & Davies, P.S. W. 1985. *Journal of Pediatrics,* 107.

Boys 2-18 years

Stages of Puberty

Ages of attainment of successive stages of pubertal sexual development are given in the Height Percentile chart.
The stage Pubic Hair 2+ represents the state of a child who shows the pubic hair appearance stage 2 but not stage 3 (see below).

The centiles for age at which this state is normally seen are given, the 97th centile being considered as the early limit, the 3rd centile as the late limit. The child's puberty stages may be plotted at successive ages (Tanner. 1962, *Growth at Adolescence*, 2nd edn). Testis sizes are judged by comparison with the Prader orchidometer (Zachmann, Prader, Kind, Haflinger & Budliger. 1974, *Helv. Paed. Acta*. 29, 61-72).

Genital (Penis) Development

Stage 1. Pre-adolescent. Testes, scrotum and penis are of about the same size and proportion as in early childhood.

Stage 2. Enlargement of scrotum and testes. Skin of scrotum reddens and changes in texture. Little or no enlargement of penis at this stage.

Stage 3. Enlargement of the penis which occurs at first mainly in length. Further growth of the testes and scrotum.

Stage 4. Increased size of penis with growth in breadth and development of glans. Testes and scrotum larger; scrotal skin darkened.

Stage 5. Genitalia adult in size and shape.

Pubic Hair Development

Stage 1. Pre-adolescent. The vellus over the pubes is not further developed than that over the abdominal wall, i.e. no pubic hair.

Stage 2. Sparse growth of long, slightly pigmented downy hair, straight or slightly curled at the base of the penis.

Stage 3. Considerably darker, coarser and more curled. The hair spreads sparsely over the junction of the pubes.

Stage 4. Hair now adult in type, but area covered is still considerably smaller than in the adult. No spread to the medial surface of thighs.

Stage 5. Adult in quantity and type with distribution of the horizontal (or classically 'feminine') pattern. Spread to medial surface of thighs but not up linea alba or elsewhere above the base of the inverse triangle (spread up linea alba occurs late and is rated stage 6).

Genital and Pubic Hair Development Stages

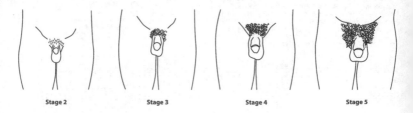

Stage 2   Stage 3   Stage 4   Stage 5

Stretched Penile Length

Measured from the pubo-penile skin junction to the tip of the glans (Shonfeld & Beebe. 1942, *Journal of Urology*, 48, 759-777).

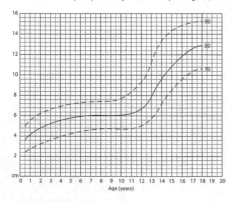

Boys 2-18 years

Endorsed By **A**ustralasian **P**aediatric **E**ndocrine **G**roup

| Surname | | Identification No. | |
| Given Names | | Date of Birth | |

Weight Percentile

Weight should be taken in the nude, or as near thereto as possible. If a surgical gown or minimum underclothing (vest and pants) is worn, then its estimated weight (about 0.1 kg) must be subtracted before weight is recorded. Weights are conventionally recorded to the last completed 0.1 kg above the age of six months. The bladder should be empty.

Body-Mass Index

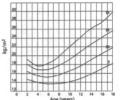

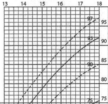

					PUBERTAL STAGES			
DATE	AGE	HEIGHT	WEIGHT	HEAD CIRCUM.	GENITAL	PUBIC HAIR	TESTES L	R

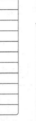

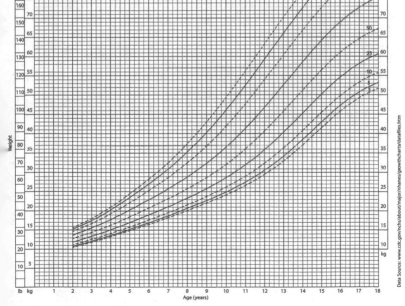

Height Percentile

Mother's Height

Father's Height

Simplified Calculation of Body Surface Area (BSA)

$$BSA\ (m^2) = \sqrt{\frac{Ht\ (cm) \times Wt\ (kg)}{3600}}$$

Reference: Mosteller, R. D. 1987, 'Simplified calculation of body surface area', *N. Engl. J. Med.*, 317: 1098.

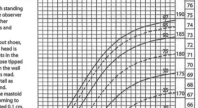

Supine Length (recommended up to the age of 3 so that there is overlap with standing height at 2 to 3) is taken on a flat surface, with the child lying on his back. One observer holds the child's head in contact with a board at the top of the table and another straightens the child's legs and turns the feet upward to be at right angles to the legs and brings a sliding board in contact with the child's heels.

Standing Height (recommended from age 2 onwards) should be taken without shoes, the child standing with his heels and back in contact with an upright wall. His head is held so that he looks straight forward with the lower borders of the eye sockets in the same horizontal plane as the external auditory meati (i.e. head not with the nose tipped upward). A right-angled block (preferably counterweighted) is then slid down the wall until its bottom surface touches the child's head and a scale fixed to the wall is read. During the measurement the child should be told to stretch his neck to be as tall as possible, though care must be taken to prevent his heels coming off the ground. Gentle but firm pressure upward should be applied by the measurer under the mastoid processes to help the child stretch. In this way the variation in height from morning to evening is minimised. Standing height should be recorded to the last completed 0.1 cm.

$C = M[1 + L.S.Z]^{1/L}$

Where C is the centile required, LMS are those parameters published by CDC and Z is the standard deviation equivalent to the centile required.

1st Centile calculated by Associate Professor Peter Davies, Children's Nutrition Research Centre, Brisbane.

Represents 50th centile height attained for an individual boy entering puberty at the average time based on longitudinal data. All other centiles are based on cross-sectional data.

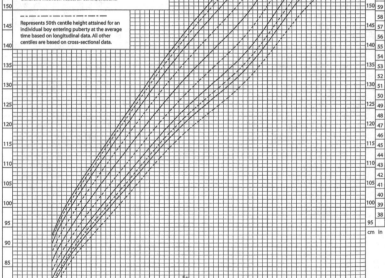

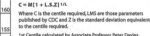

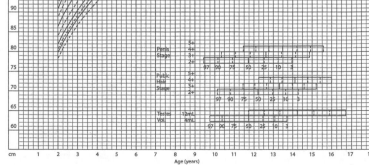

Head Circumference

Measuring Technique: The tape should be placed over the eyebrows, above the ears and over the most prominent part of the occiput taking a direct route. A paper tape is preferable to plastic, which stretches unacceptably under tension. The maximum measurement should be recorded to the nearest 0.1 cm.

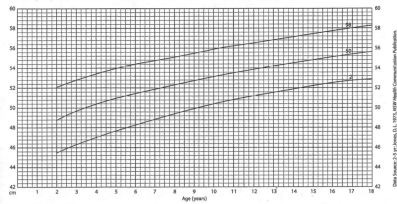

Data Source: 2–5 yr: Jones, D. L. 1973, NSW Health Communication Publication. 5–18 yr: Nellhaus, G. 1968, Pediatrics, 41:106–114.

Height Velocity

The standards are appropriate for velocity calculated over a whole year period, not less, since a smaller period requires wider limits (the 3rd and 97th centiles for a whole year being roughly appropriate for the 10th and 90th centiles over six months). The yearly velocity should be plotted at the mid-point of a year. The centiles given in black are appropriate to children of average maturational tempo, who have their peak velocity at the average age for this event. The red line is the 50th centile line for the child who is two years early in maturity and age at peak height velocity, and the green line refers to a child who is 50th centile in velocity but two years late. The arrows mark the 3rd and 97th centiles at peak velocity for early and late maturers.

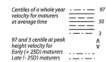

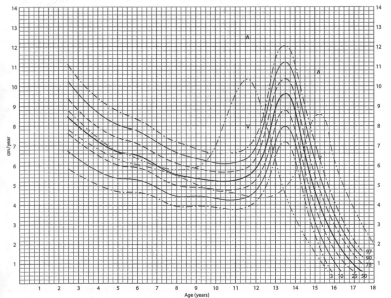

Data Source: Tanner, J. & Davies, P. S. W. 1985, Journal of Pediatrics, 107.

APPENDIX 2
Pharmacopoeia

This pharmacopoeia is reproduced directly from 'Drug doses', 13th edition, published in 2005 by the Royal Children's Hospital, Melbourne, with permission from Frank Shann. Considerable care has been taken to see that the information in this pharmacopoeia is accurate, but the user is advised to check the doses carefully. The authors shall not be responsible for any errors in this publication.

$1/100 = 1\% = 10$ mg/mL, $1/1000 = 1$ mg/mL, $1/10\,000 = 0.1$ mg/mL

Acetazolamide 5–10 mg/kg (adult 100–250 mg) 6–8 H (daily for epilepsy) oral.

Acetylcholine chloride Adult (NOT /kg): 1% instil 0.5–2 mL into anterior chamber of the eye.

Acetylcysteine Paracetamol poisoning (regardless of delay): 150 mg/kg in 5%D i.v. over 1 h; then 10 mg/kg per hour for 20 h (delay <10 h), 32 h (delay 10–16 h), 72 h (delay >16 h) and longer if still encephalopathic; oral 140 mg/kg stat, then 70 mg/kg 4 H for 72 h. Monitor serum K⁺. Give if paracetamol >1000 μmol/L (150 mg/L) at 4 h, >500 μmol/L 8 h, >250 μmol/L 12 h. Lung disease: 10% soltn 0.1 mL/kg (adult 5 mL) 6–12 H nebulised or intratracheal. Meconium ileus equivalent: 5 mL (NOT /kg) of 20% soltn 8 H oral; 60–100 mL of 50 mg/mL for 45 min PR. CF: 4–8 mg/kg 8 H oral. Eye drop 5% + hypromellose 0.35%: 1–2 drops/eye 6–8 H.

Aciclovir Neonate–12 wk: 20 mg/kg i.v. over 1 h daily (<30 wk gest), 18 H (30–32 wk), 12 H (1st wk life), 8 H (2–12 wk) for 2 wk (3 wk and CSF PCR –ve if herp enceph). >12 wk: EBV, herpes enceph, immunodef, varicella: 500 mg/m² (12 wk–12 yr) 10 mg/kg (>12 yr) 8 H i.v. over 1 h. Cutaneous herpes 250 mg/m² (12 wk–12 yr) 5 mg/kg (>12 yr) 8 H i.v. over 1 h. Genital herpes (>12 yr NOT /kg): 200 mg oral ×5/day for 10 days, then 200 mg ×2–3/day for 6 mo if reqd. Zoster (>12 yr NOT /kg): 400 mg (<2 yr) or 800 mg (≥ 2 yr) oral ×5/day for 7 days. Cold sores: 5% cream ×5/day. Eye: 3% oint ×5/day.

Activated charcoal See charcoal, activated.

Adenosine Arrhythmia: 0.1 mg/kg (adult 3 mg) stat by rapid i.v. push, incr by 0.1 mg/kg (adult 3 mg) every 2 min to max. 0.5 mg/kg (adult 18 mg). Pul hypertension: 50 mcg/kg per min (3 mg/mL at 1 mL/kg per hour) into central vein.

Adrenaline Croup: 1% 0.05 mL/kg diluted to 4 mL by inhaltn; or 1/1000 0.5 mL/kg (max. 6 mL) by inhaltn. Cardiac arrest (repeat if reqd): 0.1 mL/kg of 1/10 000 i.v. or intra-cardiac; via ETT 0.1 mL/kg of 1/1000. Anaphylaxis: 0.05–0.1 mL/kg of 1/10 000 i.v., repeat if reqd. I.m. into thigh: 0.01 mg/kg (0.01 mL/kg of 1/1000) up to 0.1 mg/kg, ×3 doses 20 min apart if reqd. I.v. infsn 0.3 mg/kg in 50 mL 5%dex–hep at 0.5–10 mL/h (0.05–1 mcg/kg per min).

Albendazole   Pinworm, threadworm, roundworm, hookworm, whipworm: 20 mg/kg (adult 400 mg) oral once (may repeat after 2 wk). *Strongyloides*, cutaneous larva migrans, *Taenia, H. nana, O. viverrini, C. sinesis:* 20 mg/kg (adult 400 mg) daily for 3 days, repeated in 3 wk. 7.5 mg/kg (adult 400 mg) 12 H for 8–30 days (neurocysticercosis); 12 H for three 28 day courses 14 days apart (hydatid).

Albumin   20%: 2–5 mL/kg i.v. 4%: 10–20 mL/kg. If no loss from plasma: dose (mL/kg) = 5 × (increase g/L)/(% albumin).

Alendronate   Adults (NOT /kg), oral. Osteoporosis 5 mg daily, or 35 mg slow-relse wkly (prevention); 10 mg daily, or 70 mg slow-relse wkly (treatment). Paget's 40 mg daily.

Alginic acid (Gaviscon single strength)   <1 yr: liquid 2 mL with feed 4 H. 1–12 yr: liquid 5–10 mL, or 1 tab after meals. >12 yr: liquid 10–20 mL, or 1–2 tab after meals.

Allopurinol   10 mg/kg (adult 300 mg) 12–24 H oral. Chemotherapy: 50–100 mg/m^2 6 H i.v., oral.

Alpha-tocopheryl acetate   One alpha-tocopheryl (at) equivalent = 1 mg d-at = 1.1 mg d-at acetate = 1.5 mg dl-at acetate = 1.5 u vit E. Abetalipoproteinaemia: 100 mg/kg (max. 4 g) daily oral. Cystic fibrosis: 45–200 mg (NOT /kg) daily oral. Newborn (high dose, toxicity reported): 10–25 mg/kg daily i.m. or i.v., 10–100 mg/kg daily oral.

Alprostadil (prostaglandin E1, PGE1)   To maintain PDA: 60 mcg/kg in 50 mL 0.9% saline 0.5–3 mL/h (10–60 ng/kg per min). Erectile dysfunction (adult NOT /kg): 2.5 mcg intracavernous inj, incr in 2.5 mcg increments if reqrd to max. 60 mcg (max. of 3 doses/wk).

Alteplase (tissue plasminogen activator)   0.1–0.6 mg/kg per hour i.v. for 6–12 h (longer if no response); keep fibrinogen >100 mg/dL (give cryoprecipitate 1 bag/5 kg), give heparin 10 u/kg per hour i.v., give fresh frozen plasma (FFP) 10 mL/kg i.v. daily in infants. Local IA infsn: 0.05 mg/kg per hour, give FFP 10 mL/kg i.v. daily. Blocked central line: 0.5 mg/2 mL (<10 kg) 2 mg/2 mL (>10 kg) per lumen left for 2–4 h, withdraw drug, flush with saline; repeat once in 24 h if reqd.

Aluminium acetate   13% soltn (Burrow's lotion): for wet compresses, or daily to molluscum contagiosum.

Aluminium hydroxide   25 mg/kg (adult 0.5–1 g) 4–6 H oral. Gel (64 mg/mL) 0.1 mL/kg 6 H oral.

Aluminium hydroxide 40 mg/mL, magnesium hydroxide 40 mg/mL, simethicone 4 mg/mL (Mylanta, Gelusil)   0.5–1 mL/kg (adult 10–20 mL) 6–8 H oral. ICU: 0.5 mL/kg 3 H oral if gastric pH <5.

Amethocaine (tetracaine)   Gel 4% in methylcellulose (RCH AnGel): 0.5 g to skin, apply occlusive dressing, wait 30–60 min, remove gel. 0.5%, 1%: 1–2 drops/eye.

Amikacin   Single daily dose i.v. or i.m. Neonate: 15 mg/kg stat, then 7.5 mg/kg (<30 wk) 10 mg/kg (30–35 wk) 15 mg/kg (term <1 wk) daily. 1 wk–10 yr: 25 mg/kg day 1, then 18 mg/kg daily. >10 yr: 20 mg/kg day 1, then 15 mg/kg (max. 1.5 g) daily. Trough level <5.0 mg/L (RCH sent to St.V's).

Amiloride   0.2 mg/kg (adult 5 mg) 12–24 H oral.

Aminocaproic acid   3 g/m^2 (adult 5 g) over 1 h i.v., then 1 g/m^2/h (adult 1–1.25 g/h). Prophylaxis: 70 mg/kg 6 H i.v., oral.

Aminophylline (100 mg aminophylline, 80 mg theophylline) Load: 10 mg/kg (max. 500 mg) i.v. over 1 h. Maintenance: 1st wk life 2.5 mg/kg i.v. over 1 h 12 H; 2nd wk life 3 mg/kg 12 H; 3 wk–12 mo ((0.12 × age in wk) + 3) mg/kg 8 H; <35 kg and >12 mo, 55 mg/kg in 50 mL 5%dex-hep at 1 mL/h (1.1 mg/kg per hour) or 6 mg/kg i.v. over 1 h 6 H; >35 kg and <17 yr, or >17 yr and smoker, 25 mg/mL at 0.028 mL/kg per hour (0.7 mg/kg per hour) or 4 mg/kg i.v. over 1 h 6 H; >17 yr non-smoker 25 mg/mL at 0.02 mL/kg per hour (0.5 mg/kg per hour) or 3 mg/kg i.v. over 1 h 6 H. Level 60–80 μmol/L (neonate), 60–110 (asthma) (×0.18 = mcg/mL).

Amiodarone I.v.: 15 mg/kg in 50 mL 5%dex (no heparin) at 5 mL/h (25 mcg/kg per min) for 4 h, then 1–3 mL/h (5–15 mcg/kg per min, max. 1.2 g/24 h). Oral: 4 mg/kg (adult 200 mg) 8 H 1 wk, 12 H 1 wk, then 12–24 H. After starting tablets, taper i.v. infsn over 5 days. Reduce dose of digoxin and warfarin. Pulseless VF or VT: 5 mg/kg i.v. over 3–5 min.

Amitriptyline hydrochloride Usually 0.5–1 mg/kg (adult 25–50 mg) 8 H oral. Enuresis: 1–1.5 mg/kg nocte.

Amoxycillin (amoxicillin) 10–25 mg/kg (adult 0.25–1 g) 8 H i.v., i.m. or oral; or 20 mg/kg 12 H oral. Severe inftn: 50 mg/kg (adult 2 g) i.v. 12 H (1st wk life), 6 H (2–4 wk), 4–6 H or constant infsn (4+ wk).

Amoxycillin (amoxicillin) and clavulanic acid Dose as for amoxicillin. 4:1 (non-Duo products) given 8 H, 7:1 (Duo) 12 H, 16:1 (XR) 12 H oral.

Amphotericin B (Fungizone) Usually 1.5 mg/kg per day (up to 2 mg/kg per day) by continuous infsn i.v. Central line: 1.5 mg/kg in 50 mL 5%dex-hep at 2 mL/h (≤46 kg); 1.5 mg/kg in 1.2 mL/kg 5%dex-hep (1.25 mg/mL) at 0.05 mL/kg per hour (>46 kg). Peripheral i.v.: usually 1.5 mg/kg in 12 mL/kg 5% dex-hep at 0.5 mL/kg per hour (higher concentrations may cause thrombophlebitis). Oral (NOT /kg): 100 mg 6 H treatment, 50 mg 6 H prophylaxis. Bladder washout: 25 mcg/mL. Cream or ointment 3%: apply 6–12 H.

Amphotericin, lipid complex (Abelcet) 2.5–5 mg/kg daily over 2 h i.v., typically for 2–4 wk.

Amphotericin, liposomal (AmBisome) 3–6 mg/kg (up to 15 mg/kg for severe infection) daily over 1–2 h i.v., typically for 2–4 wk.

Ampicillin 10–25 mg/kg (adult 0.25–1 g) 6 H i.v., i.m. or oral. Severe inftn: 50 mg/kg (max. 2 g) i.v. 12 H (1st wk life), 6 H (2–4 wk), 3–6 H or constant infsn (4+ wk).

Ampicillin 1 g + sulbactam 0.5 g 25–50 mg/kg (adult 1–2 g) of ampicillin 6 H i.m. or i.v. over 30 min.

Amrinone <4 wk old: 4 mg/kg i.v. over 1 h, then 3–5 mcg/kg per min. >4 wk: 1–3 mg/kg i.v. over 1 h, then 5–15 mcg/kg per min.

Anti-D See immunoglobulin, Rh.

Antivenom to Australian box jellyfish, snakes (black, brown, death adder, sea, taipan, tiger), spiders (funnel-web) and ticks Dose depends on amount of venom injected, not size of patient. Higher doses needed for multiple bites, severe symptoms or delayed administration. Give adrenaline 0.005 mg/kg (0.005 mL/kg of 1 in 1000) s.c. Initial dose usually 1–2 amp diluted 1/10 in Hartmann's soltn i.v. over 30 min. Monitor PT, PTT, fibrinogen, platelets; give repeatedly if symptoms or coagulopathy persist.

Antivenom to black widow spider (USA), red back spider (Australia) 1 amp i.m., may repeat in 2 h. Severe envenomation: 2 amp diluted 1/10 in Hartmann's soltn i.v. over 30 min.

Antivenom to Crotalidae (pit vipers, rattlesnakes – USA) 4–6 vials, with higher dose for more severe envenomation, diluted 1/10 in saline i.v. over 1 h, repeated 1 h later if reqd; then 2 vials 6 H for 3 doses.

Aprotinin (1 kiu = 140 ng = 0.00056 epu, 1 mg = 7143 kiu) 1 200 000 kiu/m^2 i.v. over 1 h (plus 1 200 000 kiu/m^2 in prime), then 300 000 kiu/m^2/h; half for 'low dose'. Adult (NOT /kg): 2 000 000 kiu i.v. over 1 h (plus 2 000 000 kiu in prime), then 500 000 kiu/h; half for 'low dose'. Prophylaxis: 4000 kiu/kg, then 2000 kiu/kg 6 H i.v.

Arginine hydrochloride Dose (mg) = BE × wt(kg) × 70; give 1/2 this i.v. over 1 h, then repeat if reqd.

Ascorbic acid Burn (NOT /kg): 200–500 mg daily i.v., i.m., s.c., oral. Metabolic disease (NOT /kg): 250 mg (<7 yr) 500 mg (>7 yr) daily oral. Scurvy (NOT /kg): 100 mg 8 H oral for 10 days. Urine acidification: 10–30 mg/kg 6 H.

Aspirin 10–15 mg/kg (adult 300–600 mg) 4–6 H oral. Antiplatelet: 3–5 mg/kg (max. 100 mg) daily. Kawasaki: 10 mg/kg 6 H (low dose) or 25 mg/kg 6 H (high dose) for 2 wk, then 3–5 mg/kg daily. Arthritis: 25 mg/kg (max. 2 g) 6 H for 3 days, then 15–20 mg/kg 6 H. Salicylate level (arthritis) midway between doses 0.7–2.0 mmol/L (×13.81 = mg/100 mL).

Aspirin 25 mg + dipyridamole 200 mg Adult (NOT /kg) 1 sustained release cap 12 H oral.

Atenolol Oral: 1–2 mg/kg (adult 50–100 mg) 12–24 H. I.v.: 0.05 mg/kg (adult 2.5 mg) every 5 min if reqd (max. 4 doses), then 0.1–0.2 mg/kg (adult 5–10 mg) over 10 min 12–24 H.

Atracurium besylate 0.3–0.6 mg/kg stat, then 0.1–0.2 mg/kg when reqd or 5–10 mcg/kg per min i.v.

Atropine sulfate 0.02 mg/kg (max. 0.6 mg) i.v. or i.m., then 0.01 mg/kg 4–6 H. Organophosphate poisoning: 0.05–1 mg/kg (adult 2 mg) i.v., then 0.02–0.05 mg/kg (adult 2 mg) every 15–60 min until atropinised, then 0.02–0.08 mg/kg per hour may be needed for many days. Colic: see phenobarbitone.

Azathioprine 25–75 mg/m^2 (~1–3 mg/kg) daily oral, i.v.

Azithromycin Oral (only 40% bioavailable): 15 mg/kg (adult 500 mg) on day 1 then 7.5 mg/kg (adult 250 mg) days 2–5, or 15 mg/kg (adult 500 mg) daily for 3 days. Trachoma 20 mg/kg (adult 1 g) wkly ×3; MAC prophylaxis (adult) 1.2 g wkly; Gp A strep 20 mg/kg daily ×3. i.v.: 15 mg/kg (adult 500 mg) day 1, then 5 mg/kg (adult 200 mg) daily.

Aztreonam 30 mg/kg (adult 1 g) 8 H i.v. Severe inftn: 50 mg/kg (adult 2 g) 12 H (1st wk life), 8 H (2–4 wk), 6 H or constant infsn (4+ wk).

Bacillus Calmette–Guérin (BCG) suspension, ~5 × 10^8 cfu/vial Adult: 1 vial (OncoTICE) or 3 vials (ImmuCyst) left in bladder for 2 h each wk for 6 wks, then at 3, 6, 12, 18 and 24 mo.

Bacillus Calmette–Guérin (BCG) vaccine (CSL) Live. Intradermal (1 mg/mL): 0.075 mL (<3 mo) or 0.1 mL (>3 mo) once. Percutaneous (60 mg/mL suspension): 1 drop on skin, inoculated with Heaf apparatus, once.

Bacitracin 400 u/g + neomycin 5 mg/g + polymyxin B 5000 u/g (Neosporin) Ointment or eye ointment: apply ×2–5/day. Powder: apply 6–12 H (skin inftn), every few days (burns). Eye drops: see gramicidin.

Baclofen 0.2 mg/kg (adult 5 mg) 8 H oral, incr every 3 days to 1 mg/kg (adult 25 mg, max. 50 mg) 8 H. Intrathecal infsn: 2–20 mcg/kg (max. 1000 mcg) per 24 h.

Appendices

Beclomethasone dipropionate Rotacap or aerosol (NOT /kg): 100–200 mcg (<8 yr), 150–400 mcg (>8 yr) ×2/day (rarely ×4/day). Nasal (NOT /kg): aerosol or pump (50 mcg/ spray): 1 spray 12 H (<12 yr), 2 spray 12 H (>12 yr).

Benzhexol >3 yr: 0.02 mg/kg (adult 1 mg) 8 H, incr to 0.1–0.3 mg/kg (adult 1.5–5 mg) 8 H oral.

Benzocaine 1%–20% topical: usually applied 4–6 H.

Benztropine >3 yr: 0.02 mg/kg (adult 1 mg) stat i.m. or i.v., may repeat in 15 min. 0.02–0.06 mg/kg (adult 1–3 mg) 12–24 H oral.

Benzyl benzoate 25% lotion. Scabies: apply from neck down after a hot bath, remove in bath after 24 h; repeat after 5 days. Lice: apply to infected region, wash off after 24 h; repeat after 7 days.

Benzylpenicillin See penicillin G.

Beractant (bovine surfactant, Survanta) 25 mg/mL soltn. 4 mL/kg intratracheal 2–4 doses in 48 h, each dose in 4 parts: body inclined down with head to right, body down head left, body up head right, body up head left.

Beta-carotene Porphyria: 1–5 mg/kg (adult 30–300 mg) daily oral.

Betamethasone 0.01–0.2 mg/kg daily oral. Betamethasone has no mineralocorticoid action, 1 mg = 25 mg hydrocortisone in glucocorticoid action. Gel 0.05%; cream, lotion or ointment, 0.02%, 0.05%, 0.1%: apply sparingly 8–24 H.

Betamethasone acetate 3 mg/mL with betamethasone sodium phosphate 3.9 mg/mL (Celestone Chronodose) Adult: 0.25–2 mL (NOT /kg) intramuscular, intra-articular, or intralesional injection.

Bethanecol Oral: 0.2–1 mg/kg (adult 10–50 mg) 6–8 H. S.c.: 0.05–0.1 mg/kg (adult 2.5–5 mg) 6–8 H.

Bicarbonate Slow i.v.: dose (mmol) = BE × wt/4 (<5 kg), BE × wt/6 (child), BE × wt/10 (adult). These doses correct 1/2 the base deficit. Alkalinise urine: 0.25 mmol/kg 6–12 H oral.

Bisacodyl NOT /kg: <12 mo 2.5 mg PR, 1–5 yr 5 mg PR or 5–10 mg oral, >5 yr 10 mg PR or 10–20 mg oral. Enema: 1/2 daily (6 mo–3 yr), 1 enema daily (>3 yr).

Bismuth subsalicylate 5 mg/kg (adult 240 mg) 12 H oral 30 min before meal. *H. pylori* (adult, NOT /kg): 107.7 mg ×4/day with meals and nocte for 2 wk + tetracycline 500 mg ×4/day + metronidazole 200 mg with meals and 400 mg nocte; see also omeprazole.

Blood See packed red blood cells.

Botulinum toxin type A NOT /kg: 1.25–2.5 u/site (max. 5 u/site) i.m., max. total 200 u in 30 days. Oesoph achalasia: 100 u per session divided between 4–6 sites. Hyperhidrosis: 50 u/2 mL intradermal per axilla (given in 10–15 sites).

Botulinum toxin type B NOT /kg: usual total dose 2 500–10 000 u, repeated every 3–4 mo if reqd.

Bretylium tosylate 5–10 mg/kg i.v. over 1 h, then 5–30 mcg/kg per min.

Bromocriptine mesylate 0.025 mg/kg (adult 1.25 mg) 8–12 H, incr wkly to 0.05–0.2 mg/kg (adult 2.5–10 mg) 6–12 H oral. Inhibit lactn, NOT /kg: 2.5 mg 12 H for 2 wk.

Budesonide Metered dose inhaler (NOT /kg): <12 yr 50–200 mcg 6–12 H, reducing to 100–200 mcg 12 H; >12 yr 100–600 mcg 6–12 H, reducing to 100–400 mcg 12 H. Nebuliser (NOT /kg): <12 yr 0.5–1 mg 12 H, reducing to 0.25–0.5 mg 12 H; >12 yr

1–2 mg 12 H, reducing to 0.5–1 mg 12 H. Croup: 2 mg (NOT /kg) by nebuliser. Nasal spray or aerosol (NOT /kg): 64–128 mcg/nostril 12–24 H. Crohn's dis, adult (NOT /kg): 9 mg daily for 8 wk, then reduce over 4 wk.

Bupivacaine Max dose: 2–3 mg/kg (0.4–0.6 mL/kg of 0.5%). With adrenaline: max. dose: 3–4 mg/kg (0.6–0.8 mL/kg of 0.5%). Epidural: 2 mg/kg (0.4 mL/kg 0.5%) stat intraop, then 0.25 mg/kg per hour (0.2 mL/kg per hour 0.125%) postop. Intrapleural: 0.5% 0.5 mL/kg (max. 20 mL) 8–12 H, or 0.5 mL/kg (max. 10 mL) stat then 0.1–0.25 mL/kg per hour (max. 10 mL/h). Epidural in ICU: 25 mL 0.5% + 1000 mcg (20 mL) fentanyl + saline to 100 mL at 2–8 mL/h in adult. See Pain management, chapter 4, page 60.

Caffeine citrate 2 mg citrate = 1 mg base. 1–5 mg/kg (adult 50–250 mg) of citrate 4–8 H oral, PR. Neonate: 20 mg/kg stat of citrate, then 5 mg/kg daily oral or i.v. over 30 min; weekly level 5–30 mg/L midway between doses.

Calamine Lotion: usually applied 6–8 H.

Calcifediol (25-OH D3) Deficiency: 1–2 mcg/kg daily oral.

Calciferol (vitamin D₂) See ergocalciferol.

Calcipotriol 50 mcg/g ointment: apply 12–24 H.

Calcitonin Hypercalcaemia: 4 u/kg 12–24 H i.m. or s.c., may incr up to 8 u/kg 6–12 H. Paget's: 1.5–3 u/kg (max. 160 u) ×3/wk i.m. or s.c.

Calcitriol (1,25-OH vitamin D₃) Renal failure, vit D resistant rickets: 0.02 mcg/kg daily oral, incr by 0.02 mcg/kg every 4–8 wk according to serum calcium.

Calcium (as carbonate, lactate or phosphate) NOT /kg: Neonate: 50 mg ×4–6/day; 1 mo-3 yr: 100 mg ×2–5/day oral; 4–12 yr: 300 mg ×2–3/day; >12 yr: 1000 mg ×1–2/day.

Calcium carbonate Adult NOT /kg: 840 mg 8–12 H oral.

Calcium chloride 10% soltn (0.7 mmol/mL Ca): 0.2 mL/kg (max. 10 mL) slow i.v. stat. Requirement <16 yr 2 mL/kg per day i.v. Inotrope: 0.03–0.12 mL/kg per hour (0.5–2 mmol/kg per day) undiluted via CVC.

Calcium folinate NOT /kg. 5–15 mg oral, or 1 mg i.m. or i.v. daily. Rescue starting up to 24 h after methotrexate: 10–15 mg/m² 6H for 36–48 h i.v. Methotrexate toxicity: 100–1000 mg/m² 6H i.v. Before a fluorouracil dose of 370 mg/m²: 200 mg/m² i.v. daily ×5, repeat every 3–4 wk.

Calcium gluconate 10% soltn (0.22 mmol/mL Ca): 0.5 mL/kg (max. 20 mL) slow i.v. stat. Requirement <16 yr 5 mL/kg per day i.v. Inotrope: 0.5–2 mmol/kg per day (0.1–0.4 mL/kg per hour) undiluted via CVC.

Calcium polystyrene sulfonate (Calcium Resonium) 0.3–0.6 g/kg (adult 15–30 g) 6 H NG (+ lactulose), PR.

Calfactant (Infasurf) 35 mg/mL phospholipids, 0.65 mg/mL proteins: 1.5 mL/kg intratracheal gradually over 20–30 breaths during inspiration with infant lying on one side, then another 1.5 mL/kg with infant lying on other side.

Canrenoate 3–8 mg/kg (adult 150–400 mg) daily i.v.

Captopril Beware hypotension. 0.1 mg/kg (adult 2.5–5 mg) 8 H oral, incr if reqd to max. 2 mg/kg (adult 50 mg) 8 H. Less hypotension if mixed with NG feeds given continuously (or 1–2 hrly).

Carbamazepine 2 mg/kg (adult 100 mg) 8 H oral, may incr over 2–4 wk to 5–10 mg/kg (adult 250–500 mg) 8 H. Bipolar disorder (adult, NOT /kg): 200 mg as slow-release capsule

12 H oral, incr if reqd to max. 800 mg 12 H. Level 20–40 µmol/L (×0.24 = mg/L), done Mo–Fri 1100 RCH.

Carbenicillin   382 mg tab, adult (NOT /kg): 1–2 tab 4 H oral.

Carbenoxolone sodium   Adult (NOT /kg): 20–50 mg 6 H oral. Mouth gel 2%, or 2 g granules in 40 mL water, apply 6 H.

Carbimazole   0.4 mg/kg (adult 20 mg) 8–12 H oral for 2 wk, then 0.1 mg/kg (adult 5–10 mg) 8–24 H.

Carnitine, L form   I.v.: 5–15 mg/kg (max. 1 g) 6 H. Oral: 25 mg/kg 6–12 H (max. 3 g/day).

Carob bean gum (Carobel Instant)   NOT /kg: 1 scoop (1.8 g) in 100 mL water, give 10–20 mL by spoon; or add 1/2 scoop to every 100–200 mL of milk.

Cefaclor   10–15 mg/kg (adult 250–500 mg) 8 H oral. Slow release tab 375 mg (adult, NOT /kg): 1–2 tab 12 H oral.

Cefdinir   14 mg/kg (adult 600 mg) daily (or in two divided doses) oral.

Cefditoren   4–8 mg/kg (adult 200–400 mg) 12 H oral.

Cefepime hydrochloride   25 mg/kg (adult 1 g) 12 H i.m. or i.v. over 5 min. Severe inftn: 50 mg/kg (adult 2 g) i.v. 8–12 H or constant infsn.

Cefixime   5 mg/kg (adult 200 mg) 12–24 H oral.

Cefodizime   25 mg/kg (max. 1 g) 12 H i.v. or i.m.

Cefonicid   15–50 mg/kg (adult 0.5–2 g) i.v. or i.m. daily.

Cefoperazone   25–60 mg/kg (adult 1–3 g) 6–12 H i.v. over 1 h or i.m.

Cefotaxime   25 mg/kg (adult 1 g) 12 H (<4 wk), 8 H (4+wk) i.v. Severe inftn: 50 mg/kg (adult 2–3 g) i.v. 12 H (preterm), 8 H (1st wk life), 6 H (2–4 wk), 4–6 H or constant infsn (4+ wk).

Cefotetan   25 mg/kg (adult 1 g) 12 H i.m., i.v. Severe inftn: 50 mg/kg (max. 2–3 g) 12 H or constant infsn.

Cefoxitin   25–60 mg/kg (adult 1–3 g) 12 H (1st wk life), 8 H (1–4 wk), 6–8 H (>4 wk) i.v.

Cefpirome   25–50 mg/kg (adult 1–2 g) 12 H i.v.

Cefpodoxime   5 mg/kg (adult 100–200 mg) 12 H oral.

Cefprozil   15 mg/kg (adult 500 mg) 12–24 H oral.

Ceftazidime   15–25 mg/kg (adult 0.5–1 g) 8 H i.v. or i.m. Severe inftn, CF: 50 mg/kg (max. 2 g) 12 H (1st wk life), 8 H (2–4 wk), 6 H or constant infsn (4+ wk).

Ceftibuten   10 mg/kg (adult 400 mg) daily oral.

Ceftizoxime   25–60 mg/kg (adult 1–3 g) 6–8 H i.v.

Ceftriaxone sodium   25 mg/kg (adult 1 g) 12–24 H i.v., or i.m. (in 1% lignocaine [lidocaine]). Severe inftn: 50 mg/kg (max. 2 g) daily (1st wk life), 12 H (2+ wk). Epiglottitis: 100 mg/kg (max. 2 g) stat, then 50 mg/kg (max. 2 g) after 24 h. Meningococcus prophylaxis (NOT /kg): child 125 mg, >12 yr 250 mg i.m. in 1% lignocaine [lidocaine] once.

Cefuroxime   Oral (as cefuroxime axetil): 10–15 mg/kg (adult 250–500 mg) 12 H. i.v.: 25 mg/kg (adult 1 g) 8 H. Severe inftn: 50 mg/kg (max. 2 g) i.v. 12 H (1st wk life), 8 H (2nd wk), 6 H or constant infsn (>2 wk).

Celecoxib   Usually 2 mg/kg (adult 100 mg) 12 H, or 4 mg/kg (adult 200 mg) daily oral. See Pain management, chapter 4, page 60.

Cephalexin   7.5 mg/kg (adult 250 mg) 6 H, or 15 mg/kg (adult 500 mg) 12 H oral.

Cephalothin   15–25 mg/kg (adult 0.5–1 g) 6 H i.v. or i.m. Severe inftn: 50 mg/kg (max. 2 g) i.v. 4 H or constant infsn. Irrigation fluid: 2 g/L (2 mg/mL).

Cephamandole 15–25 mg/kg (adult 0.5–1 g) 6–8 H i.v. over 10 min or i.m. Severe inftn: 40 mg/kg (adult 2 g) i.v. over 20 min 4–6 H or constant infsn.

Cephazolin 10–15 mg/kg (adult 0.5 g) 6 H i.v. or i.m. Severe inftn: 50 mg/kg (adult 2 g) i.v. 4–6 H or constant infsn. Surgical proph: 50 mg/kg i.v. at induction.

Cetirizine NOT /kg: 2.5 mg (6 mo-2 yr), 2.5–5 mg (2–5 yr), 5–10 mg (>5 yr) daily oral.

Cetylpyridinium + benzocaine Mouthwash (Cepacaine): apply 3 H prn. Not to be swallowed.

Charcoal, activaked Check bowel sounds present. 1–2 g/kg (adult 50–100 g) NE; then 0.25 g/kg haly if required. Laxative: sorbitol 1 g/kg (1.4 mL/kg of 70% once NG, may repeat xl.

Chloral hydrate Hypnotic: 50 mg/kg (max. 2 g) stat (ICU up to 100 mg/kg, max. 5 g). Sedative: 8 mg/kg 6–8 H oral or PR.

Chloramphenicol Severe inftn: 40 mg/kg (max. 2 g) stat i.v., i.m. or oral; then 25 mg/kg (max. 1 g) daily (1st wk life) 12 H (2–4 wk) 8 H (>4 wk) for 5 days, then 6 H. Eye drops, oint: apply 2–6 H. Ear: 4 drops 6 H. Serum level 20–30 mg/L at 2 h, <15 mg/L trough.

Chloroquine, base Oral: 10 mg/kg (max. 600 mg) daily ×3 days. i.m.: 4 mg/kg (max. 300 mg) 12 H for 3 days. Prophylaxis: 5 mg/kg (adult 300 mg) oral ×1/wk. Lupus, rheu arthritis: 12 mg/kg (max. 600 mg) daily, reduce to 4–8 mg/kg (max. 400 mg) daily oral.

Chlorothiazide 5–20 mg/kg (adult 0.25–1 g) 12–24 H oral, i.v.

Chlorphenamine 0.1 mg/kg (adult 4 mg) 6–8 H oral.

Chlorphenamine 1.25 mg + phenylephrine 2.5 mg in 5 mL Syrup (NOT /kg): 1.25–2.5 mL (0–1 yr), 2.5–5 ml (2–5 yr), 5–10 mL (6–12 yr), 10–15 mL (>12 yr) 6–8 H oral.

Chlorpromazine Oral or PR: 0.5–2 mg/kg (max. 100 mg) 6–8 H; up to 20 mg/kg 8 H for psychosis. I.m. (painful) or slow i.v. (beware hypotension): 0.25–1 mg/kg (usual max. 50 mg) 6–8 H.

Chlorpropamide Adult: initially 125–250 mg (NOT /kg) daily oral, max. 500 mg daily.

Chlortetracycline 3% cream or ointment: apply 8–24 H.

Cholecalciferol (vitamin D₃) 1 mcg = 40 u = 1 mcg ergocalciferol (qv). Osteodystrophy: 0.2 mcg/kg (hepatic) 15–40 mcg/kg (renal) daily oral.

Cholera toxin b subunit recombinant vaccine (Dukoral) Inactivated. 2–6 yr: dissolve granules in 75 mL water, give 3 doses in 6 wk oral, boost after 6 mo. >6 yr: dissolve granules in 150 mL water, give 2 doses in 6 wk, boost after 2 yr.

Cholestyramine NOT /kg: 1 g (<6 yr) 2–4 g (6–12 yr) 4 g (>12 yr) 4–12 H oral with feeds. 16% paste: apply 8–12 H.

Ciclosporin See cyclosporin.

Cimetidine Oral: 5–10 mg/kg (adult 300–400 mg) 6 H, or 20 mg/kg (adult 800 mg) nocte. i.v.: 10–15 mg/kg (adult 200 mg) 12 H (newborn), 6 H (>4 wk).

Ciprofloxacin 5–10 mg/kg (adult 250–500 mg) 12 H oral, 4–7 mg/kg (adult 200–300 mg) 12 H i.v. Severe inftn, or cystic fibrosis: 20 mg/kg (max. 750 mg) 12 H oral, 10 mg/kg (max. 400 mg) 8 H i.v.; higher doses used occasionally. Meningococcus proph: 15 mg/kg (max. 500 mg) once oral. Reduce dose of theophylline.

Ciprofloxacin, eye drops 0.3%. Corneal ulcer: 2 drop /15 min for 6 h then 2 drop/ 30 min for 18 h (day 1), 2 drop 1 H (day 2), 2 drop 4 H (day 3–14). Conjunctivitis: 1–2 drop 4 H; if severe 1–2 drop 2 H when awake for 2 days, then 6 H.

Cisplatin   60–100 mg/m² i.v. over 6 h every 3–4 wk ×6 cycles.

Clarithromycin   7.5–15 mg/kg (adult 250–500 mg) 12 H oral. Slow release tab, adult (NOT /kg): 0.5 g or 1 g daily.

Clindamycin   6 mg/kg (adult 150–450 mg) 6 H oral. I.v. or i.m. >28 days: 10 mg/kg (adult 600 mg) 8 H (i.v. over 30 min). Neonate: 5 mg/kg 12 H (preterm <1 wk old), 5 mg/kg 8 H (preterm >1 wk, term <1 wk), 7.5 mg/kg 8 H (term >1 wk) i.v. over 30 min. Severe inftn (>28 days): 15–20 mg/kg (adult 900 mg) 8 H i.v. over 1 h. Acne soltn 1%: apply 12 H.

Clioquinol   10 mg/g cream, 100% powder: apply 6–12 H.

Clobazam   0.1 mg/kg (adult 10 mg) daily oral, incr if reqd to max. 0.4 mg/kg (adult 20 mg) 8–12 H oral.

Clomiphene (clomifene)   Adult: 50 mg (NOT /kg) daily for 5 days oral, incr to 100 mg daily for 5 days if no ovulation.

Clomipramine   0.5–1 mg/kg (adult 25–50 mg) 12 H oral, incr if reqd to max. 2 mg/kg (adult 100 mg) 8 H.

Clonazepam   1 drop = 0.1 mg. 0.01 mg/kg (max. 0.5 mg) 12 H oral, slowly incr to 0.05 mg/kg (max. 2 mg) 6–12 H oral. Status (may be repeated), NOT /kg: neonate 0.25 mg (if ventilated), child 0.5 mg, adult 1 mg i.v.

Clonidine   Hypertension: 1–5 mcg/kg slow i.v., 1–6 mcg/kg (adult 50–300 mcg) 8–12 H oral. Migraine: start with 0.5 mcg/kg 12 H oral. Analgesia: 2.5 mcg/kg premed oral, 0.3 mcg/kg per hour i.v., 1–2 mcg/kg local block; ventld 0.5–2 mcg/kg per hour (<12 kg 1 mcg/kg per hour is 50 mcg/kg in 50 mL at 1 mL/h, >12 kg 25 mcg/kg in 50 mL at 2 mL/h) + midazolam 1 mcg/kg per min (3 mg/kg in 50 mL at 1 mL/h).

Clotrimazole   Topical: 1% cream or solution 8–12 H. Vaginal (NOT /kg): 1% cream or 100 mg tab daily for 6 days, or 2% cream or 500 mg tab daily for 3 days.

Cloxacillin   15 mg/kg (adult 500 mg) 6 H oral, i.m. or i.v. Severe inftn: 25–50 mg/kg (adult 1–2 g) i.v. 12 H (1st wk life), 8 H (2–4 wk), 4–6 H (>4 wk) or constant infsn (>4 wk).

Coagulation factor, human (Prothrombinex)   Factors 2, 9 and 10; 250 u/10 mL. 1 ml/kg slow i.v. daily. Risk of thrombosis in acute liver failure.

Coal tar, topical   0.5% incr to max. 10%, applied 6–8 H.

Cocaine   Topical: 1–3 mg/kg.

Codeine phosphate   Analgesic: 0.5–1 mg/kg (adult 15–60 mg) 4 H oral, i.m., s.c. Antitussive: 0.25–0.5 mg/kg (adult 15–30 mg) 6 H. See Pain management, chapter 4, page 58.

Co-dergocrine mesylate   Adult: usually 3.0–4.5 mg (NOT /kg) daily before meal oral or sublingual. 300 mcg (NOT /kg) daily i.m., SC or i.v. infsn.

Colchicine   Acute gout: 0.02 mg/kg (adult 1 mg) 2 H oral (max. 3 doses/day). Chronic use (gout, FMF): 0.01–0.04 mg/kg (adult 0.5–2 mg) daily oral.

Colfosceril palmitate (Exosurf Neonatal)   Soltn 13.5 mg/mL. Prophylaxis: 5 mL/kg intratracheal over 5 min immediately after birth, and at 12 h and 24 h if still ventilated. Rescue: 5 mL/kg intratracheal over 5 min, repeat in 12 h if still ventilated.

Colistin sulfomethate sodium (colistimethate sodium)   2.6 mg = 1 mg colistin base = 30000 u. i.m., or i.v. over 5 min: 40000 u/kg (adult 2 million u) 8 H, or 1.25–2.5 mg/kg of colistin base 12 H. Oral or inhaled: 30000–60000 u/kg (adult 1.5–3 million u) 8 H.

Colistin 3 mg/mL + neomycin 3.3 mg/mL   Otic: 4 drops 8 H.

Colonic lavage, macrogol-3350 105 g/L Poisoning, severe constipation: if bowel sounds present, 30 mL/kg per hour (adult 1.5 L/h) oral or NG for 2–4 h (until rectal effluent clear). Before colonoscopy: clear fluids only to noon, 1 whole 5 mg bisacodyl tab per 10 kg (adult 4 tab) at noon, wait for bowel motion (max. 6 h), then macrogol 4 g/kg (adult 210 g) over 2 h oral or NG.

Corticorelin 1–2 mcg/kg (max. 100 mcg) i.v.

Corticotropin releasing factor or hormone (CRF, CRH) See corticorelin.

Cortisone acetate 1–2.5 mg/kg 6–8 H oral. Physiological: 7.5 mg/m^2 8 H. Cortisone acetate 1 mg = hydrocortisone 1.25 mg in mineralo- and glucocorticoid action.

Co-trimoxazole (trimethoprim 1 mg + sulfamethoxazole 5 mg) TMP 1.5–3 mg/kg (adult 80–160 mg) 12 H i.v. over 1 h or oral. Renal proph: TMP 2 mg/kg (max. 80 mg) daily oral. Pneumocystis proph: TMP 5 mg/kg daily on 3 days/wk. Pneumocystis treat: TMP 250 mg/m^2 stat, then 150 mg/m^2 8 H (<11 yr) or 12 H (>10 yr) i.v. over 1 h; in renal failure dose interval (h) = serum creatinine (mmol/l) × 135 (max. 48 h); 1 h post-infsn serum TMP 5–10 mcg/mL, SMX 100–200 mcg/mL. i.v. infsn: TMP max. 1.6 mg/mL in 5% dext.

Coumarin Oral: 1–8 mg/kg (adult 50–400 mg) daily. Cream 100 mg/g: apply 8–12 H.

Cromoglycate See sodium cromoglycate.

Crotamiton 10% cream or lotion: apply ×2–3/day.

Cryoprecipitate Low factor 8: 1 u/kg incr activity 2% (half-life 12 h); usual dose 5 mL/kg or 1 bag/4 kg 12 H i.v. for 1–2 infns (muscle, joint), 3–6 infns (hip, forearm, retroperitoneal, oropharynx), 7–14 infns (intracranial). Low fibrinogen: usual dose 5 mL/kg or 1 bag/4 kg i.v. A bag is usually 20–30 mL: factor 8 ~5 u/mL and 100 u/bag, fibrinogen ~10 mg/mL and 200 mg/bag.

Cyanocobalamin (vitamin B$_{12}$) 20 mcg/kg (adult 1000 mcg) i.m. daily for 7 days then wkly (treatment), monthly (prophylaxis). I.v. dangerous in megaloblastic anaemia.

Cyclopentolate 0.5%, 1%: 1 drop/eye, repeat after 5 min. Pilocarpine 1% speeds recovery.

Cyclophosphamide A typical regimen is 600 mg/m^2 i.v. over 30 min daily for 3 days, then 600 mg/m^2 i.v. wkly or 10 mg/kg twice wkly (if leucocytes >3000/mm^3).

Cyclosporin (ciclosporin) 1–3 mcg/kg per min i.v. for 24–48 h, then 5–8 mg/kg 12 H reducing by 1 mg/kg per dose each month to 3–4 mg/kg per dose oral. Eczema, juvenile arthritis, nephrotic syndrome, psoriasis: 1.5–2.5 mg/kg 12 H. Usual target trough levels by Abbott TDx monoclonal specific assay (× 2.5 = non-specific assay level) on whole blood: 100–250 ng/mL (marrow), 300–400 ng/mL first 3 mo then 100–300 ng/mL (kidney), 200–250 first 3 mo then 100–125 (liver), 100–400 ng/mL (heart, lung).

Cyproheptadine 0.1 mg/kg (adult 4 mg) 8–12 H oral. Migraine 0.1 mg/kg (adult 4 mg), repeated in 30 min if reqd.

Cyproterone acetate 1 mg/kg (adult 50 mg) 12 H oral. Prec puberty: 25–50 mg/m^2 8–12 H oral. Hyperandrogenism: 50–100 mg daily days 5–14, with oestradiol valerate 1 mg daily days 5–25.

Cysteamine bitartrate (mercaptamine) 0.05 mg/m^2 6 H oral, incr over 6 wk to 0.33 mg/m^2/dose (<50 kg) or 0.5 mg/kg per dose (>50 kg) 6 H.

Dalteparin sodium Proph (adult): 2500–5000 u s.c. 1–2 h preop, then daily. Venous thrombosis: 100 u/kg 12 H s.c., or infuse 200 u/kg per day i.v. (anti-Xa 0.5–1 u/mL 4 h post dose). Haemodialysis: 5–10 u/kg stat, then 4–5 u/kg per hour i.v. (acute renal failure, anti-Xa 0.2–0.4 u/mL); 30–40 u/kg stat, then 10–15 u/kg per hour (chronic renal failure, anti-Xa 0.5–1 u/mL).

Danazol   2–4 mg/kg (adult 100–200 mg) 6–12 H oral.

Dantrolene   Hyperpyrexia: 1 mg/kg per min until improves (max. 10 mg/kg), then 1–2 mg/kg 6 H for 1–3 day i.v. or oral. Spasticity: 0.5 mg/kg (adult 25 mg) 6 H, incr over 2 wk if reqd to 3 mg/kg (adult 50–100 mg) 6 H oral.

Dapsone   1–2 mg/kg (adult 50–100 mg) daily oral. Derm herpet: 1–6 mg/kg (adult 50–300 mg) daily oral. See also pyrimethamine.

DDAVP   See desmopressin.

Desferrioxamine   Antidote: 10–15 mg/kg per hour i.v. for 12–24 h (max. 6 g/24 h) if Fe >60–90 µmol/l at 4 h or 8 h; some also give 5–10 g (NOT /kg) once oral. Thalassaemia (NOT /kg): 500 mg per unit blood; and 5–6 nights/wk 1–3 g in 5 mL water s.c. over 10 h, 0.5–1.5 g in 10 mL water s.c. over 5 min.

Desmopressin (DDAVP)   1 u = 1 mcg. Nasal (NOT /kg): 5–10 mcg (0.05–0.1 mL) per dose 12–24 H; enuresis 10–40 mcg nocte. I.v.: 0.5–2 mcg in 1L fluid, and replace urine output + 10% hrly (but much better to use vasopressin). Haemophilia, von Wille: 0.3 mcg/kg (adult 20 mcg) i.v. over 1 h 12–24 H. More potent and longer acting than vasopressin.

Dexamethasone   0.1–0.25 mg/kg 6 H oral, i.m. or i.v. BPD: 0.1 mg/kg 6 H for 3 days, then 8 H 3 days, 12 H 3 days, 24 H 3 days, 48 H 7 days. Cerebral oedema: 0.25–1 mg/kg (adult 10–50 mg) stat, then 0.1–0.2 mg/kg (adult 4–8 mg) 4 H i.v. reducing over 3–5 days to 0.05 mg/kg (adult 2 mg) 8–12 H. Congen adr hypopl: 0.27 mg/m^2 daily oral. Severe croup, extubtn stridor: 0.6 mg/kg (max. 12 mg) i.v. or i.m. stat, then prednisolone 1 mg/kg 8–12 H oral. Eye drops 0.1%: 1–2 drops per eye 3–8 H. Dexamethasone has no mineralocorticoid action; 1 mg = 25 mg hydrocortisone in glucocorticoid action.

Dexamphetamine   0.2 mg/kg (max. 10 mg) daily oral, incr if reqd to max. 0.6 mg/kg (max. 40 mg) 12 H.

Dexchlorpheniramine maleate   0.05 mg/kg (adult 2 mg) 6–8 H oral. Repetab (adult NOT /kg): 6 mg 12 H oral.

Dextropropoxyphene   Hydrochloride 1.3 mg/kg (adult 65 mg) or napsylate 2 mg/kg (adult 100 mg) 6 H oral.

Dextrose   Infant sedation (NOT /kg): 1 mL 50%D oral. Hypoglycaemia: 0.5 mL/kg 50%D or 2.5 mL/kg 10%D slow i.v., then incr maintenance infsn rate. Hyperkalaemia: 0.1 u/kg insulin + 2 mL/kg 50%D i.v. Neonates: 6 g/kg per day (~4 mg/kg per min) day 1, incr to 12 g/kg per day (up to 18 g/kg per day with hypoglycaemia). Infsn rate (mL/h) = (4.17 × wt × g/kg per day)/%D = (6 × wt × mg/kg per min)/%D. Dose (g/kg per day) = (mL/h × %D)/(4.17 × wt). Dose (mg/kg per min) = (mL/h × %D)/(6 × wt). mg/kg per min = g/kg per day/1.44. 0.5 ml/kg per hour of 50% = 6 g/kg per day.

Diazepam   0.1–0.4 mg/kg (adult 10–20 mg) i.v. or PR. 0.04–0.2 mg/kg (adult 2–10 mg) 8–12 H oral. Do not give by i.v. infsn (binds to PVC). Premed: 0.2–0.4 mg/kg oral, PR.

Diazoxide   Hypertension: 1–3 mg/kg (max. 150 mg) stat by rapid i.v. injection (severe hypotension may occur) repeat once if reqd, then 2–5 mg/kg i.v. 6 H. Hyperinsulinism: <12 mo 5 mg/kg 8–12 H oral; >12 mo 30–100 mg/m^2 per dose 8 H oral.

Diclofenac   1 mg/kg (adult 50 mg) 8–12 H oral, PR. Eye drops 0.1%: preop 1–5 drops over 3 h, postop 3 drops stat, then 1 drop 4–8 H. Topical gel: apply 2–4 g 6–8 H. See Pain management, chapter 4, page 59.

Dicloxacillin 15–25 mg/kg (adult 250–500 mg) 6 H oral, i.m. or i.v. Severe inftn: 25–50 mg/kg (max. 2 g) i.v. 12 H (1st wk life), 8 H (2–4 wk), 4–6 H or constant infsn (>4 wk).

Digitoxin 4 mcg/kg (max. 0.2 mg) 12 H oral for 4 days, then 1–6 mcg/kg (adult usually 0.15 mg, max. 0.3 mg) daily.

Digoxin 15 mcg/kg stat and 5 mcg/kg after 6 H, then 3–5 mcg/kg (usual max. 200 mcg i.v., 250 mcg oral) 12 H slow i.v. or oral. Level 6 h or more after dose: 1.0–2.5 nmol/L (×0.78 = ng/mL), done Mo–Sat 1400 at RCH.

Digoxin immune FAB (antibodies) I.v. over 30 min. Dose (to nearest 40 mg) = serum digoxin (nmol/L) × wt (kg) × 0.3, or mg ingested × 55. Give if >0.3 mg/kg ingested, or level >6.4 nmol/L or 5.0 ng/mL.

Dihydrocodeine 0.5–1 mg/kg 4–6 H oral.

Dihydroergotamine mesylate Adult (NOT /kg): 1 mg i.m., s.c. or i.v., repeat hrly ×2 if needed. Max 6 mg/wk.

Diltiazem 1 mg/kg (adult 60 mg) 8 H, incr if reqd to max. 3 mg/kg (adult 180 mg) 8 H oral. Slow release (adult, NOT /kg): 120–240 mg daily, or 90–180 mg 8–12 H oral.

Diphenhydramine hydrochloride 1–2 mg/kg (adult 50–100 mg) 6–8 H oral.

Diphenoxylate 2.5 mg and atropine 25 mcg tab (Lomotil) Adult (NOT /kg): 1–2 tab 6–8 H oral.

Diphtheria + pertussis (acellular) + tetanus + hepatitis B vaccine + polio (Pediarix) Inactivated. 0.5 mL at 2 mo, 4 mo, 6 mo (3 doses), and (DaPT) 18 mo.

Diphtheria + pertussis (acellular) + tetanus + hepatitis B vaccine (Infanrix Hep B) Inactivated. 0.5 mL at 2 mo, 4 mo, 6 mo (3 doses), and (without hep B) 18 mo.

Diphtheria + pertussis (acellular) + tetanus vaccine (Infanrix, Tripacel) Inactivated. 0.5 mL i.m. at 2 mo, 4 mo, 6 mo, 18 mo and 4–5 yr of age (5 doses).

Diphtheria + pertussis (whole cell) + tetanus vaccine (Triple Antigen) Inactivated. 0.5 mL i.m. at 2 mo, 4 mo, 6 mo, 18 mo and 4–5 yr of age (5 doses).

Diphtheria + tetanus vaccine, adult (ADT) Inactivated. 0.5 mL i.m. stat, 6 wk later, and 6 mo later (3 doses). Boost every 10 yr.

Diphtheria + tetanus vaccine, child <8 yr (CDT) Inactivated. 0.5 mL i.m. stat, 6 wk later, 6 mo later (3 doses). Boost with ADT.

Diphtheria vaccine, adult (CSL) Inactivated. 0.5 mL i.m. stat, 6 wk later, and 6 mo later (3 doses). Boost every 10 yr.

Diphtheria vaccine, child <8 yr (CSL) Inactivated. 0.5 mL i.m. stat, 6 wk later, and 6 mo later (3 doses). Boost with adult vaccine.

Dipyridamole 1–2 mg/kg (adult 50–100 mg) 6–8 H oral. See also aspirin + dipyridamole.

Disopyramide Oral: 1.5–4 mg/kg (adult 75–200 mg) 6 H. i.v.: 2 mg/kg (max. 150 mg) over 5 min, then 0.4 mg/kg per hour (max. 800 mg/day). Level 9–15 μmol/L (×0.3395 = mcg/mL).

Disulfiram Adult (NOT /kg): 500 mg oral daily for 1–2 wk, then 125–500 mg daily.

Dobutamine <30 kg: 15 mg/kg in 50 mL 0.9% saline with heparin 1 u/mL at 1–4 mL/h (5–20 mcg/kg per min) via CVC or periph i.v.; >30 kg: 6 mg/kg made up to 100 mL with 0.9% saline with heparin 1 u/mL at 5–20 mL/h (5–20 mcg/kg per hour).

Docusate sodium NOT /kg: 100 mg (3–10 yr), 120–240 mg (>10 yr) daily oral. Enema (5 mL 18% + 155 mL water): 30 mL (newborn), 60 mL (1–12 mo), 60–120 mL (>12 mo) PR.

Docusate sodium 100 mg + bisacodyl 10 mg <2 yr 1/2 suppos, 1–11 yr 1/2–1 suppos, >11 yr 1 suppos daily.

Docusate sodium 50 mg + sennoside 8 mg, tab >12 yr: 1–4 tab at night oral.

Domperidone Oral: 0.2–0.4 mg/kg (adult 10–20 mg) 4–8 H. Rectal suppos: adult (NOT /kg) 30–60 mg 4–8 H.

Dopamine <30 kg: 15 mg/kg in 50 mL 5%dex-hep at 1–4 mL/h (5–20 mcg/kg per min) via CVC; >30 kg: 6 mg/kg made up to 100 mL in 5%dex-hep at 5–20 mL/h (5–20 mcg/kg per hour).

Dopexamine I.v. infsn 0.5–6 mcg/kg per min.

Dornase alpha (deoxyribonuclease I) NOT /kg: usually 2.5 mg (max. 10 mg) inhaled daily (5–21 yr), 12–24 H (>21 yr).

Dothiepin (dosulepin) 0.5–1 mg/kg (adult 25–50 mg) 8–12 H oral.

Doxapram 5 mg/kg i.v. over 1 h, then 0.5–1 mg/kg per hour for 1 h (max. total dose 400 mg).

Doxercalciferol (1,25-OH D$_2$ analogue) Initially 0.2 mcg/kg (adult 10 mcg) oral, or 0.08 mcg/kg (adult 4 mcg) IV, ×3/wk at end of dialysis. Aim for blood iPTH 150–300 pg/mL.

Doxycycline >8 yr: 2 mg/kg (adult 100 mg) 12 H for 2 doses, then daily oral. Severe: 2 mg/kg 12 H. Malaria proph: 2 mg/kg (adult 100 mg) daily oral.

D-penicillamine See penicillamine

Droperidol Antiemetic: postop 0.02–0.05 mg/kg (adult 1.25 mg) 4–6 H i.m. or slow i.v., chemother 0.02–0.1 (adult 1–5 mg) 1–6 H. Psychiatry, neuroleptanalgesia, i.m. or slow i.v.: 0.1 mg/kg (adult 2.5 mg) stat, incr if reqd to max. 0.3 mg/kg (adult 15 mg) 4–6 H. Psychiatry, oral: 0.1–0.4 mg/kg (adult 5–20 mg) 4–8 H.

Econazole nitrate Topical: 1% cream, powder or lotion 8–12 H. Vaginal: 75 mg cream or 150 mg ovule twice daily.

Eformoterol (formoterol) Caps 12 mg (NOT /kg): 1 cap (5–12 yr) or 1–2 caps (adult) inhaled 12 H.

Enalapril 0.1 mg/kg (adult 2.5 mg) daily oral, incr over 2 wk if reqd to max. 0.5 mg/kg (adult 5–20 mg) 12 H.

Enoximone I.v.: 5–20 mcg/kg per min. Oral: 1–3 mg/kg (adult 50–150 mg) 8 H.

Ephedrine 0.25–1 mg/kg (adult 12.5–60 mg) 4–8 H oral, i.m., s.c. or i.v. Nasal (0.25%–1%): 1 drop each nostril 6–8 H, max. 4 days.

Epoetin alpha, beta 20–50 u/kg ×3/wk, incr to max. 240 u/kg ×1–3/wk s.c., i.v. When Hb >10 g%: 20–100 u/kg ×2–3/wk.

Epoprostenol (prostacyclin, PGI$_2$) Incompatible with all other drugs. <8 kg: 60 mcg/kg in 50 mL diluent at 0.25–0.75 mL/h (5–15 ng/kg per min) via CVC or periph i.v.; >8 kg: 500 mcg in 50 mL diluent at 0.03–0.09 mL/kg per hour (5–15 ng/kg per min). Chronic pul ht: 2 ng/kg per min i.v., incr to 20–40 ng/kg per min.

Ergocalciferol (vitamin D$_2$) 40 u = 1 mcg = 1 mcg cholecalciferol (D$_3$). Cystic fib, cholestasis: 10–20 mcg daily oral. Cirrhosis: adult 40–120 mcg daily oral. Deficiency: 50–100 mcg daily for 2 wk oral, then 10–625 mcg daily (more if severe malabs); or 2.5–5 mg (100 000–200 000 u) every 6–8 wk. Monitor serum calcium; measure alk phos and parathyroid hormone after 6–8 wk. See also doxercalciferol.

Ergometrine maleate   Adult (NOT /kg): 250–500 mcg i.m. or i.v.; 500 mcg 8 H oral, sublingual or PR.

Ergonovine maleate   See ergometrine maleate.

Ergotamine tartrate   >10 yr (NOT /kg): 2 mg sublingual stat, then 1 mg/h (max. 6 mg/episode, 10 mg/wk). Suppos (1–2 mg): 1 stat, may repeat once after 1 h.

Erythromycin   Oral or slow i.v. (max. 5 mg/kg per hour): usually 10 mg/kg (adult 250–500 mg) 6 H; severe inftn 15–25 mg/kg (adult 0.75–1 g) 6 H. Gut prokinetic: 2 mg/kg 8 H. 2% gel: apply 12 H.

Esmolol   0.5 mg/kg (500 mcg/kg) i.v. over 1 min, repeated if reqd. Infsn (undiluted 10 mg/mL soltn): 0.15–1.8 mL/kg per hour (25–300 mcg/kg per min); rarely given for >48 h.

Estradiol   See oestradiol.

Etanercept   0.4 mg/kg (max. 25 mg) twice wkly deep s.c.

Ethacrynic acid   I.v.: 0.5–1 mg/kg (adult 25–50 mg) 12–24 H. Oral: 1–4 mg/kg (adult 50–200 mg) 12–24 H.

Ethambutol hydrochloride   25 mg/kg once daily for 8 wk, then 15 mg/kg daily oral. Intermittent: 35 mg/kg ×3/wk. I.v.: 80% oral dose.

Ethamsylate   12.5 mg/kg (max. 500 mg) 6 H oral, i.m., i.v.

Ethanol, dehydrated (100%)   Vessel sclerosis: inject max. of 1 mL/kg.

Ethanolamine oleate   5% soltn, adult (NOT /kg): 1.5–5 mL per varix (max. 20 mL per treatment).

Ethionamide   TB: 15–20 mg/kg (max. 1 g) at night oral. Leprosy: 5–8 mg/kg (max. 375 mg) daily.

Ethosuximide   10 mg/kg (adult 500 mg) daily oral, incr by 50% each wk to max. 40 mg/kg (adult 2 g) daily. Trough level 0.3–0.7 mmol/L.

Etidocaine   0.5%–1.5% soltn: max. 6 mg/kg (0.6 mL/kg of 1%) parenteral, or 8 mg/kg (0.8 mL/kg of 1%) with adrenaline.

Etidronate   5–20 mg/kg daily oral (no food for 2 h before and after dose) for max. 6 mo. I.v.: 7.5 mg/kg daily for 3–7 days.

Etomidate   0.3 mg/kg slow i.v.

Factor 8 concentrate (vial 200–250 u), recombinant antihaemophilic factor (rAHF)   Joint 20 u/kg, psoas 30 u/kg, cerebral 50 u/kg. 2 × dose(u/kg) = % normal activity, e.g. 35 u/kg gives peak level of 70% normal.

Factor 8 inhibitor bypassing fraction   I.v. max. 2 u/kg per min: joint 50 u/kg 12 H, mucous mem 50 u/kg 6 H, soft tissue 100 u/kg 12 H, cerebral 100 u/kg 6–12 H.

Famciclovir   Zoster, varicella: 5 mg/kg (adult 250 mg) 8 H oral for 7 days; immunocompromised 10 mg/kg (adult 500 mg) 8 H for 10 days. Genital herpes (adult, NOT /kg): 125 mg 12 H oral for 5 days (treat), 250 mg (suppress) 12 H; immunocompromised 500 mg 12 H for 7 days (treat), 500 mg daily (suppress).

Famotidine   0.5–1 mg/kg (adult 20–40 mg) 12–24 H oral. 0.5 mg/kg (max. 20 mg) 12 H slow i.v.

Fat emulsion 20%   See lipid.

Felodipine   0.1 mg/kg (adult 2.5 mg) daily, incr if reqd to 0.5 mg/kg (adult 10 mg) daily oral.

Fenoterol   Oral: 0.1 mg/kg 6 H. Resp soltn 1 mg/mL: 0.5 mL diluted to 2 mL 3–6 H (mild), 1 mL diluted to 2 mL 1–2 H (moderate), undiluted continuous (severe, in ICU). Aerosol (200 mcg/puff): 1–2 puffs 4–8 H.

Fentanyl   Not ventltd: 1–2 mcg/kg (adult 50–100 mcg) i.m. or i.v.; infsn 2–4 mcg/kg per hour (<10 kg 100 mcg/kg in 50 mL 5%dex-hep at 1–2 mL/h; >10 kg amp 50 mcg/mL at 0.04–0.08 mL/kg per hour). Ventltd: 5–10 mcg/kg stat or 50 mcg/kg i.v. over 1 h; infuse amp 50 mcg/mL at 0.1–0.2 mL/kg per hour (5–10 mcg/kg per hour). Patch (lasts 72 h) in adult (NOT /kg): 25 mcg/h, incr if reqd by 25 mcg/h every 3 days. Epidural: 0.5 mcg/kg stat, or 0.4 mcg/kg per hour.

Ferrous salts   Prophylaxis 2 mg/kg per day elemental iron oral, treatment 6 mg/kg per day elemental iron oral. Fumarate 1 mg = 0.33 mg iron. Gluconate 1 mg = 0.12 mg iron; so Fergon (60 mg/mL gluconate) prophylaxis 0.3 mL/kg daily, treatment 1 mL/kg daily oral. Sulfate (dried) 1 mg = 0.3 mg iron; so Ferro-Gradumet (350 mg dried sulfate) prophylaxis 7 mg/kg (adult 350 mg) daily, treatment 20 mg/kg (adult 1050 mg) daily oral.

Filgrastim (granulocyte CSF)   Idiopathic or cyclic neutropenia: 5 mcg/kg daily s.c. or i.v. over 30 min. Congenital neutropenia: 12 mcg/kg daily s.c. or i.v. over 1 h. Marrow transplant: 20–30 mcg/kg daily i.v. over 4–24 h, reducing if neutrophils >1 × 10^9/L.

Flecainide   2–3 mg/kg (max. 100 mg) 12 H oral, may incr over 2 wk to 7 mg/kg (max. 200 mg) 8–12 H. I.v. over 30 min: 0.5–2 mg/kg (max. 150 mg) 12 H.

Flucloxacillin   Oral: 12.5–25 mg/kg (adult 250–500 mg) 6 H. i.m. or i.v.: 25 mg/kg (adult 1 g) 6 H. Severe inftn: 50 mg/kg (adult 2 g) i.v. 12 H (1st wk life), 8 H (2–4 wk), 6 H or constant infsn (>4 wk).

Fluconazole   6 mg/kg (adult 200 mg) stat, then 3 mg/kg (adult 100 mg) daily oral or i.v. Severe inftn: 12 mg/kg (adult 400 mg) stat, then 6–12 mg/kg (adult 200–400 mg) daily i.v.; if haemofiltered 12 mg/kg (adult 600 mg) 12 H.

Flucytosine (5-fluorocytosine)   400–1200 mg/m^2 (max. 2 g) 6 H i.v. over 30 min, or oral. Peak level 50–100 mcg/mL, trough 25–50 mcg/mL (×7.75 = umol/L).

Fludrocortisone acetate   150 mcg/m^2 daily oral. Fludrocortisone 1 mg = hydrocortisone 125 mg in mineralocorticoid activity, 10 mg in glucocorticoid.

Flumazenil   5 mcg/kg every 60 s to max. total 40 mcg/kg (adult 2 mg), then 2–10 mcg/kg per hour i.v.

Flunitrazepam   Adult (NOT /kg): 0.5–2 mg at night, oral.

Fluoxetine   0.5 mg/kg (max. 20 mg) daily, incr to max. 1 mg/kg (max. 40 mg) 12 H oral. Weekly 90 mg cap: 1 per wk.

Fluticasone   Inhaled (NOT /kg): 50–100 mcg (child), 100–500 mcg (adult) 12 H. 0.05% soltn: 1–4 sprays /nostril daily. 0.05% cream: apply sparingly daily.

Fluticasone + salmeterol   Accuhaler (NOT /kg): 100/50 (child), 250/50 or 500/50 (adult) ×1–2 inhltn 12 H. MDI (NOT /kg): 50/25 (child), 125/25 or 250/25 ×1–2 inhltn 12 H.

Fluvastatin   0.4 mg/kg (adult 20 mg) nocte oral, incr to 0.8 mg/kg (adult 40 mg) 12 H if reqd. Slow relse: 80 mg nocte.

Fluvoxamine   2 mg/kg (adult 100 mg) 8–24 H oral.

Folic acid   NOT /kg. Deficiency: 50 mcg (neonate), 0.1–0.25 mg (<4 yr), 0.5–1 mg (>4 yr) daily i.v., i.m., s.c. or oral. Metabolic disease: 5 mg/day oral. Pregnancy: 0.5 mg (high risk 4 mg) daily oral.

Folinic acid   See calcium folinate.

Follicle stimulating hormone (FSH)   Adult (NOT /kg), monitor urinary oestrogen. Anovulation: usually 50–150 iu s.c. daily for 9–12 days. Superovulation (2 wk after starting GnRH agonist): 100–225 iu/kg daily starting day 3 of cycle.

Formoterol   See eformoterol.

Foscarnet   20 mg/kg i.v. over 30 min, then 200 mg/kg per day by constant i.v. infsn (less if creatinine >0.11 mmol/l) or 60 mg/kg 8 H i.v. over 2 h. Chronic use: 90–120 mg/kg i.v. over 2 h daily.

Framycetin sulfate (Soframycin)   Subconjunctival: 500 mg in 1 mL water daily ×3 days. Bladder: 500 mg in 50 mL saline 8 H ×10 days. Eye/ear 0.5%: 2–3 drops 8 H, ointment 8 H.

Framycetin sulfate 15 mg/g + gramicidin 0.05 mg/g   Cream or ointment (Soframycin topical): apply 8–12 H.

Framycetin sulfate 5 mg + gramicidin 0.05 mg dexamethasone 0.5 mg/mL (Sofradex)   Eye/ear: 2–3 drops 6–8 H, ointment 8–12 H.

Fresh frozen plasma   Contains all clotting factors. 10–20 mL/kg i.v. 1 bag is ~230 mL.

Frusemide (furosemide)   Usually 0.5–1 mg/kg (adult 20–40 mg) 6–24 H (daily if preterm) oral, i.m., or i.v. over 20 min (max. 0.05 mg/kg per min i.v.). I.v. infsn: 0.1–1 mg/kg per hour (<20 kg 25 mg/kg in 50 mL 0.9% saline with heparin 1 u/mL at 0.2–2 mL/h; >20 kg amp 10 mg/mL at 0.01–0.1 mL/kg per hour); protect from light.

Fusidic acid   Fusidic acid (susp) absorption only 70% that of sodium fusidate (tabs). Suspension: 15–20 mg/kg (adult 750 mg) 8 H oral. For tablets and i.v., see sodium fusidate.

Gabapentin   Anticonvulsant: 10 mg/kg (adult 300 mg) once day 1 oral, 12 H day 2, 8 H day 3 then adjusted to 10–20 mg/kg (adult 300–1200 mg) 8 H. Premed: 25 mg/kg (adult 1200 mg) 1 h preop. Analgesia: 2 mg/kg (adult 100 mg) 8 H, incr if reqd to 15 mg/kg (adult 800 mg) or higher if tolerated.

Ganciclovir   5 mg/kg 12 H i.v. over 1 h for 2–3 wk; then 5 mg/kg i.v. daily, or 6 mg/kg i.v. on 6 days every wk, or 20 mg/kg (adult 1 g) 8 H oral. Congenital CMV: 7.5 mg/kg 12 H i.v. over 2 h.

Gentamicin   I.v. or i.m. 1 wk–10 yr: 8 mg/kg day 1, then 6 mg/kg daily. >10 yr: 7 mg/kg day 1, then 5 mg/kg (max. 240–360 mg) daily. Neonate, 5 mg/kg dose: <1200 g 48 H (0–7 days of life), 36 H (8–30 days), 24 H (>30 days); 1200–2500 g 36 H (0–7 days of life), 24 H (>7 days); term 24 H (0–7 days of life), then as for 1 wk–10 yr. Trough level <1.0 mg/L.

Glibenclamide   Adult (NOT /kg): initially 2.5 mg daily oral, max. 20 mg daily.

Glucagon   1 u = 1 mg. 0.04 mg/kg (adult 1–2 mg) i.v. or i.m. stat, then 10–50 mcg/kg per hour (0.5 mg/kg in 50 mL at 1–5 mL/h) i.v. Beta-blocker overdose: 0.1 mg/kg i.v. stat, then 0.3–2 mcg/kg per min.

Glucose   See dextrose.

Glucose electrolyte solution   Not dehydrated: 1 heaped teaspoon sucrose in a large cup of water (4% sucrose = 2% glucose); do NOT add salt. Dehydrated: 1 sachet of Gastrolyte in 200 mL water; give frequent small sips, or infuse through a nasogastric tube.

Glutamic acid   10–20 mg/kg (adult 0.5–1 g) oral with meals.

Glyceryl trinitrate   Adult (NOT /kg): sublingual tab 0.3–0.9 mg/dose (lasts 30–60 min); sublingual aerosol 0.4–0.8 mg/dose; slow-release buccal tab 1–10 mg 8–12 H; transdermal 0.5–5 cm of 2% ointment, or 5–15 mg patch 8–12 H. I.v. infsn 0.5–5 mcg/kg per min (<30 kg 3 mg/kg in 50 mL 5%dex-hep at 0.5–5 mL/h; >30 kg 3 mg/kg made up to 100 mL in 5%dex-hep at 1–10 mL/h). Use special non-PVC tubing.

Glycopyrrolate To reduce secretions or treat bradycardia: 5–10 mcg/kg (adult 0.2–0.4 mg) 6–8 H i.v. or i.m. with 0.05 mg/kg neostigmine: 10–15 mcg/kg i.v. Anticholinergic: 0.02–0.04 mg/kg (max 2 mg) 8 H oral.

Glycopyrronium bromide Dose as for glycopyrrolate.

Gramicidin 25 mcg/mL + neomycin 2.5 mg/mL + polymyxin B 5000 u/mL (Neosporin) Eye drops: 1–2 drops/eye every 15–30 min, reducing to 6–12 H.

Granulocyte CSF See filgastrim.

Griseofulvin (Grisovin, Fulcin) 10–20 mg/kg (adult 0.5–1 g) daily oral.

Griseofulvin, ultramicrosize (Griseostatin) 5.5–7 mg/kg (adult 330–660 mg) daily oral.

Haemophilus influenzae type b + hepatitis B vaccine (Comvax) Inactivated. 0.5 mL i.m. 2 mo, 4 mo, 12–15 mo (3 doses).

Haemophilus influenzae type b vaccine Inactivated. <12 mo: give diphtheria protein conjugate (HibTITER, ProHIBiT), or tetanus conjugate (Act-HIB, Hiberix) 0.5 mL i.m. at 2 mo, 4 mo, 6 mo and 15 mo; or meningococcal conjugate (Pedvax HIB) 0.5 mL i.m. at 2 mo, 4 mo and 15 mo. If 1st dose >18 mo: give 1 dose of HibTITER or Pedvax HIB.

Haloperidol 0.01 mg/kg (max. 0.5 mg) daily, incr up to 0.1 mg/kg 12 H i.v. or oral; up to 2 mg/kg (max. 100 mg) 12 H used rarely. Acutely disturbed: 0.1–0.2 mg/kg (adult 5–10 mg) i.m. Long-acting decanoate ester: 1–6 mg/kg i.m. every 4 wk.

Heparin 1 mg = 100 u. Low dose: 75 u/kg i.v. stat, then 500 u/kg in 50 mL 0.9% saline at 1–1.5 mL/h (10–15 u/kg per hour) i.v. Full dose: 75 u/kg (adult 5000 u) i.v. stat, then 500 u/kg in 50 mL 0.9% saline at 2–4 mL/h (20–40 u/kg per hour) <12 mo, 2–3 mL/h (20–30 u/kg per hour) child, 1.5–2 mL/h (15–20 u/kg per hour) adult; adjust to give APTT 60–85 sec, or anti-Xa 0.3–0.7 u/mL. Heparin lock: 100 u/mL.

Heparin calcium Low dose: 75 u/kg s.c. 12 H.

Hepatitis A + hepatitis B vaccine (Twinrix) Inactivated. 1–15 yr 0.5 mL, >15 yr 1 mL i.m. stat, after 1 mo, and after 6 mo (3 doses). Boost every 5 yr.

Hepatitis A vaccine (Havrix) Inactivated. 0.5 mL (child) or 1 mL (adult) i.m. stat, and after 6–12 mo (2 doses). Boost every 5 yr.

Hepatitis A vaccine (VAQTA) Inactivated. 0.5 mL (child) or 1 mL (>17 yr) i.m. stat, and after 6–18 mo (2 doses).

Hepatitis B vaccine (Engerix-B, HB Vax II) Inactivated. Engerix-B 10 mcg/dose (<10 yr), 20 mcg (>9 yr); HB Vax II 2.5 mcg/dose (<10 yr), 5 mcg (10–19 yr), 10 mcg (>19 yr), 40 mcg (dialysis) i.m. stat, after 1 mo, and after 6 mo (3 doses). Boost every 5 yr approx. See also diphtheria and *Haemophilus* vaccines.

Homatropine 2%, 5% soltn: 1–2 drop/eye 4 H.

Hydralazine 0.1–0.2 mg/kg (adult 5–10 mg) stat i.v. or i.m., then 4–6 mcg/kg per min (adult 200–300 mcg/min) i.v. Oral: 0.4 mg/kg (adult 20 mg) 12 H, slow incr to 1.5 mg/kg (usual max. 50 mg) 6–8 H.

Hydrochloric acid Use soltn of 100 mmol/L (0.1 M = 0.1 N = 100 mEq/L); give i.v. by central line only. Alkalosis: dose (mL) = BE × wt × 3 (give 1/2 this); maximum rate 2 mL/kg per hour. Blocked central line: 1.5 mL/lumen over 2–4 h.

Hydrochlorothiazide   1–1.5 mg/kg (adult 25–50 mg) 12–24 H oral.

Hydrochlorothiazide + quinapril 10/12.5, 20/12.5   Adult (NOT /kg): 10/12.5 tab daily oral, incr if reqd to 20/12.5 tab, max. two 10/12.5 tab daily.

Hydrocortisone   Usually 0.5–2 mg/kg (adult 25–50 mg) 6–8 H oral, reducing as tolerated. 0.5%, 1% cream, ointment: apply 6–12 H. 1% cream + clioquinol: apply 8–24 H. 10% rectal foam: 125 mg/dose.

Hydrocortisone sodium succinate   2–4 mg/kg 3–6 H i.m., i.v. reducing as tolerated. Physiological: 5 mg/m^2 6–8 H oral; 0.2 mg/kg 8 H i.m., i.v. Physiological, stress: 1 mg/kg 6 H i.m., i.v.

Hydrogen peroxide   10 volume (3%). Mouthwash 1 : 2 parts water. Skin or ear disinfectant 1 : 1 part water.

Hydroxocobalamin (vitamin B$_{12}$)   20 mcg/kg (adult 1000 mcg) i.m. daily for 7 days then wkly (treatment), then every 2–3 mo (prophyl); i.v. dangerous in megaloblastic anaemia. Homocystinuria, methylmalonic acidur: 1 mg daily i.m.; after response, some patients maintained on 1–10 mg daily oral.

Hydroxychloroquine sulfate   Doses as sulfate. Malaria: 10 mg/kg (max. 600 mg) daily for 3 days; prophylaxis 5 mg/kg (max. 300 mg) once a wk oral. Arthritis, SLE: 3–6.5 mg/kg (adult 200–600 mg) daily oral.

Hydroxyzine   0.5–2 mg/kg (adult 25–100 mg) 6–8 H oral. 0.5–1 mg/kg (adult 25–100 mg) 4–6 H if reqd i.m.

Hyoscine butylbromide   0.5 mg/kg (adult 20–40 mg) 6–8 H i.v., i.m. or oral.

Hyoscine hydrobromide (scopolamine hydrobromide)   6–8 mcg/kg (adult 400–600 mcg) 6–8 H i.v., i.m., s.c. Motion sickness 300 mcg tab (NOT /kg): 0.25 tab (2–7 yr), 0.5 tab (7–12 yr), 1–2 tab (>12 yr) 6–24 H oral 30 min before, may repeat in 4 h. Transdermal (1.5 mg patch): >10 yr 1 every 72 h.

Hyoscine methobromide (methscopolamine)   0.2 mg/kg (adult 2.5–5 mg) 6 H oral.

Hyoscyamine (L-atropine)   2–5 mcg/kg (adult 100–300 mcg) 4–6 H oral, sublingual, i.m. or i.v.

Ibuprofen   5–10 mg/kg (adult 200–400 mg) 4–8 H oral. Arthritis: 10 mg/kg (adult 400–800 mg) 6–8 H. Cystic fibrosis: 20–30 mg/kg 12 H. PDA: 10 mg/kg stat, then 5 mg/kg after 24 h and 48 h i.v. over 15 min. See Pain management, chapter 4, page 59.

Imipenem-cilastatin   15 mg/kg (adult 500 mg) 6 H i.v. over 30 min. Severe inftn: 25 mg/kg i.v. over 1 h (adult 1 g) 12 H (1st wk life), 8 H (2–4 wk), 6–8 H or constant infsn (4+ wk).

Imipramine   0.5–1.5 mg/kg (adult 25–75 mg) 8 H oral. Enuresis: 5–6 yr 25 mg, 7–10 yr 50 mg, >10 yr 50–75 mg nocte.

Immunoglobulin, antilymphocyte (thymocyte)   Horse (Atgam): 10–15 mg/kg daily for 3–5 days i.v. over 4 h; occasionally up to 30 mg/kg daily. Rabbit (ATG-Fresenius): 2.5–5 mg/kg daily over 4–6 h i.v.

Immunoglobulin, CMV   100–200 mg/kg i.v. over 2 h. Transplant: daily for first 3 days, wkly ×6, monthly ×6.

Immunoglobulin, diphtheria   250 u i.m. once.

Immunoglobulin, hepatitis B   400 u i.m. within 5 days of needle stick, repeat in 30 days; 100 u i.m. within 24 h birth to baby of Hep B carrier.

Immunoglobulin, normal, human   Hypogammaglobulinaemia: 10–15 mL/kg of 6% soltn (600–900 mg/kg) i.v. over 5–8 h, then 5–7.5 mL/kg (300–450 mg/kg) over 3–4 h monthly; or 0.6 mL/kg of 16% soltn (100 mg/kg) every 2–4 wk i.m. Sepsis: 0.5 g/kg i.v. over 4 h. Kawasaki, Guillain-Barré, ITP, myasth gravis, Still's dis: 35 mL/kg of 6% soltn (2 g/kg) i.v. over 16 h stat, then if required 15 mL/kg (900 mg/kg) i.v. over 8 h each month. Prevention hep A: 0.1 mL/kg (16 mg/kg) i.m. Prevention measles: 0.2 mL/kg (32 mg/kg) i.m. (repeat next day if immunocompromised).

Immunoglobulin, rabies (Hyperab, Imogam)   20 iu (0.133 mL)/kg i.m. once (1/2 infiltrated around wound), with rabies vaccine.

Immunoglobulin, respiratory syncytial virus   750 mg/kg every month i.v. (50 mg/mL: 1.5 mL/kg per hour for 15 min, 3 mL/kg per hour for 15 min, then 6 mL/kg per hour).

Immunoglobulin, Rh (anti-D)   1 mL (625iu, 125 mcg) i.m. within 72 h of exposure. Large transfusion: 0.16 mL (100iu, 20 mcg) per mL RH positive red cells (maternal serum should be anti-D positive 24–48 h after injection).

Immunoglobulin, tetanus (TIG)   I.m. preparation, prophylaxis: 250–500 iu (1–2 amp). I.v. preparation, treatment: 4000 iu (100 mL) at 0.04 mL/kg per min for 30 min, then 0.075 mL/kg per min i.v.; intrathecal usually 250 iu.

Immunoglobulin, zoster   Within 96 h of exposure: <10 kg 125 iu, 10–20 kg 250 iu, 20–30 kg 375 iu, 30–40 kg 500 iu, >40 kg 600 iu deep i.m.

Indomethacin (indometacin)   0.5–1 mg/kg (adult 25–50 mg) 8 H (max. 6 H) oral or PR. PDA: 0.1 mg/kg (<1 kg) or 0.2 mg/kg (≥1 kg) day 1, then 0.1 mg/kg daily days 2–7 oral or i.v. over 1 h. See Pain management, chapter 4, page 59.

Infliximab   Arthritis (with methotrexate): 3 mg/kg Crohn's: 5 mg/kg i.v. over 2 h then (if response) after 2 wk, 6 wk, and then 5–10 mg/kg every 8 wk.

Influenza A and B vaccine (Fluvax, Vaxigrip)   Inactivated. 0.125 mL (3 mo–2 yr), 0.25 mL (2–6 yr), 0.5 mL (>6 yr) s.c. stat and 4 wk later (2 doses). Boost annually (1 dose).

Insulin   Regular insulin i.v.: 0.05–0.2 u/kg prn, or 0.025–0.1 u/kg per hour (2.5 u/kg in 50 mL 4% albumin at 0.5–2 mL/h); later 1 u/10 g dextrose. For hyperkalaemia: 0.1 u/kg insulin and 2 mL/kg 50% dextrose i.v. In TPN: 5–25 u/250 g dextrose. s.c. insulin (onset/peak/ duration): lispro 10–15 min/1 h/2–5 h; aspart 15–20 min/1 h/3–5 h; regular 30–60 min/4 h/6–8 h; isophane (NPH) 2–4 h/4–12 h/18–24 h; zinc (Lente) 2–3 h/7–15 h/24 h; glargine 1.5 h/none/24 h; crystalline zinc (Ultralente) 4–6 h/10–30 h/24–36 h; protamine zinc 4–8 h/15–20 h/24–36 h.

Interferon alfa-2a, recombinant   Haemangioma: 1 million u/m^2 daily s.c. or i.m. incr over 4 wk to 2–3 million u/m^2 daily for 16–24 wk, then ×3/wk. Hep B, C: 3–6 million u/m^2 ×3/wk s.c. or i.m. for 4–6 mo; higher doses may be reqd in hep B.

Interferon alfa-2b, recombinant   Condylomata: 1 million unit into each lesion (max. 5) ×3/wk for 5 wk. Haemangioma: as for interferon alfa-2a. Hep B: monotherapy as for interferon alfa-2a. Hep C (adult, NOT /kg) 3 million unit ×3/wk s.c., plus ribavirin 1000 mg (1200 mg if >75 kg) daily oral, for 24–48 wk.

Interferon alfacon-1   Hepatitis C (adult, NOT /kg): usually 9 mcg (7.5 mcg if not tolerated) ×3/wk s.c. for 24 wk; if relapse 15 mcg ×3/wk s.c. for 6 mo.

Interferon alfa-n3   Warts (NOT /kg): 250 000 u injected into base of wart (max. 10 doses/session) ×2/wk for max. 8 wk.

Interferon beta-1a   Mult scler (adult, NOT /kg): Avonex 30 mcg (6 million IU) once a wk i.m., Rebif 44 mcg ×3/wk s.c.

Interferon beta-1b   Mult scler (adult, NOT /kg): 250 mcg (8 million IU) s.c. alternate days.

Interferon gamma-1b   Chronic gran dis: 1.5 mcg/kg (body area $\leq$ 0.5 m^2) or 50 mcg/m^2 (area >0.5 m^2) ×3/wk s.c..

Ipecacuanha syrup (total alkaloids 1.4 mg/mL)   1–2 mL/kg (adult 30 mL) stat oral, NG. May repeat once in 30 min.

Ipratropium bromide   Resp soltn (250 mcg/mL): 0.25–1 mL diluted to 4 mL 4–8 H; severe attack every 20 min for 3 doses, then 4–6 H. Aerosol 20 mcg/puff: 2–4 puffs 6–8 H. Nasal: 84 mcg/nostril 6–12 H.

Iron   See ferrous salts.

Iron dextran, iron polymaltose   Fe 50 mg/mL: dose (mL) = 0.05 × wt in kg × (15 – Hb in g%) i.m. (often in divided doses). I.v. infsn possible (but dangerous).

Isoconazole   Topical: 1% cream 12 H. Vaginal: 600 mg (2 tab) once.

Isoetharine   Inhaltn soltn (1%): 0.5 mL diltd to 4 mL 3–6 H (mild), 1 mL diltd to 4 mL 1–2 H (moderate), undiltd constant (severe, in ICU). Aerosol 340 mcg/puff: 1–2 puffs 4–6 H.

Isoniazid (INAH)   10 mg/kg (max. 300 mg) daily oral, i.m. or i.v. TB meningitis: 15–20 mg/kg (max. 500 mg) daily.

Isoprenaline   I.v. infsn: <33 kg 0.3 mg/kg in 50 mL 5%dex-hep at 0.5–10 mL/h (0.05–1 mcg/kg per min); >33 kg give 1/5000 (0.2 mg/mL) soltn at 0.015–0.15 mL/kg per hour (0.05–0.5 mcg/kg per min).

Isosorbide dinitrate   Sublingual: 0.1–0.2 mg/kg (max. 10 mg) 2 H or as needed. Oral: 0.5–1 mg/kg (max. 40 mg) 6 H or as needed. Slow release tab, adult (NOT /kg): 20–80 mg 12 H. I.v. infsn 0.6–2 mcg/kg per min.

Isotretinoin   Adult: 0.5–1 mg/kg daily oral for 2–4 wk, reducing if possible to 0.1–0.2 mg/kg daily for 15–20 wk. 0.05% gel: apply sparingly at night.

Ispaghula husk   Adult (NOT /kg): 1–2 teaspoonfuls 6–12 H oral. Half this dose 6–12 yr.

Isradipine   0.05 mg/kg 12 H oral, may incr after 2–4 wk gradually to 0.1–0.2 mg/kg (max. 10 mg) 12 H.

Itraconazole   2–4 mg/kg (adult 100–200 mg) 12–24 H oral after food. Trough level >0.5 mcg/mL at 10–14 days.

Ivermectin   0.15–0.4 mg/kg (adult 12–24 mg) oral every 6–12 mo.

Kanamycin   Single daily dose i.v. or i.m. Neonate: 15 mg/kg stat, then 7.5 mg/kg (<30 wk) 10 mg/kg (30–35 wk) 15 mg/kg (term <1 wk) daily. 1 wk–10 yr: 25 mg/kg day 1, then 18 mg/kg daily. >10 yr: 20 mg/kg day 1, then 15 mg/kg (max. 1.5 g) daily. Trough level <5.0 mg/L.

Ketamine   Sedation, analgesia: 2–4 mg/kg i.m., 4 mcg/kg per min i.v. Premed: 5 mg/kg oral. Anaesthesia: 5–10 mg/kg i.m., 1–2 mg/kg i.v., infsn 30 mg/kg in 50 mL 5%dex-hep at 1–4 mL/h (10–40 mcg/kg per min). Incompatible with aminophylline, magnesium and salbutamol.

Ketoconazole   Oral: 5 mg/kg (adult 200 mg) 12–24 H. 2% cream: apply 12–24 H. 2% shampoo: wash hair, apply liquid for 5 min, wash off.

Ketoprofen   1–2 mg/kg (adult 50–100 mg) 6–12 H (max. 4 mg/kg or 200 mg in 24 h) oral, i.m., PR. Slow release, adults (NOT /kg): 200 mg daily.

Appendices

Ketorolac Oral: 0.2 mg/kg (adult 10 mg) 4–6 H (max. 0.8 mg/kg per day or 40 mg/day). I.v. or i.m.: usually 0.2 mg/kg (adult 10 mg) 6 H; but may use 0.6 mg/kg (max. 30 mg) stat, then 0.2–0.4 mg/kg (max. 20 mg) 4–6 H for 5 days, then 0.2 mg/kg (max. 10 mg) 6 H. See Pain management, chapter 4, page 60.

Ketotifen Child >2 yr (NOT /kg): 1 mg 12 H oral with food. Adult (NOT /kg): 1–2 mg 12 H oral with food.

Labetalol Oral: 1–2 mg/kg (adult 50–100 mg) 12 H, may incr wkly to max. 10 mg/kg (max. 600 mg) 6 H. I.v.: 0.25–0.5 mg/kg (adult 20 mg) over 2 min repeated every 10 min if reqd, then 0.25–3 mg/kg per hour.

Lactulose 3.3 g/5 mL soltn. Laxative: 0.5 mL/kg 12–24 H oral. Hepatic coma: 1 mL/kg hrly until bowel cleared, then 6–8 H.

Lamotrigine 0.2 mg/kg (adult 25 mg) oral daily, double dose every 2 wk if reqd to max. 1–4 mg/kg (adult 50–200 mg) 12 H. Double dose if taking carbamazepine, phenobarbitone, phenytoin or primidone; halve dose if taking valproate.

Latanoprost 50 mcg/mL: 1 drop/eye daily.

L-atropine See hyoscyamine.

Levodopa + benserazide (4:1) Adult (NOT /kg): initially levodopa 100 mg 8 H oral; if not controlled, incr wkly by 100 mg/day to max. 250 mg 6 H.

Levodopa + carbidopa 250 mg/25 mg and 100 mg/10 mg tabs. Adult (NOT /kg): initially one 100/10 tab 8 H oral; if not controlled, substitute one 250/25 tab for one 100/25 tab every 2nd day; if not controlled on 250/25 8 H, incr by one 250/25 tab every 2nd day to max. 6–8 tab/day.

Levonorgestrel Contraception: 30 mcg daily oral, starting 1st day menstruation. Intra-uterine T-system 52 mg: insert within 7 days of start of menstruation, replace after 3 yr. Postcoital: 0.75 mg oral within 72 h, repeated after 12 h; or 0.5 mg + ethinyloestradiol 100 mcg oral within 72h, repeated after 12 h.

Levothyroxine 50 mcg tab. 100 mcg/m^2 rounded to nearest 1/4 tab (adult 100–200 mcg) daily oral.

Lignocaine (lidocaine) I.v.: 1% soltn 0.1 mL/kg (1 mg/kg) over 2 min, then 0.09–0.3 mL/kg per hour (15–50 mcg/kg per min); or 30 mg/kg in 50 mL 5%dex-hep at 50 mL/h for 2 min, then 1.5–15 mL/h (15–50 mcg/kg per min). Nerve block: without adrenaline max. 4 mg/kg (0.4 mL/kg of 1%), with adrenaline 7 mg/kg (0.7 mL/kg of 1%). Topical spray: max. 3–4 mg/kg (Xylocaine 10% spray pack: ~10 mg/puff). Topical 2% gel, 2.5% compound mouth paint/gel (SM-33), 2% and 4% soltn, 5% ointment, 10% dental ointment: apply 3 H prn. See Pain management, chapter 4, page 60.

Lignocaine (lidocaine) 2.5% + prilocaine 2.5% Cream (EMLA): 1.5 g/10cm^2 under occlusive dressing for 1–3 h.

Lincomycin 10 mg/kg (adult 600 mg) 8 H oral, i.m. or i.v. over 1 h. Severe inftn: 15–20 mg/kg (adult 1.2 g) i.v. over 2 h 6 H.

Lindane 1% cream, lotion. Scabies: apply from neck down, wash off after 8–12 h. Lice: rub into hair for 4 min, then wash off; repeat after 24 h (max. ×2/wk).

Liothyronine sodium (T$_3$) Oral: 0.2 mcg/kg (adult 10 mcg) 8 H, may incr to 0.4 mcg/kg (adult 20 mcg) 8 H. I.v.: 0.1–0.4 mcg/kg (adult 5–20 mcg) 8–12 H. Septic shock: 0.1–0.2 mcg/kg per hour (adult 100–200 mcg/day) i.v. infsn.

Lipid   20% emulsion: 1–3 g/kg per day i.v. (mL/h = g/kg per day × wt × 0.21).

Lisinopril   0.1 mg/kg (adult 5 mg) daily oral, may incr over 4–6 wk to 0.2–1 mg/kg (adult 10–20 mg) daily.

Lithium (salts)   5–20 mg/kg 8–24 H oral. Slow release tab 450 mg (adult, NOT /kg): 1–2 tab 12 H. Maintain trough level 0.8–1.6 mmol/L (>2 mmol/L toxic).

Loperamide   0.05–0.1 mg/kg (adult 2–4 mg) 8–12 H oral, incr if reqd to max. 0.4 mg/kg (max. 4 mg) 8 H.

Lorazepam   0.02–0.06 mg/kg (adult 1–3 mg) 8–24 H oral. I.v.: 0.05–0.2 mg/kg i.v. over 2 min, then 0.01–0.1 mg/kg per hour. .

Lypressin (lysine-8-vasopressin)   1 spray (2.5 iu) into 1 nostril 4–8 H, may incr to 1 spray both nostrils 4–8 H.

Magnesium chloride 10%   0.48 g/5 mL = Mg 1 mmol/mL. 0.4 mL/kg 12 H slow i.v. Myoc infarct (NOT /kg): 5 mL/h i.v. for 6 h, then 1 mL/h for 24–48 h. VF: 0.1–0.2 mL/kg i.v.

Magnesium hydroxide   Antacid: 10–40 mg/kg (max. 2 g) 6 H oral. Laxative: 50–100 mg/kg (max. 5 g) oral.

Magnesium sulfate   Deficiency: 50% mag sulf (2 mmol/mL) 0.2 mL/kg (max. 10 mL) 12 H i.m., slow i.v. Asthma, digoxin tachycardia, eclampsia, prem labour, pul ht: 50% 0.1 mL/kg (50 mg/kg) i.v. over 20 min, then 0.06 mL/kg per hour (30 mg/kg per hour); keep serum Mg 1.5–2.5 mmol/l (pul ht 3–4 mmol/l). Myoc infarct (NOT /kg): 50% 2.5 mL/h (5 mmol/h) i.v. for 6 h, then 0.5 mL/h (1 mmol/h) for 24–48 h. VF: 50% 0.05–0.1 mL/kg (0.1–0.2 mmol/kg) i.v. Incompatible with aminophylline, ketamine, salbutamol. Laxative: 0.5 g/kg (max. 15 g) as 10% soltn 8 H for 2 days oral.

Maldison   0.5% liquid: 20 mL to hair, wash off after 12 h.

Mannitol   0.25–0.5 g/kg i.v. (2–4 mL/kg of 12.5%, 1.25–2.5 mL/kg of 20%, 1–2 mL/kg of 25%) 2 H prn, provided serum osmolality <320–330 mmol/L.

Measles + mumps + rubella vaccine (MMRII, Priorix)   Live. >12 mo: 0.5 mL s.c.

Measles + mumps vaccine (Rimparix)   Live. >12 mo: 0.5 mL s.c. once.

Measles vaccine (Attenuvax)   Live. >12 mo: 0.5 mL s.c. once.

Mebendazole   NOT /kg: 100 mg 12 H ×3 days. Enterobiasis (NOT /kg): 100 mg once, may repeat after 2–4 wks.

Mebeverine   135 mg tab: adult (NOT /kg) 1–3 tab daily oral.

Mefenamic acid   10 mg/kg (adult 500 mg) 8 H oral.

Mefloquine   15 mg/kg (adult 750 mg) stat, then 10 mg/kg (adult 500 mg) after 6–8 h. Prophylaxis: 5 mg/kg (adult 250 mg) once a wk.

Meningococcus gp A, C, W135 and Y conjugated vaccine (Menactra)   Inactivated. >10 yr: 0.5 mL i.m.

Meningococcus gp A, C, W135 and Y vaccine (Mencevax ACWY, Menomune)   Inactivated. >2 yr: 0.5 mL s.c. Boost 1–3 yrly.

Meningococcus gp C, conjugate vaccine (Meningitec, Menjugate, NeisVac-C)   Inactivated. 0.5 mL i.m.: 3 doses at least 1 mo apart (6 wk-6 mo), 2 doses (6–12 mo), 1 dose (>12 mo).

Mercaptamine   See cysteamine bitartrate.

Meropenem   10–20 mg/kg (adult 0.5–1 g) 8 H i.v. over 5–30 min. Severe inftn: 20–40 mg/kg (adult 1–2 g) 12 H (1st wk life) 8 H (>1 wk) or constant infsn.

Metaraminol   I.v.: 0.01 mg/kg stat (repeat prn), then 0.15 mg/kg in 50 mL 5% dextrose (no heparin) at 1–10 mL/h (0.05–0.5 mcg/kg per min) and titrate dose against BP. s.c.: 0.1 mg/kg.

Methadone   Usually 0.1–0.2 mg/kg (adult 5–10 mg) 6–12 H oral, s.c. or i.m.

Methionine   50 mg/kg (max. 2.5 g) oral 4 H for 4 doses. Prophylaxis: 1 mg to paracetamol 5 mg.

Methotrexate   Leukaemia: typically 3.3 mg/m^2 i.v. daily for 4–6 wk; then 2.5 mg/kg i.v. every 2 wk, or 30 mg/m^2 oral or i.m. ×2/wk; higher doses with folinic acid rescue. Intrathecal: 12 mg/m^2 wkly for 2 wk, then monthly. Arthritis: 10–20 mg/m^2 wkly oral, i.v., i.m. or s.c. Adult psoriasis: 0.2–0.5 mg/kg wkly oral, i.v. or i.m. until response, then reduce.

Methscopolamine   See hyoscine methobromide.

Methylcellulose   Constipation: 30–60 mg/kg (adult 1.5–3 g) with at least 300 mL fluid 12 H oral.

Methylene blue   1–2 mg/kg (G6PD deficiency 0.4 mg/kg) i.v., repeated as reqd. Septic shock: 2 mg/kg stat i.v., then 0.25–2 mg/kg per hour.

Methylphenidate   0.1 mg/kg oral 8am, noon and (occasionally) 4pm; incr if reqd to max. 0.5 mg/kg per dose (adult 20 mg). Long acting: 20–60 mg (18–54 mg in US) in morning.

Methylprednisolone   Asthma: 0.5–1 mg/kg 6 H oral, i.v. or i.m. day 1, 12 H day 2, then 1 mg/kg daily, reducing to minimum effective dose. Severe croup: 4 mg/kg i.v. stat, then 1 mg/kg 8 H. Severe sepsis before antibiotics (or within 4 h of 1st dose): 30 mg/kg i.v. once. Spinal cord injury (within 8 h): 30 mg/kg stat, then 5 mg/kg per hour 2 days. Lotion 0.25%: apply sparingly 12–24 H. Methylpred 1 mg = hydrocortisone 5 mg in glucocorticoid activity, 0.5 mg in mineralocorticoid.

Methylprednisolone aceponate   0.1% cream, ointment: apply 12–24 H.

Methyltestosterone   NOT /kg: 2.5–12.5 mg/day buccal.

Methysergide maleate   0.02 mg/kg (adult 1 mg) 12 H oral, incr if reqd to max. 0.04 mg/kg (adult 2 mg) 8 H for 3–6 mo.

Metoclopramide   0.15–0.3 mg/kg (adult 10–15 mg) 6 H i.v., i.m., oral; 0.2–0.4 mg/kg (adult 10–20 mg) 8 H PR. Periop: 0.5 mg/kg (adult 15–20 mg) i.v. stat, then 0.2 mg/kg (adult 10 mg) 4–6 H if reqd. With chemother: up to 1–2 mg/kg 4 H i.v.

Metolazone   0.1–0.2 mg/kg (adult 5–10 mg) daily oral. Up to 0.5 mg/kg (adult 30 mg) daily short term.

Metoprolol   I.v.: 0.1 mg/kg (adult 5 mg) over 5 min, repeat every 5 min to max. 3 doses, then 1–5 mcg/kg per min. Oral: 1–2 mg/kg (adult 50–100 mg) 6–12 H.

Metronidazole   15 mg/kg (max. 1 g) stat, then 7.5 mg/kg (max. 1 g) 12 H in neonate (1st maintenance dose 48 h after load if <2 kg, 24 h in term baby), 8 H (4+ wk) i.v., PR or oral. Giardiasis: 30 mg/kg (adult 2 g) daily ×3 oral. Amoebiasis: 15 mg/kg (adult 750–800 mg) 8 H oral for 10 days, usually followed by diloxanide furoate 10 mg/kg (adult 500 mg) 8 H oral for 10 days. Topical gel 0.5%: apply daily. Level 60–300 μmol/mL (×0.17 mcg/mL).

Mianserin   0.2–0.5 mg/kg (adult 10–40 mg) 8 H oral.

Miconazole   7.5–15 mg/kg (adult 0.6–1.2 g) 8 H i.v. over 1 h. Topical: 2% cream, powder, lotion, tincture or gel 12–24 H. Vaginal: 2% cream or 100 mg ovule daily ×7.

Microlax enema   <12 mo 1.25 mL, 1–2 yr 2.5 mL, >2 yr 5 mL.

Midazolam   Sedation: usually 0.1–0.2 mg/kg (adult 5 mg) i.v. or i.m., up to 0.5 mg/kg used safely in children; 0.2 mg/kg (repeated in 10 min if reqd) nasal; 0.5 mg/kg (max. 20 mg) oral. Infusion (ventltd): 3 mg/kg in 50 mL 5%dex-hep at 1–4 mL/h (1–4 mcg/kg per min); fitting usually 2–4 mL/h (range 1–18 mL/h); sedatn 1 mL/h + clonidine 0.5–2 mcg/kg per hour.

Milrinone   <30 kg: 1.5 mg/kg in 50 mL 5%dex-hep, 2.5 mL over 1 h (75 mcg/kg), then 1–1.5 mL/h (0.5–0.75 mcg/kg per min). >30 kg: 1.5 mg/kg made up to 100 mL in 5%dex-hep, 5 mL over 1 h (75 mcg/kg), then 2–3 mL/h (0.5–0.75 mcg/kg per min).

Minocycline   Over 8 yr: 4 mg/kg (max. 200 mg) stat, then 2 mg/kg (max. 100 mg) 12 H oral or i.v. over 1 h.

Minoxidil   0.1 mg/kg (max. 5 mg) daily, incr to max. 0.5 mg/kg (max. 25 mg) 12–24 H oral. Male baldness: 2% soltn 1 mL 12 H to dry scalp.

Mometasone   0.1% cream or oint: apply daily. 50 mcg spray: adult 2 sprays/nostril daily.

Montelukast   NOT /kg: 4 mg (2–5 yr) 5 mg (6–14 yr) 10 mg (>14 yr) daily at bedtime, oral.

Morphine   Half-life 2–4 h i.m.: neonate 0.1 mg/kg, child 0.1–0.2 mg/kg, adult 10–20 mg; 1/2 this i.v. over 10 min. i.v. (ventltd): 0.1–0.2 mg/kg per dose (adult 5–10 mg). Infsn of 1 mg/kg in 50 mL 5%dex-hep: ventltd neonate 0.5–1.5 mL/h (10–30 mcg/kg per hour), child or adult 1–4 mL/h (20–80 mcg/kg per hour). Patient controlled: 20 mcg/kg boluses (1 mL of 1 mg/kg in 50 mL) with 5 min lockout time + (in child) 5 mcg/kg per hour. Oral double i.m. dose; slow release: start with 0.6 mg/kg 12 H and incr every 48 h if reqd. See Pain management, chapter 4, page 58.

Mumps vaccine (Mumpsvax)   Live. >12 mo: 0.5 mL s.c. once. See also measles + mumps + rubella vaccine.

Mupirocin   2% ointment: apply 8–12 H.

Nalidixic acid   15 mg/kg (adult 1 g) 6 H oral, reducing to 7.5 mg/kg (adult 500 mg) 6 H after 2 wk.

Naloxone   Postop sedatn: 0.002 mg/kg per dose (0.4 mg diluted to 20 mL, give 0.1 mL/kg per dose) repeat every 2 min ×4 if reqd, then 0.3 mg/kg in 30 mL 5%dex-hep at 1 mL/h (0.01 mg/kg per hour) i.v. Opiate overdose (including newborn): 0.01 mg/kg (max. 0.4 mg) (0.4 mg diluted to 10 mL, give 0.25 mL/kg per dose), repeated every 2 min (15 min if i.m. or s.c.) ×4 if reqd, then 0.3 mg/kg in 30 mL 5%dex-hep at 1 mL/h (0.01 mg/kg per hour) i.v.

Naltrexone   0.5 mg/kg (adult 25 mg) stat, then 1 mg/kg (adult 50 mg) daily oral.

Naproxen   1 mg = 1.1 mg naproxen sodium. >2 yr: 5–10 mg/kg (adult 250–500 mg) 8–12 H oral. Adult (NOT /kg): 500 mg 12 H PR.

Nedocromil   Inhltn: 4 mg (2 puffs) 6 H, reducing to 12 H when improved. 2% eye drops: 1 drop/eye 6–24 H.

Neomycin   1 g/m^2 4–6 H oral (max. 12 g/day). Bladder washout: 40–2000 mg/L.

Neostigmine   Reverse relaxants: 0.05–0.07 mg/kg (adult 0.5–2.5 mg) i.v.; suggested dilution: neostigmine (2.5 mg/mL) 0.5 mL + atropine (0.6 mg/mL) 0.5 mL + saline 0.5 mL, give 0.1 mL/kg i.v. Myasth gravis: 0.2–0.5 mg/kg (adult 1–2.5 mg) 2–4 H i.m., s.c.

Netilmicin   I.v. or i.m. 1 wk–10 yr: 8 mg/kg day 1, then 6 mg/kg daily. >10 yr: 7 mg/kg day 1, then 5 mg/kg (max. 240–360 mg) daily. Neonate, 5 mg/kg dose: <1200 g 48 H (0–7 days of life), 36 H (8–30 days), 24 H (>30 days); 1200–2500 g 36 H (0–7 days of life), 24 H (>7 days); term 24 H (0–7 days of life), then as for 1 wk–10 yr. Trough level <1.0 mg/L.

Nicardipine 0.4–0.8 mg/kg (adult 20–40 mg) 8 H oral. 1–3 mcg/kg per min (max. 20 mg/h) i.v.

Nicotine resin chewing gum NOT /kg: 2–4 mg chewed over 30 min when inclined to smoke; usually need 16–24 mg/day, max. 60 mg/day.

Nicotine transdermal patches Usually 21 mg, 14 mg and 7 mg per 24 h. Adult: if smoked >20 cig/day apply strongest patch daily 3–4 wk, medium patch daily 3–4 wk (initial dose if smoked ≤20 cig/day), then weakest patch daily 3–4 wk.

Nicotinic acid Hypercholesterolaemia and hypertriglyceridaemia: 5 mg/kg (adult 200 mg) 8 H, gradually incr to 20–30 mg/kg (adult 1–2 g) 8 H oral.

Nifedipine Caps 0.25–0.5 mg/kg (adult 10–20 mg) 6–8 H, tabs 0.5–1 mg/kg (adult 20–40 mg) 12 H oral or sublingual.

Nimodipine 10–15 mcg/kg per hour (adult 1 mg/h) i.v. for 2 h, then 10–45 mcg/kg per hour (adult 2 mg/h). Adult: 60 mg 4 H oral.

Nisoldipine Slow release: 0.2 mg/kg (adult 10 mg) daily oral, incr to 0.4–0.8 mg/kg (adult 20–40 mg) daily.

Nitrazepam Child epilepsy: 0.125–0.5 mg/kg 12 H oral. Hypnotic (NOT /kg): 2.5–5 mg (child) 5–10 mg (adult) nocte.

Nitric oxide 1–40 ppm (up to 80 ppm used occasionally). 0.1 L/min of 1000 ppm added to 10 L/min gas gives 10 ppm. [NO] = Cylinder [NO] × (1 − (Patient FiO_2/Supply FiO_2)). [NO] = Cylinder [NO] × NO flow/total flow.

Nitrofurantoin 1.5 mg/kg (adult 50–100 mg) 6 H oral. Prophylaxis: 1–2 mg/kg (adult 50–100 mg) at night.

Noradrenaline 0.15 mg/kg in 50 mL 5%dex-hep at 1–10 mL/h (0.05–0.5 mcg/kg per min). Flows <2 mL/h often cause swings in blood pressure.

Norethisterone Contraception: 350 mcg daily, starting 1st day of menstruation. Menorrhagia: 10 mg 3 H until bleeding stops, then 5 mg 6 H for 1 wk, then 5 mg 8 H for 2 wk.

Norethisterone + ethinyloestradiol (0.5 mg/35 mcg or 1 mg/35 mcg) 21 tab, + 7 inert tab Contraception: 1 tab daily, starting 1st day of menstruation.

Norethisterone + oestradiol patches Adult (NOT /kg): 0 mg/4 mg (Estraderm 50) patch ×2/wk for 2 wk, then 30 mg/10 mg (Estragest 250/50) patch ×2/wk for 2 wk.

Norethisterone 1 mg + mestranol 50 mcg Contraception: 1 tab daily from 5th to 25th day of menstrual cycle.

Norethisterone 1 mg + oestradiol 2 mg Adult: 1 tab daily.

Norfloxacin 10 mg/kg (adult 400 mg) 12 H oral.

Norgestimate 0.25 mg + ethinyloestradiol 0.035 mg + 7 inert tab Contraception: 1 tab daily, starting 1st day of menstruation.

Norgestrel See levonorgestrel.

Normacol granules 6 mo-5 yr 1/2 teasp 12 H, 6–10 yr 1 teasp 12 H, >10 yr 1 teasp 8 H.

Nortriptyline 0.5–1.5 mg/kg (adult 25–75 mg) 8 H oral.

NTBC (nitro-trifluoromethylbenzoyl cyclohexanedione) 0.5 mg/kg 12 H oral.

Nystatin 100 000 u <12 mo, 500 000 u (1 tab) >12 mo 6 H NG or oral. Prophylaxis: 50 000 u <12 mo, 250 000 u >12 mo 8 H. Topical: 100 000 u/g gel, cream or ointment 12 H. Vaginal: 100 000 u 12–24 H.

Oestradiol (estradiol)   NOT /kg. Menopause: transdermal patch 3.8 mg, 5.7 mg or 7.6 mg (releases 50, 75 or 100 mcg/day) apply every 7 days (add progestogen for 14 days per month if uterus intact). Osteoporosis: 1 mg patch applied wkly. Induction puberty: 0.5 mg alternate days oral, incr over 2–3 yr to 2 mg/day (add progestogen for 14 days per month when dose 1.5 mg/day or when bleeding occurs). Tall stature: 12 mg/day oral until bone age >16 yr (add progestogen for 14 days per cycle). Gonadal failure: 2 mg/day oral (add progestogen for 14 days per cycle).

Oestradiol 2 mg (×11 tab), oestradiol 2 mg + cyproterone 1 mg (×10 tab)   1 tab daily for 21 days (starting 5th day of menstruation), then 7 days with no tablet.

Oestradiol 2 mg + norethisterone 1 mg   Adult 1 tab daily.

Oestradiol 2 mg or 4 mg (×12 tab), oestradiol 1 mg (×6 tab), oestradiol 2 mg or 4 mg + norethisterone 1 mg (×10 tab)   1 tab daily, starting 5th day of menstruation. Vaginal tab 25 mcg: 1 tab daily for 2 wk, then 1 tab ×2/wk. See also norethisterone + oestradiol.

17-beta-Oestradiol   2 mg vaginal ring, replace every 3 mo.

Oestriol   Inductn puberty: 0.25 mg/day incr to 2 mg/day (+ progestogen 12 days/cycle) oral. Epiphyseal maturtn: 10 mg/day (+ progestogen 12 days/cycle). Vaginal: 0.5 mg daily, reducing to ×2/wk. Patch (Menorest) 37.5 (3.28 mg), 50 (4.33 mg), 75 (6.57 mg), 100 (8.66 mg): apply 1 patch ×2/wk (adjust dose monthly), with medroxyprogesterone acetate (if uterus intact) 10 mg × 10 days/month.

Ofloxacin   5 mg/kg (adult 200 mg) 8–12 H, or 10 mg/kg (adult 400 mg) 12 H oral or i.v. over 1 h. 0.3%: 1 drop/eye hrly for 2 days (4 H overnight), reducing to 3–6 H.

Omeprazole   Usually 0.4–0.8 mg/kg (adult 20–40 mg) 12–24 H oral. ZE synd: 1 mg/kg (adult 60 mg) 12–24 H oral, incr up to 3 mg/kg (adult 120 mg) 8 H if reqd. I.v.: 2 mg/kg (adult 80 mg) stat, then 1 mg/kg (adult 40 mg) 8–12 H. *H. pylori:* 0.8 mg/kg (adult 40 mg) daily oral with metronidazole 8 mg/kg (adult 400 mg) 8 H + amoxycillin 10 mg/kg (adult 500 mg) 8 H for 2 wk.

Ondansetron   I.v.: prophylaxis 0.15 mg/kg (adult 4 mg); treatment 0.2 mg/kg (adult 8 mg) over 5 min, or 0.2–0.5 mcg/kg per min. Oral: 0.1–0.2 mg/kg (usual max. 8 mg) 6–12 H.

Oxacillin   15–30 mg/kg 6 H oral, i.v., i.m. Severe inftn: 40 mg/kg (max. 2 g) 12 H (1st wk life), 8 H (2nd wk), 6 H or constant infsn (>2 wk).

Oxandrolone   0.1–0.2 mg/kg (adult 2.5–20 mg) daily oral. Turner's synd: 0.05–0.1 mg/kg daily.

Oxazepam   0.2–0.5 mg/kg (adult 10–30 mg) 6–8 H oral.

Oxybutynin   <5 yr: 0.2 mg/kg 8–12 H oral. >5 yr (NOT/ kg): 2.5–5 mg 8–12 H oral. Slow rel: adult 5–30 mg daily oral. Patch: adult 39 cm^2 patch ×2/wk (3.9 mg/day).

Oxycodone   0.1–0.2 mg/kg (adult 5–10 mg) 4–6 H oral, incr if reqd. Slow release: 0.6–0.9 mg/kg (adult 10 mg) 12 H oral, incr if reqd. Suppos: adult 30 mg 6–8 H PR. See Pain management, chapter 4, page 58.

Oxymorphone   Usually 0.02–0.03 mg/kg (adult 1–1.5 mg) 4–6 H i.m. or s.c. Slow i.v.: 0.01 mg/kg (adult 0.5 mg) 4–6 H. P.r.: 0.1 mg/kg (adult 5 mg) 4–6 H.

Oxytetracycline   >8 yr (NOT /kg): 250–500 mg 6 H oral, or 250–500 mg 6–12 H slow i.v.

Oxytocin   Labour (NOT /kg): 1–4 mU/min i.v., may incr to 20 mU/min max. Lactation: 1 spray (4 iu) into each nostril 5 min before infant feeds.

Packed red blood cells   4 mL/kg raises the Hb by 10 g/L (or 1 g%). Number of mL required = weight (kg) × Hb rise required (g/L) × 0.4. 1 bag is ~300 mL.

Pamidronate   Osteoporosis, OI: 3–7 mg/kg daily oral, 1.0 mg/kg (adult 15–90 mg) i.v. over 4 h daily ×3 every 4 mo, or once every 3–4 wk. Hypercalcaemia 20–50 mg/m^2 (depending on Ca level) i.v. over 4 h every 4 wk.

Pancreatic enzymes   With meals (NOT /kg): usually 1–3 Cotazyme-S Forte cap, 1–5 Pancrease cap oral. Max lipase 10 000 u/kg per day.

Pancuronium   ICU: 0.1–0.15 mg/kg i.v. prn. Theatre: 0.1 mg /kg i.v., then 0.02 mg/kg prn. Infsn: 0.25–0.75 mcg/kg per min.

Pantoprazole   1.0 mg/kg (adult 40 mg) 12–24 H oral, i.v. GI hge, adult: 80 mg stat, then 8 mg/h. ZE: 80 mg 8–12 H adjusted to achieve acid <10 mmol/L.

Papaveretum (20 mg/mL) + hyoscine (0.4 mg/mL)   0.4 mg/kg (P) + 0.008 mg/kg (H) = 0.02 mL/kg per dose i.m.

Papaveretum (Omnopon)   0.2 mg/kg i.v., 0.4 mg/kg i.m. (half-life 2–4 h). ICU: 0.3 mg/kg i.v., 0.6 mg/kg i.m.

Paracetamol   Oral or i.v.: 20 mg/kg stat, then 15 mg/kg 4 H (max. 4 g/day); child usual daily max. 90 mg/kg for 48 h, then max. 60 mg/kg. Rectal: 40 mg/kg stat, then 30 mg/kg 6 H (max. 5 g/day). Overdose: acetylcysteine. See Pain management, chapter 4, page 57.

Paraffin   Liquid: 1 mL/kg (adult 30–45 mL) daily oral. Liquid 50% + white soft 50%, ointment: apply 6–12 H.

Paraffin 65% + agar   NOT /kg: 6 mo–2 yr 5 mL, 3–5 yr 5–10 mL, >5 yr 10 mL 8–24 H oral.

Paraffin, phenolphthalein and agar (Agarol)   NOT /kg: 6 mo–2 yr 2.5 mL, 3–5 yr 2.5–5 mL, >5 yr 5 mL 8–24 H oral.

Paraldehyde   I.m.: 0.2 mL/kg (adult 10 mL) stat, then 0.1 mL/kg 4–6 H. I.v.: 0.2 mL/kg (adult 10 mL) over 15 min, then 0.02 mL/kg per hour (max. 1.5 mL/h). Rectal or NG: 0.3 mL/kg (adult 5–10 mL) diluted 1 : 10.

Penicillamine (D-penicillamine)   Arthritis: 1.5 mg/kg (adult 125 mg) 12 H oral, incr over several months to max. 3 mg/kg (adult 375 mg) 6–8 H. Wilson's dis, lead poisoning: 5–7.5 mg/kg (adult 250–500 mg) 6 H oral. Cystinuria: 7.5 mg/kg (adult 250–1000 mg) 6 H oral, titrated to urine cystine <100–200 mg/day.

Penicillin V   See phenoxymethylpenicillin.

Penicillin, benzathine   1 mg = 1250 u. Usually 25 mg/kg (max. 900 mg) i.m. once. STI: 40 mg/kg (max. 1.8 g) i.m. once. Strep proph: 25 mg/kg (max. 900 mg) i.m. 3–4 wkly, or 10 mg/kg i.m. 2 wkly.

Penicillin, benzyl (penicillin G, crystalline)   1 mg = 1667 u. 30 mg/kg 6 H. Severe inftn: 50 mg/kg (max. 2 g) i.v. 12 H (1st wk life), 6 H (2–4 wk), 4 H or constnt infsn (>4 wk).

Penicillin, procaine   1 mg = 1000 u. 25–50 mg/kg (max. 1.2–2.4 g) 12–24 H i.m. Single dose: 100 mg/kg (max. 4.8 g).

Pentamidine isethionate   3–4 mg/kg (1.7–2.3 mg/kg base) i.v. over 2 h or i.m. daily for 10–14 days (1 mg base = 1.5 mg mesylate = 1.74 mg isethionate). Neb: 600 mg/6 mL daily for 3 wk (treatment), 300 mg/3 mL every 4 wk (prophylaxis).

Pentastarch   10% soltn: 10–40 mg/kg i.v.

Pentazocine   Oral: 0.5–2.0 mg/kg (adult 25–100 mg) 3–4 H. S.c., i.m. or slow i.v.: 0.5–1 mg/kg (adult 30–60 mg) 3–4 H. P.r.: 1 mg/kg (adult 50 mg) 6–12 H.

Pentobarbital   See pentobarbitone.

Pentobarbitone   0.5–1 mg/kg (adult 30–60 mg) 6–8 H oral, i.m., slow i.v. Hypnotic: 2–4 mg/kg (adult 100–200 mg).

Permethrin   1% creme rinse (head lice): wash hair, apply creme for 10 min, wash off; may repeat in 2 wk. 5% cream (scabies): wash body, apply to whole body except face, wash off after 12–24 h.

Pethidine   0.5–1 mg/kg (adult 25–50 mg) i.v., 0.5–2 mg/kg (adult 25–100 mg) i.m. (half-life 2–4 h). Infsn: 5 mg/kg in 50 mL at 1–4 mL/h (0.1–0.4 mg/kg per hour). PCA 5 mg/kg in 50 mL: usually bolus 2 mL with lockout 5 min, optional background 0.5 mL/h.

Pheniramine   0.5–1 mg/kg (adult 25–50 mg) 6–8 H oral. Slow release tab 75 mg at night.

Phenobarbitone (phenobarbital)   Loading dose in emergency: 20–30 mg/kg i.m. or i.v. over 30 min stat. Ventilated: repeat doses of 10–15 mg/kg up to 100 mg/kg per day (beware hypotension). Usual maintenance: 5 mg/kg (adult 300 mg) daily i.v., i.m. or oral. Infant colic: 1 mg/kg 4–8 H oral. Level 80–120 umol/L (×0.23 = mcg/mL) done Mo–Fr 1100 at RCH.

Phenoxybenzamine   0.2–0.5 mg/kg (adult 10–40 mg) 8–12 H oral. Cardiac surgery: 1 mg/kg i.v. over 1–4 h stat, then 0.5 mg/kg 8–12 H i.v. over 1 h or oral.

Phenoxymethylpenicillin (penicillin V)   7.5–15 mg/kg (adult 250–500 mg) 6 H oral. Proph: 12.5 mg/kg (adult 250 mg) 12 H oral.

Phentolamine   15 mg/kg in 50 mL 5%dex-hep at 1–10 mL/h (5–50 mcg/kg per min) i.v. May accumulate (1/2-life 19 min, longer if renal impairment).

Phenylephrine   I.v.: 2–10 mcg/kg stat (adult 500 mcg), then 1–5 mcg/kg per min. S.c. or i.m.: 0.1–0.2 mg/kg (max. 10 mg). Oral: 0.2 mg/kg (max. 10 mg) 6–8 H. 0.15%, 10% eye drops: 1–2 drops/eye 6–8 H. 0.25%, 0.5% nose drops: 1–3 drops/sprays per nostril 6–8 H.

Phenyltoloxamine   1 mg/kg (adult 50 mg) 8 H oral.

Phenytoin   Loading dose in emergency: 15–20 mg/kg (max. 1.5 g) i.v. over 1 h. Initial maintenance, oral or i.v.: 2 mg /kg 12 H (preterm); 3 mg/kg 12 H (1st wk life), 8 H (2 wk–4 yr), 12 H (5–12 yr); 2 mg/kg (usual max. 100 mg) 8 H >12 yr. Level 40–80 umol/L (×0.25 = mcg/mL).

Pholcodine   0.1–0.2 mg/kg (adult 5–15 mg) 6–12 H oral.

Phosphate, potassium (1 mmol/mL)   0.1–1.5 mmol/kg per day (max. 70 mmol/day) i.v. infsn.

Phosphate, sodium   Laxative, diluted, NOT /kg: 250 mg (2–4 yr) 250–500 mg (>4 yr) 6 H oral.

Phosphate, sodium (Fleet enema)   Na 1.61 mEq/l + PO_4 4.15 mEq/l + P 1.38 mEq/l: 33 mL (2–5 yr), 66 mL (5–11 yr), 133 mL (adult) rectal.

Physostigmine   0.02 mg/kg (max. 1 mg) i.v. every 5 min until response (max. 0.1 mg/kg), then 0.5–2.0 mcg/kg per min.

Phytomenadione (vitamin K_1)   Deficiency with hge: FFP 10 mL/kg, then 0.3 mg/kg (max. 10 mg), i.m. or i.v. over 1 h. Prophylaxis in neonates (NOT /kg): 1 mg (0.1 mL) i.m. at birth; or 2 mg (0.2 mL) oral at birth, at 3–5 days, and by 4 wk (give 1/2 dose if <1.5 kg). Warfarin reversal: 0.1 mg/kg (max. 5 mg) s.c. or oral (repeat if reqd); if severe hge 0.3 mg/kg (max. 10 mg) with FFP 10 mL/kg. Mitochondrial dis (NOT /kg): 10 mg 6 H oral.

Pilocarpine   0.1 mg/kg (adult 5 mg) 4–8 H oral. 0.5%, 1%, 2%, 3%, 4% eye drops: 1–2 drops 6–12 H.

Pimecrolimus   1% cream: apply 12 H.

Pimozide   0.04 mg/kg (adult 20 mg) daily oral, incr if reqd to max. 0.4 mg/kg (adult 20 mg) daily.

Pine tar   Gel, solution: 5 mL to baby bath, 15–30 mL to adult bath; soak for 10 min.

Piperacillin   50 mg/kg (adult 2–3 g) 6–8 H i.v. Severe inftn: 75 mg/kg (adult 4 g) 8 H (1st wk life) 6 H (2–4 wk) 4–6 H (>4 wk) or constant infsn.

Piperazine   75 mg/kg (max. 4 g) oral daily for 2 days (ascaris), 7 days (pinworm).

Piroxicam   0.2–0.4 mg/kg (adult 10–20 mg) daily oral. Gel 5 mg/g: apply 1 g (3 cm) 6–8 H for up to 2 wk. See Pain management, chapter 4, page 59.

Pizotifen   NOT /kg: 0.5 mg daily oral, incr if reqd to max. 0.5 mg morning and 1 mg at night.

Platelets   10 mL/kg i.v. stat, then as reqd. 1 unit ~60 mL.

Pneumococcal vaccine, CRM conjugate (Prevenar)   Inactivated. 0.5 mL i.m. <6 mo: 2 mo, 3 mo, 4 mo, 12–15 mo (4 doses). 6–11 mo: 6 mo, 7 mo, 12–15 mo (3 doses). 12–23 mo: 2 doses 2 mo apart. >23 mo: 1 dose.

Pneumococcal vaccine, polysaccharide (Pneumovax 23)   Inactivated. >2 yr: 0.5 mL s.c. or i.m. once. Boost every 5 yr.

Podophyllotoxin   0.5% paint: apply 12 H for 3 days, then none for 4 days; 4 wk course.

Poliomyelitis vaccine, oral (Sabin)   Live. 2 drops oral at 2 mo, 4 mo and 6 mo (3 doses). Boost at 5 yr, and if going to epidemic area.

Poliomyelitis vaccine, s.c. (IPOL)   Inactivated. 0.5 mL s.c. stat, 8 wk later and 8 wk later (3 doses). Boost 12 mo later and at school entry.

Poloxamer   10% soltn: <6 mo 10drops, 6–18 mo 15drops, 18 mo–3 yr 25drops 8 H oral.

Poractant alfa (porcine surfactant, Curosurf)   Intratracheal: 200 mg/kg stat, then up to 4 doses of 100 mg/kg 12 H if required.

Potassium   Deficiency: usually 0.3 mmol/kg per hour (max. 0.4 mmol/kg per hour) for 4–6 h i.v., then 4 mmol/kg per day. Max oral dose 1 mmol/kg (<5 yr), 0.5 mmol/kg (>5 yr). Maintenance 2–4 mmol/kg per day. If peripheral i.v., max. 0.05 mmol/mL. 1 g KCl = 13.3 mmol K, 7.5% KCl = 1 mmol/mL.

Potassium guaiacolsulfonate   1–3 mg/kg (adult 50–160 mg) 4–6 H oral.

Povidone-iodine   Cream, oint, paint, soltn: apply 6–12 H.

Praziquantel   20 mg/kg oral once (tapeworm), 4 H ×3 doses (schistosomiasis), 8 H ×6 doses (other flukes), 8 H 14 days (cysticercosis).

Prazosin   5 mcg/kg (max. 0.25 mg) test dose, then 0.025–0.1 mg/kg (adult 1–5 mg) 6–12 H oral.

Prednisolone   Oral. Alopecia, autoimm liver, Crohn's, epilepsy, SLE, ulcerative col: 2 mg/kg daily, gradually reducing. Asthma: 0.5–1 mg/kg 6 H for 24 h, 12 H for the next 24 h, then 1 mg/kg daily. Croup: 1 mg/kg stat and in 12 h; severe 4 mg/kg stat, then 1 mg/kg 8–12 H. ITP: 4 mg/kg daily. Nephrotic: 60 mg/m^2 (max. 80 mg) daily, reducing over several months. Physiological: 4–5 mg/m^2 daily. Prednisolone 1 mg = hydrocortisone 4 mg in glucocorticoid activity, 0.8 mg in mineralocorticoid. See also methylprednisolone.

Prednisolone acetate 1% + phenylephrine 0.12%   1–2 drops per eye 6–12 H.

Prednisolone sodium phosphate   0.5% ear/eye drops: 1–3 drops 2–6 H.

Prednisone   Action equivalent to prednisolone.

Primaquine   Usually 0.3 mg/kg (adult 15 mg) daily for 14–21 days oral. Gameteocyte: 0.7 mg/kg (adult 45 mg) once.

Primidone   Initially 2.5 mg/kg (adult 125 mg) at night, incr if reqd to max. 15 mg/kg (adult 750 mg) 12 H oral. Trough level (phenobarbitone) 60–120 μmol/L.

Probenicid   25 mg/kg (adult 1 g) stat, then 10 mg/kg (adult 500 mg) 6 H oral.

Probucol   10 mg/kg (adult 500 mg) 12 H oral.

Procainamide   I.v.: 0.4 mg/kg per min (adult 20 mg/min) for max. 25 min, then 20–80 mcg/kg per min (max. 2 g/day). Oral: 5–8 mg/kg 4 H. Level 3–10 mcg/mL.

Procaine   Max dose 20 mg/kg (1 mL/kg of 2%).

Prochlorperazine   1 mg base = ~1.5 mg edisylate, maleate or mesylate. Only use if >10 kg. Oral (salt): 0.2 mg/kg (adult 5–10 mg) 6–8 H, slow incr if reqd to max. 0.6 mg/kg (max. 35 mg) 6 H in psychosis. I.m., slow i.v. (salt): 0.2 mg/kg (adult 12.5 mg) 8–12 H. Buccal (salt): 0.05–0.1 mg/kg (max. 6 mg) 12–24 H. PR (base): 0.2 mg/kg (adult 25 mg) 8–12 H.

Progesterone   Adult (NOT /kg). Premenst syn: 200–400 mg PV or PR 12–24 H (last 1/2 of cycle). Dysf ut hge: 5–10 mg/day i.m. for 5–10 days before menses. Prevent abrtn: 25–100 mg i.m. every 2–4 days.

Promazine   Oral: 2–4 mg/kg (adult 100–200 mg) 6 H. i.m. 0.7 mg/kg (max. 50 mg) 6–8 H.

Promethazine   Antihist, antiemetic: 0.2–0.5 mg/kg (adult 10–25 mg) 6–8 H i.v., i.m. or oral. Sedative, hypnotic: 0.5–1.5 mg/kg (adult 25–100 mg).

Propafenone   Oral: 70 mg/m^2 (adult 150 mg) 8 H, incr if reqd to max. 165 mg/m^2 (adult 300 mg) 8 H. I.v.: 2 mg/kg over 2 h, then 4 mcg/kg per min incr if reqd to max. 8 mcg/kg per min.

Propantheline   0.3–0.6 mg/kg (adult 15–30 mg) 6 H oral.

Propiverine   0.3 mg/kg (adult 15 mg) 6–12 H oral.

Propofol   Child: 2.5–3.5 mg/kg stat, then 7.5–15 mg/kg per hour i.v. Adult: 1–2.5 mg/kg stat, then 3–12 mg/kg per hour i.v.

Propoxyphene   See dextropropoxyphene.

Propranolol   I.v.: 0.02 mg/kg (adult 1 mg) test dose then 0.1 mg/kg (adult 5 mg) over 10 min (repeat ×1–3 prn), then 0.1–0.3 mg/kg (adult 5–15 mg) 3 H. Oral: 0.2–0.5 mg/kg (adult 10–25 mg) 6–12 H, slow incr to max. 1.5 mg/kg (max. 80 mg) 6–12 H if required.

Propylthiouracil   50 mg/m^2 8 H oral, reduce according to response.

Prostacyclin, PGI$_2$ See epoprostenol.

Prostaglandin E1, PGE1   See alprostadil.

Protamine   I.v. 1 mg/100 u heparin (0.5 mg/100 u if >1 h since heparin dose) slow i.v. stat; subsequent doses of protamine 1 mg/kg (max. 50 mg). 1 mg per 25 mL pump blood. Heparin 1 mg = 100 u (half-life 1–2 h).

Prothrombinex   See coagulation factor, human.

Proxymetacaine   0.5%: 1–2 drops/eye before procedure.

Pseudoephedrine 1 mg/kg (adult 60 mg) 6–8 H oral. Slow release: adult (NOT /kg) 120 mg 12 H.

Pumactant (ALEC) Preterm babies (NOT /kg): disconnect ETT, rapidly inject 100 mg in 1 mL saline via catheter at lower end ETT, flush with 2 mL air; repeat after 1 h and 24 h. Prophylaxis if unintubated: 100 mg into pharynx.

Pyrantel Threadworm: 10 mg/kg (adult 750 mg) once oral, may repeat 2 wkly ×3 doses. Roundworm, hookworm: 20 mg/kg (adult 1 g) once, may repeat in 7 days. Necator: 20 mg/kg (adult 1 g) daily ×2–3 doses.

Pyrazinamide 20–35 mg/kg (max. 1.5 g) daily oral, or 75 mg/kg (max. 3 g) ×2/wk.

Pyridostigmine Myas gravis: 1 mg/kg (adult 60 mg) 4–6 H oral, incr to max. 2–3 mg/kg (adult 120–180 mg) 4–6 H if reqd. 180 mg slow rel tab (Timespan), adult (NOT /kg): 1–3 tab 12–24 H oral. 1 mg i.v., i.m. or s.c. = 30 mg oral.

Pyridoxine With isoniazid or penicillamine (NOT /kg): 5–10 mg daily i.v. or oral. Fitting: 10–15 mg/kg daily i.v. or oral. Siderobl anaem: 2–8 mg/kg (max. 400 mg) daily i.v. or oral.

Pyrimethamine 12.5 mg and dapsone 100 mg (Maloprim) 1–4 yr 1/4 tab wkly, 5–10 yr 1/2 tab, >10 yr 1 tab.

Pyrimethamine 25 mg and sulfadoxine 500 mg (Fansidar) <4 yr 1/2 tab once, 4–8 yr 1 tab, 9–14 yr 2 tab, >14 yr 3 tab. Prophylaxis: <4 yr 1/4 tab wkly, 4–8 yr 1/2 tab, 9–14 yr 3/4 tab, >14 yr 1 tab.

Quinidine, base 10 mg/kg stat, then 5 mg/kg (max. 333 mg) 4–6 H oral. I.v.: 6.3 mg/kg (10 mg/kg of gluconate) over 2 h, then 0.0125 mg/kg per min. I.m.: 15 mg/kg stat, then 7.5 mg/kg (max. 400 mg) 8 H. NOTE: 1 mg base = 1.2 mg sulfate = 1.3 mg bisulfate = 1.6 mg gluconate.

Quinine, base Oral: 8.3 mg/kg (max. 500 mg) 8 H for 7–10 days. Parenteral: 16.7 mg/kg (20 mg/kg of dihydrochloride) i.v. over 4 h or i.m., then 8.3 mg/kg 8 H i.v. over 2 h or i. m. for 2–3 days, then 8.3 mg/kg 8 H oral for 5 days. NOTE: 1 mg base = 1.7 mg bisulfate = 1.2 mg dihydrochloride = 1.2 mg ethyl carbonate = 1.3 mg hydrobromide = 1.2 mg hydrochloride = 1.2 mg sulfate.

Ramipril 0.05 mg/kg (adult 2.5 mg) oral daily, may incr over 4–6 wk to 0.1–0.2 mg/kg (adult 5–10 mg) daily.

Ranitidine I.v.: 1 mg/kg (adult 50 mg) slowly 6–8 H, or 2 mcg/kg per min. Oral: 2–4 mg/ kg (adult 150 mg) 8–12 H, or 300 mg (adult) at night.

Ranitidine bismuth citrate 8 mg/kg (adult 400 mg) 12 H oral; to eradicate *H. pylori*, add an antibiotic.

Reserpine 0.005–0.01 mg/kg (adult 0.25–0.5 mg) 12–24 H oral.

Ribavirin Inhltn (Viratek nebulizer): 20 mg/mL at 25 mL/h (190 mcg/l of gas) for 12–18 h/ day for 3–7 days. Oral: 5–15 mg/kg 8–12 H. Hepatitis C: see interferon alfa-2b.

Riboflavin NOT /kg: 5–10 mg daily oral. Organic acidosis (NOT /kg): 50–200 mg daily oral, i.m. or i.v.

Rifampicin 10–15 mg/kg (max. 600 mg) daily oral fasting, or i.v. over 3 h (monitor AST). Prophylaxis: *N. meningitidis* 10 mg/kg daily (neonate), 10 mg/kg (max. 600 mg) 12 H for 2 days; *H. influenzae* 10 mg/kg daily (neonate), 20 mg/kg (max. 600 mg) daily for 4 days.

Risedronate Osteoporosis: 0.1 mg/kg (adult 5 mg) daily oral; slow release 35 mg (adult) weekly. Paget's: 0.5 mg/kg (adult 30 mg) daily oral.

Risperidone   0.02 mg/kg (adult 1 mg) 12 H, incr if reqd to 0.15 mg/kg (adult 2–4 mg, max. 8 mg) 12 H oral.

Rituximab   260–370 mg/m^2 by i.v. infsn wkly ×4.

Ropivacaine   4–5 mg/kg (adult max. 200–250 mg). Postop infusion 0.2–0.4 mg/kg per hour (adult 12–20 mg/h).

Roxithromycin   2.5–4 mg/kg (adult 150 mg) 12 H oral.

Rubella vaccine (Ervevax, Meruvax II) Live   >12 mo: 0.5 mL s.c. once. See also measles + mumps + rubella vaccine.

Salbutamol (and levalbuterol)   0.1–0.15 mg/kg (adult 2–4 mg) 6 H oral. Inhaltn: mild resp soltn (5 mg/mL, 0.5%) 0.5 mL diluted to 4 mL, or nebule 2.5 mg/2.5 mL 3–6 H; moderate 0.5% soltn 1 mL diluted to 4 mL, or nebule 5 mg/2.5 mL 1–2 H; severe (in ICU) 0.5% soltn undiluted continuous. Aerosol 100 mcg/puff: 1–2 puff 4–6 H. Rotahaler: 200–400 mcg 6–8 H. i.m. or s.c.: 10–20 mcg/kg (adult 500 mcg) 3–6 H. I.v. in child: amp 1 mg/mL at 0.3–0.6 mL/kg per hour (5–10 mcg/kg per min) for 1 h, then 0.06–0.12 mL/kg per hour (1–2 mcg/kg per min). Preterm labour (adult, NOT /kg): 200 mcg/mL in 5%D at 3 mL/h (10 mcg/min), incr until contractions cease (usually at 3–15 mL/h), then halve dose every 6 h; max. duration usually 48 h. I.v. infsn incompatible with aminophylline, ketamine and magnesium.

Salicylic acid   Cradle cap: 6% soltn (Egocappol) 12 H 3–5 days. Plantar warts: 15% soltn ×1–2/day, 40% medicated disc 24–48 H.

Salmeterol   Aerosol, diskhaler (NOT /kg): 50–100 mcg 12 H. See also fluticasone + salmeterol.

Scopolamine hydrobromide   See hyoscine hydrobromide.

Selenium sulfide   2.5% shampoo ×2/wk for 2 wk.

Sennoside   Tab 7.5 mg daily (NOT /kg): 6 mo–2 yr 1/2-one tab, 3–10 yr 1–2 tab, >10 yr 2–4 tab. Granules 22.5 mg/teasp, 12–24 H (NOT /kg): <6 mo 1/4–1/2 teasp, 6 mo–2 yr 1/2–1 teasp, 3–10 yr 1–2 teasp.

Simvastatin   Adult (NOT /kg): 10 mg daily oral, incr if reqd every 4 wk to max. 80 mg daily.

Sodium   Deficit (mL saline) = wt(kg) × 4 × (140 − [Na])/% saline. To increase serum Na by 0.5 mmol/L per hour (maximum safe rate), infusion rate (mL/h) = 2 × wt(kg)/(% saline infused); hours of infusion = 2 × (140 − serum Na). 4 mL/kg of X% saline raises serum Na by X mmol/L. Need 2–6 mmol/kg per day. NaCl MW = 58.45, 1 g NaCl = 17.1 mmol Na, NaCl 20% = 3.4 mmol/mL.

Sodium cromoglycate   Inhalation (Intal): 1 cap (20 mg) 6–8 H, 2 mL soltn (20 mg) 6–8 H, aerosol 1–10 mg 6–8 H. Eye drops (2%): 1–2 drops per eye 4–6 H. Oral: 5–10 mg/kg (max. 200 mg) 6 H oral. Nasal (Rynacrom): insufflator 5 mg in each nostril 6 H, spray 1 puff in each nostril 6 H.

Sodium ferric gluconate   Fe 12.5 mg/mL. 0.05 mL/kg (adult 2 mL) test dose i.v. over 1 h, then 0.25 mL/kg (adult 10 mL) i.v. over 1 h with each dialysis (usually for 8 doses).

Sodium fusidate   Tablets: 10–15 mg/kg (adult 250–500 mg) 8 H oral. IV over 2–8 h: 10 mg/kg (adult 500 mg) 8H; severe inftn 15 mg/kg (adult 750 mg). Peak level 30–200 umol/L (×0.52 = mcg/ml). For suspension, see fusidic acid.

Sodium nitroprusside   <30 kg: 3 mg/kg in 50 mL 5%dex-hep at 0.5–4 mL/h (0.5–4 mcg/kg per min) i.v. >30 kg: 3 mg/kg made to 100 mL in 5%dex-hep at 1–8 mL/h

(0.5–4 mcg/kg per min). If used for >24 h, max. rate 4 mcg/kg per min. Max total 70 mg/kg with normal renal function (or sodium thiocyanate <1725 umol/L, ×0.058 = mg/L). Protect from light.

Sodium polystyrene sulfonate (Resonium) 0.3–1 g/kg (adult 15–30 g) 6 H NG (give lactulose) or PR.

Sodium valproate 5 mg/kg (adult 200 mg) 8–12 H oral, incr if reqd to max. 20 mg/kg (adult 1 g) 8–12 H. Level 2 h after dose 300–700 μmol/L (×0.14 = mg/L).

Sorbitol 70% 0.2–0.5 mL/kg (adult 20–30 mL) 8–24 H oral. With activated charcoal: 1 g/kg (1.4 mL/kg) NG, ×1–2.

Sorbolene cream; pure, with 10% glycerin, or with 5% or 10% olive oil or peanut oil Skin moisturiser: apply prn.

Sotalol I.v.: 0.5–2 mg/kg (adult 25–120 mg) over 10 min 6 H. Oral: 1–4 mg/kg (adult 50–160 mg) 8–12 H.

Spironolactone Oral (NOT /kg): 0–10 kg 6.25 mg 12 H, 11–20 kg 12.5 mg 12 H, 21–40 kg 25 mg 12 H, over 40 kg 25 mg 8 H. Female hirsutism 50 mg 8 H. i.v.: see canrenoate.

Streptokinase (SK) Short term (myoc infarct): 30 000 u/kg (max. 1 500 000 u) i.v. over 60 min, repeat if occlusion recurs <5 days. Long term (DVT, pul emb, art thrombosis): 2 000 u/kg (max. 100 000 u) i.v. over 10 min, then 1000 u/kg per hour (max. 100 000 u/h); stop heparin and aspirin, if PTT <×2 normal at 4 h give extra 10 000 u/kg (max. 500 000 u) i.v. over 30 min, stop SK if PTT >×5 normal then give 1000 u/kg per hour. Local infsn: 50 u/kg per hour (continue heparin 10–15 u/kg per hour). Blocked i.v. cannula: 5000 u/kg in 2 mL in cannula for 2 h then remove, may repeat ×2.

Streptomycin 20–30 mg/kg (max. 1 g) i.m. daily.

Sucralfate 1 g tab (NOT /kg): 0–2 yr 1/4 tab 6 H, 3–12 yr 1/2 tab 6 H, >12 yr 1 tab 6 H oral.

Sulfadiazine 50 mg/kg (max. 2 g) 6 H slow i.v.

Sulfasalazine Active colitis: 20 mg/kg 6–12 H (max. 4 g/day) oral; remission 7.5 mg/kg (max. 0.5 g) 6–8 H, suppos (NOT /kg) adult 0.5–1 g 12 H. Arthritis: 5 mg/kg 12 H, incr if reqd to 10 mg/kg 8–12 H (max. 2 g/day).

Sulindac 4 mg/kg (adult 200 mg) 12 H oral.

Sumatriptan Oral: 1–2 mg/kg (adult 50–100 mg) stat, may repeat twice. S.c.: 0.12 mg/kg (max. 6 mg) stat, may repeat once after 1 h. Nasal: 10–20 mg, may repeat ×1 after 2 h.

Surfactant See beractant (Survanta), calfactant (Infasurf), colfosceril palmitate (Exosurf), poractant alfa (Curosurf), pumactant (ALEC).

Suxamethonium I.v.: neonate 3 mg/kg, child 2 mg/kg, adult 1 mg/kg. I.m.: double i.v. dose.

Tacrolimus I.v. infsn: 2 mg/m^2/day. Oral: 3 mg/m^2 12 H. Trough level: whole blood 10–15 ng/mL (sent to Austin daily at 1000 from RCH).

Tacrolimus ointment 2–16 yr: apply 0.03% sparingly 12 H for max. 3 wk, then daily. >16 yr: apply 0.1% sparingly 12 H for max. 3 wk, then 0.03% 12 H.

Tamoxifen Adult (NOT /kg): 20 mg daily, incr to 40 mg daily if no response after 1 mo.

Tazobactam 125 mg + piperacillin 1 g See piperacillin.

Teicoplanin 250 mg/m^2 i.v. over 30 min stat, then 125 mg/m^2 i.v. or i.m. daily. Severe inftn: 250 mg/m^2 12 H ×3 doses, then 250 mg/m^2 i.v. or i.m. daily.

Temazepam 0.3 mg/kg (adult 20–40 mg) oral.

Terbinafine 62.5 mg (<20 kg), 125 mg (20–40 kg), 250 mg (adult) daily oral. 1% cream, gel: apply 12–24 H to dry skin.

Terbutaline   Oral: 0.05–0.1 mg/kg (adult 2.5–5 mg) 6 H. S.c.: 5–10 mcg/kg (adult 0.25–0.5 mg). I.v.: child 3–6 mcg/kg per min for 1 h, then 0.4–1 mcg/kg per min; adult 0.25 mg stat over 10 min, then 1–10 mcg/kg per hour. Inhaltn: mild resp soltn (1%, 10 mg/mL) 0.25 mL diluted to 4 mL 3–6 H; moderate 0.5 mL of 1% diluted to 4 mL, or respule 5 mg/2 mL 1–2 H; severe (in ICU) undiluted continuous. Aerosol 250 mcg /puff: 1–2 puffs 4–6 H.

Terfenadine   30 mg (6–12 yr), 60 mg (adult) 12 H oral.

Testosterone   Esters (NOT /kg): 100–500 mg i.m. every 2–4 wk. Implant: 8 mg/kg (to nearest 100 mg) every 16–24 wk. Undecanoate (NOT /kg): 40 mg daily oral, incr to 80–120 mg daily. 1% gel: 5 g tube (50 mg testosterone) applied to skin daily. 30 mg buccal tablet: applied just above incisor 12 H. Testosterone level: <16 yr 5–10 nmol/L, >16 yr 10–30 nmol/L.

Tetanus toxoid (Tet-Tox)   0.5 mL i.m. stat, 6 wk later, and 6 mo later. Boost every 10 yr, or if contaminated wound. See also diphtheria (+ pertussis) + tetanus vaccines.

Tetracaine   See Amethocaine.

Tetracycline   >8 yr (NOT /kg): 250–500 mg 6 H oral. Acne (NOT /kg): 500 mg 12 H, reducing to 250 mg 12 H. Eye: apply 2–8 H. See also rolitetracycline.

Theophylline   80 mg theophylline = 100 mg aminophylline. Loading dose: 8 mg/kg (max. 500 mg) oral. Maintenance: 1st wk life 2 mg/kg 12 H; 2nd wk 3 mg/kg 12 H; 3 wk–12 mo (($0.1 \times$ age in wk) + 3) mg/kg 8 H; 1–9 yr 4 mg/kg 4–6 H, or 10 mg/kg slow rel 12 H; 10–16 yr or adult smoker 3 mg/kg 4–6 H, or 7 mg/kg 12 H slow rel; adult non-smoker 3 mg/kg 6–8 H; elderly 2 mg/kg 6–8 H. Serum level: neonate 60–80 μmol/L, asthma 60–110 ($\times0.18$ = mcg/mL), done as reqd at RCH.

Thiabendazole (tiabendazole)   25 mg/kg (max. 1.5 g) 12 H oral 3 days.

Thiopentone   2–5 mg/kg slowly stat (beware hypotension). I.v. infsn: amp 25 mg/mL at 0.04–0.2 mL/kg per hour (1–5 mg/kg per hour). Level 150–200 μmol/L ($\times0.24$ = mcg/mL).

Thrombin glue   10 000 u thrombin in 9 mL mixed with 1 mL 10% calcium chloride in syringe 1, 10 mL cryoprecipitate in syringe 2: apply to bleeding sites together. Do not inject.

Thrombin, topical   100–2000 u/mL onto bleeding surface.

Thymidine   75 g/m^2 every 4–6 wk i.v. over 24 h.

Thyroxine   See levothyroxine

Ticarcillin   50 mg/kg (adult 3 g) i.v. 6–8 H (1st wk life), 4–6 H or constant infsn (2+ wk). Cystic fibrosis: 100 mg/kg (max. 6 g) 8 H i.v.

Ticarcillin + clavulanic acid   Dose as for ticarcillin.

Tilactase   200 u/drop: 5–15 drops/L added to milk 24 h before use. 3300 u/tab: 1–3 tabs with meals oral.

Timolol   0.1 mg/kg (adult 5 mg) 8–12 H, incr to max. 0.3 mg/kg (adult 15 mg) 8 H. Eye drops (0.25%, 0.5%): 1 drop/eye 12–24 H; see also latanoprost.

Tinidazole   *Giardia, Trichomonas:* 50 mg/kg (adult 2 g) stat oral; often repeated after 48 h. Amoebiasis: 50 mg/kg (adult 2 g) daily oral for 3–5 days, usually followed by diloxanide furoate 10 mg/kg (adult 500 mg) 8 H oral for 10 days.

Tissue plasminogen activator   See alteplase.

Tobramycin   I.v. or i.m. 1 wk–10 yr: 8 mg/kg day 1, then 6 mg/kg daily. >10 yr: 7 mg/kg day 1, then 5 mg/kg (max. 240–360 mg) daily. Neonate, 5 mg/kg dose: <1200 g 48 H (0–7 days of life), 36 H (8–30 days), 24 H (>30 days); 1200–2500 g 36 H (0–7 days of life), 24 H (>7 days); term 24 H (0–7 days of life), then as for 1 wk–10 yr. Trough level

<1.0 mg/L. Inhaltn: 80 mg diluted to 4 mL 12 H; or TOBI 300 mg 12 H alternate months. Eye: 1 drop or 1 cm cream 4 H.

Tolazoline   Newborn: 1–2 mg/kg slowly stat (beware hypotension), then 2–6 mcg/kg per min (0.12–0.36 mg/kg per hour) i.v. Note: 1–2 mg/kg per hour too much (*Pediatrics* 1986; 77: 307).

Tolbutamide   Adult (NOT /kg): initially 1 g 12 H oral, often reducing to 0.5–1 g daily.

Topiramate   1 mg/kg (adult 50 mg) 12–24 H oral, incr slowly if reqd to 4–10 mg/kg (adult 100–500 mg) 12 H.

Tramadol   2–3 mg/kg (adult 50–100 mg) stat, then 1–2 mg/kg (adult 50–100 mg) 4–6 H (usual max. 400 mg/day, up to 600 mg/day) oral or i.v. over 3 min. I.v. infusion 2–8 mcg/kg per min. See Pain management, chapter 4, page 58.

Tranexamic acid   Oral: 15–25 mg/kg (adult 1–1.5 g) 8 H. I.v.: 10–15 mg/kg (adult 0.5–1 g) 8 H.

Triamcinolone   Joint, tendon (NOT /kg): 2.5–15 mg stat. i.m.: 0.05–0.2 mg/kg every 1–7 days. Cream or ointment 0.02%, 0.05%: apply sparingly 6–8 H. Triamcinolone has no mineralcorticoid action, 1 mg = 5 mg hydrocortisone in glucocorticoid action.

Triamcinolone 0.1% + neomycin 0.25% + gramicidin 0.025% + nystatin 100 000 u/g   Kenacomb ointment: apply 8–12 H. Kenacomb otic oint, drops: apply 8–12 H (2–3 drops).

Triazolam   0.005–0.01 mg/kg (adult 0.125–0.5 mg) at night oral. 30 min preop: 0.01–0.03 mg/kg (adult 0.5 mg) oral.

Trifluoperazine   0.02–0.4 mg/kg (adult 1–10 mg, occasionally 20 mg) 12 H oral. Capsule: adult 15 mg daily.

Trimethoprim   3–4 mg/kg (usual max. 150 mg) 12 H, or 6–8 mg/kg (usual max. 300 mg) daily oral or i.v. Urine prophylaxis: 1–2 mg/kg (adult 150 mg) at night oral.

Trimethoprim-sulfamethoxazole   See co-trimoxazole.

Trometamol (THAM)   mL of 0.3 M (18 g/500 mL) soltn = (wt in kg) × BE; give 1/2 this i.v. over 30 min, then repeat if reqd.

Typhoid vaccine, oral (Typh-Vax)   Live. 1 cap oral days 1, 3, 5 and (for better immunity) 7. Boost yearly.

Typhoid vaccine, parenteral, polysaccharide (Typherix, Typhim Vi)   Inactivated. >5 yr: 0.5 mL i.m. once. Boost 3 yrly.

Urea   10% cream: apply 8–12 H.

Urofollitrophin   See follicle stimulating hormone.

Urokinase   4000 u/kg i.v. over 10 min, then 4000 u/kg per hour for 12 h (start heparin 3–4 h later). Blocked cannula: instil 5000–25 000 u (NOT /kg) in 2–3 mL saline for 2–4 h. Empyema: 2 mL/kg of 1500 u/mL in saline, position head up/down and right side up/down 30 min each, then drain. Pericard eff: 10 000 u/mL (max. 20 mL), clamp 1 h, drain.

Ursodeoxycholic acid   5–10 mg/kg (adult 200–400 mg) 12 H oral.

Vancomycin   10 mg/kg (adult 500 mg) 6 H i.v. over 1 h, or 1 g 12 H in adult i.v. over 2 h. Newborn (any gestation): 10 mg/kg 8 H i.v. over 1 h. Oral: 10 mg/kg to nearest 125 mg (adult 500 mg) 6 H. Intraventric (NOT /kg): 10 mg 48 H. Trough 5–10 mg/L (peak 20–40 mg/L).

Varicella vaccine (Varilix, Varivax)   Live. 9 mo–12 yr: 0.5 mL s.c. once. >12 yr: 0.5 mL s.c. stat, and 4–8 wk later.

Vasopressin, aqueous i.m., s.c.: 2.5–10 u 6–12 H. I.v.: put 2–5 u in 1 L fluid, and replace urine output + 10% each hour. Hypotension (brain death, sepsis, post-bypass): 1 u/kg in 50 mL 5%dex-hep at 1–3 mL/h (0.02–0.06 units/kg per hour) + adrenaline 0.1–0.2 mcg/kg per min. GI hge: 6 u/kg in 50 mL at 1–5 mL/h i.v., 1 mL/h local IA. See desmopressin, lypressin.

Vasopressin, oily 2.5–5 u (NOT /kg) i.m. every 2–4 days.

Verapamil I.v.: 0.1–0.2 mg/kg (adult 5–10 mg) over 10 min, then 5 mcg/kg per min. Oral: 1–3 mg/kg (adult 80–120 mg) 8–12 H.

Vigabatrin 40 mg/kg (adult 1 g) daily oral, incr if reqd to 80–150 mg/kg (max. 4 g) daily (given in 1–2 doses).

Vitamin A High risk (NOT /kg): 100 000 iu (<8 kg), 200 000 iu (>8 kg) oral or i.m. every 4–6 mo. Severe measles: 400 000 iu (NOT /kg) once. Cystic fib: 1500 u daily (<3 yr) 5000 u daily (3–10 yr) 10 000 u daily (>10 yr) oral. >10 000 iu daily or >25 000 u per wk may be teratogenic.

Vitamin A, B, C, D compound (Pentavite, child) <3 yr (NOT /kg): 2.5 mL daily. >3 yr (NOT /kg): 5 mL daily.

Vitamin A, B, C, D compound (Pentavite, infant) <3 yr (NOT /kg): 0.15 mL daily, incr by 0.15 mL/day to 0.45 mL/day.

Vitamin B group Amp: i.v. over 30 min. Tab: 1–2/day.

Vitamin B$_{12}$ See cyanocobalamin and hydroxocobalamin.

Vitamin D$_2$ See ergocalciferol.

Vitamin D$_3$ See cholecalciferol.

Vitamin E 1 u = 1 mg. Preterm babies, Coperol E (NOT /kg): 40 u (2 drops) daily oral. CF, malabs: 50–100 u (<3 yr) 200–400 u (>3 yr) daily oral. Cholestasis: 50 u/kg daily oral, incr if reqd in 50 u/kg increments. A-beta-lipoproteinaemia: 35–70 u/kg 8 H oral. HUS: 0.25 g/m^2 6 H oral. See also alpha-tocopheryl acetate.

Vitamin K$_1$ See phytomenadione.

Vitamins, parenteral MVI-12 (for adult): 5 mL in 1 litre i.v. fluid. MVI Paediatric, added to i.v. fluid: 65% of a vial (<3 kg), 1 vial (3 kg–11 yr).

Vitaprem (RCH: Pentavite, folate, B12, C) 1 mL daily oral.

Warfarin Usually 0.2 mg/kg (adult 5 mg) stat, 0.2 mg/kg (adult 5 mg) next day providing INR <1.3, then 0.05–0.2 mg/kg (adult 2–5 mg) daily oral. INR usually 2–2.5 for prophylaxis, 2–3 for treatment. Beware drug interactions.

Whole blood 6 mL/kg raises Hb 1 g%. 1 bag = ~400 mL.

Xylometazoline <6 yr: 0.05% 1 drop or spray 8–12 H. 6–12 yr: 0.05% 2–3 drops or sprays 8–12 H. >12 yr: 0.1% 2–3 drops or sprays 6–12 H.

Yellow fever vaccine (Stamaril) Live. >12 mo: 0.5 mL s.c. once. Boost every 10 yr.

Zidovudine (AZT) Preterm: 1.5 mg/kg 12 H i.v., or 2 mg/kg 12 H oral to 2 wk, then 2 mg/kg 8 H. Term newborn: 2 mg/kg 6 H oral, 1.5 mg/kg 6 H i.v. Child: usually 180 mg/m^2 12 H oral; 120 mg/m^2 6 H i.v., or 20 mg/m^2/h i.v. (range 90–180 mg/m^2 6–8 H i.v.). Adult (NOT /kg): usually 200 mg 8 H oral, or 300 mg 12 H oral, or 150 mg 8 H i.v.

Zinc sulfate 220 mg cap = 50 mg Zn = 765 μmol Zn. Deficiency, acroderm enteropath: initially 3 mg/kg (adult 220 mg) 8–12 H oral, adjusted to achieve serum zinc 11–22 μmol/L (0.7–1.4 mg/L). Diarrhoea child (NOT /kg): 10–20 mg daily oral.

APPENDIX 3

ANTIMICROBIAL GUIDELINES

Nigel Curtis, Mike Starr and Mike South

CENTRAL NERVOUS SYSTEM/EYE

Infection	Likely organisms	Initial antimicrobials[1] ( ) = maximum dose	Duration of treatment[2] and other comments
Brain abscess	*S. milleri* and other streptococci Anaerobes Gram-negatives *S. aureus*	Flucloxacillin 50 mg/kg (2 g) iv 4H **and** Cefotaxime 50 mg/kg (2 g) iv 6H **and** Metronidazole 15 mg/kg (1 g) iv stat, then 7.5 mg/kg (500 mg) iv 8H	3 weeks minimum Penicillin hypersensitivity: substitute Flucloxacillin with Vancomycin 15 mg/kg (500 mg) iv 6H
... post-neurosurgery	As above plus *S. epidermidis*	As above but substitute Flucloxacillin with Vancomycin 15 mg/kg (500 mg) iv 6H	
Encephalitis $SA\,(m^2) = \sqrt{\dfrac{ht\,(cm) \times wt\,(kg)}{3600}}$	Herpes simplex virus Enteroviruses Arboviruses *M. pneumoniae*	Aciclovir 20 mg/kg iv 8H [age < 3 months] 500 mg/m² iv 8H [age 3 months–12 yrs] 10 mg/kg iv 8H [age > 12 yrs]	3 weeks minimum Consider macrolide antibiotic if *M. pneumoniae* suspected
Meningitis			
... over 2 months of age	*S. pneumoniae*[3] *N. meningitidis* *H. influenzae* type b[4]	Cefotaxime 50 mg/kg (2 g) iv 6H	*S. pneumoniae* 10 days *N. meningitidis* 5–7 days *H. influenzae* type b 7–10 days
... over 2 months of age and possibility of penicillin-resistant pneumococci[3] (**www.snipurl.com/vanco**)	As above	Cefotaxime 50 mg/kg (2 g) iv 6H **and** Vancomycin 15 mg/kg (500 mg) iv 6H	Penicillin or cephalosporin hypersensitivity: see footnote 5

CENTRAL NERVOUS SYSTEM / EYE (continued)			
Infection	**Likely organisms**	**Initial antimicrobials[1]** **( ) = maximum dose**	**Duration of treatment[2]** **and other comments**
. . . under 2 months of age	As above plus Group B streptococci E. coli and other Gram-negative coliforms L. monocytogenes	Cefotaxime **and** Benzylpenicillin **and** Gentamicin[6] (for first week) [See doses in 'Septicaemia (under 2 months of age)' section]	Gram-negative 3 weeks GBS / Listeria 2–3 weeks See footnote 7 re Gentamicin dosing/monitoring Substitute Benzylpenicillin with Vancomycin if possibility of penicillin-resistant pneumococci[3]
. . . with shunt infection, post-neurosurgery, head trauma or CSF leak	As for over 2 months of age plus S. epidermidis S. aureus Gram-negative coliforms incl. P. aeruginosa	Vancomycin 15 mg/kg (500 mg) iv 6H **and** Ceftazidime 50 mg/kg (2 g) iv 3H	10 days minimum
. . . contact prophylaxis	N. meningitidis	Rifampicin 10 mg/kg (600 mg) po 12H	2 days (alternatives: see table 30.3)
. . . contact prophylaxis	H. influenzae type b[4]	Rifampicin 20 mg/kg (600 mg) po 24H	4 days (alternatives: see table 30.3)
Postseptal (orbital) cellulitis	S. aureus H. influenzae spp. S. pneumoniae M. catarrhalis Gram-negatives Anaerobes	Flucloxacillin 50 mg/kg (2 g) iv 6H **and** Cefotaxime 50 mg/kg (2 g) iv 6H	10 days minimum Rule out meningitis Consider adding Metronidazole if not responding

CENTRAL NERVOUS SYSTEM / EYE (continued)

Infection	Likely organisms	Initial antimicrobials[1] ( ) = maximum dose	Duration of treatment[2] and other comments
Preseptal (periorbital) cellulitis			
... mild (outpatient)	Group A streptococci S. aureus H. influenzae spp.[4]	Amoxycillin/clavulanate [400/57 mg per 5 mL] 22.5 mg/kg (875 mg) [Amoxycillin component] = 0.3 mL/kg (11 mL) po 12H	7–10 days Consider non-infective cause in trivial cases
... moderate (inpatient)	As above	Flucloxacillin 50 mg/kg (2 g) iv 6H	
... severe, or not responding, or under 5 yrs of age and non-Hib immunised	As above plus H. influenzae type b[4]	Flucloxacillin 50 mg/kg (2 g) iv 6H *and* Cefotaxime 50 mg/kg (2 g) iv 6H	

CARDIOVASCULAR

Endocarditis			
... native valve or homograft	Viridans streptococci Other streptococci Enterococcus spp. S. aureus	Benzylpenicillin 60 mg/kg (2 g) iv 6H *and* Gentamicin 2.5 mg/kg (240 mg) iv 8H* *and* Flucloxacillin 50 mg/kg (2 g) iv 4–6H	4–6 weeks *Gentamicin 1 mg/kg (80 mg) iv 8H for 1–2 weeks when used only for synergy
... artificial valve or post surgery	As above plus S. epidermidis	Vancomycin 15 mg/kg (500 mg) iv 6H *and* Gentamicin 2.5 mg/kg (240 mg) iv 8H*	Gentamicin monitoring is generally not required when low dose is used for synergy in this setting

CARDIOVASCULAR (continued)			
Infection	Likely organisms	Initial antimicrobials[1] ( ) = maximum dose	Duration of treatment[2] and other comments
Endocarditis prophylaxis			
... for dental procedures only	Viridans streptococci S. aureus S. pneumoniae Other Gram-positive cocci Enterococcus spp.	Amoxycillin 50 mg/kg (2 g) Local anaesthetic: give po 1 hr before procedure General anaesthetic: give iv with induction	Penicillin hypersensitivity: substitute Amoxycillin with Clindamycin 20 mg/kg (600 mg) po or iv
GASTROINTESTINAL			
Diarrhoea			
... *Salmonella* spp. isolated in infant under 3 months of age or in immunocompromised	Salmonella spp.	Cefotaxime 50 mg/kg (2 g) iv 6H	3–5 days Antibiotic treatment is generally unnecessary for most other organisms
... antibiotic associated	C. difficile	Metronidazole 7.5 mg/kg (400 mg) po 8H	7–10 days
Giardiasis	G. lamblia	Metronidazole 30 mg/kg (2 g) po daily **or** Tinidazole 50 mg/kg (2 g) po	3 days Single dose
Peritonitis or ascending cholangitis	Gram-negative coliforms Anaerobes Enterococcus spp.	Ampicillin or Amoxycillin 50 mg/kg (2 g) iv 6H **and** Gentamicin 7.5 mg/kg (360 mg) iv daily [<10 yrs] 6 mg/kg (360 mg) iv daily [≥ 10 yrs] **and** Metronidazole 15 mg/kg (1 g) iv stat, then 7.5 mg/kg (500 mg) iv 8H	Up to 14 days See footnote 7 re Gentamicin dosing/monitoring

GASTROINTESTINAL (continued)

Infection	Likely organisms	Initial antimicrobials[1] ( ) = maximum dose	Duration of treatment[2] and other comments
Threadworm (Pinworm)	*Enterobius vermicularis*	Mebendazole 50 mg po [<10 kg] 100 mg po [≥10 kg]	Single dose; may need to repeat after 14 days Treat whole family
GENITOURINARY			
Urinary tract infection			
. . . over 6 months of age and not sick	*E. coli* *P. mirabilis* *K. oxytoca* Other Gram-negatives	Trimethoprim 4 mg/kg (150 mg) po 12H *or* if syrup is necessary then Co-trimoxazole [Trimethoprim/Sulphamethoxazole 8/40 mg per mL] 0.5 mL/kg (20 mL) po 12H	5 days
. . . under 6 months of age or sick or acute pyelonephritis	As above plus *Enterococcus* spp.	Benzylpenicillin 60 mg/kg (2 g) iv 6H **and** Gentamicin 7.5 mg/kg (360 mg) iv daily [< 10 yrs] 6 mg/kg (360 mg) iv daily [≥ 10 yrs] [For infants under 1 month of age, see doses in 'Septicaemia in neonate' section]	5–7 days for UTI 10–14 days for pyelonephritis See footnote 7 re Gentamicin dosing/monitoring
. . . prophylaxis	As above	Trimethoprim 2 mg/kg (150 mg) po daily *or* if syrup is necessary then Co-trimoxazole [Trimethoprim/Sulphamethoxazole 8/40 mg per mL] 0.25 mL/kg (20 mL) po daily	

RESPIRATORY			
Infection	**Likely organisms**	**Initial antimicrobials[1]** **( ) = maximum dose**	**Duration of treatment[2]** **and other comments**
Epiglottitis	H. influenzae type b[4]	Ceftriaxone 100 mg/kg (2 g) iv followed by 50 mg/kg (1 g) 24 hrs later	2 doses only
Gingivostomatitis			
. . . in immunocompromised	Herpes simplex virus	Aciclovir 500 mg/m² iv 8H [age 3 months–12 yrs] 10 mg/kg iv 8H [age > 12 yrs]	7 days Treatment is only recommended in the immunocompromised
Otitis externa			
. . . acute diffuse	S. aureus S. epidermidis P. aeruginosa Proteus spp. Klebsiella spp.	Clean ear canal Topical steroid/antibiotic [e.g. Sofradex®] drops [± insertion of wick soaked in drops if ear canal oedematous]	7 days
. . . acute localised (furuncle) ± cellulitis	S. aureus Group A streptococci	Flucloxacillin 50 mg/kg (2 g) iv 6H	7–10 days
. . . failure of first line treatment, high fever or severe persistent pain	As above plus P. aeruginosa	Ticarcillin/Clavulanate 50 mg/kg (3 g) [Ticarcillin component] iv 6H	14 days minimum Consider fungal infection
Otitis media	Viruses S. pneumoniae M. catarrhalis H. influenzae spp. Group A streptococci	Consider no antibiotics for 48 hrs if over 2 yrs of age **or** Amoxycillin 15 mg/kg (500 mg) po 8H	5 days Consider higher dose Amoxycillin 30 mg/kg (500 mg) po 8H if not responding

RESPIRATORY (continued)

Infection	Likely organisms	Initial antimicrobials[1] ( ) = maximum dose	Duration of treatment[2] and other comments
Pertussis	B. pertussis	Erythromycin 12.5 mg/kg (500 mg) po 6H **or** Clarithromycin 7.5 mg/kg (500 mg) po 12H	14 days 7 days Can be given up to 3 weeks after contact with index case
Pneumonia . . . mild (outpatient)	Viruses S. pneumoniae H. influenzae spp.	Amoxycillin 15 mg/kg (500 mg) po 8H **or** Roxithromycin 4 mg/kg (150 mg) po 12H*	7–10 days 10 days
. . . moderate (inpatient)	As above	Benzylpenicillin 60 mg/kg (2 g) iv 6H **and** consider Roxithromycin (dose as above)*	Consider admission for all children under 1 yr of age *To cover M. pneumoniae
. . . severe systemic toxicity or pneumatocoele	As above plus S. aureus Group A streptococci Gram-negatives	Flucloxacillin 50 mg/kg (2 g) iv 4H **and** Gentamicin 7.5 mg/kg (360 mg) iv daily [< 10 yrs] 6 mg/kg (360 mg) iv daily [≥ 10 yrs] **and** consider Azithromycin 15 mg/kg (500 mg) iv stat, then 5 mg/kg (200 mg) iv daily*	10 days minimum *To cover M. pneumoniae
Tonsillitis	Viruses Group A streptococci A. haemolyticum	Consider no antibiotics [particularly if < 4 yrs] **or** Phenoxymethylpenicillin [penicillin V] 250 mg po 12H [< 10 yrs] 500 mg po 12H [≥ 10 yrs]	10 days

SKIN/SOFT TISSUE/BONE			
Infection	Likely organisms	Initial antimicrobials[1] ( ) = maximum dose	Duration of treatment[2] and other comments
Adenitis	S. aureus Group A streptococci Oral anaerobes	Flucloxacillin 50 mg/kg (2 g) iv 6H	10–14 days
Bites (animal/human)	Viridans streptococci S. aureus Group A streptococci Oral anaerobes E. corrodens Pasteurella spp. (cat and dog) C. canimorsus (dog)	Amoxycillin/Clavulanate [400/57 mg per 5 mL] 22.5 mg/kg (875 mg) [Amoxycillin component] = 0.3 mL/kg (11 mL) po 12H	3–5 days for prophylaxis 7–14 days for treatment Check tetanus immunisation status consider risk and Hepatitis B and C, and HIV
. . . if severe, penetrating injuries, esp. involving joints or tendons	As above	Ticarcillin/Clavulanate 50 mg/kg (3 g) [Ticarcillin component] iv 6 H	
Cellulitis			
. . . mild (outpatient)	Group A streptococci S. aureus	Cephalexin 25 mg/kg (500 mg) po 6H *or* Cephalexin 35 mg/kg (500 mg) po 8H	5–10 days Consider adding
. . . moderate/severe (inpatient)	As above	Flucloxacillin 50 mg/kg (2 g) iv 6H	Clindamycin 10 mg/kg (600 mg) iv 6H if rapid progression suggestive of
. . . if facial cellulitis in child under 5 yrs of age and non-Hib immunised	As above plus S. pneumoniae H. influenzae spp.[4]	Flucloxacillin 50 mg/kg (≥ g) iv 6H *and* Cefotaxime 50 mg/kg (2 g) iv 6H	necrotising fasciitis or features of toxic shock syndrome

SKIN/SOFT TISSUE/BONE (continued)

Infection	Likely organisms	Initial antimicrobials[1] ( ) = maximum dose	Duration of treatment[2] and other comments
Head lice	Pediculus humanus var. capitis	1% Permethrin liquid or cream rinse	Repeat after one week
Impetigo	Group A streptococci S. aureus	Mupirocin 2% ointment top 8H if localised **or** Cephalexin 35 mg/kg (500 mg) po 8H	5–10 days
Osteomyelitis	S. aureus Group A streptococci S. pneumoniae	Flucloxacillin 50 mg/kg (2 g) iv 4–6H	3 weeks for uncomplicated cases[2]
. . . if under 5 yrs of age and non-Hib immunised	As above plus H. influenzae type b[4]	Flucloxacillin 50 mg/kg (2 g) iv 4–6H **and** Cefotaxime 50 mg/kg (2 g) iv 6–8H	
. . . in patient with sickle cell anaemia	As above plus Salmonella spp.	Flucloxacillin 50 mg/kg (2 g) iv 4–6H **and** Cefotaxime 50 mg/kg (2 g) iv 6H	
. . . with penetrating foot injury	As above plus P. aeruginosa	Ticarcillin/Clavulanate 50 mg/kg (3 g) [Ticarcillin component] iv 6H **and** Gentamicin 7.5 mg/kg (360 mg) iv daily [< 10 yrs] 6 mg/kg (360 mg) iv daily [≥ 10 yrs]	Surgical intervention important See footnote 7 re Gentamicin dosing/monitoring
Scabies	Sarcoptes scabiei	5% Permethrin cream top	One application from neck down; may need to repeat after 14 days Treat whole family

SKIN/SOFT TISSUE/BONE (continued)

Infection	Likely organisms	Initial antimicrobials[1] ( ) = maximum dose	Duration of treatment[2] and other comments
Septic arthritis	As for osteomyelitis	As for osteomyelitis	3 weeks for uncomplicated cases[2] Always consider surgical drainage
Shingles			
… in immunocompromised or involving eye	Varicella zoster virus	Aciclovir 500 mg/m² iv 8H [age 3 months–12 yrs] 10 mg/kg iv 8H [age > 12 yrs] **and** Aciclovir ointment to eye 5 times/day	7 days Shingles in immunocompetent children does not generally require treatment

SEPTICAEMIA (UNDER 2 MONTHS OF AGE)

Septicaemia (age < 2 months)			
… community-acquired infection	Group B streptococci E. coli and other Gram-negative coliforms L. monocytogenes H. influenzae spp.[4] plus those listed below for 'Septicaemia with unknown CSF'	Benzylpenicillin 60 mg/kg iv 12H [first week of life] 6H [1–4 weeks of age] 4H [> 4 weeks of age] **and** Gentamicin 2.5 mg/kg iv 12H [first week of life] 8H [> 1 week of age]	Substitute Benzylpenicillin with Flucloxacillin 50 mg/kg iv 12H [first week of life] 8H [1–4 weeks of age] 6H [> 4 weeks of age] if infection with S. aureus suspected
… if meningitis suspected	As above	Benzylpenicillin **and** Gentamicin[6] as above **and** Cefotaxime 50 mg/kg iv 12H [first week of life] 6H [> 1 week of age]	Duration depends on culture results See footnote 7 re Gentamicin dosing/monitoring
… if abdominal source suspected	As above plus Anaerobes	Benzylpenicillin **and** Gentamicin[6] as above **and** Metronidazole 15 mg/kg iv stat, then 7.5 mg/kg iv 12H	Premature neonates require special dosing consideration

SEPTICAEMIA (OVER 2 MONTHS OF AGE)

Infection	Likely organisms	Initial antimicrobials[1] ( ) = maximum dose	Duration of treatment[2] and other comments
Septicaemia with unknown CSF (www.snipurl.com/vanco)[3]	S. pneumoniae[3] N. meningitidis S. aureus Group A streptococci Gram-negatives	Flucloxacillin 50 mg/kg (2 g) iv 4H[†] **and** Cefotaxime 50 mg/kg (2 g) iv 6H	[†] Substitute Flucloxacillin with Vancomycin 15 mg/kg (500 mg) iv 6H if central line in situ or suspected MRSA
Septicaemia with unknown CSF	As above	Flucloxacillin 50 mg/kg (2 g) iv 4H[†] **and** Cefotaxime 50 mg/kg (2 g) iv 6H Gentamicin 7.5 mg/kg (360 mg) iv daily [< 10 yrs] 6 mg/kg (360 mg) iv daily [≥10 yrs]	Consider adding Clindamycin 10 mg/kg (600 mg) iv 6H if suspect Gram-positive toxic shock syndrome
... in non-Hib immunised	As above plus H. influenzae type b[4]	Flucloxacillin 50 mg/kg (2 g) iv 4H[†] **and** Cefotaxime 50 mg/kg (2 g) iv 6H	Duration depends on culture results
... in neutropenic patient	As above plus Enterococcus spp. P. aeruginosa	Ticarcillin/Clavulanate 50 mg/kg (3 g) [Ticarcillin component] iv 6H **and** Gentamicin 7.5 mg/kg (360 mg) iv daily [< 10 yrs] 6 mg/kg (360 mg) iv daily [≥ 10 yrs]	See footnote 7 re Gentamicin dosing/monitoring
... in neutropenic patient with potential line infection	As above plus Gram-positive cocci incl. S. epidermidis	Ticarcillin/clavulanate as above **and** Gentamicin as above **and** consider Vancomycin 15 mg/kg (500 mg) iv 6H	Consult local protocols and also consider anaerobic and fungal infection in neutropenic patients

NOTES TO ANTIMICROBIAL GUIDELINES

Further information available at www.snipurl.com/RCHantibiotics

These guidelines have been developed to assist doctors with their choice of initial empiric treatment. Except where specified, they do not apply to neonates or immunocompromised patients. Always ask about previous antibiotic reactions. The choice of antimicrobial, dose and frequency of administration for continuing treatment may require adjustment according to the clinical situation. The recommendations are not intended to be proscriptive and alternative regimens may also be appropriate.

1 Antimicrobial choice and dose

- Antibiotics should be changed to narrow spectrum agents once sensitivities are known.
- Dose adjustments may be necessary for neonates, and for children with renal or hepatic impairment.
- Alternative antimicrobial regimens may be more appropriate for neonates, immuno-compromised patients or others with a special infection risk (e.g. cystic fibrosis, sickle cell anaemia).
- Resistance to antimicrobials is an increasing problem worldwide. Of particular concern is the increasing incidence of penicillin-resistant pneumococci (see footnote 3). It is important to take into account local resistance patterns when using these guidelines.
- Cefotaxime can usually (except in neonates) be substituted with: Ceftriaxone 100 mg/kg (2 g) iv daily or 50 mg/kg (1 g) iv 12H.

2 Duration of treatment

Duration of treatment is given as a guide only and may vary with the clinical situation. 'Step down' from intravenous to oral treatment is appropriate in many cases. **Durations given generally refer to the minimum total intravenous and oral treatment.**

3 Penicillin-resistant pneumococci (www.snipurl.com/vanco)

The prevalence of invasive strains that are highly resistant to penicillin or cephalosporins in Melbourne remains low. Cefotaxime remains the drug of first choice for the empiric treatment of meningitis. However, vancomycin should be added if *S. pneumoniae* is suspected (www.snipurl.com/vanco). This should be stopped if sensitivity to cefotaxime is shown, as will be the case with most isolates. The prevalence of resistant strains is being monitored and this recommendation may change.

Penicillin remains the drug of first choice for the empiric treatment of suspected pneumococcal pneumonia and other non-CNS infections, regardless of susceptibility. High doses of penicillin overcome resistance in this setting and should be used for confirmed non-CNS infection caused by penicillin-resistant pneumococci.

4 Invasive *H. influenzae* type b disease

Since the introduction of *H. influenzae* type b (Hib) immunisation, there has been a dramatic decline in the incidence of invasive disease. However, in children with potential invasive disease, who are not fully immunised against Hib, therapy should include cover against Hib.

5 Treatment of meningitis in patients with hypersensitivity to penicillins or cephalosporins

In patients with a history of severe (anaphylactic) penicillin hypersensitivity, avoid cephalosporins: use chloramphenicol 25 mg/kg (1 g) iv 6H and vancomycin 15 mg/kg (500 mg) iv 6H.

6 Empiric treatment of neonatal meningitis

Gentamicin is recommended in this setting to provide double Gram-negative cover, and for synergy with benzylpenicillin against *Listeria monocytogenes* and group B streptococci.

7 Gentamicin dosing/monitoring

Once-daily administration of gentamicin is safe and effective for most patients. Certain patients, such as neonates and those with cystic fibrosis, endocarditis or renal failure, may require special dosing consideration.

The regimen for monitoring gentamicin levels is different for once-daily and 8, 12 or 18H dosing, and depends on renal function:

Once-daily dosing
- Normal renal function – if the patient is to have more than 3 doses, the trough level (pre-dose) should be checked before the third dose and then every 3 days (target level <1 mg/L).
- Abnormal renal function – trough levels may need to be checked earlier and more frequently (target level <1 mg/L).
- Renal failure – levels should be checked post-dose at 2, 12 and 24 hours, and adjusted accordingly. The results should be discussed with a specialist familiar with therapeutic drug monitoring.

8, 12 and 18 hourly dosing
- The trough level should be checked before the fourth dose and peak level 1 hour after the start of the fourth dose (target trough <2 mg/L, target peak 5–10 mg/L).
- Levels should be repeated every 3 days, or more frequently if levels are inappropriate or if renal function is abnormal.

Formulae

ETT tube size and position (p. 3)
Neonates Table 32.1 p. 435
Tube size (internal diameter) = (age/4) + 4 mm (for patients over 1 year of age)
Depth of insertion is approximately (age/2) + 12 cm from the lower lip

Anion gap (p. 76)
Anion gap = Na − bicarbonate − Cl

Bicarbonate administration (pp. 76, 83, 303)
mmol of HCO_3 required = basic deficit (mmol/L) × weight (kg) × 0.3 (child)
mmol of HCO_3 required = basic deficit (mmol/L) × weight (kg) × 0.5 (newborn)
Infuse half with cardiac monitoring, then reassess.

Dose Na replacement (p. 82)
Dose of Na^+ (mmol) = bodyweight × 0.8 × (140 − current serum Na^+)

Additives (p. 84)
Molar potassium chloride (0.75 g in 10 mL) = 1 mmol/mL of K^+ and Cl^-
Sodium chloride (20%) = 3.4 mmol/mL of Na^+ and Cl^-
Molar sodium bicarbonate (8.4%) = 1 mmol/mL of Na^+ and HCO_3^-
Calcium gluconate 10% = 0.22 mmol/mL of Ca^{2+}, which is 8.9 mg/mL of Ca^{2+}
Magnesium chloride for injection (0.48 g anhydrous in 5 mL) = 1 mmol/mL of Mg^{2+}

Conversion factors (p. 84)
Sodium chloride 1 g contains 17 mmol Na and 17 mmol Cl
Potassium chloride 1 g contains 13 mmol K and 13 mmol Cl
Sodium bicarbonate 1 g contains 12 mmol Na and 12 mmol HCO_3

Formulae (p. 84)
Anion gap = Na − (bicarbonate + Cl); normal <12
Number mmol = mEq/valence = mass (mg)/mol. wt
Sodium deficit: mL 20% NaCl = wt × 0.2 × (140 − serum Na)
Water deficit (mL) = 600 × wt (kg) × [1 − (140/Na)] (if body Na normal)
Non-catabolic anuria: urea rises of 3–5 mmol/L per day

kcal (p. 92)

$$kcal = \frac{mJ \times 1000}{4.2}$$

Estimated weight

Weight = (age + 4) × 2

Surface area (pp. 374, 564)

$$\text{Surface area (m}^2) = \sqrt{\frac{height(cm) \times weight(kg)}{3600}}$$

BMI (p. 106)

BMI = bodyweight in kg divided by the square of height in metres (kg/m^2). Standard growth charts now include BMI centile charts.

- Overweight = BMI between 85–95th centile for age and sex.
- Obesity = BMI greater than 95th centile for age and sex.

Osmolality (pp. 300, 303)

Calculated values

Serum osmolality = (Na$^+$ × 2) + glucose + urea

Adjusted Na$^+$ = plasma Na$^+$ + 0.3 × (plasma glucose − 5.5)

Normal (270 − 295 mmol/L)

Transfusion volume (pp. 372, 378)

Packed red cells (mL) = weight (kg) × Hb rise required (g/L) × 0.4

Index

Note: Bold page numbers refer to diagrams and tables.